DATE DUE

DEC 1 1 2004	

BRODART   Cat. No. 23-221

Clinical Handbook of Eating Disorders

Medical Psychiatry

Series Editor Emeritus

William A. Frosch, M.D.

Weill Medical College of Cornell University
New York, New York, U.S.A.

Advisory Board

Jonathan E. Alpert, M.D., Ph.D.
Massachusetts General Hospital and
Harvard University School of Medicine
Boston, Massachusetts, U.S.A.

Siegfried Kasper, M.D.
University Hospital for Psychiatry
and University of Vienna
Vienna, Austria

Bennett Leventhal, M.D.
University of Chicago School of Medicine
Chicago, Illinois, U.S.A.

Mark H. Rapaport, M.D.
Cedars-Sinai Medical Center
Los Angeles, California, U.S.A

ADDITIONAL VOLUMES IN PREPARATION

Clinical Handbook of Eating Disorders

An Integrated Approach

edited by
Timothy D. Brewerton
Medical University of South Carolina
Charleston, South Carolina, U.S.A.

MARCEL DEKKER, INC.   NEW YORK • BASEL

Library of Congress Cataloging-in-Publication Data
A catalog record for this book is available from the Library of Congress.

ISBN: 0-8247-4867-0

This book is printed on acid-free paper.

Headquarters
Marcel Dekker, Inc., 270 Madison Avenue, New York, NY 10016, U.S.A.
tel: 212-696-9000; fax: 212-685-4540

Distribution and Customer Service
Marcel Dekker, Inc., Cimarron Road, Monticello, New York 12701, U.S.A.
tel: 800-228-1160; fax: 845-796-1772

Eastern Hemisphere Distribution
Marcel Dekker AG, Hutgasse 4, Postfach 812, CH-4001 Basel, Switzerland
tel: 41-61-260-6300; fax: 41-61-260-6333

World Wide Web
http://www.dekker.com

The publisher offers discounts on this book when ordered in bulk quantities. For more information, write to Special Sales/Professional Marketing at the headquarters address above.

Current printing (last digit):

10 9 8 7 6 5 4 3 2 1

PRINTED IN THE UNITED STATES OF AMERICA

This book is inspired by and dedicated to all
my most important teachers—my patients.

Foreword

It is surprising that the literature on eating disorders has taken a very long time to blossom. The original descriptions of anorexia nervosa by Gull and Lasègue date back to 1874 and 1873 respectively, but there were long delays before its recognition as a diagnostic entity. In its early editions, DSM merely labelled anorexia nervosa as a gastrointestinal reaction or a feeding disturbance. It was only in 1980, in DSM-III, that the "eating disorders" category was created and the diagnostic criteria originally formulated by clinicians in the early 1970s given a seal of approval. Bulimia nervosa was first described in 1979 and correctly accorded this term in DSM-IIIR in 1987. Proposals for the recognition of a new disorder, binge eating disorder, were put forward in the early 1990s, and accorded grudging recognition in an appendix of DSM-IV in 1994.

The expansion of our field of study owes a great deal to the assiduous research carried out by clinicians and scientists during the past 40 years, but there is an additional reason not sufficiently recognised. This is the fact that anorexia nervosa is an illness which has undergone profound changes over time. It is not clear when this transformation began but the key socio-cultural changes made an impact during the 1960s or even earlier. The actual increase in the incidence of anorexia nervosa may have been fairly modest, but there has been an outburst of eating disorders as a whole. Since the first description of the syndrome of bulimia nervosa in 1979, its incidence has reached twice that of anorexia nervosa. There has been an even larger number of patients with less specified eating disorders. This proliferation explains in part why our subject matter has become more varied and complex, and has given rise to a growing clinical and scientific literature.

An important causative factor for the transformation of anorexia nervosa into related disorders, is the cult of thinness which has pervaded modern westernised and industrial societies. The components of the cult of thinness and its impact have aroused much interest. In 1988, the social historian Joan Jacobs Brumberg expressed deep concern about the social pressures promoting anorexia nervosa and other eating disorders. She listed among the culprits magazines disseminating weight reducing diets, the fashion industry catering for the slimmer figure, and television attributing sexual allure and professional success to the possession of a svelte figure. These concerns seem at face value to be entirely justified. She went further, however, in describing how Americans are competitive even about a disease and regretted what she called "an army of health professionals and a deluge of publications and conferences since the 1970s." Presumably these observations were made tongue in cheek and have fortunately not deterred Professor Brewerton and his team of contributors from producing this new handbook much needed to do justice to the growth of our subject.

The handbook aims at providing an integrated approach. The first feature of integration that immediately strikes the reader is the full cover given to the well-established disorders—not only anorexia and bulimia nervosa, but binge eating disorder (BED) as well, and sometimes obesity is thrown in for good measure. This has led the authors sometimes having to concede that there are only slender research findings available, especially in BED. For example, there are no randomised controlled trials for the evaluation of the psychological treatments and very few on pharmacological agents in this disorder. Yet this negative statement is useful because it demonstrates the gaps that remain to be filled. Similarly, the chapter on Risk Factors in the various eating disorders frankly admits that the number of studies into BED are very small, owing to the recency of defining its research criteria.

Also important in the editor's mission of integration is the convergence of the main avenues of investigation—the psychosocial, the biomedical and the study of personality. This handbook adheres therefore to the multidimensional perspective first put forward in 1982 by Garfinkel and Garner. The significance of this commitment should not be under-estimated. For example, Campbell in 1995 boldly asserted that the term "multifactorial," although popular in psychiatry, has little explanatory power and may simply serve as a cloak to conceal our ignorance. His plea was to insist on research seeking a unitary and necessary causal element as has been possible in many physical illnesses. Unfortunately this worthwhile goal remains just as elusive now as it was in 1995. It remains important practically to examine risk factors in the various fields of endeavour—sociocultural, psychological, and biomedical—because this approach ensures that no field of study is neglected. What is particularly striking in this handbook is the breadth and erudition of the chapters devoted to the biomedical approach which range from genetics and molecular biology to neuroendocrine, neuropeptide, and neurotransmitter disturbances, and finally opens the hopeful prospects of brain imaging in patients with eating disorders.

A striking feature of the handbook is a strict objectivity in assessing the relevant literature. In the overview of risk factors for each of the eating disorders, the authors rightly confine their appraisal to combinations of symptoms forming syndromes and not the symptoms themselves. Their method of establishing causality is a demanding one. They require that the factors suspected of causing an eating disorder are indeed precursors to the illness itself. Consequently they largely reject the findings of mere correlations in cross-sectional studies, and express a strong preference for prospective longitudinal studies. These are rather rare, and thus they are obliged to use "retrospective correlates," meaning factors shown to predate the onset of the disorder according to the subjects' self-report. This stark self-discipline leads to a drastic pruning of our previously cherished lists of causal factors, such as family interaction and perfectionism. We are left with the following shortened list: gender, ethnicity, higher BMI, childhood eating problems, sexual abuse, psychiatric morbidity, low self-esteem, weight concerns and dieting.

It cannot be said that the handbook is unduly rigid in insisting on objectivity. Fluidity has been maintained and one example will suffice. In recent years the concept of co-morbidity has entered the domain of psychiatric disorders, and particularly eating disorders. The term "co-morbidity" features in several chapters ranging from the co-existence of different psychiatric symptoms, to the secondary complications from nutritional disturbances in anorexia and bulimia nervosa. In his chapter, Dr. Brewerton expresses the view that co-morbidity is the rule rather than the exception, and he ingeniously finds aetiological links in the way trauma and victimisation are apt to result in a post-traumatic stress disorder, co-morbid with an eating disorder in some patients. In case this fluidity is thought to be excessive, there is a suitable corrective in the chapter dealing specifically with co-morbidity, where clear definitions and illustrations of the multiple use of this term are provided. There is also a timely warning to avoid co-morbidity that arises as an artefact from overlapping diagnostic criteria.

In the field of treatment, flexibility of approach is usually an advantage, and this is certainly illustrated in the chapter on family evaluation and therapy. The role of the family in the genesis of eating disorders remains uncertain and controversial. In this chapter the arguments are presented fairly and from a historical prospective. Justice is done to the different schools of family therapy, including the Maudsley model. Due credit is given to the systematic evaluation of family therapy through randomised control trials undertaken by the Maudsley school. The contributors believe the value of these trials, at least in anorexia nervosa. On the other hand they also recognise that there may be a place for family therapy in bulimia nervosa and binge eating disorder where such studies are sparse or non-existent. Here is another example of integration, this time between research-based and clinical approaches.

Finally, a neat example of integration is provided in the very first chapter, "Diagnostic Issues in Eating Disorders." Leaning on the work of Sing Lee in Hong Kong, the contributors propose a new approach to the diagnostic criteria for anorexia nervosa, dividing them between culture-independent criteria (e.g., deliberate food avoidance), and criteria which are culture-specific. The latter include a fear of fatness in western patients, and a different reason for food avoidance in Chinese patients, namely a desire for an enhanced spiritual or religious experience.

This *Clinical Handbook* can be warmly recommended to clinicians and clinical scientists, whether their main interest is in understanding the nature of eating disorders or treating the patients suffering from them. Dr. Brewerton is to be congratulated on designing a handbook with a coherent structure and assembling a team of authors who display both erudition and well-balanced judgement.

Gerald Russell MD, FRCP, FRCPEd., FRCPsych. (Hon.)
Emeritus Professor of Psychiatry
Consultant Psychiatrist
The Priory Hospital Hayes Grove
Bromley, Kent, England

REFERENCES

Brumberg JJ. Fasting Girls: The Emergence of Anorexia Nervosa as a Modern Disease. Cambridge, Mass: Harvard University Press, 1988.

Campbell PG. What would a causal explanation of the eating disorders look like? In: Szmukler G, Dare C, Treasure J, eds. Handbook of Eating Disorder: Theory, Treatment and Research. Chichester: Wiley, 1995:49–64.

Garfinkel PE, Garner DM. Anorexia Nervosa: A Multidimensional Perspective. New York: Brunner Mazel, 1982.

Lee S, Ho TP, Hsu LKG. Fat-phobic and non-fat phobic anorexia nervosa: a comparative study of 70 Chinese patients in Hong Kong. Psychological Medicine 1993; 23:999–1017.

Preface

Eating is a basic drive that is taken for granted by most people. However, disorders of human eating behavior, including eating and feeding disorders, have been of increasing interest and importance to clinicians over the last several decades. This has been in part due to their increasing prevalence and the realization that they are associated with marked degrees of an array of medical and psychiatric comorbidities, as well as significant mortality. Parallel to other areas in medicine, psychiatry, and psychology, progress has been swift (although never fast enough), and this book attempts to present a concise, integrated and up-to-date overview of the scientific advancement to date in this knowledge base. This perspective is designed to be of particular interest and relevance to the clinical practitioner, but it also has potential appeal for students, scholars and researchers alike. Areas covered in this book include diagnosis and assessment, developmental perspectives, epidemiology, course of illness, etiology, specific and non-specific risk factors, medical and psychiatric comorbidity, and various treatment approaches and perspectives, including speculations about future directions in the field. These topics are organized into 4 basic sections: (I) Diagnosis, Epidemiology, and Course (Chapters 1–5); (II) Risk Factors, Etiology, and Comorbidity (Chapters 6–10); (III) Psychobiology (Chapters 11–14); and (IV) Treatment (Chapters 15–23).

In Chapter 1, Dr. Blake Woodside and Richelle Twose provide a modern overview of the diagnosis and assessment of the eating disorders, not only from the perspective of an evolving DSM, which has had its limitations, but also from the perspective of selective populations, such as men, the very young, and the very old, who have eating disorders. Furthermore, the authors propose and explain the rationale for a new classification scheme for anorexia nervosa (AN) that is "culture-independent." In this chapter the authors underscore the fact that accurate diagnosis is the foundation of effective treatment interventions. In an Appendix to this chapter a very helpful outline of a sample clinical diagnostic interview that is suitable for distinguishing between AN, bulimia nervosa (BN) and binge eating disorder (BED) is provided.

In Chapter 2, Drs. Jacqueline Carter, Traci McFarlane, and Marion Olmsted extend the discussion about diagnosis into the area of assessment and review the latest information on the most common and reliable psychometric instruments used in the assessment and screening of eating disorder patients. Structured interviews, self-report instruments, and motivation to change assessment tools used in the evaluation of patients with eating disorders are covered. In addition, structured interviews and self-report instruments used in the measurement of comorbid psychopathology are reviewed, as well as some family function assessment tools.

In Chapter 3, Dr. Dasha Nichols examines feeding disorders in infancy and early childhood, such as rumination, pica, post-traumatic feeding disorder, selective or picky eating, and general food refusal, which are increasingly recognized clinically in pediatric populations. The complex interplay between genetic factors and psycho-social factors, such as problematic parent-child interactions, are discussed. Furthermore, the potential links between feeding disorders of infancy and early childhood and eating disorders that occur later in life are discussed.

In Chapter 4, Drs. Maria Råstam, Christopher Gillberg, Daphne van Hoeken and Hans Hoek review studies to date on the epidemiology of disordered eating and the formal eating disorders from a developmental perspective. Although concentrated in the second and third decades of life, disordered eating and eating disorders occur across the lifespan. In addition to age factors, gender and cultural differences are also highlighted, which shed further light on the nature-nurture interaction.

In Chapter 5, Drs. Pamela Keel and David Herzog provide an appraisal on the long-term outcome, course and mortality of these potentially life-threatening illnesses. Although much remains to be learned in this area, the known prognostic indicators for recovery and/or relapse are reviewed, as are the results on the impact of treatment on outcome.

In Chapter 6, Dr. Corinna Jacobi, Lisette Morris, and Dr. Martina de Zwaan provide a highly integrated and critically comprehensive overview of known risk factors, both specific and nonspecific, for the development of AN, BN and BED. Of particular interest to the field is the issue of causation, which serves to guide treatment. Historically, there has tended to be a polarization of thinking about etiology into classical nature vs. nurture arenas, but each pole falls short when it attempts to stand alone. Available data clearly point to an interplay of factors that cut across these classical divisions and point to an interactive model across the life span. There does not appear to be only one cause of eating disorders, any more so than there is only one cause of mood or anxiety disorders. The "action is in the inter-action," as the anonymous saying goes.

In Chapter 7, using a wealth of twin and family studies, Dr. Cindy Bulik explores an exploding area of research and its profound clinical ramifications in a chapter on the role of genetics in the eating disorders. These data underscore the importance of biological factors in the development of all types of eating disorders. However, because genetic factors do not explain 100% of the variance, they also point out the limitations of genetics as an explanatory paradigm and lend credence to the impact of important psycho-social forces in shaping these disorders, perhaps by triggering and interacting with underlying genetic and biological mechanisms.

In Chapter 8, Dr. Lisa Lilenfeld provides a comprehensive overview of axis I psychiatric comorbidity that can be associated with AN, BN and BED. Relationships with mood, anxiety, substance use, impulse control, psychotic, dissociative, somatoform, attention-deficit, and disruptive behavior disorders are all described, although the emphasis is on the most common co-occurring conditions—mood, anxiety, and substance use disorders.

In Chapter 9, Drs. Howard Steiger and Kenneth Bruce look at the increasingly recognized role of premorbid personality traits in the develop-ment and perpetuation of the eating disorders. In addition, comorbid axis II personality disorders that are typically associated with the eating disorders are examined in depth. The implications of these data for the etiology and treatment of eating disorders is a major focus of discussion in this chapter.

In Chapter 10, Drs. Pauline Powers and Yvonne Bannon examine in detail the spectrum of medical (axis III) comorbidities associated with the various eating disorders. Eating disorders are known to adversely affect literally every organ system in the body, and it behooves the clinician to be informed of these potentially irreversible and life-threatening problems. The importance of working with a team of specialists, including a primary care physician who understands and can treat these associated medical conditions is emphasized.

In Chapter 11, Dr. Howard Steiger and myself discuss neurotransmitter dysregulation in the eating disorders. Primary focus is on the monoamines (serotonin, norepinephrine, and dopamine), with special reference to seroto-nin, which has been repeatedly found to be intimately involved in the pathophysiology as well as the neuropsychopharmacology of the eating disorders. A table that links various phenomenological aspects associated with the eating disorders to each of these three neurotransmitter systems provides a helpful perspective. Just as there is no one cause of the eating disorders, there is also not just one neurotransmitter or neurochemical system involved in these complex conditions.

Likewise, in Chapter 12, Drs. Ursula Bailer and Walter Kaye review the fundamental areas of neuroendocrine and neuropeptide dysregulation in the eating disorders, which underlie many of their clinical manifestations, including core symptoms as well as their medical and psychiatric comorbidities.

In Chapter 13, Drs. Janet Treasure and Rudolph Uher review data from the emerging area of brain imaging of the eating disorders, which provide further insights into the causes and underlying brain mechanisms involved in these tenacious conditions. Although functional brain imaging of individual eating disorder cases has not reached the status of clinical application as of yet, the potential for this approach in the future and the immediate clinical implications of these group comparison studies will be expounded.

In Chapter 14, Dr. Dorothy Grice gives an overview of the role of molecular biology in elucidating the role of genes in the etiology of the eating disorders. Dr. Grice takes us beyond the traditional genetic methodology of twin, family, and adoption studies into the modern realm of genetic association analyses used to identify genes, and she provides an up-to-date appraisal of this rapidly changing field as applied to the eating disorders.

In Chapter 15, Dr. Wayne Bowers, Dr. Arnold Andersen and Kaye Evans explain the indications for and role of inpatient and partial hospitalization in the treatment of patients with eating disorders. In certain clinical situations, such as low-weight AN, or BN with severe medical and/or psychiatric comorbidity, a structured setting is often required in order to provide the level of intensity of care required to significantly impact these conditions. This chapter provides the theoretical basis and specific guidelines for this often life-saving level of treatment.

In Chapter 16, nutritionists Jillian Croll and Dr. Dianne Neumark-Sztainer expound on the basics of the practice of nutrition counseling for AN, BN, and BED. This chapter underscores the need for a multidisciplinary approach toward all of the eating disorders in which a knowledgeable nutritionist is involved. The authors guide the reader through the components of a comprehensive nutritional assessment and provide the fundamentals of nutritional rehabilitation and weight restoration/maintenance as well as their scientific basis. The authors also provide a daily food and feelings journal, as well as sample meal plans for various daily caloric intake levels.

In Chapter 17, Drs. Stephen Wonderlich, Jim Mitchell, Lorraine Swan-Kremier, Scott Crow, and Carol Peterson provide an overview of cognitive-behavioral therapy (CBT) in the treatment of the eating disorders, particularly in the outpatient setting. CBT is clearly the most extensively studied and best empirically supported psychotherapeutic approach to the eating disorders, especially for bulimic disorders, and its fundamental principles and components are expounded. The authors also provide a food and liquid monitoring form that can be used by patients to identify contextual cues (thoughts, feelings, circumstances) associated with eating disordered behaviors.

In Chapter 18, Dr. Deb Marcontell Michel and Susan Willard, M.S.W. provide an overview of family evaluation and therapy for AN, BN and BED. Basic concepts and principles of family therapy are described, as is the history of its application in the management of eating disorders. The family characteristics of individuals with eating disorders are appraised, and the components of a family evaluation are illustrated. In addition, common approaches and issues seen in the treatment of eating disorders are discussed.

In Chapter 19, Drs. Joy Jacobs, J.D., Robinson Welch, and Denise Wilfley instruct us on the principles of Interpersonal Psychotherapy (IPT) for AN, BN and BED. Originally developed for the treatment of depression, IPT has been successfully adapted to the treatment of BN and BED and has been empirically validated for these conditions. The authors review the theoretical foundations of IPT and discuss the role of interpersonal functioning in the eating disorders. The basic concepts of IPT in the treatment of eating disorders are explained, as well as its treatment structure, therapeutic stance and typical phases of evolution. Finally, the authors review data to date on outcome studies of the use of IPT in the treatment of eating disorders.

In Chapter 20, Drs. Marsha Marcus and Michele Levine bring us up to speed on the powerful principles and techniques of Dialectical Behavior Therapy (DBT) as applied to the treatment of eating disorders. The authors review the philosophy and assumptions underlying DBT and discuss the modes of treatment used in this approach. The authors also provide a DBT diary card adapted for use in patients with eating disorders.

In Chapter 21, Drs. Joanna Steinglass and Timothy Walsh update the reader on the role of psychopharmacology in the treatment of AN, BN and BED. Unlike some psychiatric disorders, psychopharmacologic treatment alone is neither sufficient nor optimal for the treatment of any of the eating disorders, so it should be ideally conceived as an adjunct to appropriate psychotherapeutic approaches. This is especially true for AN for reasons that are elucidated. In this chapter current and realistic guidelines and limitations for using psychopharmacologic agents appropriate for these and related conditions are provided.

In Chapter 22, I review the recent literature on the role of victimization in eating disorders and related psychiatric comorbidity. A host of controlled studies now clearly implicate victimization experiences, especially childhood sexual abuse and subsequent post-traumatic stress disorder (PTSD) or symptoms, as important risk factors in the development of BN, and perhaps AN, binge-purge type, BED, and severe obesity (but not AN, restricting type). In addition, victimization experiences are associated with a host of commonly seen comorbid psychiatric disorders, including mood, anxiety, substance use, dissociative, somatoform, impulse control, disruptive behavior, and personality disorders. The implications of these data for the understanding of the etiology of eating disorders and associated psychiatric comorbidity, as well as for their treatment in clinical practice, are highlighted. Specific principles or guidelines used to approach the comorbid eating disordered patient are provided.

In Chapter 23, Dr. Joel Yager relies on his extensive experience, knowledge and creative vision to speculate about future directions in the management of eating disorders. Dr. Yager explores several areas, including future directions in diagnosis, epidemiology, molecular genetic research, other biological investigations, biological interventions, psychosocial interventions, and systems of care. In addition, the impact of computers and information technology on eating disorders management is explored.

I would like to earnestly thank all of these outstanding contributors. It is my sincerest wish that the knowledge imparted to the reader will ultimately lead to more lives saved, enhanced recovery from these formidable conditions, and less suffering by patients and their loved ones. In addition, may it inspire continued research and further advances in this field, without which this book would not have been feasible.

Timothy D. Brewerton, M.D., D.F.A.P.A., F.A.E.D.

Contents

Contents

Contributors

Arnold E. Andersen   University of Iowa Hospital & Clinics, Iowa City, Iowa, U.S.A.

Ursula F. Bailer   Anorexia and Bulimia Nervosa Research Module, Western Psychiatric Institute and Clinic, University of Pittsburgh School of Medicine, Pittsburgh, Pennsylvania, U.S.A.

Yvonne Bannon   Department of Psychiatry & Behavioral Medicine, College of Medicine, University of South Florida, Tampa, Florida, U.S.A.

Wayne A. Bowers   University of Iowa Hospital & Clinics, Iowa City, Iowa, U.S.A.

Timothy D. Brewerton   Institute of Psychiatry, Medical University of South Carolina, Charleston, South Carolina, U.S.A.

Kenneth R. Bruce   Eating Disorders Program, Douglas Hospital, and McGill University, Montreal, Quebec, Canada

Cynthia M. Bulik   Department of Psychiatry, University of North Carolina, Chapel Hill, North Carolina, U.S.A.

Jacqueline C. Carter   The Eating Disorders Program, University of Toronto, Toronto, Ontario, Canada

Jillian K. Croll   Eating Disorders Institute, St. Louis Park, Minnesota, U.S.A.

Scott J. Crow   Eating Disorders Research Program, Department of Psychiatry, University of Minnesota, Minneapolis, Minnesota, U.S.A.

Martina de Zwaan   Department of Psychosomatic Medicine and Psychotherapy, Friedrich Alexander University Erlangen-Nuremberg, Erlangen, Germany

Kay Evans University of Iowa Hospital & Clinics, Iowa City, Iowa, U.S.A

Christopher Gillberg Department of Child and Adolescent Psychiatry, Göteborg University, Göteborg, Sweden, and St. George's Hospital Medical School, London, England

Dorothy Grice[*] Center for Neurobiology and Behavior, University of Pennsylvania, Philadelphia, Pennsylvania, U.S.A.

David B. Herzog Department of Psychiatry, Massachusetts General Hospital, Boston, Massachusetts, U.S.A.

Hans Wijbrand Hoek Department of Research, Parnassia, The Hague, The Netherlands, and Mailman School of Public Health, Columbia University, New York, New York, U.S.A.

Corinna Jacobi Department of Clinical Psychology and Psychotherapy II, FB I – Psychology, University of Trier, Trier, Germany

M. Joy Jacobs Center for Eating and Weight Disorders, San Diego State University/University of California San Diego Joint Doctoral Program in Clinical Psychology, San Diego, California, U.S.A.

Walter H. Kaye Western Psychiatric Institute and Clinic, University of Pittsburgh School of Medicine, Pittsburgh, Pennsylvania, U.S.A.

Pamela K. Keel Department of Psychology, Harvard University, Cambridge, Massachusetts, U.S.A.

Michele D. Levine Department of Psychiatry, Western Psychiatric Institute and Clinic, and Behavioral Medicine and Eating Disorders Program, University of Pittsburgh School of Medicine, Pittsburgh, Pennsylvania, U.S.A.

Lisa Rachelle Riso Lilenfeld Department of Psychology, Georgia State University, Atlanta, Georgia, U.S.A.

Marsha D. Marcus Department of Psychiatry, Western Psychiatric Institute and Clinic, and Behavioral Medicine and Eating Disorders Program, University of Pittsburgh School of Medicine, Pittsburgh, Pennsylvania, U.S.A.

Traci L. McFarlane The Eating Disorders Program, University of Toronto, Toronto, Ontario, Canada

---

[*]*Current affiliation*: Child and Adolescent Psychiatry, Department of Psychiatry, University of Medicine and Dentistry of New Jersey, New Jersey Medical School, Newark, New Jersey, U.S.A.

Deborah Marcontell Michel Tulane University School of Medicine, New Orleans, Louisiana, U.S.A.

James E. Mitchell Department of Neuroscience, University of North Dakota School of Medicine and Health Sciences, and the Neuropsychiatric Research Institute, Fargo, North Dakota, U.S.A.

Lisette Morris Department of Clinical Psychology and Psychotherapy, Georg-Elias-Müller Institute of Psychology, University of Göttingen, Göttingen, Germany

Dianne Neumark-Sztainer Division of Epidemiology, School of Public Health, University of Minnesota, Minneapolis, Minnesota, U.S.A.

Dasha Nicholls Head of Feeding and Eating Disorders Service, Department of Child and Adolescent Mental Health, Great Ormond Street Hospital, London, England

Marion P. Olmsted The Eating Disorders Program, University of Toronto, Toronto, Ontario, Canada

Carol B. Peterson Eating Disorders Research Program, Department of Psychiatry, University of Minnesota, Minneapolis, Minnesota, U.S.A.

Pauline S. Powers Department of Psychiatry & Behavioral Medicine, College of Medicine, University of South Florida, Tampa, Florida, U.S.A.

Maria Råstam Department of Child and Adolescent Psychiatry, Göteborg University, Göteborg, Sweden

Howard Steiger Eating Disorders Program, Douglas Hospital, Montreal, Quebec, Canada

Joanna E. Steinglass New York State Psychiatric Institute, Columbia University, New York, New York, U.S.A.

Lorraine Swan-Kremier Department of Neuroscience, University of North Dakota School of Medicine and Health Sciences, and the Neuropsychiatric Research Institute, Fargo, North Dakota, U.S.A.

Janet Treasure Department Academic Psychiatry, Thomas Guy House, London, England

Richelle Twose University of Toronto, Toronto, Ontario, Canada

Rudolf Uher Eating Disorder Unit, Institute of Psychiatry, London, England

Daphne van Hoeken   Department of Research, Parnassia, The Hague, The Netherlands

B. Timothy Walsh   Department of Clinical Psychopharmacology, New York State Psychiatric Institute, Columbia University, New York, New York, U.S.A.

R. Robinson Welch   Department of Psychiatry, Washington University School of Medicine, St. Louis, Missouri, U.S.A.

Denise E. Wilfley   Department of Psychology, Washington University School of Medicine, St. Louis, Missouri, U.S.A.

Susan G. Willard   Department of Psychiatry & Neurology, Pediatrics, Tulane University School of Medicine, New Orleans, Louisiana, U.S.A.

Stephen A. Wonderlich   Department of Neuroscience, University of North Dakota School of Medicine and Health Sciences, and the Neuropsychiatric Research Institute, Fargo, North Dakota, U.S.A.

D. Blake Woodside   Toronto General Hospital and University of Toronto, Toronto, Ontario, Canada

Joel Yager   Department of Psychiatry, University of New Mexico School of Medicine, Albuquerque, New Mexico, U.S.A.

1

Diagnostic Issues in Eating Disorders: Historical Perspectives and Thoughts for the Future

D. Blake Woodside
Toronto General Hospital and University of Toronto
Toronto, Ontario, Canada

Richelle Twose
University of Toronto
Toronto, Ontario, Canada

Diagnostic issues have always been important in the field of eating disorders, whether debating the role of gender in these conditions or examining possible etiologic factors. With recent advances in areas as diverse as culture and genetics, reexamining thinking about diagnosis in anorexia nervosa, bulimia nervosa, and binge eating disorder becomes increasingly important.

This chapter will review some of the historical issues in the diagnosis of eating disorders and examine diagnostic schemas for special populations. A final section will address some thoughts about possible revisions to the diagnostic criteria in the light of recent developments in the field. A sample clinical diagnostic interview schedule is attached as an appendix.

DIAGNOSTIC CRITERIA

Anorexia Nervosa

The essential diagnostic criteria for anorexia nervosa has undergone more gradual and subtle shifts over time relative to bulimia nervosa. The *Diag-*

nostic and Statistical Manual of Psychiatric Disorders (DSM) criteria (Table 1) are largely reflective of Russell's 1970 description of three essential factors: (a) purposeful loss of body weight, (b) amenorrhea in females, and (c) psychopathology expressed as an intense fear of becoming fat (1,2). Many of the successive alterations are merely semantic in nature.

The weight loss threshold for diagnosis of anorexia nervosa has become less strict and severe with each revision of the DSM. In the DSM-III, a loss of 25% of original body weight (or loss of original body weight plus projected weight gain if an adolescent) is required (3). In subsequent versions, this threshold falls to 15% and becomes only a "rough" guideline. In fact, the relevant text in the DSM-IIIR (Table 2) states that weighing 85% of that expected is merely an "arbitrary but useful guide" (4).

In contrast, the evolution of the requirement for amenorrhea has become increasingly stringent over time. Contrary to Russell's description (1970), the DSM-III does not list amenorrhea as part of the diagnostic criteria but merely mentions it in the relevant text on the section (3). In later versions, this aspect of the disorder becomes mandatory for diagnosis, and the nature of amenorrhea itself is further specified (4,5). However, the presence of this criterion continues to spark controversy among experts in the field, since in approximately 15% of cases menstruation ceases prior to weight loss, and in some individuals amenorrhea persists for a period of time following restorative weight gain (1). One group (6) compared women who meet all DSM-IIIR criteria for anorexia nervosa to women who met all criteria except amenorrhea and found no significant differences on a wide variety of clinical and psychometric variables. The final issue that is relevant is the increasingly common use of oral contraceptives in this population, either for contraception or as a treatment for osteoporosis. Most experts suggest that in the presence of oral contraceptive use this criterion should be waived.

TABLE 1   DSM-III Diagnostic Criteria for Anorexia Nervosa

A. Intense fear of becoming obese, which does not diminish as weight loss progresses.
B. Disturbance of body image, e.g., claiming to "feel fat" even when emaciated.
C. Weight loss of at least 25% of original body weight or, if under 18 years of age, weight loss from original body weight plus projected weight gain expected from growth charts may be combined to make the 25%.
D. Refusal to maintain body weight over a minimal normal weight for age and height.
E. No known physical illness that would account for the weight loss.

Source: American Psychiatric Association, 1980.

TABLE 2   DSM-IIIR Diagnostic Criteria for 307.10 Anorexia Nervosa

A. Refusal to maintain body weight over a minimal normal weight for age and height, e.g., weight loss leading to the maintenance of body weight 15% below that expected; or failure to make expected weight gain during period of growth, leading to body weight 15% below that expected.
B. Intense fear of gaining weight or becoming fat, even though underweight.
C. Disturbance in the way in which one's body weight, size, or shape is experienced, e.g., the person claims to "feel fat" even when emaciated, believes that one area of the body is "too fat" even when obviously underweight.
D. In females, absence of at least three consecutive menstrual cycles when otherwise expected to occur (primary or secondary amenorrhea). (A woman is considered to have amenorrhea if her periods occur only following hormone, e.g., estrogen, administration.)

Source: American Psychiatric Association, 1987.

While the usefulness of this feature appears to be less and less important, it may be some time before it is abandoned.

Successive versions of the DSM have increasingly emphasized the psychopathological aspects of the illness. For example, criterion C in the DSM-IV, (Table 3) was expanded to include a description of three different examples of how one's body weight or shape is cognitively experienced in a pathological way. Here the mental "disorder" is said to likely involve body image distortion, its disproportionate influence on self-esteem, and the failure to recognize the dangers of a low body weight (5). Denial of the illness is also included in DSM-IV for the first time. DSM-III states only in the surrounding text on the disorder that individuals with anorexia nervosa "steadfastly deny the illness and are . . . resistant to therapy" (3). The DSM-IV, however, notes "denial of the seriousness of the current low body weight" as an essential diagnostic criterion (5).

Another recent change has been the shift away from percent average weight to body mass index (BMI), which is weight in kilograms divided by height in meters squared. DSM-IV suggests a BMI of 17.5 as an appropriate standard for the diagnosis of anorexia nervosa. This change has a number of benefits both in terms of diagnostic homogeneity across different countries and with the adolescent age group. However, it does not take into account ethnocultural differences and these require further study.

The increasing importance of recognizing both the physical and psychological effects of starvation has been recognized in DSM-IV, where sections have been added identifying common associated physical and psy-

TABLE 3   DSM-IV Diagnostic Criteria for 307.1 Anorexia Nervosa

A. Refusal to maintain body weight at or above a minimally normal weight for age and height (e.g., weight loss leading to maintenance of body weight less than 85% of that expected; or failure to make expected weight gain during period of growth, leading to body weight less than 85% of that expected).
B. Intense fear of gaining weight or becoming fat, even though underweight.
C. Disturbance in the way in which one's body weight or shape is experienced, undue influence of body weight or shape on self-evaluation, or denial of the seriousness of the current low body weight.
D. In postmenarchal females, amenorrhea, i.e., the absence of at least three consecutive menstrual cycles. (A woman is considered to have amenorrhea if her periods occur only following hormone, e.g., estrogen, administration.)

Specify type:

Restricting type: During the current episode of anorexia nervosa, the person has not regularly engaged in binge eating or purging behavior (i.e., self-induced vomiting or the misuse of laxatives, diuretics, or enemas)

Binge eating/purging type: During the current episode of anoreia nervosa, the person has regularly engaged in binge eating or purging behavior (i.e., self-induced vomiting or the misuse of laxatives, diuretics, or enemas)

Source: America Psychiatric Association, 1994.

chological symptoms. This allows for increased sophistication in the diagnosis of comorbid axis I disorders, some of which may be confused with starvation effects. This allows for distinguishing between anorexia nervosa and depression, obsessive-compulsive disorder, and specific phobias.

There have been several attempts to deal with the diagnosis of comorbid bulimia nervosa and/or purging behaviors. In DSM-IIIR, if both conditions were present, both diagnoses were made. However, DSM-IV introduced a change in the way this was handled, allowing a diagnosis of anorexia nervosa to "trump" a diagnosis of bulimia nervosa. In DSM-IV, anorexia is subclassified into the restricting and binge–purge subtypes. This distinction remains somewhat controversial, particularly in the light of some of the recent genetic findings in anorexia and bulimia, which will be reviewed below. It remains to be seen as to whether this is the optimal way in which to proceed with this area of comorbidity.

Bulimia Nervosa

Bulimia was not recognized as a mental disorder in the DSM until the publication of the third edition in 1980 (Table 4) (3). This followed its identifi-

TABLE 4 DSM-III Diagnostic Criteria for Bulimia

A. Recurrent episodes of binge eating (rapid consumption of a large amount of food in a discrete period of time, usually less than 2 hours).
B. At least three of the following:
   (1) consumption of high-caloric, easily ingested food during a binge
   (2) inconspicuous eating during a binge
   (3) termination of such eating episodes by abdominal pain, sleep, social interruption, or self-induced vomiting
   (4) repeated attempts to lose weight by severely restrictive diets, self-induced vomiting, or use of cathartics or diuretics
   (5) frequent weight fluctuations greater than 10 pounds due to alternating binges and fasts
C. Awareness that the eating pattern is abnormal and fear of not being able to stop eating voluntarily.
D. Depressed mood and self-deprecating thoughts following eating binges.
E. The bulimic episodes are not due to anorexia nervosa or any known physical disorder.

Source: American Psychiatric Association, 1980.

cation by Russell during the previous year (7). The original diagnostic criteria in DSM-III were overinclusive and led to some confusion among clinicians and researchers. The publication of the DSM-IIIR and, later, the DSM-IV addressed many of the original version's shortcomings (4,5).

Bulimia, or "ox-like eating," the original term for the illness itself, paints an incomplete picture of the syndrome it is meant to characterize. It does not depict the patient's characteristic psychopathology regarding her intense fear of fatness and obsession with body shape and weight, nor the presence of compensatory behaviors that are so important in the illness. The renaming of the condition as bulimia nervosa in DSM-IV helped to clarify that the illness included important psychopathological features as well as abnormal eating.

The DSM-III criteria for bulimia is composed of both "monothetic and polythetic criteria," i.e., both essential and optional symptoms, respectively, which complicates diagnosis of this disorder (8). The subsequent elimination of the optional indicators in the DSM-IIIR (Table 5) functioned to create a more homogeneous description (and thus a homogeneous group to research/study) and greatly simplified the task of diagnosing this disorder.

The original description of binge eating in DSM-III, "the consumption of a large amount of food in a discrete period of time" (3), was insufficient to characterize this phenomenon. DSM-IIIR added the requirement for lack of

TABLE 5   DSM-IIIR Diagnostic Criteria for 307.51 Bulimia Nervosa

A. Recurrent episodes of binge eating (rapid consumption of a large amount of food in a discrete period of time).
B. A feeling of lack of control over eating behavior during the eating binges.
C. The person regularly engages in either self-induced vomiting, use of laxatives or diuretics, strict dieting and fasting, or vigorous exercise in order to prevent weight gain.
D. A minimum average of two eating binge episodes a week for at least 3 months.
E. Persistent overconcern with body shape and weight.

Source: American Psychiatric Association, 1987.

control, differentiating bingeing qualitatively from normal eating (4). Provisions governing the time restrictions defining a binge have also evolved over time. Originally, a binge was temporally restricted to "usually under two hours" (3). The DSM-IIIR, on the other hand, abandoned the requirement of a time limit, favoring a less restrictive "discrete period of time" to define the binge event (4). The most recent criteria (5) simply provide a 2-hour period as a useful guideline. More importantly, the criterion defines the context in which a binge would occur. It is characterized as an amount of food that is "definitely larger than most people would eat during a similar period of time under similar circumstances" (5). The use of this specification distinguishes binge eating from instances in which non-disordered individuals may overeat (i.e., at a holiday party).

In addition, the frequency with which binge episodes and inappropriate compensatory strategies must occur was not established until publication of the DSM-IIIR (and DSM-IV; Table 6), where a minimum of two episodes per week over 3 months is required for diagnosis (4,5). However, it is not clear that the current frequency requirement of twice per week for 3 months is meaningful (9). One group compared a sample of bulimia nervosa patients who differed only in whether they binged once or twice per week on average and found no differences across a wide spectrum of variables. It is not clear at present what frequency of bingeing is associated with the typical psychopathology of the condition.

Psychopathologically, the original diagnostic criteria for bulimia did not require the presence of a preoccupation with weight and shape. The accompanying text merely mentions that "individuals with bulimia usually exhibit great concern about their weight" (3). This statement decreased the emphasis on the individual's pathological disturbance in attitudes, beliefs, and cognitions, and their resulting distress—attributes that distinguish mental pathology. This weakness is corrected in the DSM-IIIR, where a "persis-

TABLE 6 DSM-IV Diagnostic Criteria for 307.51 Bulimia Nervosa

---

A. Recurrent episodes of binge eating. An episode of binge eating is characterized by both of the following:
- (1) eating, in a discrete period time (e.g., within any 2-hour period) an amount of food that is definitely larger than most people would eat during a similar period of time under similar circumstances
- (2) a sense of lack of control over eating during the episode (e.g., a feeling that one cannot stop eating or control what or how much one is eating)

B. Recurrent inappropriate compensatory behavior in order to prevent weight gain, such as self-induced vomiting; misuse of laxatives, diuretics, enemas, or other medications; fasting; or excessive exercise.

C. The binge eating and inappropriate compensatory behaviors both occur, on average, at least twice a week for 3 months.

D. Self-evaluation is unduly influenced by body shape and weight.

E. The disturbance does not occur exclusively during episodes of anorexia nervosa.

Specify type:

Purging type: during the current episode of bulimia nervosa, the person has regularly engaged in self-induced vomiting or the misuse of laxatives, diuretics, or enemas.

Nonpurging type: during the current episode of bulimia nervosa, the person has regularly used inappropriate compensatory behaviors, such as fasting or excessive exercise, but has not regularly engaged in self-induced vomiting or the misuse of laxatives, diuretics, or enemas.

Source: American Psychiatric Association, 1994.

tent overconcern with body shape and weight" is listed as an essential criterion required for diagnosis, thereby addressing the sufferer's abnormal attitudes (criterion E) (4). This criterion was then strengthened in DSM-IV to include wording related to evaluation of self (criterion D) (5).

The original formulation of compensatory behaviors in DSM-III focused on physiology, i.e., the relief of fullness as opposed to the psychological significance of the behavior. Induced vomiting is also mentioned last in a series of physiological factors, such as abdominal pain and sleep, that terminate a binge (criterion B) (3). Behaviors designed to counteract the effects of binge eating did not become a mandatory requirement for diagnosis until the DSM-IIIR (4), where compensatory behaviors were linked to a fear of weight gain (4) or to modulating affect, suggesting the multiple purposes of the behaviors.

In the DSM-IV, the diagnosis of bulimia nervosa becomes more specific, as the disorder is further divided into two subtypes: (a) individuals who regularly engage in self-induced vomiting, or the misuse of laxatives, diuretics, or enemas following a binge (purging subtype: BN-P), versus (b) those who compensate for binge eating primarily through the use excessive exercise or fasting (nonpurging subtype: BN-N/P). While the purging form of the illness is more common in treatment settings, the nonpurging form is reported to be more common in the community, accounting for 70% of cases (10). A careful examination for compensatory behavior in the form of dieting or exercise is necessary to distinguish this form of the illness from binge eating disorder, as will be reviewed below.

Binge Eating Disorder

Research criteria for a new syndrome, "binge eating disorder" (Table 7), are included in Appendix B "Criteria Sets and Axes Provided for Further Study" of the DSM-IV (8). However, individuals currently fulfilling criteria for this disorder would technically still fall under the "Eating Disorder Not

TABLE 7   DSM-IV Research Criteria for Binge Eating Disorder

A. Recurrent episodes of binge eating. An episode of binge eating is characterized by both of the following:
   (1) eating, in a discrete period of time (e.g., within any 2-hour period), an amount of food that is definitely larger than most people would eat in a similar time under similar circumstances
   (2) a sense of lack of control over eating during the episode (e.g., a feeling that one cannot stop eating or control what or how much one is eating)
B. The binge-eating episodes are associated with three (or more) of the following:
   (1) eating much more rapidly than normal
   (2) eating until feeling uncomfortably full
   (3) eating large amounts of food when not feeling physically hungry
   (4) eating alone because of being embarrassed by how much one is eating
   (5) feeling disgusted with oneself, depressed, or very guilty after overeating
C. Marked distress regarding binge eating is present.
D. The binge eating occurs, on average, at least 2 days a week for 6 months.
Note: The method of determining frequency differs from that used for bulimia nervosa; future research should address whether the preferred method of setting a frequency threshold is counting the number of days on which binges occur or counting the number of episodes of binge eating.
E. The binge eating is not associated with the regular use of inappropriate compensatory behaviors (e.g., purging, fasting, excessive exercise) and does not occur exclusively during the course of anorexia nervosa.

Source: American Psychiatric Association, 1994.

Otherwise Specified" (EDNOS; Table 8) category (4). Many of the suggested diagnostic criteria resemble symptoms of bulimia nervosa, except for the absence of the regular use of "inappropriate compensatory behaviors" following the binge eating (4). The proposed criteria for binge eating disorder are reminiscent of the original characterization of bulimia in the DSM-III (3,11). This is likely a reflection of the need for further study and characterization of this illness, in order to create a more uniform list of criteria and thus describe/encompass a less heterogeneous set of individuals.

The characteristics of binge eating in binge eating disorder are virtually identical to those described in bulimia nervosa, with the exception of the frequency and duration with which they occur. The time threshold for a binge is lengthened, defined in terms of entire days rather than discrete 2-hour episodes. In addition, the research criteria for binge eating disorder must be met for 6 consecutive months, rather than 3, as required for bulimia nervosa.

Individuals who qualify for diagnosis of binge eating disorder may still occasionally engage in inappropriate compensatory behaviors, but these behaviors are not regularly used to counteract weight gain from a binge (5). More research is necessary to determine the frequency/upper threshold with which these individuals may purge and still maintain the essential features of this disorder as distinct from bulimia nervosa. Perhaps the only major difference between bulimia nervosa and binge eating disorder is the presence or absence of weight consciousness (8).

TABLE 8 DSM-IV 307.50 Eating Disorder Not Otherwise Specified

1. For females, all of the criteria for anorexia nervosa are met except that the individual has regular menses.
2. All of the criteria for anorexia nervosa are met except that, despite significant weight loss, the individual's current weight is in the normal range.
3. All of the criteria for bulimia nervosa are met except that the binge eating and inappropriate compensatory mechanisms occur at a frequency of less than twice a week for a duration of less than 3 months.
4. The regular use of inappropriate compensatory behavior by an individual of normal body weight after eating small amounts of food (e.g., self-induced vomiting after the consumption of two cookies).
5. Repeatedly chewing and spitting out, but not swallowing, large amounts of food.
6. Binge eating disorder: recurrent episodes of binge eating in the absence of the regular use of inappropriate compensatory behaviors characteristic of bulimia nervosa.

Source: American Psychiatric Association, 1994.

Unlike those with bulimia nervosa or anorexia nervosa-B/P, individuals with binge eating disorder binge-eat when they are *not* physically hungry. That is, the binge eating does not occur as simply a physiological response to starvation (11).

Furthermore, the marked distress experienced by individuals with binge eating disorder occurs not only following the binge, as in bulimia nervosa and anorexia nervosa-B/P, but *during* the binge eating as well. Perhaps this is due to the potential length episode, as one binge may last an entire day.

The weight history, current weight, diet history, and present dieting behavior of these individuals varies. Again, additional research is required to determine whether these factors will be important for diagnosis. Empirical work to date suggests that these individuals have tendency to be more obese and have a history of more marked weight fluctuations than individuals who are obese and do not binge-eat. These factors are usually attributed to their numerous unsuccessful dieting attempts and intermittent periods of binge eating behavior. Furthermore, compared to obese individuals who do not binge-eat, individuals with binge eating disorder describe pathological cognitions, attitudes, and emotions, experienced as or characterized by "higher rates of self-loathing, disgust about body size, depression, anxiety, somatic concern, and interpersonal sensitivity" (5).

CLINICAL IDENTIFICATION OF EATING DISORDERS

Appendix 1 provides a sample clinical diagnostic interview for eating disorders, suitable for distinguishing between anorexia nervosa, bulimia nervosa, and binge eating disorder.

COMMON DIFFERENTIAL DIAGNOSES IN EATING DISORDERS IN ADULTS

A number of other psychiatric disturbances will periodically be confused with anorexia nervosa or bulimia nervosa. Major depression will of course lead to significant weight loss in a minority of patients. These individuals will deny any interest in weight loss itself and will most usually still be eating a wide range of foods, if in smaller quantities. When such individuals are treated they gain weight rapidly and show none of the associated psychological comorbidity of anorexia nervosa.

A rare patient will develop food-specific delusions that cause him or her to avoid eating and to lose large amounts of weight. These cases can usually be distinguished from anorexia nervosa by the presence of widespread psychotic features that include many other issues other than food, weight, and shape.

An occasional patient will present with symptoms of obsessive-compulsive disorder and rituals around food. These patients may behaviorally resemble those with anorexia nervosa and may also have extensive cognitive schemata around their eating habits. Most typically, however, they are uninterested in weight loss per se and do not have a wish to avoid food. They will experience their food avoidance as largely ego-dystonic while recognizing that their avoidance behaviors afford them a brief interval of relief from their chronic anxiety.

Choking and swallowing phobias are relatively commonly found masquerading as anorexia nervosa, as they are often associated with extreme degrees of food avoidance and very significant weight loss. In such cases, a careful history will elicit a pattern of increasing food avoidance that is not linked to an interest in reducing calories but rather to the avoidance of a class of foods, such as hard foods. Over time, the avoidance pattern will become more and more generalized. These patients also deny any fear of fatness and will typically be able to identify with some precision the exact time of onset of their food avoidance. Such patients are readily treated with systematic desensitization, although extreme cases may require an initial period of hospitalization to get the process started. A variant of this problem is the individual with a choking phobia who has lost so much weight that a duodenal feeding tube has been inserted. Often the patient will not have eaten or drunk anything by mouth for a number of years and will require extensive desensitization in order to be able to eat normally again.

SPECIAL POPULATIONS

Males

Men have been identified as suffering from eating disorders from the beginning of the English language literature, where Morton (12) presented both a male and a female case of anorexia nervosa. More recent comprehensive examinations (13–15) have demonstrated that the illnesses, when occurring in men, are essentially indistinguishable from cases occurring in women.

Diagnostic criteria for bulimia nervosa and binge eating disorder are identical in men and women. The requirement for amennorrhea must obviously be waived in men; while some authors have suggested replacing this with various substitutes (14), such as diminished sexual drive, these suggestions have not generally been adopted. At the present time it is acceptable to diagnose anorexia nervosa in a man if he meets all the other diagnostic criteria for the condition.

TABLE 9 Russell's Criteria for Anorexia Nervosa in the Young

Criteria	Symptom
Weight loss or a failure to gain weight	Avoidance of "fattening" foods
Specific psychopathology	Overvalued dread of fatness
Delayed puberty	Delay in the sequence of pubertal events, especially menarche

The Very Young

There has been some controversy attached to the possibility that children younger than 12 years might be prone to the development of eating disorders. This controversy stems in part from a debate about the capability of younger children to generate the cognitive set required to behave in an anorectic fashion. Nonetheless, there is increasing evidence that these illnesses may occur in some form in increasingly younger girls and boys.

This has led to the development of some suggested alternations to the diagnostic criteria that take into account the lack of physical and psychological development in a prepubertal child. One group (16) have provided a thorough review of this topic. Diagnostically, they comment that some revision of the usual adult criteria must be accepted. Table 9 shows Russell's (2) criteria for anorexia nervosa in the young, focusing on the presence of morbid fears of food and fatness and the failure to achieve normal developmental milestones.

The Very Old

An occasional report (17) comments on the occurrence of new eating pathology in the elderly. At the present time, no alterations in the diagnostic criteria have been proposed for this population.

EFFECTS OF CULTURE ON THE DIAGNOSIS OF ANOREXIA NERVOSA

An interesting recent line of thought is of interest to diagnosticians. For many years, clinicians would periodically report atypical cases of anorexia nervosa where weight loss was pursued, but not for the sake of thinness; these often were described as "ascetic" anorexia nervosa, referring to the most typical presentation involving a desire to live a simpler life.

In the mid-1990s, a psychiatrist in Hong Kong, Sing Lee, began to publish about his experience in treating young Chinese girls with anorexia nervosa (18–21). He noted that his patient population was roughly equally divided into two groups. The first resembled traditional Western description of anorexia nervosa, demonstrating a fear of fatness or drive for thinness accompanied by food avoidance, dieting, and significant weight loss. Most of these individuals also experienced body image distortion.

The second group, which he labeled "Chinese anorexia," clearly avoided food and lost weight—but had no interest in thinness per se, no fear of food or of fat, and no body image disturbance. These individuals attributed their food avoidance to spiritual or religious desires, such as the wish to achieve a more pure level of existence through self-denial. Lee and his colleagues proposed that the drive for thinness/fear of fatness and associated drive for thinness paradigm were actually culture-bound aspects of anorexia nervosa. In his schema, the core culture-independent aspects of the illness are deliberate food avoidance and the achievement of a very low weight, lower than normal individuals can achieve. From this viewpoint, the precise rationale or cognitive content would be culture specific, and not otherwise central to the diagnosis of the condition.

No other formal research has been done on this intriguing concept. The advantage of the concept is that it would help account for trends in incidence of anorexia across different time periods and cultures, and would allow for an understanding of the effect of the dissemination of Western, largely American culture worldwide. Clinically, in our own treatment setting we see examples of this phenomenon, both in recent immigrants from Hong Kong and in individuals from the subcontinent of India. These latter individuals often present with somatic complaints as the rationale for their food avoidance and weight loss. So abdominal pain, constipation, or swallowing difficulties become the reason for cutting out more and more foods.

The most interesting clinical observation that we could add here relates to the effect of placing such individuals in a group therapy treatment program primarily attended by women with classical North American anorexia nervosa. The inevitable outcome seems to be that over the course of 2 or 3 months the women of Chinese or Indian origin acculturate to the dominant culture of the program, gradually abandoning their original rationale for food avoidance and developing a fear of fatness, a drive for thinness, and body image distortion! It is of course not certain that this represents an improvement, although it does allow for a more homogeneous group.

The other advantage of this approach to the diagnosis of anorexia nervosa is that it dovetails neatly with some of the information becoming available about the genetic influences on the disorder, as will be reviewed below.

TABLE 10 Proposed Culture-Independent Diagnostic Criteria for Anorexia Nervosa

---

1. Core symptoms (present across cultures)
   (a) Deliberate food avoidance
   The individual purposefully reduces his or her food intake without needing to do so. This may be achieved by cutting back on portion sizes, eliminating certain foods or restricting the range of foods eaten. This behavior may be overt or hidden.
   (b) Achievement of a low weight
   The individual achieves a weight representing the 5th percentile for his or her gender, age, and ethnocultural group. In adolescents, the individual has a previously normal pattern of weight gain with age, which has changed to a pattern of being below the 5th percentile for age, gender, and ethnocultural group.
   (c) Denial of severity
   The individual minimizes the severity of the condition.
2. Culture-specific symptoms
   Individuals in specific ethnocultural groups may display similar sets of cognitions surrounding their food avoidance behaviors, which are not required for the diagnosis. Some examples include:
   (a) Western. The food avoidance is usually accompanied by a fear of fatness and an interest in calorie-reduced dieting to lose weight. This interest in a low weight may simply be expressed as a fear of being too heavy or as an interest in a more "healthy" lifestyle. The pattern of eating typically involves the avoidance of high-calorie foods or foods that are associated with weight gain. A body image distortion is often present whereby the individual perceives himself or herself as larger than he or she actually is.
   (b) Chinese (Mainland). The food avoidance is usually associated with a desire for an enhanced spiritual or religious experience. Food avoidance is framed as self-denial or strengthening. Weight loss is not desired per se but may be presented as evidence of adherence to the spiritual beliefs driving the process. The food avoidance includes most foods but few foods are cut out entirely.
   (c) Indian subcontinent. The food avoidance is associated with physical symptoms in the abdomen or thorax that the person associates with eating. Bloating, constipation, abdominal pain, or difficulty in swallowing are often cited as rationales for not eating. Weight loss is not desired but is often presented as evidence of the seriousness of the physical problem. Specific patterns of food avoidance are generally related to the nature of the physical symptoms endorsed as the cause of the food avoidance.

Table 10 presents a preliminary attempt to construct a set of diagnostic criteria according to these culturally sensitive principles. In this schema, the core requirements are deliberate food avoidance and the achievement of a very low weight by the standards of the culture involved. The content of the cognitive set become culture-specific associated symptoms and are no longer core elements of the diagnosis. Such a schema would represent a marked shift in thinking, especially for Western clinicians and researchers, but deserves some consideration.

EFFECT OF GENETIC CAUSALITY ON DIAGNOSIS IN EATING DISORDERS

Some information has recently been reported concerning the heritable genetic components of both anorexia nervosa and bulimia nervosa that may be relevant in the diagnoses of these conditions. The Price Foundation collaborative group has recently published some preliminary results of their studies in this area (22,23). Their findings on anorexia nervosa show significant association between the restricting form of the illness and high perfectionism to a site on chromsome 1. The addition of increasing levels of bingeing or purging symptoms reduces the magnitude of the finding, suggesting that on a genetic basis, the restricting form of the illness has some characteristics distinct from the binge–purge form. The report of a significant finding for a separate area of the genome (chromosome 10) adds to the evidence that there may be distinct genetic liabilities for the type of dietary restriction associated with anorexia nervosa and the purging of bulimia nervosa.

Further work in this area may lead to a totally new diagnostic schema that is related to the genetic etiology of the conditions.

CONCLUSION

The field of diagnosis in eating disorders faces many challenges in the next few years. These relate primarily to the presentation of novel data concerning the cultural and genetic determinants of the conditions. These data have the potential to dramatically alter the way in which we view the nature of the psychiatric diagnostic labels for these conditions.

It seems likely that the next revision of DSM will include formal diagnostic criteria for binge eating disorder. However, the relationship between this condition and the other eating disorders remains unclear. As well, the ED-NOS classification could benefit from some clarification, possibly along the lines of "AN-like" and "BN-like."

Such changes, while difficult to adapt to, will in the long run allow for a greater understanding of the nature of the illnesses.

APPENDIX 1   Sample Clinical Interview Format

1. Introduction and overview
- patient's view of the problem
- overall course of the development of the illness

2. Weight history
- height
- current weight
- highest-ever weight
- lowest weight since onset of illness
- typical weight ranges
- ideal weight

3. Typical daily intake
- breakfast
- lunch
- snacks
- dinner

Quantify amounts, types of food eaten and liquid consumed—is fluid avoided or restricted?

- foods avoided
- safe foods
- diet products

4. Bingeing
- carefully define and distinguish from overeating
- onset, frequency, initiating and ameliorating factors
- specific details of a typical binge
- usual response
- nocturnal binges, odd binges, stealing

5. Purging
For all of: vomiting, laxatives, diuretics, diet pills, thyroid, exercise:
- onset, frequency, initiating and ameliorating factors
- ipecac
- surgery
- consumption of inedible items

6. Complications of starvation/bingeing and purging
- endocrine (menses)
- metabolic (K^+, Hgb, ECG)

- Dermatological (skin, hair, nails)
- Gastrointestinal (bloating, early satiety, parotid swelling, dental caries, hematemesis, hematochezia, bowel function)
- cardiac (palpitations, edema)
- psychological
  sleep pattern
  concentration
  food preoccupation
  mood

7. **Medical history**
   - significant illnesses
   - current medications

8. **Past treatment history**

9. **Past psychiatric history**
   - Axis I screen

10. **Family history**
    - includes family/genetic history

11. **Personal and developmental history**
    - includes screen for sexual abuse

12. **Relationship history**

REFERENCES

1. Fairburn CG, Garner DM. Diagnostic criteria for anorexia nervosa and bulimia nervosa: the importance of attitudes to shape and weight. In: Garner DM, Garfinkel PE, eds. Diagnostic Issues in Anorexia Nervosa and Bulimia Nervosa. New York: Brunner/Mazel, 1988.

2. Russell GFM. Premenarchal anorexia nervosa and its sequelae. J Psychiat Res 1985; 19:363–369.

3. American Psychiatric Association. Diagnostic and Statistical Manual of Mental Disorders. 3rd ed. Washington, DC.

4. American Psychiatric Association. Diagnostic and Statistical Manual of Mental Disorders. 3rd ed. Revised. Washington, DC.

5. American Psychiatric Association. Diagnostic and Statistical Manual of Mental Disorders. 4th ed. Washington, DC.

6. Garfinkel PE, Lin E, Goering P, Spegg C, Goldbloom D, Kennedy S, Kaplan A,

Woodside DB. Purging and non-purging forms of bulimia nervosa in a community sample. Int J Eating Disord 1996; 20:23–231.

7. Russell GFM. Bulimia nervosa: an ominous variant of anorexia nervosa. Psychol Med 1979; 9:429–448.

8. Pope HG Jr, Hudson JI, Spitzer RL, Williams JBW. Revisions in DSM-III criteria for bulimia nervosa. In: Garner DM, Garfinkel PE, eds. Diagnostic Issues in Anorexia Nervosa and Bulimia Nervosa. New York: Brunner/Mazel, 1988:80–111.

9. Garfinkel PE, Lin E, Goering P, Spegg C, Goldbloom D, Kennedy S, Kaplan A, Woodside DB. Bulimia nervosa in a Canadian community sample. Am J Psychiatry 1995; 152:1052–1058.

10. Garfinkel PE, Lin E, Goering P, Spegg C, Goldbloom D, Kennedy S, Kaplan A, Woodside DB. Is amenorrhea necessary for the diagnosis of anorexia nervosa? Br J Psychiatry 1996; 168:500–506.

11. Keys A, Brozek J, Henschel A, Mickelsen O, Taylor HL. The Biology of Human Starvation, Vol. 1. Minneapolis: University of Minnesota Press, 1950.

12. Morton R. Phthisologica: Or a Treatise of Consumption. London: S Smith and B Walford, 1694.

13. Woodside DB, Garfinkel PE, Lin E, Goering P, Kaplan AS, Goldbloom DS, Kennedy SH. Men with full and partial syndrome eating disorders: community comparisons with non–eating disordered men and eating disordered women. Am J Psychiatry 2001; 158:570–574.

14. Crisp AH, Burns T. Primary anorexia nervosa in the male and female: a comparison of clinical features and prognosis. In: Andersen AA, ed. Males with Eating Disorders. New York: Brunner/Mazel, 1990:77–99.

15. Andersen A. Males with Eating Disorders. New York: Brunner/Mazel, 1990.

16. Treasure J, Thompson P. Anorexia nervosa in childhood. Br J Hosp Med 1988; 40:362–369.

17. Pobee, Kodwo A, LaPalio, Lawrence R. Anorexia nervosa in the elderly: a multidisciplinary diagnosis. Clin Gerontologist 1996; 16:3–9.

18. Lee S, Ho TP, Hsu LKG. Fat phobic and non-fat phobic anorexia nervosa: a comparative study of 70 Chinese patients in Hong Kong. Psychol Med 1993; 23:999–1017.

19. Lee S. How abnormal is the desire for slimness? A survey of eating attitudes and behaviour among Chinese undergraduates in Hong Kong. Psychol Med 1993; 23(2):437–451.

20. Lee S, Ho TP, Hsu LKG. Fat phobic and non-fat phobic anorexia nervosa—a comparative study of 70 Chinese patients in Hong Kong. Psychol Med 1993; 23:999–1004.

21. Hsu, George L, Lee, Sing. Is weight phobia always necessary for a diagnosis of anorexia nervosa? Am J Psychiatry 1993; 150:1466–1471.

22. Grice DE, Halmi KA, Fichter MM, Strober M, Woodside DB, Treasure JT, Kaplan AS, Magistretti PJ, Goldman D, Kaye WH, Bulik CM, Berrettini WH. Evidence for a susceptibility gene for restricting anorexia nervosa on chromosome 1. Am J Hum Genet 2002; 70:787–792.

23. Bulik CM, Devlin B, Bacanu SA, Thornton L, Klump KL, Fichter MM, Halmi KA, Kaplan AS, Strober M, Woodside DB, Bergen AW, Ganjei K, Crow S, Mitchell J, Rotondo A, Mauri M, Cassano G, Keel P, Berrettini WH, Kaye WH. Significant linkage on chromosome 10p in families with bulimia nervosa. Am J Hum Genet 2003; 72:200–207.

2

Psychometric Assessment of Eating Disorders

Jacqueline C. Carter, Traci L. McFarlane,
and Marion P. Olmsted
University of Toronto
Toronto, Ontario, Canada

Comprehensive psychometric assessment is essential for diagnosis, case formulation, treatment planning, and assessment of progress. The use of valid and reliable measures is also vital to clinical research. Certain distinctive features of eating disorders can make the clinical assessment process challenging. Individuals with eating disorders have a reputation for minimizing the seriousness of their symptoms. This is likely related to feelings of ambivalence about changing certain valued features of the disorder (e.g., food restriction, low weight). It may also be attributable to the shame and secrecy surrounding some eating-disordered behaviors (e.g., binge eating and vomiting). These factors can lead to denial or distortion in self-report (1). For these reasons, the establishment of a trusting relationship is a prerequisite to eliciting accurate information from eating disorder patients (2). The assessor should communicate an empathic awareness of the mixed feelings many individuals experience about acknowledging certain symptoms, considering change, or starting treatment. In addition, incorporating the principles of motivational viewing into the assessment process can be useful (3). Taking a collaborative approach and focusing on the aspects of the illness that are experienced as distressing to the patient may be particularly helpful.

The purpose of this chapter is to describe psychometric measures of the specific and general psychopathology of eating disorders. It is beyond the scope of the chapter to review all existing measures. For the assessment of specific psychopathology, we have decided to focus on widely used tests that were designed to be used as screening instruments in nonclinical populations as well as measures designed to measure clinical eating disorders. The focus is on more comprehensive measures, but selected measures of specific constructs (e.g., motivation to change) are discussed as well. Both structured interviews and self-report instruments are covered. For a detailed review of other eating disorder assessment methods, see Allison (4). With respect to general psychopathology, there are a multitude of well-established measures of common associated symptoms, including depression, anxiety, self-esteem, and interpersonal difficulties. The interested reader is referred to Groth-Marnat (5) for more information about general psychological assessment. The present chapter focuses on the tests that we would recommend for the purposes of treatment planning and measuring treatment outcome in persons with eating disorders. The areas covered are in line with the American Psychiatric Association Practice Guidelines for eating disorders (6). Both adult and child/adolescent measures are discussed. A clinical interview is also an important component of the assessment process and is necessary to obtain a psychiatric history and make a diagnosis. This aspect of assessment is covered in Chapter 1 of this volume on diagnosis.

SPECIFIC PSYCHOPATHOLOGY

Specific psychopathology refers to features that are distinctive to eating disorders. The clinical features of the two recognized eating disorders, anorexia nervosa (AN) and bulimia nervosa (BN), overlap significantly. The central features of BN are binge eating and inappropriate compensatory behaviors to prevent weight gain. In the fourth edition of the *Diagnostic and Statistical Manual of Mental Disorders* (DSM-IV; 7), binge eating has two defining characteristics: (a) the consumption of a large amount of food given the circumstances; and (b) a sense of loss of control. Compensatory behaviors are divided into two categories: purging and nonpurging. Purging techniques include self-induced vomiting and laxative or diuretic misuse. Nonpurging compensatory behaviors include strict dieting, fasting, and excessive exercise. The central features of AN are extreme food restriction and a refusal to maintain body weight at or above a minimally normal weight for age and height (i.e., body mass index ≤ 17.5). Approximately half of those presenting with AN also report binge eating and/or purging. Undue influence of body shape and weight on self-evaluation is common to both disorders. Binge eating disorder, a provisional diagnostic category in the DSM-IV, is characterized by recurrent binge eating in the absence of compensatory behaviors.

Structured Interviews

Structured interviews have the advantage of affording a more detailed examination of symptoms as compared with self-report inventories as they allow the opportunity for probing and clarification. On the other hand, interviews rely on the subject's self-report and the results may therefore still be influenced by recall bias, denial, or minimization of symptoms (8). A number of structured interviews to measure eating disorder symptoms have been developed. Examples include the Clinical Eating Disorder Rating Instrument (9) and the Structured Interview for Anorexia and Bulimia (10). However, these instruments have not been widely used, and very little information is available on their psychometric properties. Two of the most widely used structured interviews for the assessment of eating disorders are the Eating Disorder Examination (11) and the Yale-Brown-Cornell Eating Disorder Scale (12,13). The eating disorder section of the Structured Clinical Interview for DSM-IV (SCID; 14,15) has also been widely employed to make eating disorder diagnoses in clinical research. It will be discussed later in this chapter under "General Psychopathology."

Eating Disorder Examination (EDE; 11)

The EDE is considered by many investigators to be the best available method for assessing the specific psychopathology of eating disorders (e.g., 16). The EDE consists of four subscales: Restraint, Shape Concern, Weight Concern, and Eating Concern. The subscale scores range from 0 (no pathology) to 6 (extreme pathology). Individual item scores provide either frequency or severity rating for key behavioral or attitudinal aspects of eating disorders. In addition, there are individual items to assess the presence and frequency of key behaviors, including binge eating and weight control behaviors, over the previous 28 days. To allow DSM-IV diagnoses, certain items assess the previous 2 months as well. Operationalized diagnostic criteria are provided in the interview manual (11). The EDE is investigator based (meaning that key terms are defined by the interviewer, not the respondent) and requires properly trained assessors. It may take up to an hour to administer. At the outset, the interviewer refers to a calendar and helps the subject identify key events to enhance recall of the time period being examined. All key concepts are defined in the manual, and explicit instructions are given as to how to rate each item. The judgment as to whether an episode of eating is a "large amount" is made by the interviewer.

The EDE has been demonstrated to be a reliable and valid instrument. The internal consistency of the four subscales is satisfactory (17). High interrater reliability (18,19) and good test–retest reliability have been found

(20) in different settings. In addition, the EDE has been demonstrated to have good criterion-related validity (17,19) and convergent validity (18). Normative data for AN, BN, and normal controls are available (11). A children's version of the EDE interview has been developed (21).

Yale-Brown-Cornell Eating Disorder Scale (YBC-EDS; 12)

The YBC-EDS is a clinician-rated semistructured interview designed to measure eating disorder symptom severity. Target symptoms are preoccupations and rituals. Preoccupations are defined as "ideas, thoughts, images or impulses that repeatedly enter your mind; they may seem to occur against your will." Rituals are defined as "behaviors or acts that you feel driven to perform." Target symptoms are identified and assessed in terms of time occupied by symptoms, interference with functioning, distress caused by symptoms, and degree of control over symptoms. Items are rated on a 0 (none/not present) to 4 (extreme) scale. The four preoccupation items and the four ritual items are added to obtain preoccupation and ritual subtotals. The sum of these yields a total score. The YBC-EDS is not intended for use as a diagnostic instrument.

The YBC-EDS has been demonstrated to have high interrater reliability and good internal consistency (12). Its convergent validity was established by comparing scores on the YBC-EDS with scores on other validated measures of eating disorder symptoms (12).

Self-Report Instruments

Self-report instruments offer a number of advantages over structured interview measures. They are completely standardized, require little or no formal training to administer, are economical, and may be completed in a group format. On the other hand, Wilson (16) identified a number of shortcomings shared by most self-report measures of eating disorder features, including the lack of a specific time frame and the failure to ask directly about the frequency of key eating disorder behaviors. In addition, most fail to define key terms such as "binge eating."

Numerous measures of certain aspects of eating disorder psychopathology are available, e.g., the Restraint Scale (22), the Three Factor Eating Questionnaire which primarily measures restraint and disinhibition (23), and the Binge Eating Scale (24). For the purposes of this chapter, we will concentrate on comprehensive measures that cover a broad range of the core cognitive and behavioral features of eating disorders. Selected measures of specific constructs (e.g., motivation to change, body image) will also be discussed. The following self-report measures may be used as screening instruments in nonclinical samples or as measures of eating disorder symptom severity for clinical or research purposes. None are intended to be the sole basis for making a diagnosis, although they may be a useful adjunct to a diagnostic interview.

Eating Attitudes Test (EAT; 25,26)

The EAT is a self-report questionnaire that was developed to measure the symptoms of AN in adults and older adolescents (16 years and older) (27). The original EAT consisted of 40 items; an abbreviated 26-item version was later derived through factor analysis (EAT-26; 26). Each item is rated on a 6-point Likert scale ranging from "never" to "always." The most symptomatic answer receives a score of 3, the next adjacent response a score of 2, and so on. The three least symptomatic responses receive a score of 0. No specific time frame is given. In addition to a total score, the EAT-26 yields three subscales: Dieting, Bulimia/Food Preoccupation, and Oral Control. The EAT-26 total score is highly correlated with the EAT-40 total score and the 14 eliminated items were found to be redundant (26). A children's version of the EAT-26 intended for use with those younger than 16 years has been developed (ChEAT; 28).

The EAT has been widely employed as a screening instrument in epidemiological research to identify suspected cases of eating disorders. For screening purposes, a total score above 20 on the EAT-26 is the recommended cutoff. On average, most studies have found the EAT-26 to have a relatively low positive predictive value (e.g., 29,30). That is, a significant proportion of those scoring above 20 do not have clinical eating disorders upon diagnostic interview. Regarding the rate of false negatives, one study reported that 1% of low scorers (i.e., <20) were subsequently identified as cases.

Carter and Moss (31) reported the test–retest reliability of the EAT-40 over a 2- to 3-week period to be 0.84. Both the EAT and EAT-26 have been found to correlate moderately to highly with other measures of eating-disordered attitudes and behavior (e.g., 32–35). Gross et al. (32) found that the EAT-40 differentiated BN subjects from normal controls. However, it has not been found to differentiate between AN and BN (36). The test–retest reliability coefficient for the 26-item children's version of the EAT following a 3-week interval has been found to be 0.81 and it has been shown to have good internal consistency (28). Scores on the 26-item ChEAT have been shown to correlate significantly with measures of weight management behavior and body dissatisfaction among middle-school girls (37).

Eating Disorder Inventory (EDI; 38)

The EDI is a widely used self-report measure of symptoms commonly associated with AN and BN. It comprises three subscales that assess attitudes and behaviors concerning eating, weight, and shape (Drive for Thinness,

Bulimia, Body Dissatisfaction), and five subscales that measure psychological constructs clinically relevant to the eating disorders (Ineffectiveness, Perfectionism, Interpersonal Distrust, Interoceptive Awareness, Maturity Fears). A second edition of the EDI (EDI-2) has been published that retains the original 64 items and adds 27 items comprising three additional subscales: Asceticism, Impulse Regulation, and Social Insecurity (27). Items are rated using a 6-point scale ranging from "never" to "always." The EDI does not specify a time frame for responding to the items. Raw subscale scores are plotted on profile forms to allow comparison with norms for eating disorder patients (N = 889) and a female college student control group (N = 205). The EDI is suitable for those 12 years and older. Criterion-related and construct validity for the eight original EDI subscales have been well documented (e.g., 32,38–40). Wear and Pratz (41) obtained 3-week test–retest reliability coefficients above 0.80 for all of the original subscales except Maturity Fears. A cutoff score of 14 on the Drive for Thinness subscale has been recommended for screening purposes (27). However, this measure is most useful as a measure of eating disorder symptom severity for clinical or research purposes.

Kids Eating Disorders Survey (KEDS; 42,43)

The Kids Eating Disorders Survey (KEDS) is a 12-item screening questionnaire designed for eating-disordered behaviors and attitudes among latency-age and early adolescent children. Detailed scoring instructions have been published elsewhere (44). The KEDS assesses the presence or absence of weight loss dieting; fasting; self-induced vomiting; excessive exercise; use of diet pills, diuretics, and laxatives; as well as binge eating, with a detailed definition of binge eating provided. Body dissatisfaction is measured through the use of figure drawings. Respondents are asked to select a current and an ideal figure drawing. The body dissatisfaction score is the difference between the two drawings. The KEDS has been shown to have good internal consistency (Chronbach's α = 0.73) and total score test–retest reliability after an average interval of four months of 0.83 (43).

Revised Bulimia Test (BULIT-R; 45)

The BULIT-R is a 36-item questionnaire that was developed to measure the symptoms of BN. It contains 28 items that are scored and 8 unscored items that ask about weight control behavior. Items are rated using a five-choice multiple-choice format. The BULIT-R has been found to have high internal consistency (Cronbach's coefficient α = 0.97) and a 2-month test–retest reliability of 0.95 (45). It also has demonstrated concurrent and criterion-related validity (46). Thelen et al. (45) reported norms of bulimia nervosa (N = 24) and female control (N = 116) participants. The BULIT-R may be employed as a screening instrument or as a measure of symptom severity. A cutoff score of 85 has been recommended for screening purposes (45).

Eating Disorder Examination Questionnaire (EDE-Q; 47)

The self-report version of the EDE, the EDE-Q, was designed to address some of the shortcomings of self-report instruments (47). Like the EDE, the 36-item EDE-Q has a 28-day time frame and asks directly about the frequency of key eating disorder behaviors. It is intended for use with older adolescents and adults. Its items are closely based on the corresponding questions from the EDE interview and it uses the same 7-point rating scheme. The EDE-Q also generates four subscale scores (Restraint, Eating Concern, Shape Concern, and Weight Concern) as well as a global score that is the average of the four subscales. Respondents rate each item on a 7-point rating scale (i.e., 0–6) indicating the number of days out of 28 on which particular behaviors, attitudes, or feelings occurred. Scores of 4, 5, or 6 are interpreted as more likely to be of clinical severity.

There have been several studies on the psychometric properties of the EDE-Q. Luce and Crowther (48) reported 2-week test–retest reliability coefficients ranging from 0.81 to 0.94 across the four subscales and 0.57 to 0.70 for items measuring the frequency of key behaviors. Given the 28-day time frame of the EDE-Q, the somewhat lower stability of the behavioral items may reflect fluctuations in symptom frequency.

Five studies have examined the convergent validity of the EDE-Q by comparing it with the EDE interview (47,49–52). In general, good agreement was found across all subscales. There was also good agreement in most studies for the assessment of self-induced vomiting and laxative misuse, but significant differences were found for the frequency of binge eating. Finally, Wilson et al. (53) reported discriminant validity data on the EDE-Q. In this study, several EDE-Q items were shown to discriminate between obese binge eaters and nonbinge eaters. The self-report version appears to be an adequate substitute for the EDE interview in the assessment of most eating disorder features. A children's version has been developed, and adolescent norms for this version have recently been published (54). The EDE-Q is particularly useful as a self-report measure of the frequency of key behaviors for clinical or research purposes.

Mizes Anorectic Cognitions Scale (MACS-R; 55)

The MACS-R is designed to measure attitudes and beliefs commonly associated with eating disorders. Items are rated on a 5-point Likert scale ranging from "strongly disagree" to "strongly agree." Three subscales were derived through factor analysis: (a) self-control and self-esteem; (b) weight and approval; and (c) rigid weight regulation and fear of weight gain (56). Test–retest reliability was found to be 0.78 over a 2-month interval for the original version and the coefficient α was 0.90 for the revised version. The test–retest reliability of the revised scale has not been studied. A number of studies support the concurrent and discriminant validity of the MACS, and it has been shown to be sensitive to change with treatment (57). This measure may be useful for elucidating eating disorder cognitions and measuring cognitive change with treatment.

The Shape- and Weight-Based Self-Esteem Inventory (SAWBS; 58)

Determining self-worth based on an assessment of the body (i.e., shape- and weight-related self-esteem) is the core cognitive psychopathology in eating disorders (59), and it has been shown to predict relapse in BN (60). The SAWBS Inventory is a self-report measure that involves completing a pie diagram to measure shape- and weight-related self-esteem in adults. An adolescent version has also been developed by the authors to be used with adolescents aged 13–18 years (61). Participants are asked to select from a list of personal attributes the ones that are important in terms of how they felt about themselves (e.g., weight and shape, personality, intimate relationships) over the past 4 weeks. A second step involves rank ordering each attribute. Then participants are asked to divide a circle into pieces such that the size of each piece reflects how much their self-esteem is based on each of the ranked attributes. The shape- and weight-based self-esteem score is the angle of the shape and weight piece of the pie. The researchers found a mean angle of 58° for the weight and shape wedge in their sample of non-eating disordered women. They also found that greater evaluation of the self on the basis of weight and shape was related to higher levels of depression and lower levels of overall self-esteem. In another study, Geller et al. (62) found that eating-disordered patients reported greater weight-based self-esteem (mean angle 145°) than both a psychiatric control group (mean angle 63°) and a student control group (mean angle 59°). Overall, the SAWBS Inventory has been shown to have good psychometric properties in both adults and adolescents, including test–retest reliability after a 1-week interval of 0.81 and 0.77, respectively (58,61,62).

Motivation to Change

As previously mentioned, individuals with eating disorders are typically ambivalent about recovery. This is related to the ego-syntonic nature of certain feature of eating disorders (e.g., dietary restriction and weight control). The development and validation of measures to assess readiness to change in eating disorders is still at an early stage.

University of Rhode Island Change Assessment Scale (URICA; 63,64)

This widely used 32-item self-report measure of readiness to change (also commonly referred to as The Stages of Change Questionnaire) was originally developed to assess motivation to change among substance abusers. However, since its item do not refer to any specific behaviors but rather to "problems that need changing," it has been used in different populations, including eating disorders (e.g., 65). It has four subscales corresponding to four stages of change: Precontemplation (e.g., "As far as I'm concerned, I don't have any problems that need changing"), Contemplation (e.g., "It might be worthwhile to work on my problem"), Action (e.g., "I am really working hard to change"), and Maintenance (e.g., "I am working to prevent myself from having a relapse of my problem"). Items are rated on a 5-point Likert scale ranging from "strongly agree" to "strongly disagree" and a mean score is yielded for each subscale. One limitation of using this questionnaire to measure readiness to change in eating disorders is that the scores are not easily interpreted because the items do not refer to disorder-specific behaviors or attitudes.

Anorexia Nervosa Stage of Change Questionnaire (ANSOCQ; 66)

The ANSOCQ is a newly developed measure of motivation to change that is based on the stages-of-change model but is tailored to the specific symptoms of AN. It is designed to measure readiness to reach a normal weight, to cease extreme weight-control behaviors, to eat normally, and to consume avoided foods. Each item contains five statements corresponding to five stages of change: Precontemplation (e.g., "As far as I'm concerned, I do not need to gain weight"), Contemplation (e.g., "In some ways, I think I might be better off if I gained weight"), Preparation (e.g., "I have decided that I will attempt to gain weight"), Action (e.g., "At the moment I am putting in a lot of effort of gain weight"), and Maintenance (e.g., "I am working to maintain the weight gains I have made"). For each item, respondents are asked to select the statement that best describes their current attitude or behavior. The ANSOCQ has been demonstrated to have good internal consistency and 1-week test–retest reliability as well as acceptable concurrent and predictive validity (66). This instrument may be useful in assessing the impact of level of motivation to change on treatment outcome in eating disorders as well as in assessing the effectiveness of motivational enhancement interventions. Further study of this measure is needed.

Concerns About Change Questionnaire (CAC; 67)

The CAC is a 112-item self-report measure of fears about change that is still under development. It was designed to apply to all psychiatric conditions including eating disorders, anxiety disorders, and substance abuse. Respondents are asked to rate on a 5-point scale the extent to which each item applies to them. The questionnaire comprises 17 rational subscales (e.g., Unable to Change, Fear of Risks, Fear of Maturity, Fear of Sexuality, Fear of the Process of Change, Fear of Loss of Accomplishment, Fear of Interpersonal Loss). The internal consistency of the subscales is high (0.80–0.91). Although it requires further validation, this measure may be useful in determining the functional significance of the eating disorder and the obstacles to recovery.

GENERAL PSYCHOPATHOLOGY

General psychopathology refers to features that are shared with other psychiatric conditions. In eating disorders, commonly associated psychopathology includes depression, anxiety, low self-esteem, interpersonal problems, and personality disturbance. In addition, features of obsessive-compulsive disorder, substance abuse, posttraumatic stress disorder, and dissociative disorder may be present. Such concerns may represent premorbid conditions, or may indeed be caused or exacerbated by the eating disorder itself. Many of these symptoms have been shown to improve with successful management of the eating disorder. Patients who are severely depressed or severely anxious may need to be stabilized before undertaking a specialized symptom-focused eating disorder treatment program. Many comorbid concerns are entangled with the eating disorder and will need to be addressed during the eating disorder treatment (e.g., obsessive-compulsive disorder), while longstanding interpersonal and personality disturbances may require additional treatment after the eating disorder has been resolved. Numerous well-established measures of general psychopathology exist, and it is beyond the scope of this chapter to review them all. We will describe the instruments that we recommend for clinical and research purposes.

Structured Interviews

Structured Clinical Interview for DSM-IV (SCID; 14,15)

The SCID is a widely used semistructured interview for making DSM-IV axis I and axis II (personality disorder) diagnoses. It incorporates the use of obligatory questions, operational diagnostic criteria, a categorical system for rating symptoms, and an algorithm for arriving at a final diagnosis. In addition, it allows the interviewer to probe and restate questions, challenge the respondent, and ask for further clarification. The SCID can take between 1 and 3 hours to administer. Although it was originally developed for use in research by trained clinicians, research staff with varying levels of prior clinical experience can be trained to reliably administer the SCID. The users guides for the SCID-I and SCID-II provide basic training information. In addition, there is an 11-hour videotape training program that includes examples of interviews with patients. The SCID for Dissociative Disorders (SCID-D; 68) was developed to enable clinically trained interviewers to assess the nature and severity of the five dissociative symptoms (amnesia, depersonalization, derealization, identity confusion, and identity alteration) and to diagnose the presence of DSM-IV dissociative disorders. The reliability and validity of the SCID I and II as well as the SCID-D have been documented in several studies (68–71). Additional information about SCID training can be found at www.scid4.org.

Diagnostic Interview for Children and Adolescents (DICA; 72,73)

The DICA is a semistructured interview designed to determine the presence or absence of symptoms and other criteria required for DSM-IV lifetime diagnoses in children and adolescents. There are three separate interviews designed for children (6–12 years), adolescents (13–18 years), and parents. The interview is designed to be administered by highly trained interviewers and takes between 1–2 hours to complete. Although results vary depending on the disorder, high test–retest reliability and moderate convergent validity have been demonstrated (74,75).

Yale-Brown Obsessive Compulsive Scale (Y-BOCS; 76,77)

The Y-BOCS is a 10-item semistructured interview measure of obsessive-compulsive symptoms. It was not designed for use as a diagnostic instrument. Each item is rated from 0 (no symptoms) to 4 (extreme symptoms). The total Y-BOCS score is the sum of items 1–10 (range, 0–40). There are separate subtotals for the severity of obsessions (items 1–5) and compulsions (items 6–10). Symptoms are assessed in terms of how much of the respondent's time they occupy, the extent to which they interfere with normal functioning, the degree of subjective distress they cause, and the extent to which they are actively resisted by the patient and can be controlled by the patient. The Y-BOCS has been documented to have strong psychometric properties. It shows good internal consistency (76,78), excellent interrater reliability (76,78), and acceptable test–retest reliability (78). Evidence for its convergent validity has been established in studies that compared the Y-BOCS total score with other standard self-report and behavioral measures of obsessive-compulsive disorder (77–79). A self-report version of the Y-BOCS has been developed and has been shown to be highly correlated with the YBOCS interview (80,81).

There is also a children's version of the Y-BOCS that has been shown to be reliable and valid (82).

Clinician-Administered PTSD Scale (CAPS; 83)

The CAPS is a 34-item semistructured interview designed to measure the 17 symptoms of PTSD according to the DSM-IIIR (84). Each symptom is rated on a 5-point scale in terms of frequency and intensity. The CAPS yields two total scores, one for frequency and one for intensity, as well as two subscores for each of the reexperiencing, avoidance, and arousal subscales. It may be used to make current and lifetime PTSD diagnoses and also for measuring the severity of PTSD symptomatology. The CAPS shows high interrater reliability, test–retest reliability, and internal consistency (83,85,86). It has also been shown to have good concurrent validity, as indicated by significant correlations with self-report measures of PTSD (83).

SELF-REPORT QUESTIONNAIRES

Depression

Beck Depression Inventory, Second Edition (BDI-II; 87)

The BDI-II is a 21-item self-report instrument for measuring the severity of depression in adults and adolescents 13 years and older. The BDI-II was developed as an indicator of the presence and degree of depressive symptoms consistent with the DSM-IV criteria. Respondents are asked to endorse symptoms that apply to them during the past 2 weeks. Scores of 0–13 reflect minimal depression, 14–19 mild depression, 20–28 moderate depression, and scores of 29 or more severe depression. This measure is easily administered and scored. However, because depression is associated with suicidal risk in eating-disordered patients it should be interpreted by a professional with appropriate clinical training and experience. Moreover, the clinician should pay particular attention to the responses to item 2 (pessimism) and item 9 (suicidal thoughts or wishes) as indicators of possible suicide risk. The BDI-II has been shown to have sound psychometric properties, including coefficient α values of 0.92 for patients and 0.93 for college students, and test–retest reliability after a 1-week interval of 0.93 (87).

Depression Anxiety and Stress Scales (DASS; 88,89)

This self-report measure is available either in a 42-item or a 21-item version. The DASS has the advantage of assessing and discriminating between depression (e.g., "I felt down-hearted and blue") and anxiety symptoms (e.g., "I found myself getting agitated"), as well as a more general stress dimension. Participants are asked to respond to each statement using a 4-

point scale ranging from 0 (did not apply to me at all) to 3 (applied to me very much or most of the time) using the time frame of "over the past week." The factor structure and reliability of the DASS have been established in clinical populations, and it has been shown to have very good concurrent and discriminant validity (90).

Anxiety

Beck Anxiety Inventory (BAI; 91)

The BAI is a 21-item self-report measure of anxiety symptoms. The BAI asks respondents to rate symptoms that have bothered them over the past week using a 4-point scale ranging from 0 (not at all) to 4 (severely). This measure places an emphasis on symptoms of physical hyperarousal (e.g., numbness or tingling, heart pounding or racing, difficulty breathing). The BAI has sound psychometric properties (91) and has also demonstrated treatment sensitivity (92). This is a useful measure to screen for the presence and severity of anxiety symptoms.

The BAI and the DASS (described under depression) can be used to screen for the presence and degree of physical hyperarousal indicating anxiety and general stress. However, to identify specific anxiety disorders more specialized measures are required. It is beyond the scope of this chapter to review all possible means of identifying and measuring specific anxiety disorders. Some suggestions include the Fear Questionnaire (93) to measure the severity of common phobias, the Panic Disorder Severity Scale (94) to assess panic disorder severity in patients already diagnosed with panic disorder, the Penn State Worry Questionnaire (95) to measure the tendency to worry excessively indicative of generalized anxiety disorder, the Social Phobia Inventory (96) to measure the fear, avoidance, and physiological arousal associated with social phobia, and the Yale-Brown Obsessive-Compulsive Scale (81). For more information about these and other scales, the reader is referred to Antony et al. (97) for a comprehensive review of anxiety-related assessment measures.

Self-Esteem

Rosenberg Self-Esteem Scale (RSES; 98,99)

This is a 10-item self-report inventory that assesses self-esteem in adolescents and adults. This measure is significantly correlated with measures of depression and neuroticism (98,99), and other measures of self-esteem (100). The RSES has strong construct, convergent, and discriminant validity (99,101) and has been shown to predict outcome in the management of bulimia nervosa (102). Respondents are asked to strongly agree, agree, disagree, or strongly disagree to a series of statements about the self (e.g., "I feel I do not have much to be proud of") considering how they "usually feel." Scores range from 10 (extremely low self-esteem) to 40 (extremely high self-esteem). In a recent study of 100 respondents, it was shown that eating-disordered participants scored significantly lower (mean score 22) than both chronic dieters (mean score 31) and a student control group (mean score 33) in terms of trait self-esteem as measured by the RSES (103).

Substance Abuse

Michigan Alcoholism Screening Test (MAST; 104)

The MAST is a 25-item self-report questionnaire that was developed to detect alcohol-related problems in adults. The MAST can be used clinically with individual patients, both for diagnosis and as a means of providing a short but comprehensive profile of the medical, psychological, and social functions that are interfered with by the use of alcohol (105). The scale has been shown to have high internal consistency (106), satisfactory test–retest reliability, and good convergent validity (107).

Adolescent Drinking Index (ADI; 108)

The ADI is a 24-item self-report measure that was developed to screen for alcohol-related problems in adolescents (12–17 years old). The ADI is designed to identify adolescents who should be referred for further alcohol evaluation or treatment. The instrument contains two subscales: self-medicating problem drinking and aggressive, rebellious drinking behavior. The ADI has high internal consistency, good test–retest reliability, and has demonstrated convergent and discriminant validity (108,109).

Drug Abuse Screening Test (DAST; 110)

The DAST is a 20-item self-report measure designed to detect drug abuse in adults during the past year. This measure has high internal consistency, and good concurrent and discriminant validity (110,111). There is also an adolescent version of this measure that has demonstrated sound psychometric properties in adolescents aged 13–19 years (112).

Other Psychological Symptoms

Dissociative Experiences Scale (DES; 113,114)

The DES is a self-report questionnaire that was developed to measure normal and pathological dissociative phenomena in adults (18 years and older). The original DES consists of 28 descriptions of dissociative experiences. Respondents are asked to indicate on a visual analog scale what percentage of the time each experience occurs to them in their daily life. Subscales include amnesia, depersonalization-derealization, and absorption experiences. The total score is an average of each response.

The scale has been shown to have good psychometric properties including a coefficient α of 0.96 and test–retest reliability of 0.93 for the total score (115). In addition, the DES has demonstrated convergent and predictive validity (116) and can be used as a screening measure to identify dissociative disorders in a clinical population (117). There is also an adolescent version of the scale (Adolescent Dissociative Experiences Scale; 118) that has been shown to have sound psychometric qualities in adolescents aged 12–18 (118–120).

Brief Symptom Inventory (BSI; 121)

The BSI is a 53-item self-report symptom inventory designed to measure a range of psychological symptoms. It is essentially a brief form of the Symptom Checklist-90-R (122). The BSI is useful to screen for a wide variety of psychological symptoms in clinical and research settings where time is limited. Respondents are asked to indicate how much a problem has distressed or bothered them during the past 7 days. Each item of the BSI is rated on a 5-point scale ranging from 0 (not at all distressed) to 4 (extremely distressed). There are nine subscales (i.e., Somatization, Obsessive-compulsive, Interpersonal Sensitivity, Depression, Anxiety, Hostility, Phobic Anxiety, Paranoid Ideation, and Psychoticism) and three global indices (i.e., global severity index, positive symptom total, positive symptom distress index) (121). The α coefficients for all nine subscales are very good, ranging from a low of 0.71 on the Psychoticism dimension to a high of 0.85 on Depression. Test–retest reliability after a 2-week interval was high for the global indices scales, ranging from 0.80 to 0.90 (121,123,124). Norms are provided for adults (i.e., nonpatients and psychiatric patients) and for adolescents (aged 13–19) (121).

PTSD Symptom Scale—Self-Report (PSS; 125,126)

The PSS-SR is a 17-item self-report scale designed to measure the presence and frequency of PTSD symptoms over the previous 2 weeks in individuals with a known trauma history. Its items correspond to the 17 DSM-IIIR diagnostic criteria for PTSD. Each item is rated from 0 (not at all) to 3 (very much). The total severity score is the sum of the severity ratings for the 17 items. The PSS-SR has been shown to have satisfactory internal consistency, high test–retest reliability, and good convergent validity with the SCID PTSD module (125). For diagnostic purposes, the PSS-SR should be used in combination with a diagnostic interview.

Interpersonal Functioning and Personality

Inventory of Interpersonal Problems (IIP; 127)

The IIP is available as a 32- or 64-item self-report instrument that identifies salient interpersonal difficulties that may have important clinical implications. This measure evaluates overall interpersonal difficulty, and also assesses eight specific domains of interpersonal functioning (i.e., domineering/controlling, vindictive/self-centered, cold/distant, socially inhibited, nonassertive, overly accommodating, self-sacrificing, intrusive/needy). The eight subscales are organized around two major factors: control/submission (dominance) and positive/negative valence (affiliation). Items are divided into two sections: one section begins with "The following are things you find hard to do with other people" (e.g., join in on groups, confront people with problems that come up); the other section begins with "The following are things that you do too much" (e.g., I am overly generous to other people, I argue with other people too much). Response options range from "not at all" to "extremely." Both the IIP-64 and the IIP-32 have moderate to high internal consistency for the total scales corresponding to 0.96 and 0.93, respectively, and both have test–retest reliability after a 1-week interval of 0.78 in a nonclinical sample. Test–retest reliability is higher in clinical samples. Normative information is based on adults aged 18–89 (127,128).

Dimensional Assessment of Personality Pathology—Basic Questionnaire (DAPP-BQ; 129)

The DAPP-BQ is a 290-item self-report questionnaire developed to assess dimensions of personality pathology. It is composed of 18 subscales derived through factor analysis corresponding to easily interpreted and theoretically meaningful personality patterns. The DAPP-BQ scales are internally consistent; estimates of coefficient α for the scales range from 0.87 to 0.94. It also has demonstrated good convergence with other self-report measures of personality traits (e.g., 130,131). Norms for a general adult population control group are available (129). This instrument was used in a recent study of personality pathology in patients with eating disorders (132). For a detailed discussion of the assessment of personality disorder, the reader is referred to Clark and Harrison (133).

Family Functioning

Disturbances in family functioning are common in the eating disorders, and family therapy has been found to be helpful, particularly for younger patients (134). Therefore, it can be useful to include a measure of family functioning in the assessment battery. For a detailed discussion of self-report instruments for family assessment, see Skinner (135). We recommend using one of the following measures.

Family Environment Scale (FES; 136)

The FES is a 90-item true–false self-report measure designed to assess an individual's perceptions of the current social environment or climate of his or her whole family unit. It may be administered to individuals 12 years and older. Ten subscales reflecting three dimensions of family functioning were derived through factor analysis: (a) Interpersonal Relationships (i.e., Cohesion, Conflict, and Expressiveness subscales); (b) Personal Growth (i.e., Independence, Achievement Orientation, Intellectual-Cultural Orientation, Active Recreational Orientation, and Moral-Religious Emphasis subscales); and (c) System Maintenance (i.e., Family Organization and Control subscales). The 10 subscales have been shown to be internally consistent with Cronbach's α coefficients ranging from 0.61 to 0.78. Adequate test–retest reliability for a 2-month interval has also been demonstrated (136), and its criterion-related validity has been established in numerous studies (137). The manual presents normative data for normal and distressed families.

Family Assessment Measure (FAM-III; 138,139)

The FAM-III is a self-report measure of family functioning that was designed to measure both family strengths and weaknesses from the perspective of different family members. It may be administered to family members who are at least 10 years old. The basic processes assessed by the FAM-III include Task Accomplishment, Role Performance, Communication, Affective Expression, Involvement, Control, and Values and Norms. The FAM-III consists of three subscales: a 50-item General Scale examining the overall family system; a 42-item Dyadic Relationships Scale measuring the quality of relationships between specific pairs in the family; and a 42-item Self-Rating Scale assessing an individual's perception of his or her functioning in the family. It takes about 30–40 minutes to administer. The FAM-III subscales have been shown to have good internal consistency (α coefficients of 0.86–0.95) and adequate 12-day test–retest reliability (median correlations of 0.57–0.66) (138). FAM-III scores have been shown to differentiate between clinical and nonclinical families (140,141). Studies of its construct validity have found that the FAM-III is highly correlated with other measures of family functioning including the FES (142,143). The manual presents norms and interpretative guidelines.

SUMMARY AND RECOMMENDATIONS

This chapter has provided an overview of psychometric instruments relevant to the assessment of eating disorders that can be used clinically and/or in research. A comprehensive assessment should include measures of specific eating disorder features as well as measures of general psychopathology. We have described measures of eating disorder symptoms that may be used as screening instruments as well as those designed to measure clinical eating disorders. Recommended measures of general psychopathology were also discussed.

In specialist treatment settings, we would recommend using the EDE to measure core diagnostic features plus an additional dimensional self-report measure of the severity of eating disorder symptomatology (e.g., EDI) to measure specific psychopathology. For the measurement of general psychopathology, at a minimum we would suggest including a self-report measure of depression, anxiety, self-esteem, interpersonal difficulties, and family functioning. Including a measure of motivation to change may also be helpful in tailoring the treatment plan to the patient's level of readiness to change. For example, patients who are not ready to make behavioral changes may be referred to a purely psychoeducational intervention. Providing patients with feedback about their test results is another important element of the clinical assessment process but is beyond the scope of this chapter. It goes without saying that such feedback should be provided by qualified professionals. In primary care settings, a screening instrument (e.g., EAT or KEDS) may be useful in determining whether a referral for specialist treatment should be considered.

REFERENCES

1. Vitousek K, Daly J, Heiser C. Reconstructing the internal world of the eating-disordered individual: overcoming denial and distortion in self-report. Int J Eat Disord 1991; 10:647–666.
2. Crowther JH, Sherwood NE. Assessment. In: Garner DM, Garfinkel PE, eds. Handbook of Treatment for Eating Disorders. New York: Guilford Press, 1997: 34–39.
3. Miller WR, Rollnick S. Motivational Interviewing. 2d ed. New York: Guilford Press, 2002.
4. Allison DB. Handbook of Assessment Methods for Eating Behaviors and Weight-Related Problems—Measures, Theory and Research. Thousand Oaks, CA: Sage Publications, 1995.
5. Groth-Marnat G. Handbook of Psychological Assessment. 3d ed. New York: John Wiley and Sons, 1996.
6. American Psychiatric Association. Practice guidelines for the treatment of patients with eating disorders. Am J Psychiatry 2000; 157:1–39.
7. American Psychiatric Association. Diagnostic and Statistical Manual of Mental Disorders. 4th ed. Washington, DC, 1994.
8. Pike KM, Loeb K, Walsh BT. Binge eating and purging. In: Allison DB, ed.

Handbook of Assessment Methods for Eating Behaviors and Weight-Related Problems: Measures, Theory and Research. Thousand Oaks, CA: Sage Publications, 1995:303–346.

9. Palmer R, Christie M, Cordle C, Davies D, et al. The Clinical Eating Disorder Rating Instrument (CEDRI): a preliminary description. Int J Eat Disord 1987; 6:9–16.

10. Fichter MM, Elton M, Engel K, Meyer A-E, et al. Structured Interview for Anorexia and Bulimia Nervosa (SIAB): development of a new instrument for the assessment of eating disorders. Int J Eat Disord 1991; 10:571–592.

11. Fairburn CG, Cooper Z. The Eating Disorder Examination. In: Fairburn CG, Wilson GT, eds. Binge Eating: Nature, Assessment and Treatment. 12th ed. New York: Guilford Press, 1993:317–360.

12. Mazure CM, Halmi KA, Sunday SR, Romano SJ, Einhorn AM. The Yale-Brown-Cornell Eating Disorder Scale: development, use, reliability and validation. J Psychosom Res 1994; 28:425–445.

13. Sunday SR, Halmi KA, Einhorn A. The Yale-Brown-Cornell Eating Disorder Scale: a new scale to assess eating disorder symptomatology. Int J Eat Disord 1995; 18:237–245.

14. First MB, Gibbon M, Spitzer RL, Williams JB. User's Guide for the Structured Clinical Interview for DSM-IV Axis I Disorders. New York: Biometrics Research, 1996.

15. First MB, Gibbon M, Spitzer RL, Williams JB, Benjamin LS. User's Guide for the Structured Clinical Interview for DSM-IV Axis II Personality Disorders. Washington, DC: American Psychiatric Press, 1997.

16. Wilson GT. Assessment of binge eating. In: Fairburn CG, Wilson GT, eds. Binge Eating: Nature, Assessment and Treatment. New York: Guilford Press, 1993:317–360.

17. Cooper Z, Cooper PJ, Fairburn CG. The validity of the Eating Disorder Examination and its subscales. Br J Psychiatry 1989; 154:807–812.

18. Rosen JC, Vara L, Wendt S, Leitenberg H. Validity studies of the Eating Disorder Examination. Int J Eat Disord 1990; 9:519–528.

19. Wilson GT, Smith D. Assessment of bulimia nervosa: an evaluation of the Eating Disorder Examination. Int J Eat Disord 1989; 8:173–179.

20. Rizvi SL, Peterson CB, Crow SJ, Agras WS. Test–retest reliability of the Eating Disorder Examination. Int J Eat Disord 2000; 28:311–316.

21. Bryant-Waugh RJ, Cooper PJ, Taylor CL, Lask BD. The use of the Eating Disorder Examination with children: a pilot study. Int J Eat Disord 1996; 19: 391–397.

22. Herman CP, Polivy J. Restrained eating. In: Stunkard AJ, ed. Obesity. Philadelphia: W.B. Saunders, 1980:208–225.

23. Stunkard AJ, Messick S. The three factor eating questionnaire to measure dietary restraint, disinhibition and hunger. J Psychosom Res 1985; 29:71–81.

24. Gormally J, Black S, Daston S, Rardin D. The assessement of binge eating severity among obese persons. Addict Behav 1982; 7:47–55.

25. Garner DM, Garfinkel PE. The Eating Attitudes Test: an index of the symptoms of anorexia nervosa. Psychol Med 1979; 9:273–279.

26. Garner DM, Olmsted MP, Bohr Y, Garfinkel PE. The Eating Attitudes Test: psychometric features and clinical correlates. Psychol Med 1982; 12:871–878.

27. Garner DM. Eating Disorder Inventory-2 professional manual. Odessa, FL: Psychological Assessment Resources, 1991.

28. Maloney M, McGuire J, Daniels S. Reliability testing of a children's version of the Eating Attitudes Test. J Am Acad Child Adol Psychiatry 1988; 5:541–543.

29. Johnson-Sabine E, Wood K, Patton G, Mann A, Wakeling A. Abnormal eating attitudes in London schoolgirls: a prospective epidemiological study. Psychol Med 1988; 18:615–622.

30. Meadows GN, Palmer RL, Newball EUM, Kenrick JMT. Eating attitudes and disorder in young women: a general practice based survey. Psychol Med 1986; 16:351–357.

31. Carter PI, Moss RA. Screening for anorexia and bulimia nervosa in a college population: problems and limitations. Addict Behav 1984; 9:417–419.

32. Gross J, Rosen JC, Leitenberg H, Willmuth ME. Validity of the Eating Attitudes Test and the Eating Disorder Inventory in bulimia nervosa. J Consult Clin Psychol 1986; 54:875–876.

33. Henderson M, Freeman CPL. A self-rating scale for bulimia: the "BITE." Br J Psychiatry 1987; 150:18–24.

34. Mizes JS. Personality characteristics of bulimics and non–eating disordered female controls: a cognitive behavioral perspective. Int J Eat Disord 1988; 7:541–550.

35. Smith MC, Thelen MH. Development and validation of a test for bulimia. J Consult Clin Psychol 1984; 52:863–872.

36. Williamson DA, Cubic BA, Gleaves DH. Equivalence of body image disturbances in anorexia and bulimia nervosa. J Abnorm Psychol 1993; 102:1–4.

37. Smolak L, Levine MP. Psychometric properties of the Children's Eating Attitudes Test. Int J Eat Disord 1994; 16:275–282.

38. Garner DM, Olmsted MP, Polivy J. Development and validation of a multidimensional Eating Disorder Inventory for anorexia nervosa and bulimia. Int J Eat Disord 1983; 2:15–34.

39. Garner DM, Olmsted MP. The Eating Disorder Inventory Manual. Odessa, FL: Psychological Assessment Resources, 1984.

40. Schoemaker C, Verbank M, Breteler R, van der Staak C. The discriminant validity of the Eating Disorder Inventory-2. Br J Clin Psychol 1997; 36:627–629.

41. Wear RW, Pratz O. Test–retest reliability of the Eating Disorder Inventory. Int J Eat Disord 1987; 6:767–769.

42. Childress AC, Jarrell MP, Brewerton TD. The Kids' Eating Disorders Survey (KEDS): Internal consistency, component analysis, and reliability. Eating Disorders: J Treat Prev 1993; 1:123–133.

43. Childress AC, Brewerton TD, Hodges EL, Jarrell MP. The Kids' Eating Disorders Survey (KEDS): a study of middle school students. J Am Acad Child Adol Psychiatry 1993; 32:843–850.

44. Brewerton TD. The use and scoring of the Kids' Eating Disorders Survey (KEDS). Eating Disorders: J Treat Prev 2001; 9:71–74.
45. Thelen MH, Farmer J, Wonderlich S, Smith M. A revision of the bulimia test: the BULIT-R. Psychol Assess 1991; 3:119–124.
46. Welch G, Thompson L, Hall A. The BULIT-R: its reliability and clinical validity as a screening tool for DSM-III-R bulimia nervosa in a female tertiary education population. Int J Eat Disord 1993; 14:95–105.
47. Fairburn CG, Beglin SJ. Assessment of eating disorders: interview or self-report questionnaire. Int J Eat Disord 1994; 16:363–370.
48. Luce KH, Crowther JH. The reliability of the Eating Disorder Examination—Self-Report Questionnaire Version (EDE-Q). Int J Eat Disord 1999; 25:349–351.
49. Black CMD, Wilson GT. Assessment of eating disorders: Interview versus questionnaire. Int J Eat Disord 1996; 20:43–50.
50. Carter JC, Aime A, Mills J. Assessment of bulimia nervosa: a comparison of interview and self-report questionnaire methods. Int J Eat Disord 2001; 30:187–192.
51. Grilo CM, Masheb RM, Wilson GT. A comparison of different methods for assessing the features of eating disorders in patients with binge eating disorder. J Consult Clin Psychol 2001; 69:317–322.
52. Wilfley DE, Schwartz MB, Spurrel EB, Fairburn CG. Assessing the specific psychopathology of binge eating disorder: interview or self-report? Behav Res Ther 1997; 35:1151–1159.
53. Wilson GT, Nonas CA, Rosenblum GD. Assessment of binge eating in obese patients. Int J Eat Disord 1993; 8:173–179.
54. Carter JC, Stewart DA, Fairburn CG. Eating Disorder Examination Questionnaire: norms for young adolescent girls. Behav Res Ther 2001; 39:625–632.
55. Mizes JS, Christiano B, Madison J, Post G, Seime R, Varnado P. Development of the Mizes Anorectic Cognitions Questionnaire Revised: psychometric properties and factor structure in a large sample of eating disorders patients. Int J Eat Disord 2000; 28:415–421.
56. Mizes JS. Construct validity and factor stability of the Anorectic Cognitions Questionnaire. Addict Behav 1991; 16:89–93.
57. Mizes JS. Validity of the Mizes Anorectic Cognitions Scale: a comparison between anorectics, bulimics and psychiatric controls. Addict Behav 1992; 17:283–289.
58. Geller J, Johnson C, Madsen K. The role of shape and weight in self-concept: the shape and weight based self-esteem inventory. Cog Ther Res 1997; 21:5–24.
59. Cooper Z, Fairburn CG. Confusion over the core psychopathology of bulimia nervosa. Int J Eat Disord 1993; 13:385–389.
60. Fairburn CG, Peveler RC, Jones R, Hope RA, Doll HA. Predictors of 12-month outcome in bulimia nervosa and the influence of attitudes to shape and weight. J Consult Clin Psychol 1993; 61:696–698.
61. Geller J, Srikameswaran S, Cockell S, Zaitsoff Z. Assessment of shape- and weight-based self-esteem in adolescents. Int J Eat Disord 2000; 28:339–345.

62. Geller J, Johnson C, Madsen K, Goldner EM, Remick RA, Birmingham CL. Shape and weight-based self-esteem and the eating disorders. Int J Eat Disord 1998; 24:285–298.
63. McConnaughy EA, DiClemente CC, Prochaska JO, Velicer WF. Stages of change in psychotherapy: a follow-up report. Psychotherapy 1983; 26:494–503.
64. McConnaughy EA, Prochaska JO, Velicer WF. Stages of change in psychotherapy: measurement and sample profiles. Psychotherapy 1983; 20:368–375.
65. Ward A, Troop N, Todd G, Treasure J. To change or not to change—"how" is the question. Br J Med Psychol 1996; 69:139–146.
66. Rieger E, Touyz S, Schotte D, Beumont P, Russell J, Clarke S, Kohn M, Griffiths R. Development of an instrument to assess readiness to recover in anorexia nervosa. Int J Eat Disord 2000; 28:387–396.
67. Vitousek K, DeViva J, Slay J, Manke F. Concerns about change in the eating and anxiety disorders. Paper presented at the Annual Meeting of the American Psychological Association, New York, 1995.
68. Steinberg M. Structured Clinical Interview for DSM-IV Dissociative Disorders (SCID-D). revised. Washington, DC: American Psychiatric Press, 1994.
69. First MB, Spitzer RL, Gibbon M, Williams JB, et al. The Structured Clinical Interview for the DSM-III-R Personality Disorders (SCID-II): Part II. Multisite test–retest reliability study. J Person Disord 1995; 9:92–104.
70. Spitzer RL, Williams JB, Gibbon M, First MB. The Structured Clinical Interview for DSM-III-R: History, rationale and description. Arch Gen Psychiatry 1992; 49:624–629.
71. Williams JB, Gibbon M, First M, Spitzer RL. The Structured Clinical Interview for DSM-III-R (SCID II): Multisite test–retest reliability. Arch Gen Psychiatry 1992; 49:630–636.
72. Herjanic B, Reich W. Development of a structured psychiatric interview for children: agreement between child and parent on individual symptoms. J Abnorm Child Psychol 1982; 10: 307–324.
73. Reich W. Dignostic interview for children and adolescents (DICA). J Am Acad Child Adol Psychiatry 2000; 39:59–66.
74. De la Osa N, Ezpeleta L, Oomenech JM, Navarro JB, Losilla JM. Convergent and discriminant validity of the structured diagnostic interview for children and adolescents (DICA-R). Psychol Spain 1997; 1:37–44.
75. Welner Z, Reich W, Herjanic B, Jung KG, Amado H. Reliability, validity and parent–child agreement studies of the diagnostic interview for children and adolescents (DICA). J Am Acad Child Adol Psychiatry 1987; 5:649–653.
76. Goodman WK, Price LH, Rasmussen SA, Mazure C, Fleischmann RL, Hill CL, Heninger GR, Charney DS. The Yale-Brown Obsessive Compulsive Scale, I. Development, use, and reliability. Arch Gen Psychiatry 1989; 46:1006–1011.
77. Goodman WK, Price LH, Rasmussen SA, Mazure C, Delgado P, Heninger GR, Charney DS. The Yale-Brown Obsessive Compulsive Scale, II. Validity. Arch Gen Psychiatry 1989; 46:1012–1016.
78. Woody SR, Steketee G, Chambless DL. Reliability and validity of the Yale-Brown Obsessive-Compulsive Scale. Behav Res Ther 1995; 33:597–605.

79. Kim SW, Dysken MW, Kuskowski M. The Yale-Brown Obsessive-Compulsive Scale: a reliability and validity study. Psychiatry Res 1990; 34:99–106.
80. Rosenfeld R, Dar R, Anderson D, Kobak KA, Greist JH. A computer-administered version of the Yale-Brown Obsessive Compulsive Scale. Psychol Assess 1992; 4:329–332.
81. Steketee G, Frost R, Bogart K. The Yale-Brown Obsessive Compulsive Scale: interview versus self-report. Behav Res Ther 1996; 34:675–684.
82. Scahill L, Riddle MA, McSwiggin-Hardin M, Ort SI, King RA, Goodman WK, Cicchetti D, Leckman JF. J Am Acad Child Adol Psychiatry 1997; 36:844–852.
83. Blake DD, Weathers FW, Nagy LM, Kaloupek DG, Klauminzer G, Charney DS, Keane TM. A clinician rating scale for assessing current and lifetime PTSD: the CAPS-1. Behav Therapist 1990; 13:187–188.
84. American Psychiatric Association. Diagnostic and Statistical Manual of Mental Disorders. 3d ed. revised. Washington, DC, 1987.
85. Weathers FW, Keane TW, Davidson JRT. Clinician-Administered PTSD Scale: a review of the first ten years of research. Depression Anxiety 2001; 13: 132–156.
86. Blanchard EB, Hickling EJ, Taylor AE, Forneris CA, Loos W, Jaccard J. Effects of varying scoring rules of the Clinician-Administered PTSD Scale (CAPS) for the diagnosis of posttraumatic stress disorder in motor vehicle accident victims. Behav Res Ther 1995; 33:471–475.
87. Beck AT, Steer RA, Brown GK. The Beck Depression Inventory Manual, 2d ed. San Antonio, TX: Psychological Corporation Harcourt Brace & Company, 1996.
88. Lovibond SH, Lovibond PF. Manual for the Depression and Anxiety Stress Scales. 2d ed. Sydney, Australia: Psychological Foundation of Australia, 1995.
89. Lovibond SH, Lovibond PF. The structure of negative emotional states: Comparison of the Depression Anxiety Stress Scales (DASS) with the Beck Depression and Anxiety Inventories. Behav Res Ther 1995; 33:335–342.
90. Antony MM, Bieling PJ, Cox BJ, Enns MW, Swinson RP. Psychometric properties of the 42-item and 21-item versions of the Depression Anxiety Stress Scales in clinical groups and a community sample. Psychol Assess 1998; 10:176–181.
91. Beck AT, Epstein N, Brown G, Steer RA. An inventory for measuring clinical anxiety: psychometric properties. J Consult Clin Psychol 1988; 56:893–897.
92. de Beurs E, Wilson KA, Chambless DL, Goldstein AJ, Feske U. Convergent and divergent validity of the Beck Anxiety Inventory for patients with panic disorder and agoraphobia. Depression Anxiety 1997; 6:140–146.
93. Marks IM, Mathews AM. Brief standard self-rating for phobic patients. Behav Res Ther 1979; 17:263–267.
94. Shear MK, Brown TA, Sholomskas DE, Barlow DH, Gorman JM, Woods SW, Cloitre M. Panic Disorder Severity Scale (PDSS). Pittsburgh: Department of Psychiatry, University of Pittsburgh School of Medicine, 1992.
95. Meyer TJ, Miller ML, Metzger RL, Borkovec TD. Development and validation of the Penn State Worry Questionnaire. Behav Res Ther 1990; 28:487–495.

96. Connor KM, Davidson JRT, Churchill LE, Sherwood A, Foa E, Wesler RH. Psychometric properties of the Social Phobia Inventory (SPIN). Br J Psychiatry 2000; 176:379–386.
97. Antony MM, Orsillo SM, Roemer L. Practitioner's Guide to Empirically Based Measures of Anxiety. New York: Plenum Publishers, 2001.
98. Rosenberg M. Society and the Adolescent Self-image. Princeton, NJ: Princeton University Press, 1965.
99. Rosenberg M. Conceiving the Self. New York: Basic Books, 1979.
100. Demo DH. The measurement of self-esteem: refining our methods. J Personality Social Psychol 1985; 48:1490–1502.
101. Wylie RC. Measures of Self-concept. Lincoln: University of Nebraska Press, 1989.
102. Fairburn CG, Kirk J, O'Connor M, Anastasiades P, Cooper PJ. Prognostic factors in bulimia nervosa. Br J Clin Psychol 1987; 26:223–224.
103. McFarlane T, McCabe RE, Jarry J, Olmsted MP, Polivy J. Weight-related and shape-related self-evaluation in eating-disordered and non-eating-disordered women. Int J Eat Disord 2001; 29:328–335.
104. Selzer ML. The Michigan Alcoholism Screening Test: the quest for a new diagnostic instrument. Am J Psychiatry 1971; 127:1653–1658.
105. Brady JP, Foulks EF, Childress AR, Pertschuk M. The Michigan Alcoholism Screening Tests as a survey instrument. J Oper Psychiatry 1982; 13:27–31.
106. Thurber S, Snow M, Lewis D, Hodgson JM. Item characteristics of the Michigan Alcoholism Screening Test. J Clin Psychol 2001; 57:139–144.
107. Hedlund JL, Vieweg BW. The Michigan Alcoholism Screening Test (MAST): a comprehensive review. J Oper Psychiatry 1984; 15:55–65.
108. Harrell AV, Wirtz PW. The Adolescent Drinking Index Professional Manual. Odessa, FL: Psychological Assessment Resources, 1985.
109. Harrell AV, Wirtz PW. Screening for adolescent problem drinking: validation of a multidimensional instrument for case identification. Psychol Assess 1989; 1:61–63.
110. Skinner HA. The Drug Abuse Screening Test. Addict Behav 1982; 7:363–371.
111. Gavin DR, Ross HE, Skinner HA. Diagnostic validity of the Drug Abuse Screening Test in the assessment of DSM-III drug disorders. Br J Addict 1989; 84:301–307.
112. Martino S, Grilo CM, Fehon DC. Development of the Drug Abuse Screening Test for Adolescents (DAST-A). Addict Behav 2000; 25:57–70.
113. Bernstein EM, Putnam FW. Development, reliability, and validity of a dissociation scale. J Ner Men Dis 1986; 174:727–735.
114. Carlson EB, Putnam FW. An update of the Dissociative Experiences Scale. Dissociation: Progr Dissoc Disord 1993; 6:16–27.
115. Dubester KA, Braun BG. Psychometric properties of the Dissociative Experiences Scale. J Nerv Ment Dis 1995; 183:231–235.
116. van Ijzendoorn MH, Schuengel C. The measurement of dissociation in normal and clinical populations: meta-analytic validation of the Dissociative Experiences Scale (DES). Clin Psychol Rev 1996; 16:365–382.

117. Draijer N, Boon S. The validation of the Dissociative Experiences Scale against the criterion of the SDIC-D, using receiver operating characteristics (ROC) analysis. Dissociation: Progr Dissoc Disord 1993; 6:28–37.

118. Armstrong JG, Putnam FW, Carlson EB, Libero DZ, Smith SR. Development and validation of a measure of adolescent dissociation: the Adolescent Dissociative Experiences Scale. J Nerv Men Dis 1997; 185:491–497.

119. Farrington A, Waller G, Smerden J, Faupel AW. The Adolescent Dissociative Experiences Scale: psychometric properties and difference in scores across age groups. J Nerv Ment Dis 2001; 189:722–727.

120. Smith SR, Carlson EB. Reliability and validity of the Adolescent Dissociative Experiences Scale. Dissociation: Progr Dissoc Disord 1996; 9:125–129.

121. Derogatis LR. Brief Symptom Inventory: Administration, Scoring and Procedures Manual. 3d ed. Minneapolis: National Computer Systems, 1993.

122. Derogatis LR. Symptom Checklist 90-R: Administration, Scoring and Procedures Manual. Minneapolis: National Computer Systems, 1994.

123. Croog SH, Levine S, Testa MA, Brown B, Bulpitt CJ, Jenkins CD, Klerman GL, Williams CH. The effects of antihypertensive therapy on quality of life. N Engl J Med 1986; 314:1657–1664.

124. Derogatis LR. BSI Bibliography. Minneapolis: National Computer Systems, 1993.

125. Foa EB, Riggs DS, Dancu CV, Rothbaum BO. Reliability and validity of a brief instrument for assessing post-traumatic stress disorder. J Traum Stress 1993; 6:459–473.

126. Coffey SF, Dansky BS, Falsetti SA, Saladin ME, Brady KT. Screening for PTSD in a substance abuse sample: psychometric properties of a modified version of the PTSD Symptom Scale Self-Report. J Traum Stress 1998; 11:393–399.

127. Horowitz LM, Alden LE, Wiggins JS, Pincus AL. Inventory of Interpersonal Problems Manual. United States: The Psychological Corporation, 2000.

128. Horowitz LM, Rosenberg SE, Baer BA, Ureno G, Villasenor VS. Inventory of Interpersonal Problems: psychometric properties and clinical applications. J Consult Clin Psychol 1988; 56:885–892.

129. Livesley WJ, Jackson DW, Schroeder ML. Dimensions of personality pathology. Can J Psychiatry 1991; 36:557–562.

130. Clark LA, Livesley WJ, Schroeder ML, Irish S. The structure of maladaptive personality traits: convergent validity between two systems. Psychol Assess 1996; 8:294–303.

131. Schroeder ML, Wormworth JA, Livesley WJ. Dimensions of personality disorder and their relationship to the big five dimensions of personality. Psychol Assess 1992; 4:47–53.

132. Goldner EM, Srikameswaran S, Schhroeder ML, Livesley WJ, Birmingham CL. Dimensional assessment of personality pathology in patients with eating disorders. Psychiatry Res 1999; 85:151–159.

133. Clark LA, Harrison JA. Assessment Instruments. In: Livesley, WJ ed. Handbook of Personality Disorders. New York: Guilford Press, 2001.

134. Eisler I, Dare C, Russell GFM, Szmukler G, le Grange D, Dodge E. Family and

individual therapy in anorexia nervosa: A 5-year follow-up. Arch Gen Psychiatry 1997; 54:1025–1030.

135. Skinner HA. Self-report instruments for family assessment. In: Jacob T ed. Family Interaction and Psychopathology. New York: Plenum Publishers Co, 1987.

136. Moos R, Moos B. Family Environment Scale Manual. Palo Alto, CA: Consulting Psychologists Press, 1981.

137. Grotevant HD, Carlson CI. Family Assessment: A Guide to Methods and Measures. New York: Guilford Press, 1989.

138. Skinner HA, Steinhauer PD, Santa-Barbara J. Family Assessment Measure-III. Toronto: Multi Health Systems, 1995.

139. Skinner HA, Steinhauer PD, Sitarenios G. Family Assessment Measure (FAM) and process model of family functioning. J Fam Ther 2000; 22:190–210.

140. Forman B. Assessing perceived patterns of behavior exchange in relationships. J Clin Psychol 1988; 44:972–981.

141. Skinner HA, Steinhauer PD, Santa-Barbara J. The Family Assessment Measure. Can J Comm Men Health 1983; 2:91–105.

142. Bloom BL. A factor analysis of self-report measures of family functioning. Fam Proc 1985; 24:225–239.

143. Jacob T. The role of the time frame in the assessment of family functioning. J Marital Fam Ther 1995; 21:281–286.

3

Feeding Disorders in Infancy and Early Childhood

Dasha Nicholls
Great Ormond Street Hospital
London, England

This chapter examines the range of feeding problems from birth to early childhood from a theoretical and clinical perspective. Feeding problems are usually understood as being part of a relationship and never simply located within the child. Feeding problems are usually defined as starting before the age of 6 years and are rarely, if ever, defined in terms of subjective anxieties of the child but usually in terms of observed behavior or adults' descriptions. A feeding difficulty becomes a problem when it is associated with additional developmental, medical, or emotional problems. The boundary between a feeding problem, often parent defined, and a disorder, often professionally defined, is indistinct. Most cases presenting to a hospital setting have a multifactorial cause and maintenance involving medical, developmental, social, and psychological factors; and in these cases it is unlikely that the children will simply grow out of the problem without help. The difficulty of negotiating issues of independence and control with their caregivers can result in conflict, and these problems are often labeled as behavioral. This chapter will give an overview of issues relating to diagnosis and classification, control and responsibility, and assessment, with reference to texts from which further information can be sought.

RECOGNITION AND CLASSIFICATION

DSM-IV distinguishes three feeding disorders: two specific subtypes—pica and rumination—and a broader diagnostic category of "feeding disorder of infancy and early childhood." Each will be considered in turn.

Pica

Pica describes the persistent eating of nonnutritive substances over an extended period of time (more than a month) (see Table 1 for diagnostic criteria). It is usually only diagnosed separately if of such severity that specific intervention is required, such as when medical complications occur as a result of toxicity. The type of substance eaten tends to vary with age and developmental capacity of the child. For example, younger children may eat paint, string, or hair; older children leaves and pebbles; and adolescents clay or soil. Pica is associated with developmental disorders, including learning disability and pervasive developmental disorders, where its severity is related to the degree of disability. Poverty, neglect, and lack of supervision increase the risk for pica in vulnerable individuals. Epidemiological data on pica are limited, and the ingestion of nonnutritive substances may be quite common in preschool children and should not be considered abnormal unless persistent and severe. In a sample of 472 children attending pediatric clinics, Stein et al. found that pica was associated with parasomnias such as sleepwalking, nightmares, night terrors, and head banging or rocking in sleep (1). Case reports have suggested a role for selective serotonin reuptake inhibitors in the management of pica (2).

Rumination

Rumination is a syndrome characterized by the effortless regurgitation of recently ingested food (see Table 2 for diagnostic criteria). It has been linked

---

TABLE 1   Diagnostic Criteria for Pica

A. There is persistent eating of nonnutritive substances for a period of at least 1 month.
B. The eating of nonnutritive substances is inappropriate to the developmental level.
C. The eating behavior is not part of a culturally sanctioned practice.
D. If the eating behavior occurs exclusively during the course of another mental disorder (e.g., mental retardation, pervasive developmental disorder, schizophrenia), it is sufficiently severe to warrant independent clinical attention.

TABLE 2 Diagnostic Criteria for Rumination Disorder

A. There is repeated regurgitation and rechewing of food for a period of at least 1 month following a period of normal functioning.
B. The behavior is not due to an associated gastrointestinal or other general medical condition (e.g., esophageal reflux).
C. The behavior does not occur exclusively during the course of anorexia nervosa or bulimia nervosa. If the symptoms occur exclusively during the course of mental retardation or a pervasive developmental disorder, they are sufficiently severe to warrant independent clinical attention.

to severe medical and psychosocial conditions, including malnutrition, aspiration pneumonia, and complete social withdrawal, and is seen in three distinct populations: infants; individuals with psychiatric and neurological disorders, particularly developmental disabilities; and adults who do not have overt psychiatric or neurological disorders (3). The hallmark of rumination, which separates it from other disorders of the upper gastrointestinal tract (such as gastroesophageal reflux disease), is that in rumination the stomach contents appear in the mouth without retching or nausea. The subject appears to make a conscious decision on how to handle the regurgitated food, and the experience seems to be pleasurable. It usually occurs very soon after a meal and tends to last for 1–2 hours.

Rumination is relatively rare but potentially fatal when it occurs in infants. It is thought to be a form of self-stimulation in this age group. Observation of rumination is all that is needed to make the diagnosis, although often rumination ceases as soon as the infant notices the observer. Parents may not report the symptom spontaneously but may recognize it when described. The infant who ruminates may not retain enough nutrients and may develop potentially lethal malnutrition, a complication that seldom, if ever, occurs in older ruminators. Sensory and/or emotional deprivation are both associated with rumination in children, which may explain the increased incidence of rumination in institutionalized children, infants in intensive care units, and normal infants with attachment disorders. In infant rumination, the aim of treatment is to provide a nurturing environment and comforting care to the infant, and to help the mother improve her ability to recognize and respond sensitively to her infant's physical and emotional needs. In mentally handicapped children, providing a nurturing caregiver may not be sufficient and behavioral therapy may be necessary.

In older children rumination can be associated with weight loss and vomiting (4), and treatment includes nutritional support in combination with medication, cognitive and relaxation techniques, and pain management.

Cases may present to gastroenterologists rather than to mental health practitioners. A collaborative approach can be very effective, e.g., combining the
use of medication to reduce acid damage to the esophagus, with psychological
therapy aimed at identifying situations and emotions that trigger the symptoms. A multidisciplinary team approach is associated with satisfactory
recovery in most patients.

Feeding Disorder of Infancy and Early Childhood

These two specific feeding disorders aside, there remain a number of feeding
and eating behaviors in childhood and early adolescence that are currently
classified under the generic diagnosis of "feeding disorders of infancy and
early childhood" (see Table 3 for diagnostic criteria). The classification of
feeding disorders has been hampered by a lack of knowledge about feeding
behaviors in healthy, typically developing children, thus making the boundaries between normal, problem, and disordered feeding hard to identify. In
addition, reported feeding problems are common. More than 50% of parents
report one problem feeding behavior and more than 20% report multiple
problems (5) in children aged 9 months to 7 years. Trying to get children to eat
food during structured mealtimes appears to provide the most tension for
parents. Problem feeding is more likely to be reported among the children of
parents using strategies such as coaxing, threatening, making multiple meals,
and force feeding (5). In this study, psychosocial variables such as marital
status, socioeconomic status, or the child's birth order were not significantly
associated with reported frequency and number of feeding problems.

Bax [quoted in (6)] has suggested that the fact that feeding and feeding
problems are covered so extensively in the child rearing literature in part
explains the relative neglect of scientific research in the area. For example,
information about typical length of mealtimes in infants and toddlers has only
recently been established, from which a definition of slow eating was derived
(7). In this study more than 30 minutes was considered slow. The relative

---

TABLE 3 Diagnostic Criteria for Feeding Disorder of Infancy or Early Childhood

A. There is a feeding disturbance as manifested by persistent failure to eat
   adequately with significant failure to gain weight or significant loss of
   weight over at least 1 month.
B. The disturbance is not due to an associated gastrointestinal or other general
   medical condition (e.g., esophageal reflux).
C. The disturbance is not better accounted for by another mental disorder (e.g.,
   rumination disorder) or by lack of available food.
D. The onset is before age 6 years.

---

paucity of knowledge about the range of normal feeding behaviors has led to an overreliance on parental report of feeding as problematic in order to define disorder. An exception is the work of Dahl and colleagues in Sweden, who studied a sample of infants aged 3–12 months (8) and published follow-up findings up to primary school age. Problem feeding was defined on the basis of parent and nurse reports, had to be present for more than 1 month, and had to have responded to medical and psychological advice and treatment. She identified 50 infants fulfilling these criteria (a prevalence of 1.4%). The majority (82%) were underweight for their age. Three main problem categories were distinguished: refusal to eat (56%), colic (18%), and vomiting (16%), with 10% miscellaneous others.

Feeding Disorders Presenting to Clinical Services

A number of different approaches have been taken in attempts to classify feeding disorders based on children presenting to clinical services. There is no international consensus on how to name these feeding problems or how they should be classified. Furthermore, although there is an extensive literature relating to feeding problems of infancy and early childhood (usually pre-school), there is a very little published work about feeding and eating problems presenting in middle childhood.

The way in which feeding disorders are categorized tends to depend on the professional context in which they have presented, and the terms used are those that have been found to be meaningful in a clinical context. For example, taking a medical perspective, Burklow (9) proposed a coding system for complex feeding disorders based on combinations of five categories: structural abnormalities, neurological conditions, behavioral issues, cardiorespiratory problems, and metabolic dysfunction. In this scheme behavioral issues were defined very broadly to include feeding difficulties arising from psychosocial difficulties, negative feeding behavior shaped and maintained by reinforcement, and/or emotional difficulties (e.g., phobias, depression). Using this system, 85% of cases were classified in the behavioral category, suggesting that a biobehavioral conceptualization may be more appropriate. Skuse and Wolke (6) identify the main feeding problems as colic; gastroesophageal reflux; oral–motor dysfunction in high-risk neonates; tactile hypersensitivity; oral–motor dysfunction and failure to thrive; and psychodynamic feeding problems. For a comprehensive list of possible causes of feeding problems, see (10).

Speech and language therapists tend to consider the presence or absence of oromotor dysfunction a key factor (11), grouping feeding problems according to dysfunctional or disorganized feeding (12). Dysfunctional feeding patterns tend not to resolve over time and are associated with other neurological diagnoses and motor difficulties. Disorganized feeding either resolves over time or is related to subsequent sensory problems. It can be helpful to think separately about motor and sensory problems, although inevitably the two interact.

There are a number of psychological classifications, and these depend on particular approaches and whether the child, the parent, or the child–parent interaction is the basis for defining the problem. A symptom-based approach to classification can be helpful in behavioral management, e.g., problems with texture, quantity, and range (13). Harris et al. (14) take an even more pragmatic approach, simply identifying two types of food refusal that may occur separately or together, i.e., refusal to take in sufficient calories and refusal to ingest a sufficient range of foods.

From a psychodynamic perspective, Chatoor and colleagues have described a number of feeding problems based on attachment–separation theory, the best characterized of which are infantile anorexia (15) and post-traumatic feeding disorder of infancy (PTFD) (16). This approach emphasizes the difficulties infants have distinguishing somatic sensations such as hunger and satiety from emotional feelings such as sadness, anger, and frustration. The term infantile anorexia derives from Bruch's early descriptions of patients with anorexia nervosa, and relates to the interpersonal nature of the infant's struggle to have his or her needs met. Infant–mother relationships in this group of infants have been characterized by a lack of reciprocity, conflict, and a struggle for control in which food refusal is central (see below). In PTFD, children are distinguished by showing increased resistance during feeding interactions and a marked resistance to swallowing food. This may be an infantile precursor to what had been termed "functional dysphagia" (17), in which children identify a specific fear of swallowing, often associated with a history of choking.

Finally, attempts have been made to classify parental responses to feeding in recognition of the role that managing the "balance of power" (18) has in feeding problems. Birch and colleagues identified three types of parenting styles applicable to feeding: highly controlling, *laissez-faire*, and responsive. Highly controlling and *laissez-faire* parenting may interfere with self-regulation of children's feeding behaviors. Perhaps most importantly in this context is the association between highly controlling parenting and maternal eating disorders (19), and the link to feeding problems in their offspring (20,21). Maternal feeding practices and perceptions of their child's eating have also been linked subsequent overweight (22).

One study of classification is particularly noteworthy in terms of its research methodology. Crist et al. (5), used a feeding screening questionnaire, the Behavioral Pediatrics Feeding Assessment Scale (BPFAS), to empirically derive subtypes of feeding problem from a sample of 96 control and 249 clinically referred subjects. Using a principal-components analysis, they identified the following factors, which accounted for 55% of the total variance for the combined clinical and normative groups.

Factor 1: Picky Eaters

This factor essentially represents the willingness of children to try new foods and the variety of food groups that the child accepts. This continuum of feeding problems runs from the "picky eating" pattern, common during the toddler years, to the more severe end of the spectrum where children have narrowed their food selection to the extent that they are consuming insufficient amounts of key vitamins and minerals. Reau et al. (7) found an association between picky eating and length of meal times and speculated that lengthened meal times might reflect underlying oral–motor dysfunction in some cases. Recently Jacobi et al. (23) aimed to clarify and validate the nature of picky eating by examining the relationship between parental report of picky eating and objective behavioral measures, and also looked at both parent and child precursors of picky eating. This study is important because it attempts to clarify the relationship between parent-reported problem feeding and observed disorder. Of 29 cases classified as "picky" on the basis of parent report, objective measures confirmed a lower number and variety of foods consumed, predominantly the avoidance of vegetables. These authors found no association between picky eating and slow eating. Picky eating, sometimes to quite an extreme degree, is commonly found in children with autistic spectrum disorders. This type of feeding pattern has also been termed *selective eating* (24) or *perseverative feeding disorder* (14), both of which convey the extreme selectivity in preferred foods and resistance to trying new foods [food neophobia (25)]. Overall caloric intake is often adequate for these children, and growth and development are usually normal (26). Rydell et al. (27) found that at primary school age choosiness was not related to gender, social class, or ethnic background. The choosy children had modestly elevated levels of externalizing, hyperactive, and internalizing behavior. More pronounced choosiness was found in those with a history of refusal to eat in infancy or at preschool age. These children had more problem behaviors in other areas than less choosy children.

Factor 2: Toddler Refusal—General

The behaviors identified with this factor included whining or crying, tantrums, and spitting out food. This refusal pattern was associated with younger children and appeared to be more general in nature as opposed to food specific, and may be linked to other types of oppositional behavior. Parent training approaches may be the most fruitful.

Factor 3: Toddler Refusal—Textured Foods

The behaviors that loaded on this factor included problems chewing food; eating only ground, soft food; letting food sit in the mouth without swallowing it; and choking or gagging. This type of refusal behavior appeared to relate closely to making the transition from soft to chewy foods, and appeared to reflect the individual child's difficulty in handling textured foods or the selective refusal of textured foods rather than a general disruption of mealtime behavior. Clinical experience suggests some overlap between this factor and picky eating, and where the two co-occur the picky eating may be more persistent. Problems with textured food are also found in children with neurodevelopmental disorders, such as autism. Facial and oral hypersensitivity can be found along with neurological difficulties such as epilepsy, and is also associated with situations where oral desensitization has failed to occur. The most commonly encountered instance of this is in children who have been tube fed. Normally children experience a wide range of oral stimulation, at various phases putting almost anything and everything in their mouths. If a child has had no experience of the taste, temperature, touch, or smell of food for an extended period, the reintroduction of oral feeding may not be pleasurable. To prevent feeding problems from developing while on enteral feeding, children should be encouraged to maintain feeding skills, engage in textured messy/food play, and maintain patterns of feeding and social aspects of feeding, e.g., sitting at the table for regular meals with others.

Factor 4: Older Children Refusal—General

This factor included behaviors associated with older children, such as delaying eating by talking, trying to negotiate what food he or she will eat, getting up from the table during meals, and refusing to eat much during a meal but requesting food immediately after the meal. Much of the nutritional intake of these children was gained through snacking between meals. Although these behaviors lengthen the mealtime, they would seem to reflect general disruptive behavior, rather than possible oral–motor difficulties.

Factor 5: Stallers

This factor was not as well defined as others. The authors assigned the term "stallers" because the feature of "letting food sit in the mouth without swallowing it" was common to all cases. It was associated with a preference for fluids over food (e.g., would rather drink than eat; drinks milk). This feeding pattern may be similar to restrictive eating, a term that Bryant-Waugh and Lask (28) have used to describe children with a constitutionally small appetite, who show limited interest in food, don't eat much, and who grow and develop normally in the lower centiles for weight and height. This type of feeding pattern could therefore be considered a normal variant. Clinical presentation is often due to anxiety about growth, and there may be a long history of attempts to feed the child more that he or she can manage. Indeed, feeding practices such as coercion to eat, excessive anxiety about weight gain, and conflict over food can precipitate food refusal, vomiting, and failure to thrive.

None of the five groups outlined above would seem to identify a single factor reflecting the more serious condition of failure to thrive, which describes a pattern of faltering development as a result of poor weight gain. It may be that failure to thrive can result from any of the feeding problems described above, if sufficiently severe, and/or other factors contribute to exacerbation of feeding problems, such as the use of coercion or other negative parent–child interactions. Although malnutrition is the end point, disentangling the complex contributions of child, parent, and their interactions is not always straightforward. For example, the dichotomy of organic versus nonorganic failure to thrive is used less often since the contribution of subtle differences in sucking, chewing, and swallowing were noted in a group of children identified as having nonorganic failure to thrive (29). Nonetheless, failure to thrive can be, but is not always, associated with other evidence of neglect and deprivation.

This way of grouping feeding problems is not dissimilar to other attempts at classification but has the advantage of being empirically derived. However, there are a number of limitations. First, only 55% of the variance was accounted for by these five factors. Second, larger sample sizes would be needed to determine whether any of these patterns of feeding behavior were more common for specific medical conditions than for others. Perhaps surprisingly, only one prospective study has examined the role of early feeding problems in the development of subsequent onset of eating disorders (30), although feeding problems have been identified as a risk factor from retrospective studies (31,32) and there is increasing interest in developmental precursors of subsequent problem eating. In Marchi and Cohen's study, 659 children and their mothers were interviewed three times between 1 and 21 years of age. Picky eating in early childhood was found to predict symptoms of anorexia nervosa in later adolescence (30). The authors defined picky eating by the presence of three of the following (maternally reported) behaviors of the child: "does not eat enough," "is often or very often choosy about food," "usually eats slowly," "is usually not interested in food." This concept of picky eating is therefore broader than that defined above, in which only choosiness is a feature. Disinterest in food is a characteristic most often associated with restrictive eating, classifiable in the "stallers" group above.

What evidence there is suggests that the nature of feeding problems found in children with and without medical conditions do not differ significantly in type but only in frequency or intensity (5,33). For a review of diagnosis and treatment of feeding difficulties in children with developmental difficulties see Schwarz et al. (34), and for feeding difficulties associated with illness see Harris et al. (35).

Enteral Feeding

Increasingly children presenting to clinical services have been started on enteral feeding for any of a number of reasons and are having difficulty making the transition from tube feeding to oral feeding. Enteral feeding is a passive experience for the child. Problems created by enteral feeding include reduction of appetite and thirst leading to lack of recognition of hunger and thirst drive; absence of normal response to the sight or smell of food, e.g., salivation, lack of pleasure; reduction of opportunities to practice routine and skills required for oral feeding, such as the use of cutlery; and fear and revulsion at certain textures, tastes, and smells. Each of these difficulties may be present to a greater or lesser degree. It is unrealistic to expect a child to start oral feeding simply by withdrawing enteral feeds. Psychological approaches may consider a program of desensitization to anxiety-provoking textures and foods, as well as the establishment of normal mealtime behaviors in order to expose the child to food and to encourage feeding. Play with food must be modeled by caregivers in a relaxed, nonpressurizing manner. Self-feeding by mouthing, kissing, and licking food should be encouraged. Reduction of enteral feeds should be attempted once feeding skills have been established and a small but measured amount of food or drink is taken by mouth on a daily basis. A window of hunger and thirst may be created by tube feeding the child overnight or spacing bolus feeds. Enteral feeds should be reduced slowly and gradually under the supervision of a dietitian, in conjunction with the child's medical care and with regular weight checks. To prevent feeding problems developing while on enteral feeding, children should be encouraged to maintain feeding skills, engage in textured/messy food play, and maintain patterns of feeding and social aspects of feeding, such as sitting at the table for regular mealtimes with others.

FROM FEEDING TO EATING DISORDERS: ISSUES OF CONTROL AND SELF-REGULATION

The term "feeding disorder" suggests an interactional component between the caregiver and child, whereas "eating disorder" implies autonomy of self-regulation and care. Typically developing children vary enormously in the degree of dependence they exhibit around food, and this becomes particularly emphasized in the context of illness or disability, when the capacity of the child to follow normal trajectories toward self-regulation are delayed or deviated. Thus, a preschool child might be described as "eating" if he or she shows an ability to select food appropriate to the energy needs, respond to hunger and satiety, and exhibit socially adaptive eating behavior. By contrast, a 12-year-old girl with anorexia nervosa may, during the course of her illness, become fully dependent on her parents to choose appropriate food, determine her nutritional needs, and even feed her. In practice, therefore, the age at which feeding ends and eating begins is far from clear. Despite this, feeding problems are traditionally considered separately from eating problems and eating disorders. One consequence of this separation is the relatively limited examination to date of the continuities and discontinuities between the two. Recently, there has been an increase in interest in the association between the two, opening new avenues of investigation toward a developmental understanding of problem eating in later life.

Understanding the transition from feeding to eating requires a consideration of how control and responsibility around food intake are determined and negotiated in both a developmental and a systemic context. This process of transfer of responsibility for eating from caregiver to child is a careful balance of timing and encouragement—too much parental regulation and the child may rebel; too much autonomy for the child and he or she may not be able to cope. As such the transition from feeding to eating is highly susceptible to tension and conflict, particularly over issues of autonomy and control. It is also a point of communication between a child and a parent, and can be a means for communicating distress or anxiety.

Thus, learning to manage control over self and others is an important developmental task. The dynamic nature of who "holds" control and responsibility in a wide range of different areas forms a major part of the complex, changing relationship between parents and children. For example, our views and expectations of the appropriateness and ability of children to accept responsibility for themselves, and of the nature and degree of the control their parents might exert, vary widely according to developmental and individual considerations. At each developmental stage food can represent a vehicle for the exploration and regulation of basic needs. For example, in infancy food is the main medium through which a child can seek reassurance that his or her needs will be met reliably and predictably. In the toddler years, characterized by the learning of new skills and the making of first choices, the child is seeking mastery, with help at hand for disasters. The responses of parents, caretakers, and other significant others have an impact on the child's developmental progress and ability to successfully manage conflicts, dilemmas, and tasks at each stage. For example, the caregiver has to tolerate the frustration and mess of the toddler's failed attempts at mastery. The individual child's personal style is in part understood against the backdrop of family members' responses and communication, which is in turn considered against its own wider social and cultural background.

Control is a central theme in feeding and eating disorders, and can be considered from many different perspectives, e.g., within individuals, within relationships, culturally, systemically, developmentally, and across generations. Birch and Fisher have emphasized the role of parental attempts to control and restrict access to foods in the development of food preferences (36). Not only can parental control of food intake be counterproductive in terms of enhancing rather than reducing preferences for "bad" foods, but it can also, if habitual, influence the child's capacity for self-regulation of food intake. "Child feeding practices that encourage or restrict children's consumption of foods may decrease the extent to which children use their internal signals of satiety and hunger as a basis for adjusting energy intake" (36, p. 544).

Much of Birch and colleagues work has focused on the development of childhood overweight, but we know too that parental eating disorders may be associated with a wish for control, which in turn can impact on child development. Stein et al. (19) looked at whether parental (in this case maternal) control is specific to eating disorders and whether attempts at control with the child are specific to feeding behavior. They found that mothers with eating disorders were more controlling, both verbally and in actions, than mothers with depression or control mothers, and this was related to dietary restraint. However, rather than maternal attempts at control being restricted to mealtimes, they found that control was most likely to be exercised during the child's play. The significance of this finding is the impact of controlling parental behavior on child development outside the narrow domain of feeding and eating. The specificity of parental overcontrol to eating disorder subjects is of particular note. In Fairburn and colleagues' cognitive behavioral theory of the maintenance of anorexia nervosa, the need for control of eating is a central theme. They argue "that an extreme need to control eating is the central feature of the disorder, and that in Western societies a tendency to judge self-worth in terms of shape and weight is superimposed on this need for self control" (Fairburn et al., 1999).

The number of systematic controlled studies in this important area is relatively small (19,37–39). The available evidence suggests that children of mothers with eating disorders are at increased risk of disturbance, but that the risk is not invariable and depends on a variety of factors. Further research is needed to understand how the need for control is internalized, as well as the role of early experiences of control and self-regulation. In particular, a number of studies have suggested that some aspects of parental influence on eating behaviors are gender specific. Jacobi et al. (23) found the impact of maternal eating disorders and disturbances to be much stronger than that of fathers and that it was specifically directed at their daughters. Maternal restraint was predictive of worries about weight in 8-year-old daughters, and high maternal BMI was predictive of weight control behaviors in daughters but not sons.

Although mothers with eating disorders may be at the extreme end of the spectrum, the link between parental eating concern and reported childhood feeding problem is evident from a number of studies as well as from clinical experience. For example, in a community sample of 397 children whose parents were questioned when their child was 13 months and 5 years of age, problematical or maladaptive eating habits of the children were found to be connected to those of their parents (40). The mother's poor ability to enjoy eating and high tendency to snack regardless of hunger, as well as the father's difficulty in weight regulation, significantly predicted persistent poor eating in their children.

While there is increasing recognition of the association between parental eating behavior and child eating behavior, far less is known about the long-term course of feeding disorders and later problems both in eating and in other aspects of control and self-regulation. We are increasingly aware from clinical experience that a number of feeding problems can persist into later life. Examples are children who are tube fed, in whom increased survival may also be a factor in some patient groups; children with selective (picky) eating, which can persist into adolescence (26) and even adulthood; and food phobias.

The mechanism by which feeding problems may be linked to eating disorders or other types of eating problem in adolescence or adulthood is at this time somewhat speculative. Issues of control and of the development of specific cognitions relating to beliefs about self and others may play a part. Our capacity to distinguish eating disorder cognitions in younger children may enhance our understanding in this area. True eating disorders can be understood as disorders characterized by grossly disordered or chaotic eating behavior associated with morbid preoccupation with body weight and shape. In children as young as 7, true eating disorders have been described and can be distinguished from children of comparable age with other types of food avoidance. For these disorders, anorexia nervosa and bulimia nervosa, the overall clinical presentation is similar to that in adults, with some important distinctions that reflect developmental and gender-based differences in expression rather than differences in the disorder per se (41). Using the childhood version of the Eating Disorders Examination (EDE) (42,43), Cooper et al. (38) have shown that early-onset patients with anorexia nervosa had comparable scores to later-onset patients on all subscales apart from Eating Concern, but that AN patients were clearly distinguishable from those with other types of eating problems. It is these other types of eating problems presenting in childhood, not classifiable as eating disorders, that are of uncertain nosological status (44). In particular, a few of the subjects in the Cooper et al. study were difficult to classify and what at first appeared to be an atypical feeding/eating problem later become more characteristic of anorexia nervosa. A few may be diagnosed as "eating disorder not otherwise specified," and a proportion whose food avoidance dates back to younger than 6 years would meet criteria for "feeding disorder of infancy and early childhood." There remain a number of children who present clinically with disordered eating who do not fit into any of the current classification systems. This heterogeneous group of patients need further systematic investigation. Food avoidance emotional disorder (45), psychogenic vomiting, food phobias, and functional dysphagia are just some of the terms that have been used to describe problem eating behaviors in this age group (41). We have suggested that these can be usefully thought about in relation to associated psychopathology. For example, children with food avoidance emotional disorder or psychogenic vomiting often have other medically unexplained symptoms, and their parents may attribute weight loss to an undiagnosed physical disorder. As such, classification as a somatization disorder may be appropriate. Some children develop specific circumscribed fears in relation to food, which are associated with specific cognitions. Generalized anxiety, unrelated to food, may also be present. In these cases anxiety management techniques in combination with family work can be effective once nutritional intake has been reestablished, and hence classification as anxiety disorder, a specific phobia, or obsessive-compulsive disorder may be appropriate depending on clinical presentation. What each of these problems has in common with feeding and eating disorders is a need to specifically address the nutritional as well as the emotional needs of the child.

ASSESSMENT OF FEEDING PROBLEMS

All eating and feeding problems have biological, psychological, and social contributing factors. Assessment is one of the most important aspects of any approach to management and can in itself be a powerful intervention. It should be based on a theoretical or conceptual model, and encompass biological, psychological, behavioral, and social components. As already mentioned, both a developmental and a systemic understanding should be emphasized. Thus, the level of understanding will change if the child only, the child and mother, the child and parents, or the whole family are seen. In addition, a cultural understanding may be needed if the significance of the problem is to be understood. This is true of basic parameters such as the interpretation of height and weight data, and becomes even more complex when it comes to understanding issues of control and responsibility. Any assessment protocol will need to be comprehensive enough to gather relevant information to address the range of feeding problems thus far described and is likely to require the skills of a multidisciplinary team and a multidimensional approach. Assessment aims to identify the relative contributions of physical, emotional, behavioral, and cognitive contributions to the maintenance of the feeding problem in a developmental and systemic framework (Fig. 1).

History and Development of the Feeding Problem

A thorough history should be gathered from the parents/caregivers. A good starting point is usually the time when someone first became aware that there might be a problem, although it is helpful to then go back and review feeding from birth. This is often done by means of a semistructured questionnaire administered to parents, of which a number have been published (5,14,46). Finally the child's current general functioning should also be assessed (including school and social functioning). From the history factors that may have been associated with onset can be identified, such as medical treatment; a traumatic incident such as choking, loss events, or moves; a developmental problem; a medical condition; beliefs about feeding and parental roles; or any combination of these. Factors associated with onset can then be usefully differentiated from factors that appear to maintain the problem, such as continued medical problems/treatment causing discomfort

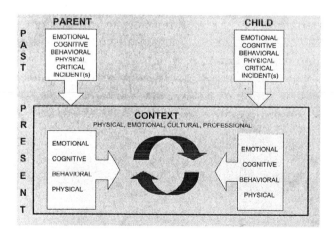

FIGURE 1 Conceptual model for the maintenance of "vicious cycles" within feeding problems. Assessment aims to identify the relative contributions of physical, emotional, behavioral, and cognitive contributions to the maintenance of the feeding problem within a developmental and systemic framework.

or loss of appetite, ongoing emotional problems such as fear of choking again, and factors such as heightened anxiety at mealtimes or poor parental management/mealtime conflict.

Physical Assessment

In addition to aiding diagnosis and management decisions, information obtained from physical assessments can be a powerful tool for both sufferers and parents/caregivers. Furthermore, medical concerns are often the main cause for concern or the reason that the problem has been taken seriously. The commonest causes for concern are significant weight loss or weight gain, failure to gain weight or height appropriately for age and stage of development, or a single low or high BMI or other weight-to-height ratio index measurement (outside 3rd or 97th centile for age). The potentially irreversible effects of malnutrition on physical, psychological, and emotional growth and development in infants and children are well described. Monitoring of growth and development should continue until the child is growing and developing along appropriate centiles. Weight and height charts are of more value for monitoring change than for assessing the significance of a single measurement. More importantly, growth charts emphasize the rate of expected weight gain for a child. Over the past few years many countries have published BMI centiles for children, e.g., (47–49), which will enable nutritional status to be more conveniently and routinely assessed.

It is important that the presence of unidentified and untreated or partially treated physical symptoms, such as esophageal reflux or problems with swallowing as a result of oromotor dyscontrol, be assessed.

Assessment of Developmental Issues

We have found it useful to take a personal history including important events in the child's life. This can be drawn on a time line that can then be placed next to the one with weight and eating history, enabling potential links to be explored more easily. The personal history should also include a developmental history, including early feeding, milestones, the child's medical history, plus any past history of emotional and/or behavioral problems.

Assessment of Systemic Context

Assessment of systemic context involves gathering information about the family, its wider context, and the family's past contact with health professionals. In addition to gathering information about family history of weight and shape issues as well as family medical and psychiatric history, the aim is to identify strengths, resources, and sources of support. This can be done through drawing a family tree involving any members of the family who live at home. It is important to gain some impression of the family's social context, their ethnic background, and any relevant associated beliefs and practices. With regard to the eating difficulty, we would routinely ask all members of the family how they understand it and how it affects them. Finally, we ask parents what they have tried in terms of managing the problem and who or what they have found helpful in the past. This will also allow a picture of help seeking and professional networks to be identified.

Behavioral and Emotional Assessment

In younger children it may be useful to observe the feeding behavior, and video material can be used therapeutically to demonstrate specific behaviors, interactions, and later to show change. Observation will identify whether food intake is limited in quantity or range, and if there is excessive, irregular, or chaotic food intake or abnormal practices such as vomiting or purging. In addition, patterns of behavior, such as inability to accommodate normal variations in eating patterns and dietary content, which can manifest as mealtime conflicts, can be identified, as can peer group interaction, social withdrawal, social isolation, and reluctance to engage in peer activities.

In addition, assessment is needed regarding the emotional well-being of the child, as well as to establish the level of anxiety surrounding the feeding/eating relationship for the child, for the parents/caregivers, and for the professionals involved. The child's view should be sought if he or she is old enough to talk. Otherwise low mood, mood swings, and anxiety, including panic attacks and specific food phobias, may be observable. In young children, play and artwork may help to identify feelings of aggression, sadness, and fear. There are also a number of responses evident in feedback from children and adults with Asperger's syndrome suggesting that these children may be vulnerable to being overwhelmed with sensory input and consequent anxiety, fear, and panic. This may be associated with unusual cognitions regarding the effects of food or beliefs designed to limit the anxiety, such as only eating from orange packets. This set of emotional responses and coping with new foods is on a continuum with that seen in extremely picky eaters, especially as they grow older and develop beliefs about the potential harm that food may represent.

Observation of the feeding relationship also allows identification of the few cases in which feeding practices have reached a point of coercion or become abusive in some other way. Examples include the restriction of food, harsh and punitive responses, and neglect. Recognition of these difficulties will inform other aspects of assessment and a formulation reached within the framework outlined above.

A final part of the assessment process is to ascertain where the child and the parents are up to in terms of their wish to change, to assess their perception of their own ability to achieve change, and to assess their understanding of the process by which change can be achieved.

Other professionals may be needed in the assessment process, e.g., other physicians, nurse specialists, speech and language therapists, dietitians, occupational therapists, social workers, and play specialists. Liaison with the child's professional network outside the hospital will give an indication of previous treatment strategies that have been tried and of the extent to which professional concerns play a part in the context of the problem.

The assessment process allows more than a diagnosis to be established. It encompasses a risk assessment in terms of physical compromise, vulnerability to abuse or neglect, and risk of aggression/violence to others. It enables determination of the impact of the feeding problem on the child's development and general functioning as well as on the family. Expectations of treatment are ascertained, together with some provisional information about level of motivation and readiness to change. A formulation can be made within the framework outlines and this formulation shared with the family as a starting point for a collaborative approach to the problem.

MANAGEMENT OF FEEDING PROBLEMS

It is beyond the scope of this text to comprehensively consider the management of feeding problems, although a number of useful publications exist outlining approaches based on behavioral, psychodynamic, and family-based approaches (50). Evidence-based treatments in this area are scarce, hampered in part by the difficulties in classification of this heterogeneous group of children and families, as discussed above. In addition, different treatment approaches reflect the fact that children with feeding difficulties are seen by a variety of professionals in a variety of settings, including pediatric or mental health settings. Most commonly feeding problems present in primary care to general practitioners and other health care professionals, from whom more complex cases will be referred to nutritional and dietetic services or specialized pediatric services, particularly gastroenterology. In addition, the common co-occurrence of feeding disorders and other developmental difficulties means that child development clinics regularly see children with feeding problems. Psychology services may be involved early on if behavioral and interactional aspects of the feeding problem are clear. Specialist feeding teams tend to be multidisciplinary and involve many or all of the professionals outlined above, i.e., medical, nursing, nutritional, and psychological expertise. For example, a multidisciplinary team has been shown to be more effective in achieving weight gain in cases of nonorganic failure to thrive than treatment in a primary care setting (51).

A guiding principle of treatment is that it should enable oral feeding at whatever developmental and physical level the child is capable. This means supporting parents/caregivers to do the work of feeding, and supplying them with the necessary information and skills this entails. It may be that oral feeding is contraindicated and in these cases intervention should focus on supporting the caregivers with this decision. As our conceptual framework suggests, it may be easier to address maintaining factors than causal factors, although the formulation should identify significant contributory factors in the past for both child and parents, and any medical conditions should be clarified and managed, e.g., reflux, choking, or aspirations due to dysphagia problems or to allergy/intolerance, before proceeding to further work.

Although treatment is specific to the problem and to the child and family, a number of elements are, in our view, essential. Treatment of young people with feeding and eating disorders works best when it is collaborative and based on a comprehensive, multidisciplinary assessment. Treatment should be appropriate to level of complexity. Treatment should be responsive to the developmental stage, physically and psychologically, of the child and take into account both the degree of independence the child has within the family and the resources within the family to support the child. In other words, the treatment should fit the patient. Finally, assessment and treatment approaches must be reviewed, developed, and evaluated.

OUTCOME

Remarkably little is known of the outcome of feeding disorders in the Western world, although the effects of malnutrition are well documented from studies in developing countries. In one of very few studies, the developmental sequelae of infant failure to thrive were examined in 42 unreferred 6-year-olds with a history of severe failure to thrive at age 1 year. At 6 years, children with a history of failure to thrive were considerably smaller than matched comparisons in terms of body mass index and height and weight centiles. Failure-to-thrive patients had more limited quantitative and memory skills than controls, but there were no significant differences in general cognitive functioning once maternal IQ was taken into consideration (53). In this small series, therefore, there was little evidence of adverse effects of early malnutrition on cognitive functioning by school age. The most comprehensive follow-up study to date has been that of Dahl and colleagues, who followed 25 of their sample of infant problem eaters. At primary school age, those who had initial refusal to eat continued to present more eating problems both at home and at school than controls but were otherwise no different on measures of general behavior, somatic health, or growth. Whether these problem eating behaviors persisted into adolescence and possible associations with later eating disorders or problems with weight regulation is unknown.

For selective (picky) eating that has persisted into late childhood or adolescence, in our sample of 20 children only those who had had specific intervention improved their range of foods (26). These were selected cases referred to a specialist service and the generalizability of these findings is unclear. For anorexia nervosa, only a few studies have reported long-term follow-up in younger patients only, although many studies include some young patients (52). Overall, outcome in childhood-onset anorexia nervosa is roughly equivalent to later-onset disorders.

SUMMARY

A developmental framework encompassing the range of feeding and eating problems from childhood to adulthood is needed, as increasing evidence of continuities between feeding and eating problems are found. A small but expanding literature is emerging identifying relationships between early feeding difficulties and later eating concerns, and in the mechanisms for systemic and transgenerational influence of food-related beliefs and cognitions. Central to this are issues of control and the development of self-regulation, concepts that go far beyond the feeding behavior in terms of their importance and impact on child development.

There are still many areas where knowledge is lacking, in terms of both theoretical understanding and treatment approaches. In particular, issues of classification remain far from resolved, nor is it clear in which conceptual framework feeding problems are best classified and understood. This hampers many aspects of further research. The relationship between parent-defined feeding problems from primary care and community samples and cases of feeding "disorder" presenting clinically needs further consideration. Treatment and outcome studies are needed.

ACKNOWLEDGMENT

My thanks to Catherine Dendy for her comments and conceptual framework.

REFERENCES

1. Stein MA, Mendelsohn J, Obermeyer WH, Amromin J, Benca R. Sleep and behavior problems in school-aged children. Pediatrics 2001; 107(4):E60.

2. Stein DJ, Bouwer C, Van Heerden B. Pica and the obsessive-compulsive spectrum disorders. S Afr Med J 1996; 86(suppl 12):1582–1586.

3. Olden KW. Rumination. Curr Treat Options Gastroenterol 2001; 4(4):351–358.

4. Khan S, Hyman PE, Cocjin J, Di Lorenzo C. Rumination syndrome in adolescents. J Pediatr 2000; 136(4):528–531.

5. Crist W, Napier-Phillips A. Mealtime behaviors of young children: a comparison of normative and clinical data. J Dev Behav Pediatr 2001; 22(5):279–286.

6. Skuse D, Wolke D. The nature and consequences of feeding problems in infancy. In: Cooper P, Stein A, eds. Feeding Problems and Eating Disorders in Children and Adolescents. Reading: Harwood Academic, 1992:1–25.

7. Reau NR, Senturia YD, Lebailly SA, Christoffel KK. Infant and toddler feeding patterns and problems: normative data and a new direction. Pediatric Practice Research Group. J Dev Behav Pediatr 1996; 17(3):149–153.

8. Dahl M, Sundelin C. Early feeding problems in an affluent society. I. Categories and clinical signs. Acta Paediatr Scand 1986; 75(3):370–379.

9. Burklow KA, Phelps AN, Schultz JR, McConnell K, Rudolph C. Classifying complex pediatric feeding disorders. J Pediatr Gastroenterol Nutr 1998; 27(2):143–147.

10. Rudolph CD. Feeding disorders in infants and children. J Pediatr 1994; 125 (6 Pt 2):S116–S124.

11. Wickendon M. The development and disruption of feeding skills: how speech and language therapists can help. In: Southall A, Schwartz A, eds. Feeding Problems in Children: A Practical Guide. Abingdon, Oxford: Radcliffe Medical Press, 2000:3–23.

12. Palmer MM, Crawley K, Blanco IA. Neonatal Oral-Motor Assessment scale: a reliability study. J Perinatol 1993; 13(1):28–35.

13. Douglas J. Behavioural approaches to the assessment and management of feeding problems in young children. In: Southall A, Schwartz A, eds. Feeding Problems in Children: A Practical Guide. Abingdon, Oxford: Radcliffe Medical Press, 2000:42–57.

14. Harris G, Booth IW. The nature and management of eating problems in preschool children. In: Cooper PJ, Stein A, eds. Feeding Problems and Eating Disorders in Children and Adolescents. Monographs in Clinical Pediatrics No 5. Reading: Harwood Academic, 1992:61–85.

15. Chatoor I, Hirsch R, Ganiban J, Persinger M, Hamburger E. Diagnosing infantile anorexia: the observation of mother–infant interactions. J Am Acad Child Adolesc Psychiatry 1998; 37(9):959–967.

16. Chatoor I, Ganiban J, Harrison J, Hirsch R. Observation of feeding in the diagnosis of posttraumatic feeding disorder of infancy. J Am Acad Child Adolesc Psychiatry 2001; 40(5):595–602.

17. Koon R. Conversion dysphagia in children. Psychosomatics 1983; 24:182–184.

18. Birch LL, Fisher JA. Appetite and eating behavior in children. Pediatr Clin North Am 1995; 42(4):931–953.

19. Stein A, Woolley H, Murray L, Cooper P, Cooper S, Noble F, et al. Influence

of psychiatric disorder on the controlling behaviour of mothers with 1-year-old infants. A study of women with maternal eating disorder, postnatal depression and a healthy comparison group. Br J Psychiatry 2001; 179:157–162.

20. Whelan E, Cooper PJ. The association between childhood feeding problems and maternal eating disorder: a community study. Psychol Med 2000; 30(1):69–77.

21. McCann JB, Stein A, Fairburn CG, Dunger DB. Eating habits and attitudes of mothers of children with non-organic failure to thrive. Arch Dis Child 1994; 70(3):234–236.

22. Birch LL, Fisher JO. Mothers' child-feeding practices influence daughters' eating and weight. Am J Clin Nutr 2000; 71(5):1054–1061.

23. Jacobi C, Agras WS, Hammer L. Predicting children's reported eating disturbances at 8 years of age. J Am Acad Child Adolesc Psychiatry 2001; 40(3):364–372.

24. Bryant-Waugh R. Overview of the eating disorders. In: Lask B, Bryant-Waugh R, eds. Anorexia nervosa and related eating disorders in childhood and adolescence. Hove, East Sussex: Psychology Press, 2000:27–40.

25. Pliner P, Loewen ER. Temperament and food neophobia in children and their mothers. Appetite 1997; 28:239–254.

26. Nicholls D, Christie D, Randall L, Lask B. Selective eating: symptom, disorder or normal variant? Clin Child Psychol Psychiatry 2001; 6(2):257–270.

27. Rydell AM, Dahl M, Sundelin C. Characteristics of school children who are choosy eaters. J Genet Psychol 1995; 156(2):217–229.

28. Bryant-Waugh R, Lask B. Eating disorders in children. J Child Psychol Psychiatry 1995; 36(2):191–202.

29. Reilly SM, Skuse DH, Wolke D, Stevenson J. Oral–motor dysfunction in children who fail to thrive: organic or non-organic? Dev Med Child Neurol 1999; 41(2):115–122.

30. Marchi M, Cohen P. Early childhood eating behaviors and adolescent eating disorders. J Am Acad Child Adol Psychiatry 1990; 29(1):112–117.

31. Rastam M. Anorexia nervosa in 51 Swedish adolescents: premorbid problems and comorbidity. J Am Acad Child Adol Psychiatry 1992; 31(5):819–829.

32. Jacobs BW, Isaacs S. Pre-pubertal anorexia nervosa: a retrospective controlled study. J Child Psychol Psychiatry 1986; 27(2):237–250.

33. Stark LJ, Jelalian E, Powers SW, Mulvihill MM, Opipari LC, Bowen A, et al. Parent and child mealtime behavior in families of children with cystic fibrosis. J Pediatr 2000; 136(2):195–200.

34. Schwarz SM, Corredor J, Fisher-Medina J, Cohen J, Rabinowitz S. Diagnosis and treatment of feeding disorders in children with developmental disabilities. Pediatrics 2001; 108(3):671–676.

35. Harris G, Blissett J, Johnson R. Food refusal associated with illness. Child Psychol Psychiatry Rev 2000; 5(4):148–156.

36. Birch LL, Fisher JO. Development of eating behaviors among children and adolescents. Pediatrics 1998; 101(3 Pt 2):539–549.

37. Patel P, Wheatcroft R, Park RJ, Stein A. The children of mothers with eating disorders. Clin Child Fam Psychol Rev 2002; 5(1):1–19.

38. Cooper PJ, Watkins B, Bryant-Waugh R, Lask B. The nosological status of early onset anorexia nervosa. Psychol Med 2002; 32(5):873–880.
39. Agras S, Hammer L, McNicholas F. A prospective study of the influence of eating-disordered mothers on their children. Int J Eat Disord 1999; 25(3):253–262.
40. Saarilehto S, Keskinen S, Lapinleimu H, Helenius H, Simell O. Connections between parental eating attitudes and children's meagre eating: questionnaire findings. Acta Paediatr 2001; 90(3):333–338.
41. Nicholls D, Bryant-Waugh R. Children and young adolescents. In: Treasure J, Schmidt U, van Furth E, eds. Handbook of Eating Disorders. Chichester: John Wiley and Sons, 2003:415–433.
42. Fairburn CG, Cooper Z. The eating disorders examination. 12th ed. In: Fairburn CG, Wilson GT, eds. Binge Eating: Nature, Assessment and Treatment. New York: Guilford Press, 1993:317–332.
43. Bryant-Waugh R, Cooper P, Taylor C, Lask B. The use of the Eating Disorder Examination with children: a pilot study. Int J Eat Disord 1996; 19(4):391–397.
44. Nicholls D, Chater R, Lask B. Children into DSM IV don't go: a comparison of classification systems for eating disorders in childhood and early adolescence. Int J Eat Disord 2000; 28(3):317–324.
45. Higgs JF, Goodyer IM, Birch J. Anorexia nervosa and food avoidance emotional disorder. Arch Dis Child 1989; 64:346–351.
46. Birch LL, Fisher JO, Grimm-Thomas K, Markey CN, Sawyer R, Johnson SL. Confirmatory factor analysis of the Child Feeding Questionnaire: a measure of parental attitudes, beliefs and practices about child feeding and obesity proneness. Appetite 2001; 36(3):201–210.
47. Cole TJ, Freeman JV, Preece MA. Body mass index reference curves for the UK, 1990. Arch Dis Child 1995; 73(1):25–29.
48. Williams S. Body Mass Index reference curves derived from a New Zealand birth cohort. N Z Med J 2000; 113(1114):308–311.
49. Luciano A, Bressan F, Zoppi G. Body mass index reference curves for children aged 3–19 years from Verona, Italy. Eur J Clin Nut 1997; 51(1):6–10.
50. Southall A, Schwartz A. Feeding Problems in Children: A Practical Guide. Abingdon, Oxford: Radcliffe Medical Press, 2000.
51. Bithoney WG, McJunkin J, Michalek J, Snyder J, Egan H, Epstein D. The effect of a multidisciplinary team approach on weight gain in nonorganic failure-to-thrive children. J Dev Behav Pediatr 1991; 12(4):254–258.
52. Steinhausen HC. Outcome of anorexia nervosa in the younger patient. J Child Psychol Psychiatry 1997; 38(3):271–276.
53. Boddy J, Skuse D, Andrews B. The developmental sequelae of nonorganic failure to thrive. J Child Psychol Psychiatry Nov 2000; 41(8):1003–1014.

4

Epidemiology of Eating Disorders and Disordered Eating: A Developmental Overview

Maria Råstam
Göteborg University, Göteborg, Sweden

Christopher Gillberg
Göteborg University, Göteborg, Sweden,
and St. George's Hospital Medical School,
London, England

Daphne van Hoeken
Parnassia, The Hague, The Netherlands

Hans Wijbrand Hoek
Parnassia, The Hague, The Netherlands,
and Mailman School of Public Health, Columbia University,
New York, New York, U.S.A.

How common are the eating disorders? The social and economic burden for the individual and the society makes the epidemiology of eating disorders an important issue. Furthermore, studies of representative samples of eating disorders are the soundest base for the examination of etiologic factors and outcome. The most consistent finding across time and studies seems to be that anorexia nervosa predominantly affects adolescent girls.

How do the eating disorders develop over time? Do they belong to a spectrum with disordered eating at one end and anorexia and bulimia nervosa at the other, with the partial syndromes of anorexia and bulimia nervosa

71

in the middle? How often does disordered eating develop into a (partial) eating disorder? Most individuals with anorexia nervosa develop bulimia nervosa or a partial syndrome of anorexia or bulimia nervosa in the course of their recovery (1). There are no data as to how often those subjects with a diagnosis of Eating Disorders–Not Otherwise Specified (ED-NOS) progress to the full syndrome of anorexia or bulimia nervosa.

Epidemiological studies have to counter a number of methodological problems (2,3). Problems specific to the eating disorders are their low prevalence and the tendency of eating disorder subjects to conceal their illness and avoid professional help (4). These make it necessary to study a very large number of subjects from the general population in order to reach enough differential power for the cases. This is highly time and cost intensive. Several strategies have been used to circumvent this problem, in particular case register and other record-based studies, two-stage studies, and studies of special populations.

The limitations of record-based studies are considerable (4). Register-based frequencies represent cases detected in inpatient and, occasionally, outpatient care. Treated patients represent only a minority of all cases. Findings from case registers and hospital records are of more value to treatment planning than for generating hypotheses on the etiology of disease because there is no direct access to the subjects and the additional information that is available is usually limited and of a demographic nature only.

At present a two-stage screening approach is the most widely accepted procedure for case identification. First a large population is screened for the likelihood of an eating disorder by means of a screening questionnaire, identifying an at-risk population (first stage). Then definite cases are established using a personal interview on subjects from this at-risk population as well as on a randomly selected sample of those not at risk (second stage) (5). Methodological problems of two-stage studies are poor response rates, sensitivity and specificity of the screening instrument, and the often restricted size of the interviewed groups, particularly those not at risk (6).

Studies of special populations address a particular segment of the general population, selected a priori for being at increased risk, such as female high school or university students, athletes, or a particular age cohort. The major methodological problem associated with this type of study is the specificity of the findings to the selected subset of the general population.

EATING DISORDERS

Classification

In the sections on anorexia nervosa and bulimia nervosa only studies using strict definitions of these eating disorders (meeting Russell, DSM, or ICD criteria) are discussed. Another category, the ED-NOS, is a mixed category. It includes heterogeneity of patients who do not meet all criteria for ano- rexia nervosa or bulimia nervosa but who have symptoms severe enough to qualify them as having a clinically significant eating disorder. In DSM-IV (7) a provision was made for a separate eating disorder category to be researched further, the binge eating disorder (BED). Only limited epidemio- logical information is available on ED-NOS and BED to date. The epi- demiology of eating disorders has been reviewed before, e.g., Hoek (3), Hsu (4), Van Hoeken et al. (8), and Hoek et al. (9).

Disordered Eating

Dieting is very common among young women and is considered a major risk factor for disordered eating and the development of eating disorders (10,11). Fairburn and colleagues compared subjects with bulimia nervosa (12), BED (13), and anorexia nervosa (14) with each other, with healthy control sub- jects without an eating disorder (general risk factors), and with subjects with other psychiatric disorders (specific risk factors), recruited from general practices in Oxfordshire, England. After screening with self-report ques- tionnaires, a retrospective risk factor interview was carried out that ad- dressed the premorbid period. The results suggest that both bulimia nervosa and BED are most likely to develop in dieters who are at risk of obesity and psychiatric disorder in general (12,13). Disordered eating in teenagers may be an important future health risk. In a community-based longitudinal investigation in New York State, 10% of girls and 1% of boys (out of 717 individuals, 51% female) were diagnosed with DSM-IV eating disorder diagnosis in adolescence. Compared to those without an eating disorder diagnosis, they had significantly more physical problems and anxiety and depressive disorders during early adolescence. Furthermore, data indicated that problems with eating or weight during adolescence may be associated with physical and mental health problems during early adulthood, regard- less of whether the full syndrome of an eating disorder had been present or not (15).

In Sweden in 1880, a health survey of schools for girls (from the upper classes) showed that 35% of 3000 adolescent girls had "chlorosis," defined as being pale, weak, and anemic with no or irregular menstruations. The cause was ascribed to the half starvation recommended for girls of that so- cial standing. The illness was reported occasionally to be epidemic in higher school grades (16). Nowadays even young children have grasped the ideal of a thin female body. In a British study, one of five 9-year-old girls was dieting, and, although more common in heavier girls, dieting was not restricted to that group (17). In a study of 318 girls and boys aged 9–

12 years (18), 45% wanted to lose weight, significantly more girls than boys. Dieting occurred in 37% (Table 1), and 6.9% had high scores on the Children's Eating Attitudes Test (ChEAT), indicating disordered eating. Trying to replicate the Maloney study on children in the same age range in Israel, Sasson and coworkers (19) found 8.8% high scorers on the ChEAT.

In a cross-sectional self-report study of eating attitudes and behaviors in girls attending junior high and high schools in Toronto, Ottawa, and Hamilton (20), one in five girls were dieting (Table 1). Bingeing and purging at a frequency consistent with a diagnosis of DSM-IV bulimia nervosa occurred in 4.9%. Disordered eating attitudes and behaviors tended to increase gradually throughout adolescence, especially in heavier teenagers (20). Table 1 summarizes one-stage (or the first stage of two) surveys of disordered eating in children and adolescents with a participation rate of at least 70%.

In a questionnaire study (28), 35% out of 1241 Swedish schoolgirls aged 14–18 years were dieting. A follow-up of 130 females with dieting plus mental problems gave an accumulated prevalence of 1.2% of anorexia nervosa for the whole female population (29). In South Carolina (22), 3129 middle school students (out of 4282) completed a self-report questionnaire, the Kids' Eating Disorders Survey (KEDS). Dieting and disordered eating was found to be fairly common in 9-to 16-year-olds (Table 1). In a second stage, designed to validate the screening tool, altogether 165 subjects, a mixture of high scorers on the KEDS and randomly selected students, were personally interviewed. One subject fulfilled criteria for DSM-IIIR anorexia nervosa and 22 for ED-NOS.

With the new male body ideal in the media, young men have become increasingly engaged in body building and the use of anabolic steroids (30, 31). Many of these young men are reminiscent of young females with anorexia nervosa in their compulsive pursuit of more training and a specific body image. Still, generally, teenage girls diet because they feel fat whereas most boys who diet are fat (32).

In a representative sample of 4746 adolescents from 31 Minnesota public schools, about 6% were self-reported vegetarians (33). The vegetarians were more likely than nonvegetarians to be female and to be involved in weight control behaviors, including some with an eating disorder. Some individuals may use vegetarianism as a disguise for dieting. In a community-based study on teenage-onset anorexia nervosa, 25% introduced their diet as vegetarianism (34), and during a 10 year follow-up period altogether 41% had a vegetarian phase (1). One cannot exclude the possibility that for some individuals a drastic change of diet per se might be a risk for the development of an eating disorder.

TABLE 1 Surveys of Disordered Eating in School Years

Study	Subjects Source	Age	N	Methods Screening	Disordered Eating Dieting %	Bingeing %	Vomiting %	Laxatives %	Diuretics %	Diet pills %
Whitaker et al., 1989[a] (21)	schoolgirls	13–18	2544	EAT-26	63(18)[b]	6	8	2	0.9	17
	schoolboys		2555	ESI	18(5)[b]	19	2	0.8	0.6	2
Maloney et al., 1989 (18)	schoolchildren	9–12	318	ChEAT	37	10.4	1.3			
Childress et al., 1993[a] (22)	schoolgirls	9–16	1599	KEDS	42.6	6.5	5.6	2.3	2.2	3.6
	schoolboys		1530		19.7	26.3	3.9	0.7	0.8	1.1
Steinhausen et al., 1997[a] (23)	school girls	14–17	276	EDE-S	10.1	1.1	3.6	1.8		
	schoolboys		307		3.6	0.7	0.7	0.3		
Nakamura et al., 1999 (24)	schoolgirls	15–18	2685	EAT-26	57.5 (11.3)[b]			9.6	1.4	4.8
Nobakht & Dezhkam, 2000[a] (25)	schoolgirls	15–18	3100	EAT-26	16.7		1.5		2.5	
Koskelainen et al., 2001 (26)	schoolgirls	13–17	725	9-item questionnaire	17		4			
	schoolboys		733		3		2			
Jones et al., 2001 (20)	schoolgirls	12–18	1739	EAT-26, EDI, DSED	23	15	8.2	1.1	0.6	2.4
Carter et al., 2001 (27)	schoolgirls	12–14	808	EDE-Q		8	4	1	0.4	

For Tables 1–4: ANIS, Anorexia Nervosa Inventory Scale; BCDS, Bulimic Cognitive Distortions Scale; ChEAT, Childrens Eating Attitudes Test-26; DIS, Diagnostic Interview Schedule; DSED, Diagnostic Survey for Eating Disorders; EAT-26, Eating Attitudes Test-26; EDE, Eating Disorder Examination; EDE-Q, Eating Disorder Examination–Questionnaire; EDE-S, Eating Disorder Examination–Screening Version; EDI, Eating Disorder Inventory; KEDS, Kids' Eating Disorders Survey.
[a] first stage of two-stage study.

Anorexia Nervosa

Prevalence

The current standard for prevalence studies of eating disorders are studies employing a two-stage selection of cases. Table 2 summarizes the two-stage surveys of anorexia nervosa in young females. All researchers have succeeded in obtaining high response rates of 85% or more, except Meadows et al. (38), who obtained a response rate of 70%. Those two-stage surveys that identified cases found a prevalence rate of strictly defined anorexia nervosa of between 0.2% and 0.8% of young females, with an average prevalence of 0.3%. These rates are possibly minimal estimates. Most studies found much higher prevalence rates for partial syndromes of anorexia nervosa. One two-stage study (23) screened 607 14- to 17-year-olds with a wide battery of questionnaires. The surveys was completed by 583 participants. The first stage reported on eating behaviors in teenagers (Table 1). In a second stage, 399 parents of screen-positive and control subjects were interviewed. The adolescents were not examined. At the first screening a clinical eating disorder was suspected in two cases, one a girl with anorexia and the other a girl with bulimia nervosa, and this was confirmed in parents' interviews. No more clinically significant eating disorders were found.

Two other studies give prevalence figures for the entire population. In a general-practice study in the Netherlands, Hoek (46) found a raw point prevalence rate of 18.4 per 100,000 of the total population (95% CI 12.7–26.8) on January 1, 1985. Lucas et al. (47) used a very extensive case finding method. It included all medical records of health care providers, general practitioners, and specialists in Rochester, Minnesota. They also screened records mentioning related diagnostic terms for possible undetected cases. They found an overall sex-and age-adjusted point prevalence of 149.5 per 100,000 (95% CI 119.3–179.7) on January 1, 1985. A main explanation for this difference can be found in the inclusion of probable and possible cases by Lucas et al. Definite cases constituted only 39% (82 of 208) of all incident cases identified in the period 1935–1989 (48). Applying this rate to the point prevalence of 149.5 gives an estimated point prevalence of 58.9 per 100,000 for definite cases in Rochester, Minnesota on January 1, 1985. The remaining difference with the point prevalence reported by Hoek (46) could be explained by the greater variety of medical sources searched by Lucas et al. (47).

Incidence

Incidence rate differences between groups are better clues to etiology than prevalence rate differences because they refer to recently started disease (49). The incidence studies of anorexia nervosa have used psychiatric case

TABLE 2 Two-Stage Surveys of Prevalence of Anorexia Nervosa in Young Females

| Study | Subjects | | | | Methods | | Prevalence |
	Source	Age	N	Screening	Criteria	%
Button & Whitehouse, 1981 (35)	college students	16–22	446	EAT	Feighner	0.2
Szmukler, 1983 (36)	private schools	14–19	1331	EAT	Russell	0.8
	state schools	14–19	1676	EAT	Russell	0.2
King, 1989 (37)	general practice	16–35	539	EAT	Russell	0
Meadows et al., 1986 (38)	general practice	18–22	584	EAT	DSM-III	0.2[a]
Johnson-Sabine et al., 1988 (39)	schoolgirls	14–16	1010	EAT	Russell	0
Råstam et al., 1989 (40)	schoolgirls	15	2136	growth chart + questionnaire	DSM-IIIR	0.70
Whitaker et al., 1990 (41)	highschool girls	13–18	2544	EAT	DSM-III	0.3
Whitehouse et al., 1992 (42)	general practice	16–35	540	questionnaire	DSM-IIIR	0.2
Rathner & Messner, 1993 (43)	schoolgirls + case register	11–20	517	EAT	DSM-IIIR	0.58
Wlodarczyk-Bisaga & Dolan, 1996 (44)	schoolgirls	14–16	747	EAT	DSM-IIIR	0
Steinhausen et al., 1997 (23)	schoolgirls	14–17	276	EDE-S	DSM-IIIR	0.7
Nobakht & Dezhkam, 2000 (25)	schoolgirls	15–18	3100	EAT	DSM-IV	0.9
Gual et al., 2002 (45)	schoolgirls	12–21	2862	EAT	DSM-IV	0.3

[a] Not found by screening (EAT score below threshold).

registers, medical records of hospitals in a circumscribed area, registrations by general practitioners, or medical records of health care providers in a community. Table 3 summarizes the results of the studies on the incidence of anorexia nervosa that report overall rates for a general population sample. The overall rates vary considerably, ranging from 0.10 in a hospital-records-based study in Sweden in the 1930's to 12.0 in a medical-records-based study in the USA in the 1980's, both per 100,000 population per year.

Incidence rates derived from general practices on average represent more recently started eating disorders than those based on other medical records. There were two studies of this type. In the study by Hoek and colleagues (58),

TABLE 3   Incidence of Anorexia Nervosa per Year per 100,000 Population

Study	Region	Source	Period	Incidence
Theander,	Southern Sweden	hospital records	1931–1940	0.10
1970 (50)			1941–1950	0.20
			1951–1960	0.45
			(1931–1960)	(0.24)
Willi et al.,	Zurich	hospital records	1956–1958	0.38
1983 (51),			1963–1965	0.55
1990 (52)			1973–1975	1.12
			1983–1985	1.43
Jones et al.,	Monroe Country	case register +	1960–1969	0.37
1980 (53)		hospital records	1970–1976	0.64
Kendell et al.,	Northeast Scotland	case register	1960–1969	1.60
1973 (54)				
Szmukler et al.,	Northeast Scotland	case register	1978–1982	4.06
1986 (55)				
Kendell et al.,	Camberwell	case register	1965–1971	0.66
1973 (54)				
Hoek & Brook,	Assen	case register	1974–1982	5.0
1985 (56)				
Møller-Madsen	Denmark	case register	1970	0.42
& Nystrup,			1988	1.36
1992 (57)			1989	1.17
Lucas et al.,	Rochester, MN	medical records	1935–1949	9.1
1999 (48)			1950–1959	4.3
			1960–1969	7.0
			1970–1979	7.9
			1980–1989	12.0
			(1935–1989)	(8.3)
Hoek et al.,	Netherlands	gen. practitioners	1985–1989	8.1
1995 (58)				
Turnbull et al.,	England, Wales	gen. practitioners	1993	4.2
1996 (59)				

general practitioners using DSM-IIIR criteria have recorded the rate of eating disorders in a large (1985: $N = 151,781$), representative sample (1.1%) of the Dutch population. The incidence rate of anorexia nervosa was 8.1 per 100,000 person years (95% CI 6.1–10.2) during 1985–1989. During the study period 63% of the incident cases were referred to mental health care, accounting for an incidence rate of anorexia nervosa in mental health care of 5.1 per year per 100,000 population. Turnbull et al. (59) searched the UK General Practice Research Database (GPRD), covering 550 general practitioners and 4 million patients, for first diagnoses of anorexia in the period 1988–1993. A randomly selected subset of cases was checked with DSM-IV criteria, from which estimates for adjusted incidence rates were made. For anorexia nervosa they found an age-and sex-adjusted incidence rate of 4.2 (95% CI 3.4–5.0) per 100,000 population in 1993.

Lucas et al. (47,48) used the most extensive case finding method (see the section on prevalence). Over the period 1935–1989, they report an over all age-and sex-adjusted incidence rate of anorexia nervosa of 8.3 per 100,000 person-years (95% CI 7.1–9.4).

Age and Sex

Earlier reports indicate a peak incidence in the late teens (55,60), whereas later studies indicate a peak age of onset between 14 and 15 years (61). Adolescent onset points to the role of pubertal changes such as body composition changes (62) and the rapid rise in estrogen levels (63). The psychological and social changes of adolescence have been shown to be important (14,39). The trend toward an earlier menarche suggests that the peak onset age might be even earlier (64). Incidence rates of anorexia nervosa are highest for females 15–19 years old. These constitute approximately 40% of all identified cases and 60% of female cases. For example, Lucas et al. (48) report an incidence rate of 73.9 per 100,000 person-years for 15- to 19-year-old women during the period 1935–1989, with a continual rise since the 1930s to a top rate of 135.7 for the period 1980–1989. On an overall female rate of 15.0 per 100,000 population per year, Lucas et al. (48) report a rate of 9.5 for 30- to 39-year-old women, 5.9 for 40- to 49-year-old women, 1.8 for 50- to 59-year-old women, and 0.0 for women 60 years and older.

The majority of male incidence rates reported were below 0.5 per 100,000 population per year, e.g., Turnbull et al. (59). In those studies where it is reported, the female-to-male ratio usually is around 11:1, e.g., Hoek et al. (58).

Time Trends

In spite of some reports of an increased rate of anorexia nervosa from the mid-1960s to the mid-1980s in certain regions (48), there is no consensus that anorexia nervosa prevalence generally has increased over the corresponding time period. Case register studies prior to the 1980s show at most a slight increase over time of incident anorexia nervosa cases (3). The studies done in the 1980s show widely diverging incidence rates. Most likely there is a methodological explanation for these differences. The main problem lies in the need for long study periods. This results in a sensitivity of these studies to minor changes in absolute incidence numbers and in methods, e.g., variations in registration policy, demographic differences between populations, faulty inclusion of readmissions, the particular method of detection used, or the availability of services (65–67).

From the studies that have used long study periods, it may now be concluded that there is an upward trend in the incidence of anorexia nervosa since the 1950s. The increase is most substantial in females 15–24 years of age. Lucas et al. (48) found that the age-adjusted incidence rates of anorexia nervosa in females 15–24 years old showed a highly significant linear increasing trend from 1935 to 1989, with an estimated rate of increase of 1.03 per 100,000 person-years per calendar year. In 10- to 14-year-old girls a rise in incidence was observed for each decade since the 1950s. The rates for men and for women 25 and older remained relatively low.

All record-based studies will grossly underestimate the true incidence because not all patients will be referred to mental health care or become hospitalized (68). The increase in incidence rates of registered cases implies at least that there is an increased demand for health care facilities for anorexia nervosa.

Bulimia Nervosa

Prevalence

In 1990 Fairburn and Beglin gave a review of the prevalence studies on bulimia nervosa (6). This landmark review yielded the generally accepted prevalence rate of 1% of young females with bulimia nervosa according to DSM criteria. Table 4 summarizes two-stage surveys of bulimia nervosa in young females that have been published since the review by Fairburn and Beglin. Despite the different classifications used—DSM-III (72) versus DSM-IIIR (73)—and different types of prevalence rates provided [lifetime prevalence, e.g., Bushnell et al. (69), versus point prevalence, e.g., Rathner and Messner (43)], the aggregated prevalence rate according to DSM criteria remains 1%. The prevalence of subclinical eating disorders is substantially higher than that of full-syndrome bulimia nervosa, e.g., Whitehouse et al. (42): 1.5% for full-syndrome and 5.4% for partial-syndrome bulimia nervosa.

The results of three studies not using a two-stage procedure for case finding are reported here as well because they are likely to represent the entire population of women. Garfinkel et al. (74) assessed eating disorders in a ran-

TABLE 4 Two-Stage Surveys of Prevalence of Bulimia Nervosa in Young Females

Study	Subjects			Methods		Prevalence %
	Source	Age	N	Screening	Criteria	
Whitaker et al., 1990 (41)	highschool girls	13–18	2544	EAT	DSM-III	4.2
Bushnell et al., 1990 (69)	household census	18–24		DIS	DSM-III	4.5
		25–44 (18–44)	(777)			2.0 (2.6)
Szabó and Túry, 1991 (70)	schoolgirls	14–18	416	EAT, BCDS ANIS	DSM-III DSM-IIIR	0 0
	college girls	19–36	224	EAT, BCDS, ANIS	DSM-III DSM-IIIR	4.0 1.3
Whitehouse et al., 1992 (42)	general practice	16–35	540	questionnaire	DSM-IIIR	1.5
Rathner & Messner, 1993 (43)	schoolgirls + case register	11–20	517	EAT	DSM-IIIR	0
Wlodarczyk-Bisaga & Dolan, 1996 (44)	schoolgirls	14–16	747	EAT	DSM-IIIR	0
Santonastaso et al., 1996 (71)	schoolgirls	16	359	EAT	DSM-IV	0.5
Steinhausen et al., 1997 (23)	schoolgirls	14–17	276	EDE-S	DSM-IIIR	0.5
Notakht & Dezhkam, 2000 (25)	schoolgirls	15–18	3100	EAT	DSM-IV	3.2
Gual et al., 2002 (45)	schoolgirls	12–21	2862	EAT	DSM-IV	0.8

dom, stratified, nonclinical community sample, using a structured interview for the whole sample. They reported a lifetime prevalence for bulimia nervosa of 1.1% in women and of 0.1% in men aged 15–65, using DSM-IIIR criteria. This is a study of a representative sample of women in the United States and provides a good estimate of the lifetime prevalence of bulimia nervosa in the United States. Another study from the United States designed for examining the relationship among assault, bulimia nervosa, and BED (DSM-IV criteria) by interviewing by telephone a national representative sample of 3006 women yielded a prevalence for bulimia nervosa of 2.4% (75). In a study by Soundy et al. (76), no attempt was made to determine prevalence rates for bulimia nervosa because they considered the information about how long symptoms had persisted and the long duration (mean 39.8 months) of symptoms before diagnosis to be too unreliable.

Incidence

There have been few incidence studies of bulimia nervosa. The most obvious reason is the lack of criteria for bulimia nervosa in the past. Most case registers use the International Classification of Diseases, currently ICD-10 (77). The ICD-9 (78) and previous versions did not provide a separate code for bulimia nervosa. Bulimia nervosa has been distinguished as a separate disorder by Russell in 1979 (79) and DSM-III in 1980 (72). Before 1980 the term "bulimia" in medical records designated symptoms of heterogeneous conditions manifested by overeating, but not the syndrome as it is known today. Therefore, it is difficult to examine trends in the incidence of bulimia nervosa or a possible shift from anorexia nervosa to bulimia nervosa, which might have influenced the previously described incidence rates of anorexia nervosa.

   Three studies are of main interest: those of Soundy et al. (76), Hoek et al. (58), and Turnbull et al. (59). Soundy and colleagues used methodology similar to that in the long-term anorexia nervosa study by Lucas et al. (47) screening all medical records of health care providers, general practitioners, and specialists in Rochester, Minnesota over the period 1980–1990 for a clinical diagnosis of bulimia nervosa as well as for related symptoms (76). Hoek and colleagues studied the incidence rate of bulimia nervosa using DSM-IIIR criteria in a large general-practice study representative of the Dutch population, covering the period 1985–1989 (58). Turnbull and colleagues screened the General Practice Research Database (GPRD), covering a large, representative sample of the English and Welsh population, for first diagnoses of anorexia nervosa and bulimia nervosa in 1993 (59). The three studies all report an annual incidence of bulimia nervosa around 12 per 100,000 population: 13.5 for Soundy et al., 11.5 for Hoek et al., and 12.2 for Turnbull et al.

Another general-population study of a relatively small population (lower than 50,000 inhabitants) is of some interest because it was based on a homogeneous population from a small Danish island (80). The Danish Psychiatric Case Register and the local records of in-and outpatients were screened, psychiatrists and physicians in primary care were interviewed, as were all school medical officers. In the period 1985–1989, the average annual incidence of bulimia nervosa was 6.8 per 100,000 population.

Age and Sex

Soundy et al. (76) report an incidence of bulimia nervosa of 26.5 for females and of 0.8 for males per 100,000 population, yielding a female-to-male ratio of 33:1. Hoek et al. (58) report similar rates of 21.9 for females and 0.8 for males per 100,000 population, yielding a female-to-male ratio of 27:1. For the highest risk group of 20- to 24-year-old females, rates close to 82 per 100,000 are found: 82.7 for Soundy et al. and 82.1 for Hoek et al. Hoek et al. report a rate of 8.3 per 100,000 for women aged 35–64. Turnbull et al. (59) report an annual incidence of 1.7 per 100,000 people (men and women) aged 40 and over.

Time Trends

Soundy et al. (76) found yearly incidence rates to rise sharply from 7.4 per 100,000 females in 1980 to 49.7 in 1983, and then remain relatively constant at around 30 per 100,000 females. This would seem to be related to the publication, and following implementation in the field, of DSM-III in 1980 (72), introducing bulimia nervosa as an official diagnostic category. Hoek et al. (58) report a nonsignificant trend for the incidence rates of bulimia nervosa to increase by 15% each year in the period 1985–1989. Turnbull et al. (59) noted a highly significant, threefold increase in bulimia nervosa incidence rates for women aged 10–39 in the period 1988–1993, increasing from 14.6 in 1988 to 51.7 in 1993. These incidence rates of bulimia nervosa can only serve as minimal estimates of the true incidence rate. The reasons are the lack of data, the greater taboo surrounding bulimia nervosa, and its smaller perceptibility in comparison with anorexia nervosa.

Eating Disorders NOS

ED-NOS [DSM-IV (7)] refers to a mixed category of individuals who do not meet all criteria for anorexia nervosa or bulimia nervosa, but who have symptoms severe enough to qualify them as having a clinically significant eating disorder. The heterogeneity of the category makes comparison of rates between studies difficult.

In a two-stage cohort study of Australian students, initially aged 14–15 years over 3 years with 6-month intervals (11), 3.3% of all girls and 0.3% of all boys had partial syndromes of an eating disorder at the start of the study. Girls who engaged in severe dieting (8%) had an 18-fold increase in the risk of developing an eating disorder within 6 months compared with nondieters. Of course, severe dieting may already be a sign of an eating disorder under way. Moderate dieting, present in 60% of all girls, was associated with a fivefold increase in risk for eating disorder. General psychiatric symptomatology as a separate factor increased the risk for an eating disorder seven times. All together, 6.6% of all girls and 1.2% of the boys were classified as having an eating disorder at least once during the study.

Binge Eating Disorder

One example of ED-NOS is binge eating disorder (BED), which has the status of "Diagnostic Category in Need of Further Research" in the DSM-IV (7). BED is characterized by eating large amounts of food with no sense of control and no use of compensatory behaviors to avoid the weight gain that is a common consequence. Weight concern and worry about body shape seem to be a clinical feature of BED, regardless of BMI (81,82). Studies, including a two-stage community study (83), support BED as a diagnosis distinct from bulimia nervosa of the purging type. Furthermore, BED seems to have a different outcome than nonpurging bulimia nervosa, suggesting a distinction between nonpurging bulimia nervosa and BED. A general problem with the comparison of studies of BED—and bulimia nervosa for that matter—lies in the definition of a binge. Studies differ in the way a binge is defined, resulting in subject groups that are not fully comparable.

We know of only one prevalence study using a two-stage case identification procedure in the general population. Cotrufo et al. (84) identified two cases of BED in a group of 919 females aged 13–19 years, giving a prevalence rate of 0.2%. The low rate may be due to the relatively young age of the investigated population. Also, the sample size is rather small for a low-frequency disorder.

In a telephone survey, Dansky et al. (75) found DSM-IV BED to be present in 1% of 3006 adult females. Hay (85) conducted interviews to determine the prevalence of bulimic-type eating disorders on all subjects in a large general-population sample (3001 interviews). The mean age of the cases was 35.2 years. Using DSM-IV criteria, a point prevalence for BED of 1% was found. Using a broader definition by Fairburn and Cooper (86), the prevalence was estimated at 2.5%. A weakness of the study was that diagnoses were based on a very limited number of questions (two gating questions and three additional probes). No information was given regarding the sensitivity and specificity of the instrument.

Time Trends

To study the prevalence of binge eating and weight control practices in West Germany over time, 2130 adult subjects were examined in 1997 and compared with 1773 adults in 1990 (87). Participation was almost 70%. The same self-report questionnaire was used in 1990 and in 1997 (complemented with a personal interview for a subsample in 1997). The prevalence for BED dropped from 1.5% in 1990 to 0.7% in 1997 in women and from 2.4% to 1.5% in men. The prevalence for bulimia nervosa dropped from 2.4% to 1.1% in women and from 2.0% to 1.1% in men. None of the differences were statistically significant.

SOME DEMOGRAPHIC VARIABLES

Social Class

Most psychiatric disorders show a higher prevalence in the lower socio-economic classes. It is difficult to determine whether this is the result of the social selection process or whether it is caused by social factors (88).

For anorexia nervosa, there has been a traditional belief of an upper social class preponderance. In reviewing the evidence, Gard and Freeman (89) concluded that the relationship between anorexia nervosa and high socio-economic status is unproven, due to data collection biases including sample size, clinical status, and referral patterns. A recent study on a large comprehensive clinical database, covering 692 referrals to a U.K. national specialist center in 33 years' time, challenges this conclusion: McLelland and Crisp (90) found referrals for anorexia nervosa from the two highest social classes to be almost twice as high as expected. They present evidence that their findings are unrelated to differences in clinical features or in access to their service. In a two-stage survey of all 15-year-olds in the city of Göteborg, Sweden, the subjects with anorexia nervosa did not differ from a sex-, age-, and school-matched comparison group concerning social class (91).

For bulimia nervosa, Gard and Freeman (89) conclude that—similar to most psychiatric disorders—there seems to be preponderance in the lower socio-economic groups.

Level of Industrialization

It is commonly thought that anorexia nervosa is a Western illness: there appears to be a developmental gradient across countries, with a predominance in industrialized, developed countries, linking the disorder to an affluent society (3). This gradient has been hypothesized to be connected with the sociocultural theory. This theory holds that eating disorders are promoted by a "Western" culture favoring slimness as a beauty ideal for females. By consequence eating disorders would be less prevalent in underdeveloped, non-Western cultures. Unfortunately, to date few developing countries have the facilities and means to arrive at reliable epidemiological data.

According to a recent extensive review of studies from the Far East (92), body dissatisfaction and dieting rates were similar to those in the West. Dieting occurred in more than 60% of females in Japan; prevalence rates were around 0.03% for anorexia nervosa and ranged from 1.9% to 2.9% for bulimia nervosa. Community studies in China found the anorexia nervosa prevalence to be 0.01%, and bulimia nervosa rates ranged from 0.5% to 1.3%. The very low rate of anorexia nervosa in the Far East may seem surprising. It could be due to a slightly different behavioral phenotype of the syndrome, including cases masquerading as bulimia nervosa. Reports from Eastern Europe are very scant. In Hungary and Poland two-stage studies have been conducted; see Tables 2 and 4 (44,70). A questionnaire lifestyle study of 453 medical students between 1995 and 1999 in Slovakia showed excessive underweight (BMI = 17.5 or lower) in 1.0% of men and 2.8% of women (93), suggesting a possible eating disorder. In Iran, Nobakht and Dezhkam (25) examined disordered eating with EAT-26 in 3100 female students, with no attrition (Table 1). Of 749 high scorers, 99.8% completed another self-report questionnaire to assess DMS-IV eating disorder diagnoses. Accumulated prevalence for full-syndrome anorexia nervosa was 0.9%, for the partial syndrome 1.84%, and for full-syndrome bulimia nervosa 3.23%, for the partial syndrome 4.79%. Comparing 59 Iranian female students living in Tehran to 45 female students of Iranian descent living in Los Angeles, Abdollahi and Mann (94) found similar amounts of self-reported disordered eating in the two samples. In a population of 351 secondary school girls in Cairo, Egypt, 11.4% scored positively on the Eating Attitude Test (EAT) Questionnaire and were subsequently interviewed (95). Three cases fulfilled Russell's criteria for a diagnosis of bulimia nervosa (1.2%), and an additional 12 individuals (3.4%) were deemed to have a partial syndrome of bulimia nervosa.

Girls and women born in countries with a low prevalence of anorexia nervosa seem to have an increased risk of developing the disorder after moving to a high-frequency region (96,97). Some recent publications cast doubts on the validity of the sociocultural theory, at least for anorexia nervosa (98,99). For example, Hoek et al. (100) found an incidence of anorexia nervosa on the Caribbean island of Curaçao within the lower range of rates reported in Western countries.

Level of Urbanization

Hoek et al. (58) report that the incidence of bulimia nervosa is three to five times higher in urbanized areas and cities than in rural areas, whereas anorexia nervosa is found with almost equal frequency in areas with different degrees of urbanization. The drift hypothesis, relating urbanization differences to migration for educational reasons, is rejected because the differences remain after adjusting for age. Other social factors involved might be an increased pressure to be slender and decreased social control in urbanized areas. If these hold true, this would imply that anorexia nervosa is less sensitive to social factors than bulimia nervosa, has a more biological origin, and is more driven by other factors such as a tendency toward asceticism and compulsive behavior.

Occupation

Some occupations appear to be linked to an increased risk of the development of an eating disorder (101). Typical examples are professions in the world of fashion (102) and ballet (2). We do not know whether this is a causal factor or rather the result of disturbed attitudes around body and shape. In other words, are preanorectics attracted by the ballet world, or are the requirements of the profession conducive to the development of anorexia nervosa?

According to a meta-analysis of 34 studies, elite athletes had a higher risk of eating disorders than nonathletes. On the other hand, nonelite athletes were more satisfied with their bodies than controls, and they seemed to have a reduced risk of eating disorders (103). In a recent study of 181 elite women runners in the United Kingdom (104), 7 (4%) had anorexia nervosa, 2 individuals (1%) had bulimia nervosa, and 20 (11%) females had an ED-NOS.

CONCLUSIONS

For anorexia nervosa an average prevalence rate of 0.3% was found for young girls. Although Soundy et al. (76) caution for the possibility of unreliable information, figures of an average prevalence rate of bulimia nervosa of 1% in women and of 0.1% in men seem accurate. A tentative conclusion is that the prevalence of BED is more likely to be 1% than 4% or more.

Assuming that even the studies with the most complete case finding methods yield an underestimate of the true incidence, as state of the art we conclude that the overall incidence of anorexia nervosa is at least 8 per 100,000 population per year and the incidence of bulimia nervosa is at least 12 per 100,000 population per year. The incidence rate of anorexia nervosa has increased during the past 50 years, particularly in females aged 10–24 years. The registered incidence of bulimia nervosa has increased, at least during the first 5 years after bulimia nervosa was added to the DSM-III (72). For BED not enough incidence information is available to summarize.

Little is known about how many people with or without (a combination of) known risk factors develop an eating disorder over time. Dieting seems a general nonspecific risk factor, increasing the risk of developing an eating disorder by about fivefold.

COMMENTS

The value of epidemiology lies in its particular methodology that gives rise to population-based disease rates and ratios. When properly established, these rates and ratios provide a scientific basis on the community level for treatment planning and etiological model building. Epidemiological information is needed to examine and extend on clinical observations.

The basic epidemiological measures are incidence and prevalence rates. For the purpose of treatment planning, there is an ongoing need for prevalence information at the local level. For reasons of time and cost efficiency, this is best done by monitoring existing health care consumption registers. Attention must be paid to the interpretation of changing consumption rates in relation to changes in health care recruitment and admission policy. When the adequacy or accuracy of case definition and registration is questioned, efforts are needed to improve registration.

For the purpose of etiological model building, the mere determination of prevalence and incidence rates is not enough. Although more is becoming known on general and specific risk factors for the onset of an eating disorder there still is an impressive gap. Furthermore, the developmental mechanisms of these factors are largely unknown. The general conclusion is that dieting behavior plays a role in the pathogenesis of anorexia nervosa, bulimia nervosa, and BED. However, not all dieters proceed to develop an eating disorder. A prospective follow-up study of initially healthy dieters sampled from the general population may shed light on the mechanisms that turn dieting into an eating disorder.

To circumvent the power and cost problems caused by the relatively low rates of eating disorders in the general population, a few suggestions for the design of economically feasible studies providing generalizable, reliable results on risk factors and mechanisms are given:

> There is a need for prospective, follow-up designs using initially healthy subjects at high risk for developing an eating disorder, such as young girls, dieters, and participants in weight-restricted sports, including ballet. Depending on the question to be answered, these could be matched on sex, age, and socio-economic status with initially healthy intermediate-and low-risk groups.

For lower risk groups, such as males or older persons, a prospective design is too cost inefficient and a case-control design is more appropriate. Cases should be collected at as low a level of entry into the health care system as possible, preferably primary care. Same-sex siblings and other same-sex persons matched for age-and socio-economic status could be of use as controls. To facilitate hypothesis testing and the exchange of knowledge and ideas, the formation of a multicenter database of these rare cases would mean a great improvement.

For both prospective follow-up studies and case-control studies of eating disorders, a comprehensive assessment of biological, psychological, familial, and social variables is needed. The factors and mechanisms studied should be based on findings from previous research such as that by Fairburn et al. (12). To decide on the effect of weight-and shape-centered beauty ideals on the frequency of eating disorders, studies are needed that compare the distribution of eating disorders between groups differing in weight- and shape-related attitudes.

Finally, an issue to be solved for epidemiological studies on eating disorders is the reliance on a categorical approach of caseness, particularly for the "newer" diagnoses of bulimia nervosa, the ED-NOS, and BED. By focusing on incident clinical cases and ignoring atypical or subclinical cases, etiological reasoning may miss the crucial developmental elements in what have been called "broad-spectrum" disorders.

SUMMARY

The average prevalence rate for young girls is 0.3% for anorexia nervosa and 1% for bulimia nervosa. The overall incidence is at least 8 per 100,000 person-years for anorexia nervosa and 12 per 100,000 person-years for bulimia nervosa.

The incidence rate of anorexia nervosa has increased during the past 50 years, particularly in females 10–24 years old. The registered incidence of bulimia nervosa has increased, at least during the first 5 years after bulimia nervosa was introduced in the DSM-III.

There is a need for prospective, follow-up designs using initially healthy subjects at high risk for developing an eating disorder. Depending on the question to be answered, these could be matched on sex, age, and socio-economic status with initially healthy intermediate-and low-risk groups.

Detailed and reliable registration of case definition, demographic, and other characteristics of the patient, symptoms, and concomitants of the disease or disorder remain of the utmost importance to advance evidence-based treatment and prevention.

REFERENCES

1. Wentz E, Gillberg C, Gillberg IC, Råstam M. Ten-year follow-up of adolescent-onset anorexia nervosa: psychiatric disorders and overall functioning scales. J Child Psychol Psychiatry 2001; 42:613–622.
2. Szmukler GI. The epidemiology of anorexia nervosa and bulimia. J Psychiatr Res 1985; 19:143–153.
3. Hoek HW, van Hoeken D. Review of the prevalence and incidence of eating disorders. Int J Eat Disord 2003; 34:383–396.
4. Hsu LKG. Epidemiology of the eating disorders. Psychiatric Clin North Am 1996; 19:681–700.
5. Williams P, Tarnopolsky A, Hand D. Case definition and case identification in psychiatric epidemiology: review and assessment. Psychol Med 1980; 10:101–114.
6. Fairburn CG, Beglin SJ. Studies of the epidemiology of bulimia nervosa. Am J Psychiatry 1990; 147:401–408.
7. American Psychiatric Association. Diagnostic and Statistical Manual of Mental Disorders. 4th ed. Washington, DC, 1994.
8. van Hoeken D, Lucas AR, Hoek HW. Epidemiology. In: Hoek HW, Treasure JL, Katzman MA, eds. Neurobiology in the Treatment of Eating Disorders. Chichester: John Wiley and Sons, 1998:97–126.
9. Hoek HW, van Hoeken D, Katzman MA. Epidemiology and cultural aspects of eating disorders: a review. In: Maj M, Halmi K, Lopez-Ibor JJ, Sartorius N, eds. Eating Disorders. Vol. 6. Chichester: John Wiley and Sons, 2003:75–104.
10. Patton GC, Johnson-Sabine E, Wood K, Mann AH, Wakeling A. Abnormal eating attitudes in London schoolgirls—a prospective epidemiological study: outcome at twelve month follow-up. Psychol Med 1990; 20:383–394.
11. Patton GC, Selzer R, Coffey C, Carlin JB, Wolfe R. Onset of adolescent eating disorders: population based cohort study over 3 years. BMJ 1999; 318:765–768.
12. Fairburn CG, Welch SL, Doll HA, Davies BA, O'Connor ME. Risk factors for bulimia nervosa: a community-based case-control study. Arch Gen Psychiatry 1997; 54:509–517.
13. Fairburn CG, Doll HA, Welch SL, Hay PJ, Davies BA, O'Connor ME. Risk factors for binge eating disorder: a community-based case-control study. Arch Gen Psychiatry 1998; 55:425–432.
14. Fairburn CG, Cooper Z, Doll HA, Welch SL. Risk factors for anorexia nervosa: three integrated case-control comparisons. Arch Gen Psychiatry 1999; 56:468–476.
15. Johnson JG, Cohen P, Kasen S, Brook JS. Eating disorders during adolescence and the risk for physical and mental disorders during early adulthood. Arch Gen Psychiatry 2002; 59:545–552.

16. Johannisson K. The Dark Continent. Stockholm: Nordstedts Förlag, 1994: 131.
17. Hill AJ, Draper E, Stack J. A weight on children's minds: body shape dissatisfactions at 9-years old. Int J Obes Relat Metab Disord 1994; 18:383–389.
18. Maloney MJ, McGuire J, Daniels SR, Specker B. Dieting behavior and eating attitudes in children. Pediatrics 1989; 84:482–489.
19. Sasson A, Lewin C, Roth D. Dieting behavior and eating attitudes in Israeli children. Int J Eat Disord 1995; 17:67–72.
20. Jones JM, Bennett S, Olmsted MP, Lawson ML, Rodin G. Disordered eating attitudes and behaviours in teenaged girls: a school-based study. CMAJ 2001; 165:547–552.
21. Whitaker A, Davies M, Shaffer D, Johnson J, Abrams S, Walsh BT, Kalikow K. The struggle to be thin: a survey of anorexic and bulimic symptoms in a non-referred adolescent population. Psychol Med 1989; 19:143–163.
22. Childress AC, Brewerton TD, Hodges EL, Jarrell MP. The Kids' Eating Disorders Survey (KEDS): a study of middle school students. J Am Acad Child Adol Psychiatry 1993; 32:843–850.
23. Steinhausen HC, Winkler C, Meier M. Eating disorders in adolescence in a Swiss epidemiological study. Int J Eat Disord 1997; 22:147–151.
24. Nakamura K, Hoshino Y, Watanabe A, Honda K, Niwa S, Tominaga K, Shimai S, Yamamoto M. Eating problems in female Japanese high school students: a prevalence study. Int J Eat Disord 1999; 26:91–95.
25. Nobakht M, Dezhkam M. An epidemiological study of eating disorders in Iran. Int J Eat Disord 2000; 28:265–271.
26. Koskelainen M, Sourander A, Helenius H. Dieting and weight concerns among Finnish adolescents. Nord J Psychiatry 2001; 55:427–431.
27. Carter JC, Stewart DA, Fairburn CG. Eating disorder examination questionnaire: norms for young adolescent girls. Behav Res Ther 2001; 39:625–632.
28. Nylander I. The feeling of being fat and dieting in a school population. An epidemiologic interview investigation. Acta Sociomed Scand 1971; 3:17–26.
29. Schleimer K. Dieting in teenage schoolgirls. A longitudinal prospective study. Acta Paediatr Scand Suppl 1983; 312:1–54.
30. Irving LM, Wall M, Neumark-Sztainer D, Story M. Steroid use among adolescents: findings from Project EAT. J Adol Health 2002; 30:243–252.
31. Labre MP. Adolescent boys and the muscular male body ideal. J Adol Health 2002; 30:233–242.
32. Lau B, Alsaker FD. Dieting behavior in Norwegian adolescents. Scand J Psychol 2001; 42:25–32.
33. Perry CL, McGuire MT, Neumark-Sztainer D, Story M. Characteristics of vegetarian adolescents in a multiethnic urban population. J Adol Health 2001; 29:406–416.
34. Råstam M. Anorexia nervosa in 51 Swedish adolescents: premorbid problems and comorbidity. J Am Acad Child Adol Psychiatry 1992; 31:819–829.
35. Button EJ, Whitehouse A. Subclinical anorexia nervosa. Psychol Med 1981; 11:509–516.

36. Szmukler GI. Weight and Food Preoccupation in a Population of English Schoolgirls. Columbus, Ohio: Ross, 1983.
37. King MB. Eating disorders in a general practice population. Prevalence, characteristics and follow-up at 12 to 18 months. Psychol Med Monogr Suppl 1989; 14:1–34.
38. Meadows GN, Palmer RL, Newball EUM, Kenrick JMT. Eating attitudes and disorder in young women: a general practice based survey. Psychol Med 1986; 16:351–357.
39. Johnson-Sabine E, Wood K, Patton G, Mann A, Wakeling A. Abnormal eating attitudes in London schoolgirls—a prospective epidemiological study: factors associated with abnormal response on screening questionnaires. Psychol Med 1988; 18:615–622.
40. Råstam M, Gillberg C, Garton M. Anorexia nervosa in a Swedish urban region. A population-based study. Br J Psychiatry 1989; 155:642–646.
41. Whitaker A, Johnson J, Shaffer D, Rapoport JL, Kalikow K, Walsh BT, Davies M, Braiman S, Dolinsky A. Uncommon troubles in young people: prevalence estimates of selected psychiatric disorders in a nonreferred adolescent population. Arch Gen Psychiatry 1990; 47:487–496.
42. Whitehouse AM, Cooper PJ, Vize CV, Hill C, Vogel L. Prevalence of eating disorders in three Cambridge general practices: hidden and conspicuous morbidity. Br J Gen Pract 1992; 42:57–60.
43. Rathner G, Messner K. Detection of eating disorders in a small rural town: an epidemiological study. Psychol Med 1993; 23:175–184.
44. Wlodarczyk-Bisaga K, Dolan B. A two-stage epidemiological study of abnormal eating attitudes and their prospective risk factors in Polish schoolgirls. Psychol Med 1996; 26:1021–1032.
45. Gual P, Perez-Gaspar M, Martinez-Gonzalez MA, Lahortiga F, de Irala-Estevez J, Cervera-Enguix S. Self-esteem, personality, and eating disorders: baseline assessment of a prospective population-based cohort. Int J Eat Disord 2002; 31:261–273.
46. Hoek HW. The incidence and prevalence of anorexia nervosa and bulimia nervosa in primary care. Psychol Med 1991; 21:455–460.
47. Lucas AR, Beard CM, O'Fallon WM, Kurland LT. 50-year trends in the incidence of anorexia nervosa in Rochester, Minn.: a population-based study. Am J Psychiatry 1991; 148:917–922.
48. Lucas AR, Crowson CS, O'Fallon WM, Melton LJ III. The ups and downs of anorexia nervosa. Int J Eat Disord 1999; 26:397–405.
49. Eaton WW, Tien AY, Poeschla BD. Epidemiology of schizophrenia. In: den Boer JA, Westenberg HGM, van Praag HM, eds. Advances in the Neurobiology of Schizophrenia. Chichester: John Wiley and Sons, 1995:27–57.
50. Theander S. Anorexia nervosa. A psychiatric investigation of 94 female patients. Acta Psychiatr Scand Suppl 1970; 214:1–194.
51. Willi J, Grossmann S. Epidemiology of anorexia nervosa in a defined region of Switzerland. Am J Psychiatry 1983; 140:564–567.
52. Willi J, Giacometti G, Limacher B. Update on the epidemiology of anorexia

nervosa in a defined region of Switzerland. Am J Psychiatry 1990; 147:1514–1517.

53. Jones DJ, Fox MM, Babigian HM, Hutton HE. Epidemiology of anorexia nervosa in Monroe County, New York: 1960–1976. Psychosom Med 1980; 42:551–558.
54. Kendell RE, Hall DJ, Hailey A, Babigian HM. The epidemiology of anorexia nervosa. Psychol Med 1973; 3:200–203.
55. Szmukler G, McCance C, McCrone L, Hunter D. Anorexia nervosa: a psychiatric case register study from Aberdeen. Psychol Med 1986; 16:49–58.
56. Hoek HW, Brook FG. Patterns of care of anorexia nervosa. J Psychiatr Res 1985; 19:155–160.
57. Møller-Madsen S, Nystrup J. Incidence of anorexia nervosa in Denmark. Acta Psychiatr Scand 1992; 86:197–200.
58. Hoek HW, Bartelds AIM, Bosveld JJF, van der Graaf Y, Limpens VEL, Maiwald M, Spaaij CJK. Impact of urbanization on detection rates of eating disorders. Am J Psychiatry 1995; 152:1272–1278.
59. Turnbull S, Ward A, Treasure J, Jick H, Derby L. The demand for eating disorder care. An epidemiological study using the General Practice Research Database. Br J Psychiatry 1996; 169:705–712.
60. Crisp AH, Palmer RL, Kalucy RS. How common is anorexia nervosa? A prevalence study. Br J Psychiatry 1976; 128:549–554.
61. Casper RC. Introduction to special issue. J Youth Adol 1996; 25:413–418.
62. Swenne I. Changes in body weight and body mass index (BMI) in teenage girls prior to the onset and diagnosis of an eating disorder. Acta Paediatrica 2001; 90:677–681.
63. Young JK. Estrogen and the etiology of anorexia nervosa. Neurosci Biobehav Rev 1991; 15:327–331.
64. Kaplowitz PB, Slora EJ, Wasserman RC, Pedlow SE, Herman-Giddens ME. Earlier onset of puberty in girls: relation to increased body mass index and race. Pediatrics 2001; 108:347–353.
65. Wakeling A. Epidemiology of anorexia nervosa. Psychiatry Res 1996; 62:3–9.
66. Williams P, King M. The "epidemic' of anorexia nervosa: another medical myth? Lancet 1987; 1:205–207.
67. Fombonne E. Anorexia nervosa. No evidence of an increase. Br J Psychiatry 1995; 166:462–471.
68. Gillberg C, Råstam M, Gillberg IC. Anorexia nervosa: who sees the patients and who do the patients see? Acta Paediatrica 1994; 83:967–971.
69. Bushnell JA, Wells JE, Hornblow AR, Oakley-Browne MA, Joyce P. Prevalence of three bulimia syndromes in the general population. Psychol Med 1990; 20:671–680.
70. Szabo P, Tury F. The prevalence of bulimia nervosa in a Hungarian college and secondary school population. Psychother Psychosom 1991; 56:43–47.
71. Santonastaso P, Zanetti T, Sala A, Favaretto G, Vidotto G, Favaro A. Prevalence of eating disorders in Italy: a survey on a sample of 16-year-old female students. Psychother Psychosom 1996; 65:158–162.

72. American Psychiatric Association. Diagnostic and Statistical Manual of Mental Disorders. 3d ed. Washington, DC,1980.
73. American Psychiatric Association. Diagnostic and Statistical Manual of Mental Disorders. 3d ed. revised. Washington, DC,1987.
74. Garfinkel PE, Lin E, Goering P, Spegg C, Goldbloom DS, Kennedy S, Kaplan AS, Woodside DB. Bulimia nervosa in a Canadian community sample: prevalence and comparison of subgroups. Am J Psychiatry 1995; 152:1052–1058.
75. Dansky BS, Brewerton TD, Kilpatrick DG, O'Neil PM. The National Women's Study: relationship of victimization and posttraumatic stress disorder to bulimia nervosa. Int J Eat Disord 1997; 21:213–228.
76. Soundy TJ, Lucas AR, Suman VJ, Melton LJ III. Bulimia nervosa in Rochester, Minnesota from 1980 to 1990. Psychol Med 1995; 25:1065–1071.
77. World Health Organization. The ICD-10 Classification of Mental and Behavioural Disorders: Clinial Descriptions and Diagnostic Guidelines. Geneva, 1992.
78. World Health Organization. The ICD-9 Classification of Mental and Behavioral Disorders. Clinical Descriptions and Diagnostic Guidelines. Geneva, 1979.
79. Russell G. Bulimia nervosa: an ominous variant of anorexia nervosa. Psychol Med 1979; 9:429–448.
80. Pagsberg AK, Wang AR. Epidemiology of anorexia nervosa and bulimia nervosa in Bornholm County, Denmark, 1970–1989. Acta Psychiatr Scand 1994; 90:259–265.
81. Schwitzer AM, Rodriguez LE, Thomas C, Salimi L. The eating disorders NOS diagnostic profile among college women. J Am Coll Health 2001; 49:157–166.
82. Striegel-Moore RH, Cachelin FM, Dohm FA, Pike KM, Wilfley DE, Fairburn CG. Comparisonof binge eating disorder and bulimia nervosa in a community sample. Int J Eat Disord 2001; 29:157–165.
83. Hay P, Fairburn C. The validity of the DSM-IV scheme for classifying bulimic eating disorders. Int J Eat Disord 1998; 23:7–15.
84. Cotrufo P, Barretta V, Monteleone P, Maj M. Full-syndrome, partial-syndrome and subclinical eating disorders: an epidemiological study of female students in Southern Italy. Acta Psychiatr Scand 1998; 98:112–115.
85. Hay P. The epidemiology of eating disorder behaviors: an Australian community-based survey. Int J Eat Disord 1998; 23:371–382.
86. Fairburn CG, Cooper Z. The Eating Disorder Examination. 12th ed. In: Fairburn CG, Wilson GT, eds. Binge Eating: Nature, Assessment and Treatment. New York: Guilford Press, 1993:317–360.
87. Westenhoefer J. Prevalence of eating disorders and weight control practices in Germany in 1990 and 1997. Int J Eat Disord 2001; 29:477–481.
88. Dohrenwend BP, Levav I, Shrout PE, Schwartz S, Naveh G, Link BG, Skodol AE, Stueve A. Socioeconomic status and psychiatric disorders: the causation-selection issue. Science 1992; 255:946–952.
89. Gard MCE, Freeman CP. The dismantling of a myth: a review of eating disorders and socioeconomic status. Int J Eat Disord 1996; 20:1–12.

90. McClelland L, Crisp A. Anorexia nervosa and social class. Int J Eat Disord 2001; 29:150–156.

91. Råstam M, Gillberg C. The family background in anorexia nervosa: a population-based study. J Am Acad Child Adol Psychiatry 1991; 30:283–289.

92. Tsai G. Eating disorders in the Far East. Eat Weight Disord 2000; 5:183–197.

93. Baska T, Straka S, Madar R. Smoking and some life-style changes in medical students—Slovakia, 1995–1999. Cent Eur J Public Health 2001; 9:147–149.

94. Abdollahi P, Mann T. Eating disorder symptoms and body image concerns in Iran: comparisons between Iranian women in Iran and in America. Int J Eat Disord 2001; 30:259–268.

95. Nasser M. Screening for abnormal eating attitudes in a population of Egyptian secondary school girls. Soc Psychiatry Psychiatr Epidemiol 1994; 29:25–30.

96. Nasser M. Comparative study of the prevalence of abnormal eating attitudes among Arab female students of both London and Cairo Universities. Psychol Med 1986; 16:621–625.

97. Dolan B, Lacey JH, Evans C. Eating behaviour and attitudes to weight and shape in British women from three ethnic groups. Br J Psychiatry 1990; 157:523–528.

98. Nasser M. Culture and Weight Consciousness. London: Routledge, 1997.

99. Nasser M, Katzman MA, Gordon RA, eds. Eating disorders and cultures in transition. London: Routledge, 2001.

100. Hoek HW, van Harten PN, van Hoeken D, Susser E. Lack of relation between culture and anorexia nervosa: results of an incidence study on Curaçao. N Engl J Med 1998; 338:1231–1232.

101. Vandereycken W, Hoek HW. Are eating disorders culture-bound syndromes? In: Halmi KA, ed. Psychobiology and Treatment of Anorexia Nervosa and Bulimia Nervosa. Washington, DC: American Psychiatric Press, 1993:19–36.

102. Santonastaso P, Mondini S, Favaro A. Are fashion models a group at risk for eating disorders and substance abuse? Psychother Psychosom 2002; 71:168–172.

103. Smolak L, Murnen SK, Ruble AE. Female athletes and eating problems: a meta-analysis. Int J Eat Disord 2000; 27:371–380.

104. Hulley AJ, Hill AJ. Eating disorders and health in elite women distance runners. Int J Eat Disord 2001; 30:312–317.

5

Long-Term Outcome, Course of Illness, and Mortality in Anorexia Nervosa, Bulimia Nervosa, and Binge Eating Disorder

Pamela K. Keel
Harvard University
Cambridge, Massachusetts, U.S.A.

David B. Herzog
Massachusetts General Hospital
Boston, Massachusetts, U.S.A.

Research on the long-term course and outcome of eating disorders (anorexia nervosa, bulimia nervosa, and binge eating disorder) has the potential to improve the treatment, diagnosis, and understanding of these disorders. In order to evaluate the efficacy of treatment interventions it is important to understand both the natural course of illness and the course following intervention. Distinctions between disorders can be revealed by differential treatment response as well as differences in course and outcome over time. Finally, accurate distinctions between disorders will ultimately contribute to revealing their etiology. For example, attempts to reveal the underlying genetic bases of eating disorders require the accurate distinction of phenotypes. The purpose of this chapter is to review and compare data concerning the long-term course and outcome of anorexia nervosa, bulimia nervosa, and binge eating disorder across the following outcome domains: mortality, recovery, relapse, cross-over, prognostic variables, and treatment utilization. Because of differences in when specific eating disorders have been introduced to the psychiatric nomenclature (ranging from 1873 to 1994), significant discrepancies exist in the amount of data available to describe outcome for anorexia nervosa, bulimia nervosa, and binge eating disorder.

ANOREXIA NERVOSA

Mortality

Anorexia nervosa has been associated with one of the highest risks of premature death among psychiatric disorders (1). Estimates of crude mortality rates across outcome studies suggest that 5–5.9% of patients diagnosed with anorexia nervosa will suffer a fatal outcome (2,3), with a 5.6% crude mortality rate per decade (4). Standardized mortality ratios (representing the ratio of the observed number of deaths to the expected number of deaths in a matched population) have ranged from 1.32 (4b) to 12.82 (4c) with most studies reporting significantly elevated risk of premature death. Earlier studies tended to report starvation as the cause of death; conversely, more recent studies have reported suicide as a leading cause of death in anorexia nervosa (5). This shift may reflect several coinciding secular trends. First, the diagnostic criteria for anorexia nervosa shifted from requiring a loss of 25% of prior body weight to weight 15% below that expected for age and height. For most individuals who develop anorexia nervosa during adolescence, the shift effectively decreased the weight loss required to be diagnosed with anorexia nervosa. Similarly, epidemiological data have demonstrated that weight of patients presenting for treatment of anorexia nervosa has increased over time (6), reflecting both the change in diagnostic criteria and the possibility of earlier intervention. Finally, there may have been secular improvements in techniques employed to refeed undernourished patients. Few predictors of fatal outcome have been revealed. These have included low weight (7,8), poor psychosocial function (9,10), longer duration of follow-up (2,10), and severity of alcohol use disorders (10).

Recovery

Although longer duration of follow-up has been associated with increased risk of death, it is also associated with higher rates of recovery (2,11). Prospective, longitudinal analyses of anorexia nervosa course suggest that recovery increases at a slow and steady rate, with continued recovery occurring years after intake (11) or treatment (12). Collapsing recovery rates across studies of varying durations of follow-up, Steinhausen (2) reported that approximately 46% of patients recover, 33% improve (but remain symptomatic), and 20% remain chronically ill.

Relapse

Unlike mortality and recovery, which can be investigated in outcome studies, relapse can only be assessed by studies of eating disorder course. Thus, fewer studies have elucidated this important variable. Morgan and Russell (13) reported that 51% of patients hospitalized for anorexia nervosa required readmission over the course of follow-up. Herzog and colleagues (11) reported that 40% of women with anorexia nervosa who achieve full recovery later relapsed. Finally, Strober et al. (12) reported that approximately 30% of women who had achieved weight recovery during hospitalization relapsed after discharge, and they recorded even lower rates of relapse among women considered partially recovered (9.8%) or fully recovered (0%) over follow-up. These latter data indicate that the definition of recovery (or remission) has a significant effect on the likelihood of relapse. A common pattern among patients with anorexia nervosa is to experience improvement in weight (a sign of recovery) as a consequence of the development of binge eating episodes (a sign of cross-over).

Cross-over

A recent report from a prospective longitudinal study of eating disorders indicated that the majority of women with the restricting subtype of anorexia nervosa develop symptoms of binge eating and purging over time (14). These findings are consistent with the restraint hypothesis (15), which posits that dietary restriction increases susceptibility to develop binge eating episodes. For some patients with anorexia nervosa, binge eating and purging occur at low weight and the person continues to suffer from anorexia nervosa. For others, binge eating results in weight gain and the binge–purge behaviors are maintained at normal weight representing cross-over from anorexia nervosa to bulimia nervosa. Across follow-up studies, approximately 10–15% of individuals presenting with anorexia nervosa cross over and develop bulimia nervosa(16).

Prognostic Factors

Table 1 presents prognostic factors adapted from a recent review of outcome in anorexia nervosa (2). As can be seen from Table 1, no prognostic factor has been unambiguously associated with prognosis in anorexia nervosa. However, there is a clear trend in the nature of the contradictory results. Studies finding a specific direction of association are most often contradicted

TABLE 1   Prognostic Indicators of Favorable Course or Outcome in Anorexia
Nervosa

	Direction of association (*N*)		
Variable	Positive	Negative	Insignificant
Age of onset or presentation	2	12	14
Duration of symptoms	0	14	7
Severity of symptoms	1	22	12
Personality disturbance	8	6	2
Treatment	0	7	7

Note: Data are adapted from Steinhausen (2) to allow comparison with data from Keel and
Mitchell (19) updated in Table 2.

by studies finding no significant association rather than an equal number of
studies finding an association in the opposite direction. For example, 12
studies have suggested that an older age of onset is associated with worse
prognosis in anorexia nervosa, and 14 studies suggest no significant association. Conversely, only 2 suggest that an older age of onset is associated with
favorable prognosis in anorexia nervosa. Similarly, 14 studies suggest that a
longer duration of symptoms prior to presentation is associated with poor
prognosis in anorexia nervosa, and 7 studies suggest no significant association. Conversely, no studies suggest that a longer duration of symptoms is
associated with favorable prognosis in anorexia nervosa. This pattern suggests that contradictory findings are most likely attributable to differences in
statistical power among studies.

   One seeming contradiction among prognostic indicators is the association between age of onset and duration of symptoms. If one develops an
eating disorder at a younger age, then one may have better prognosis.
However, if the duration of symptoms prior to presentation is longer, then
this is associated with worse prognosis. These findings may reveal the impact
of delay in seeking help. That is, an early age of onset is predictive of better
course and outcome only if there is a short delay before seeking treatment.

Treatment Utilization

In Germany, Fichter and colleagues (17) reported that 63% of women
received further inpatient treatment following baseline inpatient care for anorexia nervosa. Levels of outpatient care were also high, with approximately
89% of women receiving some form of outpatient care during follow-up
(among a subset of women for whom data were available). This treatment

comprised an average of 69.3 individuals sessions, 5.0 group sessions, and 0.4 family session. In the United States, Striegel-Moore et al. (18) reported that female patients with anorexia nervosa utilized an average of 26.0 days of inpatient care and 17.0 days of outpatient care during one year. Male patients utilized an average of 15.6 and 9.2 days of inpatient and outpatient care per year, respectively.

BULIMIA NERVOSA

Mortality

A crude mortality rate of 0.3% has been reported across follow-up studies of bulimia nervosa (19). However, this value might represent an underestimate given the relatively short duration of follow-up across studies and the low ascertainment rates for several studies. Few studies have calculated standardized mortality ratios for bulimia nervosa, and no original report has found a standardized mortality ratio that differed significantly from 1. In a recent meta-analysis of mortality in eating disorders, Nielsen (4) reported a significantly elevated SMR for bulimia nervosa. However, this analysis included studies reporting mortality among "bulimic patients" comprising both normal-weight bulimia nervosa and the binge–purge subtype of anorexia nervosa. In a recent examination of mortality in eating disorders, Keel et al. (10) found that mortality was similarly elevated for both the restricting and binge–purge subtypes of anorexia nervosa but was not elevated in bulimia nervosa. As the ascertainment methods and duration of follow-up were uniform across diagnostic categories, this study provides the strongest evidence that bulimia nervosa is not associated with increased risk of premature death. Causes of premature death have primarily included suicide and automobile accidents (19). Because risk of death does not appear to be elevated in bulimia nervosa, no predictors of fatal outcome have been revealed.

Recovery

Prospective, longitudinal analyses of bulimia nervosa course (11,20) suggest that the majority of patients recover from their eating disorder at some point during the course of follow-up. Combining results across outcome studies of varying durations of follow-up, Keel and Mitchell (19) reported that approximately 50% of individuals presenting with bulimia nervosa recover and maintain their recovery, 30% are improved but maintain partial syndromes, and 20% continue to meet full criteria for bulimia nervosa. Follow-up studies of longer duration (21,22) suggest that rates of full bulimia nervosa drop to 10% by 10 years follow-up.

Relapse

Rates of relapse have ranged from 26% to 50% across follow-up studies of bulimia nervosa (19,23,24), with definitions of "recovery" explaining the majority of variance in these estimates. Similar to the patterns observed with anorexia nervosa, more stringent definitions of recovery are associated with lower relapse rates than less stringent definitions (25,26). This pattern raises the question of whether studies are assessing relapse or simple symptom fluctuation. Despite considerable differences in methodology across studies, relapse rates converge around 30% (19), suggesting that approximately one-third of women who initially recover from their eating disorder suffer a resurgence of their bulimic symptoms.

Crossover

Across follow-up studies, between 0% and 7% crossover from bulimia nervosa to anorexia nervosa (19,24). However, it remains unclear whether these represent new-onset cases of anorexia nervosa or relapse from previous episodes of anorexia nervosa that had crossed over to bulimia nervosa. Crossover to binge eating disorder also seems low, ranging from 0% to 1.1% (19,21,24). A recent paper concerning the predictive validity of bulimia nervosa as a diagnostic category (27) reported that over time women with bulimia nervosa were more likely to continue to suffer from bulimia nervosa than the other recognized eating disorders of the DSM. Although approximately 10% reported a brief history of binge eating in the absence of inappropriate compensatory behavior, all but one of these women experienced full remission of her eating disorder, suggesting that this symptom pattern represented a phase of recovery rather than development of a distinct eating disorder. Conversely, approximately 10% of women suffered from a purging disorder, characterized by recurrent purging in the absence of objectively large binge episodes at normal weight. The likelihood of suffering from a purging disorder did not differ significantly from the likelihood of suffering from bulimia nervosa at long-term follow-up and was significantly more likely than suffering from binge eating disorder (27). Thus, to the extent that cross-over occurs in bulimia nervosa, it seems to involve crossing over to a purging disorder.

Prognostic Factors

Table 2 presents prognostic factors updated from a recent review of outcome in bulimia nervosa (19). As can be seen from the Table 2, few prognostic factors have been replicated across studies. Similar to the pattern observed in Table 1, most often findings diverge along the lines of a significant association

TABLE 2 Prognostic Indicators of Favorable Course or Outcome in Bulimia
Nervosa

	Direction of association (N)		
Variable	Positive	Negative	Insignificant
Age of onset or presentation	1	1	9
Duration of symptoms	0	6	3
Severity of symptoms	0	4	9
Personality disturbance	0	6	4
Treatment	8	0	9

Note: Data are updated from Keel and Mitchell (19) with findings from studies of follow-up
duration 5 years (21,24,43).

in one direction versus no significant association. For example, six studies
reported that longer duration of symptoms prior to presentation was associated with poor prognosis in bulimia nervosa, and three studies found no
significant association. However, no studies reported that a longer duration
of symptoms was associated with favorable prognosis in bulimia nervosa.
Similarly, six studies suggested that personality disturbance was associated
with poor prognosis, and four studies found no significant association, but no
studies reported that personality disturbances were associated with favorable
outcome. Despite this pattern for duration of symptoms and personality
disturbance, the number of studies suggesting no significant associations is
greater than the number of studies suggesting significant associations for the
remaining variables, including the impact of treatment. However, a recent
investigation (20) has demonstrated an association between baseline treatment and long-term course in bulimia nervosa, suggesting that cognitive
behavioral therapy may speed recovery (28).

Treatment Utilization

Although most women who suffer from bulimia nervosa may never seek treatment (23,29), treatment utilization is high among those who do. In Germany,
Fichter et al. (24) reported that 67% of women received further inpatient
treatment following baseline inpatient care for bulimia nervosa. Levels of
outpatient care were also high, with approximately 83% of women receiving
some form of outpatient care during follow-up (among a subset of women for
whom data were available). This treatment comprised an average of 59.2
individuals sessions, 10.9 group sessions, and 0.7 family session (24). In the
United States, Striegel-Moore et al. (18) reported that female patients with
bulimia nervosa utilized an average of 14.7 days of inpatient care and 15.6

days of outpatient care during one year. Male patients utilized an average of 21.7 and 9.1 days of inpatient and outpatient care per year, respectively. Although inpatient care did not differ between female and male patients, women received significantly more outpatient care (18).

BINGE EATING DISORDER

Since the introduction of binge eating disorder in the DSM-IV (30), a number of treatment studies have been published and several have provided short-term and intermediate follow-up data (31–36). However, relatively little is known concerning long-term course and outcome. At this point, two studies (23,37) have characterized course and outcome for this disorder at 5 or more years following presentation. Because of the limited number of long-term follow-up studies, the results of these two studies will be reviewed individually below.

Fichter et al. (37) reported one death among 68 patients treated for binge eating disorder at 6 year follow-up for a crude mortality rate of 1.5%. Fairburn et al. (23) reported no deaths in his cohort of 48 individuals with binge eating disorder recruited from the community. Rates of full binge eating disorder at follow-up were 4% (23) and 5.9% (37), with 57.4% (37) to 82% (23) reported as improved or recovered. Fairburn et al. (23) reported that relapse occurred in 4–10% of recovered individuals across various points of follow-up. Cross-over to anorexia nervosa did not occur, and cross-over to bulimia nervosa was rare, ranging from 3% (23) to 7.4% (37). Neither article reported on predictors of long-term course or outcome. Fichter and colleagues (37) reported that 66% of the binge eating disorder patients received further inpatient treatment following baseline inpatient care for binge eating disorder. Conversely, Fairburn and colleagues (23) reported that as few as 3% of individuals with binge eating disorder received treatment for an eating disorder during the course of follow-up, resulting in a total of 8% ever having received treatment.

COMPARISON OF EATING DISORDERS

Anorexia Nervosa and Bulimia Nervosa

Few studies have been designed to evaluate the course or outcome of more than one eating disorder. Thus, comparisons of anorexia nervosa and bulimia nervosa are significantly limited by methodological differences across studies. However, certain similarities and differences emerge despite this limitation.

Both within studies (10,17) and across studies (2,19), anorexia nervosa appears to be associated with significantly increased risk of premature death and bulimia nervosa is not. Suicide has been noted as a common cause of death for both disorders. Interestingly, rates and lethality of suicide attempts have not differed between women with anorexia nervosa versus bulimia nervosa (38). Thus, suicide attempts appear to be more likely to result in death among women suffering from anorexia nervosa. One possible explanation for this difference is that starvation compromises the health of individuals with anorexia nervosa, leaving them less likely to survive a suicide attempt.

Within studies (11,17), anorexia nervosa has been associated with both lower and slower rates of recovery in comparison with bulimia nervosa. However, collapsing results across studies suggests a similar distribution of recovery, improvement, and chronicity across syndromes (2,19). However, this latter comparison is flawed because follow-up studies for anorexia nervosa have a significantly longer duration of follow-up in comparison with follow-up studies of bulimia nervosa, and longer duration of follow-up is associated with higher rates of recovery for both syndromes (2,21). Thus, the apparent similarity in results between disorders across studies is likely an artifact of differences in duration of follow-up.

Despite differing rates of recovery, relapse rates were surprisingly similar between anorexia nervosa and bulimia nervosa within one study of long-term course (21). However, the relationship between relapse and chronicity likely differs between disorders. Because a higher percentage of women with bulimia nervosa than women with anorexia nervosa recover at some point during the course of follow-up, a higher percentage of women who are ill at follow-up in bulimia nervosa outcome studies represent women who have recovered and relapsed. Thus, for women with bulimia nervosa, chronicity appears to be characterized by considerable symptom fluctuation. Conversely, a smaller percentage of women recover from anorexia nervosa; thus, a smaller percentage of women who remain ill are women who achieved even brief periods of remission. Thus, chronicity within anorexia nervosa is marked by a more steady course of illness. This difference may also be reflected in the nature of the core features of these syndromes. For anorexia nervosa, the core symptom represents the absence of a behavior—eating. Conversely, for bulimia nervosa, the core symptoms represent the presence of a set of behaviors—binge eating and purging. Thus, in order to develop anorexia nervosa an individual must demonstrate persistence in not eating. Conversely, a woman can develop bulimia nervosa by having relatively normal eating behaviors interrupted by episodes of abnormal eating behaviors. For these reasons, the nature of a chronic course may differ markedly between these disorders.

Patterns of cross-over also differ markedly between anorexia nervosa and bulimia nervosa. Approximately 10–50% of women with anorexia nervosa cross over and develop bulimia nervosa, and approximately 30% of women with bulimia nervosa report a prior history of anorexia nervosa.

Conversely, only 0–7% of women with bulimia nervosa have been reported to cross over and develop anorexia nervosa. This pattern likely reflects both the psychological and physiological consequences of the core features of each disorder. Specifically, intense dietary restriction and weight loss likely increase risk for developing binge eating episodes. Conversely, the presence of objectively large binge eating episodes likely protects against low weight. Indeed, comparisons of the subtypes of anorexia nervosa suggest that binge eating is associated with higher weight.

We found better evidence for prognostic factors for anorexia nervosa than for bulimia nervosa. However, this is likely a function of the difference in the number and size of outcome studies for the two disorders. An early age of onset was associated with improved prognosis in anorexia nervosa but was unassociated with prognosis in bulimia nervosa. This may reflect the differences in age of onset between the syndromes. Currently, the most effective treatments for anorexia nervosa involve family interventions. This is likely to be more useful for young adolescent patients who reside with their parents. Thus, little is known about the effective treatment of older patients with anorexia nervosa. Conversely, bulimia nervosa develops during young adulthood, and efficacious treatments have focused on outpatient cognitive behavioral therapy and antidepressant medications that are likely to work well across the developmental range of late adolescence to middle age.

For both anorexia nervosa and bulimia nervosa, longer duration of symptoms prior to presentation predicts worse outcome. However, as has been discussed before (19), this finding is somewhat tautological as it essentially reveals that chronicity predicts itself rather than elucidating what specific factors contribute to a chronic course.

Severity of symptoms appears to be associated with prognosis in anorexia nervosa but not bulimia nervosa. This result may reflect our supposition that chronicity in anorexia nervosa is associated with a steady course whereas chronicity in bulimia nervosa is associated with considerable symptom fluctuation. If this is true, then a single measure of symptom severity in bulimia nervosa would have relatively low reliability and thus would have limited ability to predict prognosis.

Personality disturbances have been associated with worse prognosis for both anorexia nervosa and bulimia nervosa. However, the nature of personality disturbances has differed. For anorexia nervosa, obsessive-compulsive personality features are associated with worse prognosis. Conversely, for bulimia nervosa, borderline and marked impulsiveness have been associated with worse prognosis. These likely reflect differences in the core symptoms of these disorders. Anorexia nervosa is marked by rigid adherence to dietary restriction enabling maintenance of weight significantly below what would be expected for height and age. Conversely, bulimia nervosa is marked by recurrent loss of control over eating. As described above, these differences are also reflected in course among those who remain chronically ill.

The association between treatment and long-term course and outcome has differed between anorexia nervosa and bulimia nervosa. Although treatment has not demonstrated significant associations with long-term outcome in bulimia nervosa (21), it has been associated with differential course (20). Thus, treatments that have demonstrated efficacy for bulimia nervosa appear to speed recovery and be associated with improved long-term course. Conversely, few treatments have demonstrated efficacy for anorexia nervosa largely due to a relative dearth of controlled-treatment outcome studies in anorexia nervosa (39). Controlled-treatment studies have been initiated for anorexia nervosa; however, insufficient time has passed to evaluate the long-term impact of treatment on course or outcome.

Our analyses of data reported by Striegel-Moore and colleagues (18) reveal that women with anorexia nervosa spent significantly more days and money in inpatient treatment than women with bulimia nervosa, 26.0 days and 17,384 dollars versus 14.7 days and 9088 dollars, respectively [$t(196) = 3.55; p < 0.001$ for inpatient days, and $t(196) = 3.22, p < 0.01$ for inpatient cost]. However, no significant differences in days or cost of outpatient treatment existed between women with anorexia nervosa and those with bulimia nervosa 17.0 days and 2344 dollars versus 15.6 days and 1882 dollars, respectively [$t(1229) = 1.17; p > 0.05$ for outpatient days, and $t(1229) = 1.95; p > 0.05$ for outpatient cost]. However, these data were limited by insurance company coverage and do not necessarily indicate clinical need. Compared to women with bulimia nervosa, women with anorexia nervosa utilized significantly more inpatient treatment during the course of follow-up but not individual outpatient treatment or treatment with antidepressants or anxiolytics (40). Across women with eating disorders, treatment utilization was predicted by the following variables in a multivariate analysis: lower Global Assessment of Function scores (measuring both greater symptom severity and worse psychosocial function), personality disorder, and comorbid lifetime mood disorders (40).

Notably, in the National Insurance Claims Database study (18), the number of individuals receiving eating disorder treatment was quite small relative to the number of individuals in the database. Only 0.06% of female patients in the database (1194 of 2,005,760) were treated for anorexia nervosa, bulimia nervosa, or both. Considering the prevalence rates for anorexia nervosa and bulimia nervosa in the DSM-IV, this suggests that the majority of women with these eating disorders do not receive treatment for their eating disorder over the course of a year. Similarly, Fairburn et al. (23) reported that only 28% of individuals with bulimia nervosa received treatment during the course of follow-up, resulting in a total of 40% ever receiving treatment for an eating disorder.

Bulimia Nervosa and Binge Eating Disorder

Inconsistent results for the comparison of bulimia nervosa and binge eating disorder outcome have been presented in the literature. Fairburn and colleagues (23) found that rates of recovery were higher in women diagnosed with binge eating disorder than women with bulimia nervosa. However, Fichter and colleagues (37) failed to find differences in outcome between these two syndromes. Variance in sample ascertainment may account for the contradictory findings between these two studies. One study recruited women from treatment (37), and the other recruited women from the community (23).

CONCLUSIONS

In the introduction, we noted that data on long-term course and outcome could improve our treatment, diagnosis, and understanding of eating disorders. Such data support the predictive validity of distinguishing between anorexia nervosa and bulimia nervosa. These disorders appear to be associated with different rates of mortality, recovery, relapse, cross-over, and distinct sets of prognostic indicators (including differential treatment response). While promising treatments have been identified for bulimia nervosa, significant work remains for anorexia nervosa. Current controlled treatment outcome studies for anorexia nervosa should be designed to facilitate repeated follow-up assessments.

While few studies have assessed the long-term outcome of bulimia nervosa and binge eating disorder, even fewer have examined the natural history of these disorders at long-term follow-up. Almost all longitudinal studies of eating disorders (including those on anorexia nervosa) are based on treatment seeking samples, even though the majority of women with eating disorders may not seek treatment (23,29). The reliance on treatment seeking samples introduces certain biases in study results. For example, Fairburn et al. (29) reported higher rates of comorbid disorders in women seeking treatment for bulimia nervosa than in women with bulimia nervosa from the community. This is referred to as Berkson's bias (41) and represents the increased likelihood of comorbidity among treatment-seeking individuals compared to individuals who do not seek treatment. Indeed, this bias likely explains the prospective treatment utilization was predicted by greater severity of eating disorder symptoms, comorbid mood disorders, and comorbid personality disorders (40). Thus, follow-up studies of treatment seeking samples may present a more dire description of outcome due to Berkson's bias. Furthermore, relying on treatment seeking samples prevents description of disorders' natural course as treatment may increase rates of recovery (42) or speed time to recovery (20,28).

The distinct personality disturbances associated with prognosis in anorexia versus bulimia nervosa could be examined for their etiological significance. Specifically, symptoms that appear to be associated with the maintenance of eating disorder symptoms may play a role in their initiation. Most risk factor research has failed to elucidate specific risk factors for eating disorders that are distinct from risk factors for other forms of psychopathological conditions. Evidence that obsessive-compulsive features are associated with anorexia nervosa prognosis whereas impulsive-borderline features are associated with bulimia nervosa prognosis offers the opportunity to reveal risk factors that may be specific to type of eating disorder. Improved understanding of the etiologic development of eating disorders holds the promise of their prevention.

REFERENCES

Note: The following references were included in the original reports of prognostic indicators for anorexia nervosa and bulimia nervosa presented in Tables 1 and 2: (2,11–13,17,19,22,26,42,44–124).

1. Harris EC, Barraclough B. Excess mortality in mental disorder. Brit J Psychiatry 1998; 17:11–53.
2. Steinhausen H-C. The Outcome of Anorexia Nervosa in the 20th Century. Am J Psychiatry 2002; 159(8):1284–1293.
3. Sullivan PF. Mortality in anorexia nervosa. Am J Psychiatry 1995; 152:1073–1074.
4a. Nielsen S. Epidemiology and mortality in eating disorders. Eating Disorders 2001; 24:201–214.
4b. Crisp AH, Callander JS, Halek C, Hsu LKG. Long-term mortality in anorexia nervosa. Brit J Psychiatry 1992; 161:104–107.
4c. Eckert E, Halmi KA, Marchi P, Grove W, Crosby R. Ten-year follow-up study of anorexia nervosa: clinical course and outcome. Psychol Med 1995; 25:143–156.
5. Nielsen S, Moller-Madsen S, Isager T, Jorgensen J, Pagsberg K, Theander S. Standardized mortality in eating disorders: a quantitative summary of previously published and new evidence. J Psychosom Res 1998; 44:413–434.
6. Eagles JM, Johnston MI, Hunter D, Lobban M, Millar HR. Increasing incidence of anorexia nervosa in the female population of northeast Scotland. Am J Psychiatry 1995; 152:1266–1271.
7. Patton GC. Mortality in eating disorders. Psychol Med 1988; 18:947–951.
8. Herzog W, Deter HC, Fiehn W, Petzold E. Medical findings and predictors of

long-term physical outcome in anorexia nervosa: a prospective, 12-year follow-up study. Psychol Med 1997; 27:269–279.

9. Engel K, Wittern M, Hentze M, Meyer AE. Long-term stability of anorexia nervosa treatments: Follow-up study of 218 patients. Psychiatric Dev 1989; 4:395–407.

10. Keel PK, Dorer DJ, Eddy KT, Franko DL, Charatan DL, Herzog DB, Predictors of mortality in eating disorders. Arch Gen Psychiatry 2003; 60:179–183.

11. Herzog D, Dorer DJ, Keel PK, Selwyn SE, Ekeblad ER, Flores A, Greenwood DN, Burwell RA, Keller MB. Recovery and relapse in anorexia and bulimia nervosa: a 7.5-year follow-up study. J Am Acad Child Adol Psychiatry 1999; 38:829–837.

12. Strober M, Freeman R, Morrell W. The long-term course of servere anorexia nervosa in adolescents: survival analysis of recovery, relapse, and outcome predictors over 10–15 years in a prospective study. Int J Eat Disord 1997; 22:339–360.

13. Morgan H, Russell GFM. Value of family background and clinical features as predictors of long-term outcome in anorexia nervosa: four-year follow-up study of 41 patients. Psychol Med 1975; 5:355–371.

14. Eddy KT, Keel PK, Dorer DJ, Delinsky SS, Franko DL, Herzog DB. Longitudinal comparison of anorexia nervosa subtypes. Int J Eat Disord 2002; 31:191–201.

15. Polivy J, Herman CP. Dieting and binging: a causal analysis. Am Psychologist 1985; 40:193–201.

16. Herzog DB, Keller MB, Lavori PW. Outcome in anorexia nervosa and bulimia nervosa: a review of the literature. J Nerv Ment Dis 1988; 176:131–143.

17. Fichter M, Quadlieg N. Six-year course and outcome of anorexia nervosa. Int J Eating Disord 1999; 26:359–385.

18. Striegel-Moore RH, Leslie D, Petrill SA, Garvin V, Rosenheck RA. One-year use and cost of inpatient and outpatient services among female and male patients with an eating disorder: evidence from a national database of health insurance claims. Int J Eat Disord 2000; 27:381–389.

19. Keel PK, Mitchell JE. Outcome in bulimia nervosa. Am J Psychiatry 1997; 154(3):313–321.

20. Miller KB, Keel PK, Crow SJ, Thuras P, Mitchell JE: Treatment and treatment response predict the long-term course of bulimia nervosa. Submitted.

21. Keel PK, Mitchell JE, Miller KB, Davis TL, Crow SJ. Long-term outcome of bulimia nervosa. Arch Gen Psychiatry 1999; 56:63–69.

22. Collings S, King M. Ten-year follow-up of 50 patients with bulimia nervosa. Br J Psychiatry 1994; 164:80–87.

23. Fairburn CG, Cooper Z, Doll HA, Norman P, O'Conner M. The natural course of bulimia nervosa and binge eating disorder in young women. Arch Gen Psychiatry 2000; 57:659–665.

24. Fichter MM, Quadflieg N. Six-year course of bulimia nervosa. Int J Eat Disord 1997; 22:361–384.

25. Field AE, Herzog DB, Keller MB, West J, Nussbaum K, Colditz GA. Distinguishing recovery from remission in a cohort of bulimic women: how should asymptomatic periods be described? J Clin Epidemiol 1997; 50:1339–1345.

26. Olmsted M, Kaplan AS, Rockert W. Rate and prediction of relapse in bulimia nervosa. Am J Psychiatry 1994; 151:738–743.

27. Keel PK, Mitchell JE, Miller KB, Davis TL, Crow SJ. Predictive validity of bulimia nervosa. Am J Psychiatry 2000; 157:136–138.

28. Keel PK, Mitchell JE, Davis TL, Crow SJ. The long-term impact of treatment in women diagnosed with bulimia nervosa. Int J Eat Disord 2002; 31:151–158.

29. Fairburn CG, Welch SL, Norman PA, O'Connor ME, Doll HA. Bias and bulimia nervosa: how typical are clinic cases? Am J Psychiatry 1996; 153:386–391.

30. American Psychiatric Association. Diagnostic and Statistical Manual for Mental Disorders. 4th ed. Washington, DC, 1994.

31. Cachelin FM, Striegel-Moore RH, Elder KA, Pike KM, Wilfley DE, Fairburn CG. Natural course of a community sample of women with binge eating disorder. Int J Eat Disord 1999; 25:45–54.

32. Agras WS, Telch CF, Arnow B, Eldredge K, Marnell M. One-year follow-up of cognitive-behavioral therapy for obese individuals with binge eating disorder. J Consult Clin Psychol 1997; 64:343–347.

33. Devlin MJ, Goldfein JA, Carino JS, Wolk SL. Open treatment of overweight binge eaters with phentermine and fluoxetine as an adjunct to cognitive-behavioral therapy. Int J Eat Disord 2000; 28:325–332.

34. Peterson CB, Mitchell JE, Engbloom S, Nugent S, Pederson MM, Crow SJ, Thuras P. Self-help versus therapist-led group cognitive-behavioral treatment of binge eating disorder and follow-up. Int J Eat Disord 2001; 30:363–374.

35. Ricca V, Mannucci E, Mezzani B, Moretti S, Di Bernardo M, Bertelli M, Rotella CM, Faravelli C. Fluoxetine and fluvoxamine combined with individual cognitive-behaviour therapy in binge eating disorder: a one-year follow-up study. Psychother Psychosom 2001; 70:298–306.

36. Ciano R, Rocco PL, Angarano A, Biasin E, Balestrieri M. Group-analytic and psychoeducational therapies for binge-eating disorder: an exploratory study on efficacy and persistence of effects. Psychother Res 2002; 12:231–239.

37. Fichter MM, Quadflieg N, Gnutzman A. Binge eating disorder: treatment outcome over a 6-year course. J Psychosom Res 1998; 44:385–405.

38. Franko DL, Keel PK, Dorer DJ, Renn R, Eddy KT, Herzog DB. Suicidality in eating disorders: data from a 12-year longitudinal study. Submitted.

39. Peterson CB, Mitchell JE. Psychological and pharmacological treatment of eating disorders: a review of research findings. J Clin Psychol 1999; 55:685–697.

40. Keel PK, Dorer DJ, Eddy KT, Delinsky SS, Franko DL, Blais MB, Keller MB, Herzog DB. Predictors of treatment utilization among women with anorexia and bulimia nervosa. Am J Psychiatry 2002; 159:140–142.

41. Berkson J. Limitations of the application of fourfold table analysis to hospital data. Biometrics 1946; 2:47–53.
42. Fairburn C, Norman PA, Welch SL, O'Connor ME, Doll HA, Peveler RC. A prospective study of outcome in bulimia nervosa and the long-term effects of three psychological treatments. Arch Gen Psychiatry 1995; 52:304–312.
43. Rcas D, Williamson DA, Martin CK, Zucker NL. Duration of illness predicts outcome for bulimia nervosa: a long-term follow-up study. Int J Eat Disord 2000; 27:428–434.
44. Abraham S, Mira M, Llewellyn-Jones D. Bulimia: a study of outcome. Int J Eat Disord 1983; 2:175–180.
45. Agras W, Rossiter EM, Arnow B, Telch CF, Raeburn SD, Bruce B, Koran LM. One-year follow-up of psychosocial and pharmacologic treatments for bulimia nervosa. J Clin Psychiatry 1994; 55:179–183.
46. Beaumont P, George GCW, Smart DE. "Dieters" and "vomiters and purgers" in anorexia nervosa. Psychol Med 1976; 6:617–622.
47. Blitzer J, Rollins N, Blackwell A. Children who starve themselves: anorexia nervosa. Pcychosom Med 1961; 23:369–383.
48. Brotman A, Herzog DB, Hamburg P. Long-term course in 14 bulimic patients treated with psychotherapy. J Clin Psychiatry 1988; 49:157–160.
49. Browning C, Miller SI. Anorexia nervosa: a study in prognosis and management. Am J Psychiatry 1968; 124:1128–1132.
50. Bryant-Waugh R, Knibbs J, Fosson A, Kaminski Z, Lask B. Long-term follow-up of patients with early onset anorexia nervosa. Arch Dis Child 1988; 63:5–9.
51. Burns T, Crisp AH. Outcome of anorexia nervosa in males. Br J Psychiatry 1984; 145:319–325.
52. Casper R, Jabine LN. An eight-year follow-up: outcome from adolescent compared to adult-onset anorexia nervosa. J Youth Adol 1996; 25:499–517.
53. Dally P, Sargant W. Treatment and outcome of anorexia nervosa. Br Med J 1966; 2:793–795.
54. Dally P. Anorexia Nervosa. London: Heinemann, 1969.
55. Deter H, Herzog W, Petzold E. The Heidelberg–Mannheim study: long-term follow-up of anorexia nervosa patients at the University Medical Center— background and preliminary result. In: Herzog W, Deter HC, Vandereycken W, eds. The Course of Eating Disorders: Long-Term Follow-up Studies of Anorexia and Bulimia Nervosa. Berlin: Springer-Verlag, 1992:71–84.
56. Edelstein C, Yager J, Gitlin M, Landsverk J. A clinical study of anti-depressant medications in the treatment of bulimia. Psychiatr Med 1989; 7:111–121.
57. Fahy T, Eisler I, Russell GFM. Personality disorder and treatment response in bulimia nervosa. Br J Psychiatry 1993; 162:765–770.
58. Fahy T, Eisler I. Impusivity and eating disorders. Br J Psychiatry 1993; 162: 193–197.
59. Fairburn C, Peveler RC, Jones R, Hope RA, Doll HA. Predictors of 12-month outcome in bulimia nervosa and the influence of attitudes to shape and weight. J Consult Clin Psychol 1993; 61:686–698.

60. Fairburn C, Kirk J, O'Connor M, Cooper PJ. A comparison of two psychological treatments for bulimia nervosa. Behav Res Ther 1986; 24:629–643.

61. Fairburn C, Jones R, Peveler RC, Hope RA, O'Connor M. Psychotherapy and bulimia nervosa: longer-term effects of interpersonal psychotherapy, behavior therapy, and cognitive behavior therapy. Arch Gen Psychiatry 1993; 50:419–428.

62. Fallon B, Walsh T, Sadik C, Saoud JB, Lukasik V. Outcome and clinical course in inpatient bulimic women: a 2-to 9-year follow-up study. J Clin Psychiatry 1991; 52:272–278.

63. Fichter MM, Quadflieg N, Rief W. Longer-term course (6-year) course of bulimia nervosa. Neuropsychopharmacology 1994; 10:772S.

64. Fichter M, Quadfleig N, Rief W. Course of multi-impulsive bulimia. Psychol Med 1994; 24:591–604.

65. Frazier S. Anorexia nervosa. Dis Nerv Syst 1965; 26:155–159.

66. Garfinkel P, Moldofsky H, Garner DM. The outcome of anorexia nervosa: significance of clinical features, body image and behavior modification. In: Vigersky R, ed. Anorexia Nervosa. New York: Raven Press, 1977:315–329.

67. Giles T, Young RR, Young DE. Behavioral treatment of severe bulimia. Behav Ther 1985; 16:393–405.

68. Goetz P, Succop RA, Reinhart JB, Miller A. Anorexia nervosa in children: a follow-up study. Am J Orthopsychiatry 1977; 47:597–603.

69. Greenfeld D, Anyan WR, Hobart M, Quinlan DM, Plantes M. Insight into illness and outcome in anorexia nervosa. Int J Eat Disord 1991; 10:101–109.

70. Hall A, Slim E, Hawker F, Salmond C. Anorexia nervosa—long-term outcome in 50 female patients. Br J Psychiatry 1984; 145:407–413.

71. Halmi K, Brodland G, Loney J. Prognosis in anorexia nervosa. Ann Intern Med 1973; 78:907–909.

72. Halmi K, Bordland G, Rigas C. A follow-up study of seventy-nine patients with anorexia nervosa: an evaluation of prognostic factors and diagnostic criteria. In: Winokur G, Roff M, Wirt RD, eds. Life History Research in Psychopathology. Vol. 4. Minneapolis: University of Minnesota Press, 1976:290 300.

73. Hawley R. The outcome of anorexia nervosa in younger subjects. Br J Psychiatry 1985; 146:657–660.

74. Herpetz-Dahlmann B, Wewetzer C, Schulz E, Remschmidt H. Course and outcome in adolescent anorexia nervosa. Int J Eat Disord 1996; 19:335–345.

75. Herzog D, Sacks NR, Keller MB, Lavori PW, von Ranson KB, Gray HM. Patterns and predictors of recovery in anorexia nervosa and bulimia nervosa. J Am Acad Child Adol Psychiatry 1993; 32:835–842.

76. Herzog T, Hartmann A, Sandholz A, Stammer H. Prognostic factors in outpatient psychotherapy of bulimia. Psychother Psychosom 1991; 56:48–55.

77. Higgs J, Goodyer IM, Birch J. Anorexia nervosa and food avoidance emotional disorder. Arch Dis Child 1989; 64:346–351.

78. Hsu L, Holder D. Bulimia nervosa: treatment and short-term outcome. Psychol Med 1986; 16:65–70.

79. Hsu L, Crisp AH, Harding B. Outcome of anorexia nervosa. Lancet 1979; 1: 61–65.
80. Hudson J, Pope HG, Keck PE, McElroy SL. Treatment of bulimia nervosa with trazodone: short-term response and long-term follow-up. Clin Neuropharmacol 1989; 12(suppl 1):S38–S46.
81. Jarman F, Rickards WS, Hudson L. Late adolescent outcome of early-onset anorexia nervosa. J Paediatr Child Health 1991; 27:221–227.
82. Johnson C, Tobin DL, Dennis A. Differences in treatment outcome between borderline and nonborderline bulimics at one-year follow-up. Int J Eat Disord 1990; 9:617–627.
83. Johnson-Sabine E, Reiss D, Dayson D. Bulimia nervosa: a 5-year follow-up study. Psychol Med 1992; 22:951–959.
84. Kalucy R, Crisp AH, Harding B. A study of 56 families with anorexia nervosa. Br J Med Psychol 1977; 50:381–395.
85. Kay D, Shapira K. The prognosis in anorexia nervosa. In: Meyer J, Feldman H, eds. Anorexia Nervosa. Stuttgart: Thieme-Verlag, 1965:113–127.
86. Keller M, Herzog DB, Lavori PW, Ott IL, Bradburn IS, Mahoney EM. High rates of chronicity and rapidity of relapse in patients with bulimia nervosa and depression. Arch Gen Psychiatry 1989; 46:480–481.
87. Kreipe R, Churchill BH, Strauss J. Long-term outcome of adolescents with anorexia nervosa. Am J Dis Child 1989; 143:1322–1327.
88. Lacey J. Bulimia nervosa, binge eating, and psychogenic vomiting: a controlled treatment study and long-term outcome. Br Med J 1983; 286:1609–1613.
89. Laessle R, Beumont PJV, Butow P, Lennerts W, O'Connor M, Pirke KM, Touyz SW, Waadt S. A comparison of nutritional management with stress management in the treatment of bulimia nervosa. Br J Psychiatry 1991; 159: 250–261.
90. Lesser L, Ashenden BJ, Debushey M, Eisenberg L. Anorexia nervosa in children. Am J Orthopsychiatry 1960; 30:572–580.
91. Martin F. The treatment and outcome of anorexia nervosa in adolescents: a prospective study and five-year follow-up. J Psychiatr Res 1985; 19:509–514.
92. Mitchell J, Davis L, Goff G, Pyle R. A follow-up study of patients with bulimia. Int J Eating Disord 1986; 5:441–450.
93. Mitchell J, Pyle RL, Hatsukami D, Goff G, Glotter D, Harper J. A 2–5 year follow-up study of patients treated for bulimia. Int J Eating Disord 1988; 8:157–165.
94. Morgan H, Purgold J, Welbourne J. Management and outcome in anorexia nervosa—a standardized prognostic study. Br J Psychiatry 1983; 143:282–287.
95. Nash E, Colborn AL. Outcome of hospitalized anorexics and bulimics in Cape Town, 1979–1989. S Afr Med J 1994; 84:74–79.
96. Niederhoff H, Wiesler B, Kuenzer W. Somatisch orientierte Behandlung der Anorexia nervosa. Monatsschr Kinderheilkd 1975; 123:343–344.
97. Norman D, Herzog DB, Chauncey S. A one-year outcome study of bulimia:

psychological and eating symptom changes in a treatment and non-treatment group. Int J Eating Disord 1986; 5:47–57.

98. Nussbaum M, Shenner IR, Baird D, Saravay S. Follow-up investigation in patients with anorexia nervosa. J Pediatrics 1985; 106:835–840.
99. Pyle R, Mitchell JE, Eckert ED, Hatsukami D, Pomeroy C, Zimmerman R. Maintenance treatment and 6-month outcome for bulimic patients who respond to initial treatment. Am J Psychiatry 1990; 147:871–875.
100. Ratnasuriya R, Eisler I, Szmukler GI, Russell GFM. Anorexia nervosa: outcome and prognostic factors after 20 years. Br J Psychiatry 1991; 158:465–502.
101. Remschmidt H, Wienand F, Wewetzer C. Der Langzeitverlauf der Anorexia nervosa. Monatsschr Kinderheilkd 1988; 136:726–731.
102. Rollins N, Blackwell A. The treatment of anorexia nervosa in children and adolescents: stage 1. J Child Psychol Psychiatry 1968; 9:81–91.
103. Rosenvinge J, Mouland SO. Outcome and prognosis of anorexia nervosa: a retrospective study of 41 subjects. Br J Psychiatry 1990; 156:92–97.
104. Rossiter E, Agras WS, Telch CF, Schneider JA. Cluster B personality disorder characteristics predict outcome in the treatment of bulimia nervosa. Int J Eating Disord 1993; 13:349–357.
105. Saccomani L, Savoini M, Cirrincione M, Ravera G. Long-term outcome of children and adolescents with anorexia nervosa: study of comorbidity. J Psychosom Res 1998; 44:565–571.
106. Santonastaso P, Favaretto G, Canton G. Anorexia nervosa in Italy: clinical features and outcome in a long-term follow-up study. Psychopathology 1987; 20:8–17.
107. Santonastaso P, Pantano M, Panarotto L, Silvestri A. A follow-up study on anorexia nervosa: clinical features and diagnostic outcome. Eur Psychiatry 1991; 6:177–185.
108. Schulze U, Neudorfli A, Krill A, Warnke A, Remschmidt H, Herpertz-Dahlmann B. Verlauf und Heilungserfolg der fruhen Anorexia nervosa. Z Kinder Jugendpsychiatr 1997; 25:5–16.
109. Seidensticker J, Tzagournis M. Anorexia nervosa—clinical features and long-term follow-up. J Chronic Dis 1980; 21:366–367.
110. Steiner H, Mazer C, Litt IF. Compliance and outcome in anorexia nervosa. West J Med 1990; 157:133–139.
111. Steinhausen H, Glanville K. Retrospective and prospective follow-up of adolescent anorexia nervosa. Acta Psychiatr Scand 1983; 68:1–10.
112. Steinhausen H, Seidel R. Outcome in adolescent eating disorders. Int J Eat Disord 1993; 14:487–496.
113. Surzenberger S, Cantwell PD, Burroughs J, Salkin B, Green JK. A follow-up study of adolescent psychiatric inpatients with anorexia nervosa. J Am Acad Child Psychiatry 1977; 16:703–715.
114. Swift W, Kalin NH, Wamboldt FS, Kaslow N, Ritholz M. Depression in bulimia at 2- to 5-year follow-up. Psychiatry Res 1985; 16:111–122.
115. Thackwray D, Smith MC, Bodfish JW, Meyers AW. A comparison of be-

havioral and cognitive–behavioral interventions for bulimia nervosa. J Consult Clin Psychol 1993; 61:639–645.

116. Theander S. Anorexia nervosa: a psychiatric investigation of 94 female patients. Acta Psychiatr Scand Suppl 1970; 214:1–194.

117. Thiel A, Zuger M, Jacoby GE, Schussler G. Thirty-month outcome in patients with anorexia or bulimia nervosa and concomitant obsessive-compulsive disorder. Am J Psychiatry 1998; 155:244–249.

118. Toner B, Garfield PE, Garner DM. Long-term follow-up of anorexia nervosa. Psychosom Med 1986; 48:520–529.

119. Walford G, McCune N. Long-term outcome in early-onset anorexia nervosa. Br J Psychiatry 1991; 159:383–389.

120. Walsh B, Hadigan CM, Devlin MJ, Gladis M, Roose SP. Long-term outcome of antidepressant treatment for bulimia nervosa. Am J Psychiatry 1991; 148:1206–1212.

121. Warren W. A study of anorexia nervosa in young girls. J Child Psychol Psychiatry 1968; 9:27–40.

122. Willi J, Hagemann R. Langzeitverlaufe von Anorexia nervosa. Schweizerische Med Wochenschrift 1976; 106:1459–1465.

123. Willi J, Limacher B, Nussbaum P. Zehnjahres-Katamnese der 1973–75 im Kanton Zurich erstmals hospitalisierten Anorexien. Schweizerische Med Wochenschrift 1989; 119:147–159.

124. Wonderlich S, Fullerton D, Swift W, Klein MH. Five-year outcome from eating disorders relevance of personality disorders. Int J Eating Disord 1994; 15:233–243.

6

An Overview of Risk Factors for Anorexia Nervosa, Bulimia Nervosa, and Binge Eating Disorder

Corinna Jacobi
University of Trier
Trier, Germany

Lisette Morris
Universlty of Göttingen
Göttingen, Germany

Martina de Zwaan
Friedrich Alexander University Erlangen-Nuremberg
Erlangen, Germany

In the field of eating disorders, more than 30 variables have been reported as risk factors for the development of an eating disorder (Table 1). Among these variables, risk has been assessed from different perspectives: reported risk factors include social, familial, psychological, developmental, and biological factors. For many of these factors, the question of whether they occurred prior to the onset of the eating disorder has not yet been definitively answered. Therefore, it is impossible to determine whether they are symptoms, maintaining factors, consequences, or "scars" of the disorder.

The inconsistent use of the term risk factor as well as the lack of precise definitions led Kraemer and coworkers to set out a conceptual basis for a typology of risk factors (1,2). This theoretical framework forms the basis of our overview on risk factors for eating disorders.

TABLE 1   Potential Risk Factors for Eating Disorders

General and social factors
- Gender
- Race/ethnicity
- Participation in weight-related social or professional subculture

Familial factors
- Parental obesity
  - Parental psychopathology
  - Family interaction/communication style, EE

Developmental factors
- Adolescent age
- Premorbid obesity/higher BMI
- Childhood picky eating/problem eating/pica
- Childhood feeding and digestive problems
- Teasing/critical comments about weight and shape
- Early pubertal maturation
- Childhood anxiety disorders

Adverse life events
- Sexual abuse/physical abuse
- Other stressful/adverse life events

Psychological and behavioral factors
- Dieting, restrained eating, overconcern with weight and shape, body dissatisfaction/negative body image, high drive for thinness
- Low interoceptive awareness
- Low self-esteem
- Perfectionism, obsessive-compulsiveness, OCPD
- Depression, anxiety disorders, substance/alcohol abuse problems, affective instability
- Others: attachment style, self-awareness, high-level exercise

Biological factors
- Genetic factors
- Neuroendocrine and metabolic disturbances
- Changes in receptor density
- EEG changes
- Changes in regulation of hunger and satiety

In the past, risk and etiological factors for eating disorders have either been proposed from a specific theoretical perspective (e.g., biological, cognitive-behavioral, psychodynamic) or from an integrative perspective (e.g., biopsychosocial model). Factors in these models can be based on both clinical experience and empirical data, but the empirical foundation can vary from very strong to very weak and can comprise a wide range of methods and definitions for risk and etiologic factors. In contrast, the risk factor approach applied here to risk factors for eating disorders is primarily descriptive and data-oriented, refrains from making dynamic assumptions about interactions of factors, and should be regarded as a precursor to a more complex model.

The purpose of this chapter is to summarize findings on risk factors for eating disorders (anorexia nervosa, bulimia nervosa, binge eating disorder) on the basis of the risk factor approach outlined by Kraemer et al. (1). More specifically, we will compare potential risk factors from longitudinal and cross-sectional studies, establish the status of each of the potential risk factors discussed in the literature for the different eating disorder syndromes, and discuss additional risk factor characteristics (i.e., specificity, potency).

OVERVIEW OF BASIC RISK FACTOR CONCEPTS

In the conceptual papers previously noted (1,2), a risk factor is considered to be a measurable characteristic of each subject in a specified population, which precedes the outcome of interest and which can be shown to divide the population into a high- and a low-risk group. The probability of the outcome in the high-risk group must be shown to be greater than in the low-risk group. Beyond a statistically significant association between risk factor and outcome, the clinical significance of a risk factor should be indicated by the magnitude of the association, called the "potency" of the factor.

If, in the defined population, an association between the factor and the outcome can be shown, the factor is called a *correlate* (see Table 2 for a summary of definitions and identification methods). Any correlate measured concomitantly with or after the outcome may potentially be a concomitant or consequence of the outcome (i.e., a symptom or scar). Only if a correlate can be demonstrated to *precede* the outcome is the term "risk factor" justified. To establish a factor's status as a risk factor, precedence is a crucial criterion. A risk factor that can be shown to change spontaneously within a subject (e.g., age, weight) or to be changed by intervention (such as medication or psychotherapy) is called a *variable risk factor*. A risk factor that cannot be demonstrated to change or be changed (e.g., race, gender, year of birth) is called a *fixed marker*. A variable risk factor for which it can be shown that manipulation changes the risk of the outcome (e.g., onset of disorder) is called a *causal risk factor*. If that cannot be shown, it is called a *variable marker*.

Because precedence is a crucial criterion of a risk factor, the majority of risk factors can only be assessed in longitudinal studies. Exceptions are fixed markers taken from medical records or birth registers documented before the onset of the eating disorder. On the other hand, the majority of factors assessed in cross-sectional studies (e.g., epidemiological studies, case-control studies, family studies) are correlates. Exceptions are, again, some fixed markers, such as race or gender. The status of variable markers and

TABLE 2 Risk Factor Typology and Identification Method

Term	Definition	Study design
Noncorrelate	No significant association between factor and outcome (onset)	Cross-sectional and longitudinal studies
Correlate	Statistically significant association between factor and outcome	Cross-sectional studies: epidemiological studies, case-control studies, family history studies
Risk factor	Significant statistical and clinical association between factor and outcome; precedence	Longitudinal studies
Fixed marker	Risk factor that cannot be changed or change spontaneously	Cross-sectional studies using data from medical records or birth registers, longitudinal studies (including twin and genetic studies)
Variable risk factor	Risk factor that can be changed or can change spontaneously	Longitudinal studies
Variable marker	Variable risk factor, manipulation does not change the risk of outcome	Randomized clinical trial (preventive or therapeutic intervention study)
Causal risk factor	Variable risk factor, manipulation changes the risk of outcome	Randomized clinical trial (preventive or therapeutic intervention study)

causal risk factors can only be established in randomized clinical trials (prevention or intervention studies) which confirm that the modification of the factors leads to a change in the risk of the outcome (e.g., onset of the disorder).

In spite of their limitations, cross-sectional studies may constitute an important first step on the way to testing specific risk (or causal) factors in longitudinal studies (3,4). Especially cross-sectional studies that assess putative risk factors retrospectively may lead to different hypotheses compared to those that do not. Although retrospective assessment of risk factor information is problematic because of retrospective recall or memory biases, we decided to differentiate between cross-sectional studies with retrospective risk factor assessment and those without. For the former category the additional term *retrospective correlate* was coined for factors shown to predate the onset of the disorder according to subjects' self-report. This procedure allowed us to compare these results with the results of studies in which risk factor terminology is optimally realized.

METHOD

The methodology of our approach has been described in detail in Jacobi et al. (5). Therefore, only the most important methodological issues are summarized here.

For the identification of studies, a detailed computerized and manual literature search of empirical studies of potential risk factors for the *onset* of eating disorders was conducted through April 2002. Approximately 5000 abstracts were screened; about 300 (cross-sectional and longitudinal) studies were finally selected for inclusion in the review.

The following inclusion/exclusion criteria were imposed: For the majority of the factors examined, only studies with a control group (normal or unaffected control group) were included in the review; studies comparing different eating disorder groups alone were excluded. To establish specificity an additional clinical group was required. The minimal sample size in the studies was 10 subjects per cell. The follow-up interval for longitudinal studies had to be at least 1 year to allow enough time for symptoms of eating disturbances or disorders to change or emerge. Because the focus of our overview was placed on risk factors for eating disorder *syndromes*, longitudinal studies solely addressing (dimensional) disturbances or symptoms via questionnaires (e.g., Eating Disorders Inventory, EDI) were not included.

Factors from the included studies were first classified according to the Kraemer et al. (1) typology as outlined above. Factors were also classified with regard to outcome status, i.e., they were categorized according to whether they were associated with or predicted (a) *full*-syndrome anorexia nervosa, bulimia nervosa, or binge eating disorder, or (b) *partial*-syndrome eating disorders, otherwise defined "eating disturbances," or mixed outcomes of syndromes and symptoms.

Finally, a third level of classification was applied to establish additional risk factor characteristics (e.g., specificity, potency):

We classified a factor as a *specific* risk factor for one of the three diagnostic categories of eating disorders if it predicted the outcome only for this group but not for the clinical comparison group.

Risk factor potency was determined on the basis of the following indicators generally reported in the original studies: effect sizes based on Cohen's delta (ordinal risk factors) and the proportion of subjects with the risk factor in the low- vs. high-risk group (binary risk factors) (6). These were then transformed into one common potency indicator, the area under the curve (AUC) statistic. The AUC estimates the probability that a person with an eating disorder will have a higher value on an ordinal risk factor or be more likely to have a binary risk factor than a person without an eating disorder. The standards used to categorize the AUC reflect Cohen's standards for effect sizes (ES).

CHARACTERISTICS OF LONGITUDINAL RISK FACTOR STUDIES FOR EATING DISORDERS

Because longitudinal studies represent the "gold standard" of risk factor research, the main characteristics of the included studies are described here in more detail. In the following sections, we will then summarize the results of both longitudinal and cross-sectional risk factor research according to the diagnostic syndromes anorexia nervosa, bulimia nervosa, and binge eating disorder. For anorexia and bulimia nervosa, these results will also be presented graphically by ordering risk factors and retrospective correlates along a timeline according to their chronological emergence (Figs. 1 and 2).

Twenty-eight longitudinal studies were found. Thirteen of these were excluded from our overview because of too few cases, insufficient information on risk factors and reported methodology, lack of controlling for initial eating disorder symptoms, too broad outcome measures, or too short follow-up intervals.

In spite of large samples sizes, the majority of longitudinal studies have only identified risk factors for a *mixture of full DSM syndromes* of anorexia nervosa and bulimia nervosa and/or *partial syndromes* or eating disorders not otherwise specified (ED-NOS; 7–15). In six studies, the outcome samples were high-risk samples usually defined as scoring above the Eating Attitudes Test 26 (EAT-26) cutoff (16–21).

A closer examination of the outcomes in longitudinal studies reveals that the focus is on bulimic and binge eating syndromes while reports of anorexic syndromes as outcomes were much less common. Taken together, only 27 cases of anorexia nervosa out of a total of 12,776 subjects in the 15 studies emerged during the follow-up periods.

Samples in the studies consist mostly of adolescents between 12 and 15 years; three studies assess infants or younger children (8,11,12), two studies young adults (17,15). In nine studies the samples included females only, in six the samples consisted of both males and females. The duration of follow-ups varied from 1 to 18 years. Due to differences in the primary aims of the studies, the number and broadness of included potential risk factors, and the definitions and assessment of risk status or caseness (symptomatic/asymptomatic; cases/noncases; high/moderate/low risk) varies significantly: seven

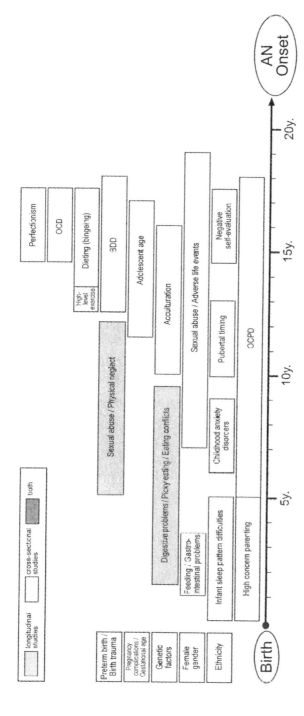

FIGURE 1 Risk factors, fixed and variable markers, and retrospective correlates for anorexia nervosa.

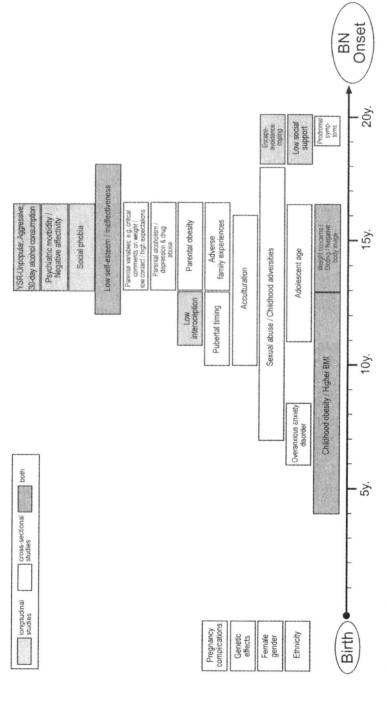

FIGURE 2 Risk factors, fixed and variable markers, and retrospective correlates for bulimia nervosa.

studies assess eating disorder symptoms and syndromes with structured diagnostic interviews, eight studies rely solely on questionnaire cutoffs or score combinations.

RISK FACTORS FOR ANOREXIA NERVOSA

Psychosocial Risk Factors

Gender

In both clinical and nonclinical samples, anorexia and bulimia nervosa have been observed to occur predominantly in females (14,15,22–25): population-based studies estimate a female-to-male ratio of 10:1 (26,27). Since gender is an immutable characteristic and asymmetrical gender distributions have been found for other mental disorders, e.g., (28), female status is classifiable as a nonspecific fixed marker for both anorexia and bulimia nervosa.

Ethnicity

Though eating disorders have been traditionally regarded as a predominantly Caucasian issue [see review by Striegel-Moore and Smolak (29)], a literature survey from Crago et al. (30) revealed a more complex ethnic distribution pattern: native Americans were noted as having higher rates of eating disorders than Caucasians, whereas equal rates were reported for Hispanics and lower rates for Asians and blacks. The results from two further studies also point to lower rates of anorexia and bulimia nervosa among Asians (31,32). Therefore, non-Asian ethnicity can be classified as a fixed marker of currently unknown specificity.

Acculturation

An association between the level of acculturation within ethnic minorities and the presence of eating disorder symptoms has been reported in a number of cross-sectional studies (33–35). On the basis of the assumption that acculturation predates onset of eating disorders symptoms, it is classified as a retrospective correlate of unknown specificity.

Age

In both clinical and population-based surveys, the peak incidence of eating disorders has been found in the age range from adolescence to early adulthood (36). The magnitude of the age-associated increase in risk depends on which age groups are compared. As yet, direct comparisons of eating disorder rates in latency age samples with later adolescent samples have not been made. In the Kraemer typology age is classified as a variable risk factor and, because of its relationship to other psychiatric disorders, age is categorized as nonspecific.

Weight concerns/Dieting/Negative Body Image

Cross-Sectional Evidence. The association between dieting and eating disorders is probably one of the most often quoted in theories on the etiology of eating disorders. Because the relationship between dieting and eating disorders seems to be particularly strong for patients who binge, i.e., patients with anorexia nervosa bingeing–purging subtype and bulimia nervosa, and less strong for restricting anorexic patients, the results will be summarized in the respective section of psychosocial risk factors for bulimia nervosa. Based on cross-sectional studies, dieting behavior appears to be a retrospective correlate of the bingeing–purging subtype of anorexia nervosa. Its specificity is unclear, since comparisons with other clinical groups have not been reported.

Longitudinal Evidence. Because most of the newly emerging cases in longitudinal studies were bulimic or partial bulimic cases, sometimes mixed with a few anorexic cases, longitudinal evidence for a relationship between weight concerns or dieting and anorexia nervosa is scarce. Only Marchi and Cohen (12) found that elevations on a measure of anorexic symptoms during childhood predicted adolescent anorexia nervosa or symptoms of anorexia. Accordingly, weight concerns, negative body image, and dieting are tentatively classified as variable risk factors for anorexia nervosa, which need replication. The specificity of these factors has not yet been addressed.

General Psychiatric Disturbance/Negative Emotionality

Cross-Sectional Evidence. Previous theories on the development of eating disorders as well as a large body of research on comorbidity have stressed the role of other psychiatric disorders (e.g., affective disorders, substance abuse disorders, anxiety disorders, personality disorders) as underlying and/or associated conditions in clinical samples of anorexic and bulimic patients [for reviews, see, for example, (37,38)]. Chronology of the onset of the comorbid disorders, however, has only been explicitly addressed in two cross-sectional comorbidity studies.

Rastam (39) examined premorbid physical and developmental problems and premorbid personality disorders obtained via a semistructured interview carried out with the mothers of an adolescent sample of anorexic patients and control probands. The total number of premorbid personality disorders was significantly higher in the anorexic patients (66% vs. 27%). Of the individual personality disorder diagnoses, only premorbid obsessive-compulsive personality disorder (OCPD) occurred significantly more often in anorexic patients than in the control probands (35% vs. 4%).

Bulik et al. (40) compared prevalence and onset of comorbid childhood anxiety disorders in two eating-disordered groups (women with anorexia and bulimia nervosa), a clinical control group (women with major depression), and a healthy control group $N = 98$. Rates of lifetime anxiety disorders were highest in the three clinical groups (48–60%) but they were also found in controls (30%). The prevalence of obsessive-compulsive disorder (OCD) and separation anxiety disorder was highest in the anorexic group, overanxious disorder highest in the anorexic and bulimic groups, and panic disorder highest in the anorexia nervosa and major depression groups. Ninety percent of anorexic women and 71% of depressed women with lifetime anxiety disorders reported that the onset of their anxiety disorder predated the onset of their other disorder.

Based on logistic regressions, the authors interpret their findings as supporting the hypothesis that overanxious disorder of childhood is a nonspecific risk factor for later psychopathology (eating or affective disorders) and that the relationship with anorexia nervosa is particularly strong. It has also been shown that OCD may be a specific risk factor for anorexia nervosa (40).

No information could be obtained as to the rates of the specific anxiety disorders preceding the eating disorders in this study. When the rates of *any* lifetime anxiety disorder were compared in the three patient groups, the rates in anorexic and bulimic versus depressed patients were almost twice as high: 54% of anorexic patients, 53% of bulimic patients, and 34% of depressed patients endorsed the presence of an anxiety disorder predating the onset of their other disorder.

Taken together, cross-sectional evidence for comorbid disorders predating the onset of anorexia nervosa is limited to childhood overanxious disorder, OCD, and OCPD. These disorders are therefore classified a *retrospective correlates* for anorexia. As the evidence for the correlate status of these anxiety disorders is limited to one study, additional studies are needed to replicate these results and also to examine the role of other comorbid disorders (e.g., affective and substance use disorders).

Longitudinal Evidence. Seven longitudinal studies included general psychiatric morbidity, psychopathology, or, more specifically, negative emotionality as potential predictors of eating disorders (10,13,14,16,19–21). In only one of these studies (21) was anorexia detected at follow-up; only one case was identified. It therefore seems premature to classify psychiatric morbidity or negative emotionality as a risk factor for the full syndrome of anorexia nervosa.

Sexual Abuse

Cross-Sectional Evidence. Sexual abuse in childhood, adolescence, or adulthood has been discussed as a risk factor for eating disorders in many studies as well as in early (41) and more recent reviews (38). All but one study are cross-sectional in nature. The studies included here were not restricted to childhood abuse but included sexual abuse at a later age as well. This procedure was elected, as a valid distinction between childhood and adolescent sexual abuse often proved impossible due to methodological inconsistencies and divergent definitions in the cross-sectional studies.

In general, cross-sectional studies comparing homogeneous diagnostic groups of anorexic patients to controls are rare. The few controlled studies primarily comprise a mixture of anorexic and bulimic clinical samples. Whereas some studies found higher rates of sexual abuse in these mixed samples, in others elevated rates seemed to be linked to binge eating–type anorexic patients (42–44). However, no information was given in these studies on the onset of the eating disorder and the first occurrence of sexual abuse.

In the study by Webster and Palmer (45), on set of eating disorders occurred in 74% of the eating-disordered subjects after age 16 years. However, no differences were found in the rates of sexual abuse occurring before age 16 when comparing four clinical groups [anorexia nervosa (AN), bulimia nervosa (BN), mixed AN/BN, major depression] to a nonmorbid comparison group. One study with clinical samples explicitly assessed the precedence of the abuse relative to the eating disorders (46). Comparing three patient groups (AN, BN, and depressive patients) and a control group, they found that the rates of abuse did not differ significantly between the three patient groups (42.9%/27.1%/40.0%), but that all of the clinical groups had significantly higher rates of sexual abuse than the control group (6.7%).

Taken together, the evidence for the classification of sexual abuse as a retrospective correlate of anorexia nervosa is based on one study only with retrospective assessment. Replication studies are therefore needed urgently.

Longitudinal Evidence. To date, only one longitudinal study has addressed the role of sexual abuse as a risk factor for eating disorders (8). Because only one patient developed anorexia nervosa at follow-up, the results will be reported in the respective section of risk factors for bulimia.

Adverse Life Events

Cross-Sectional Evidence. Only a few studies have investigated the relationship between stressful life events and the onset of an eating disorder. With one exception, these studies are again all *cross-sectional* in nature. Among studies comparing eating-disordered patients solely to normal controls, the results are not consistent: the percentages of (recovered) anorexic and bulimic patients, who had experienced a severe event before the onset of their eating disorder, did not differ markedly from the percentage of normal controls with severe events in the study by Troop and Treasure (47).

Schmidt et al. (48), comparing anorexic and bulimic patients, and community controls, found no differences in the proportion of patients with at least one severe event, but found that significantly more anorexic and bulimic patients had experienced what was called a "major difficulty"; in addition, "pudicity" problems were found more frequently in anorexic patients than in the other groups. Also, Rastam and Gillberg, (49) comparing a mixed clinical and population sample of 51 anorexic patients with a matched control group, did not find differences with respect to chronic life events but rather with respect to recent (3 months before onset of the disorder) major events such as loss of first-degree relatives (14% of anorexic vs. 0% of controls).

Among studies that also included a psychiatric control group, the studies by Horesh et al. found that adverse life events differentiated significantly between anorexic patients and healthy controls (50) and between a mixed group of anorexic and bulimic patients and healthy controls (51). More distinct differences in comparison to psychiatric controls could only be found for inappropriate parental pressures (51). Gowers et al. found an intermediate rate of negative life events for anorexic patients between that of psychiatric patients and community controls (52).

Taken together, there is some evidence that anorexic patients experience more severe life events before the onset of their eating disorder than healthy control subjects, although the evidence is not as consistent as for the role of sexual abuse. There is also some evidence that this relationship is not specific to patients with eating disorders but applies to psychiatric patients in general. In all of the studies investigating the role of life events in precipitating eating disorders, the events were reported to have occurred prior to the onset of the eating disorders. Therefore, general adverse life events are classified as nonspecific retrospective correlates.

Longitudinal Evidence. No longitudinal evidence for a relationship between adverse life events and the subsequent development of anorexia nervosa exists.

Early Childhood Eating and Digestive Problems

Cross-Sectional Evidence. One case-control study found retrospectively assessed early feeding and severe gastrointestinal problems to be extremely frequent in anorectic patients (found in 90%). Rates were almost two times higher than in the matched control group (49). Early childhood feeding and digestive problems are therefore classified as retrospective correlates of unclear specificity.

Longitudinal Evidence. The first longitudinal study including a sample of younger children found digestive problems and picky eating to be prospectively related to subsequent anorexic symptoms and anorexic symptoms to be related to later full diagnoses of anorexia nervosa (12).

The second longitudinal study also found a range of early childhood eating problems, assessed between ages 1 and 10, to predict eating disorder diagnoses in early and late adolescence and young adulthood: eating conflicts, struggles around meals, and unpleasant meals in childhood predicted later diagnoses of anorexia nervosa (11). On the basis of these studies, picky eating, anorexic symptoms in childhood, digestive and other early eating-related problems as well as eating conflicts, struggles around meals, and unpleasant meals are classified as variable risk factors for anorexia nervosa or anorexic symptoms. The specificity of these eating and digestive problems has not yet been tested. Given the small number of studies, replication studies are needed.

Family Interaction/Family Functioning/Attachment Styles

Cross-Sectional Evidence. Historically, the role of dysfunctional family interaction styles was put forward in theories on the development of eating disorders (53,54). Characteristics of the patient–family relationships of eating disordered patients include problematical family structures, interaction, or communication styles (e.g., overprotection, enmeshment) and attachment styles.

In the majority of studies, e.g., (55–59), both anorexic and bulimic patients describe different aspects of their family structure (interaction, communication, cohesion, affective expression, attachment disturbances, etc.) as more disturbed, conflictual, pathological, or dysfunctional than normal controls across different family assessment measures. However, the issue of precedence to the eating disorders was not addressed in any of these studies. Furthermore, similar patterns of family interaction or family functioning have been found in connection with other disorders, indicating a possibly nonspecific nature of these disturbances.

To date, family variables for the time span prior to onset of the eating disorders have been assessed retrospectively in only three studies: childhood and family background as well as the specificity of these possible characteristics were addressed retrospectively in the study by Webster and Palmer (45). Three groups of eating-disordered patients (AN, BN, mixed AN/BN) were compared with a group of women with major depression and a nonmorbid comparison group using a semistructured interview measure of childhood care before age 17. When compared with the nonmorbid group, patients with anorexia nervosa showed no significant differences on any of the variables studied (e.g., parental indifference, control and care, antipathy, discord in family).

Shoebridge and Gowers (60) addressed overprotection or high-concern parenting in anorexia nervosa as part of a cross-sectional case-control study. High-concern parenting was assessed by a structured clinical interview carried out with the mothers covering the first 5 years of the child's life. Two or more high-concern attitudes and behaviors were almost four times more common in mothers of anorexic patients than in mothers of controls. In addition, infant sleep pattern difficulties were significantly more common in anorexic patients than in controls. In the same sample, a more than threefold higher frequency of obstetric losses was found prior to the birth of the future anorexic patients compared with controls. The findings concerning parenting may therefore also reflect an adaptive parental behavior to a severe life event and may not be generalizable to a different sample or different (e.g., adolescent) age group. The presence of two or more variables of high-concern parenting is classified as retrospective correlate of unclear specificity.

The community-based studies by Fairburn et al. (61–63) compared three groups of eating-disordered patients (patients with a history of anorexia nervosa, with bulimia nervosa, and with binge eating disorder) with general psychiatric patients and healthy controls. A large number of putative risk factors (including variables of parental interaction) were assessed by an interview focusing on the period before the onset of the eating disorders. For most of the retrospectively assessed variables of parental interaction (arguments, criticism, high expectations, underinvolvement, minimal affection, low care, and high overprotection) the (previously) anorexic patients showed elevated rates when compared with normal controls (63). However, in comparison with the psychiatric controls, none of these variables turned out to be specifically predictive of anorexia nervosa.

These factors together with high-concern parenting are therefore classified as nonspecific retrospective correlates.

Longitudinal Evidence. As anorexia nervosa was not included as an outcome in any of the longitudinal studies assessing variables of family interaction, no evidence for these variables as risk factors for anorexia nervosa exists.

Family History/Family Psychopathology

Cross-Sectional Evidence. To date, a large body of cross-sectional research has examined the role of familial psychiatric disorders as a risk factor for eating disorders utilizing both the family history and the family study methods. The results of eight cross-sectional studies comparing the familial psychopathology of anorexic patients with relatives of either healthy or psychiatric controls can be summarized as follows [for details, see Jacobi et al. (5)].

The majority of these studies suggest elevated rates of psychiatric disorders in first-degree relatives of anorexic patients. The evidence is particularly strong for rates of eating disorders (AN and BN), affective disorders, some anxiety disorders (panic, generalized anxiety disorder, OCD), and OCPD, and rather weak for rates of substance abuse disorders. However, the chronology of the onset of anorexia nervosa in relation to the respective psychiatric disorders in the families was not addressed in any of these studies.

Selected parental psychiatric disorders (parental depression, alcoholism, and drug abuse) occurring prior to the onset of the child's anorexia nervosa were assessed retrospectively in the risk factor study by Fairburn et al. (63) as part of the environmental domain risk factor. For none of these parental psychiatric disorders were significantly elevated rates found in the previously anorexic patients in comparison with healthy and psychiatric controls. These variables therefore remain correlates.

Longitudinal Evidence.   No longitudinal evidence for the role of family psychopathology as a risk factor for anorexia nervosa exists.

Low Self-Esteem/Negative Self-Concept/Ineffectiveness

Cross-Sectional Evidence.   Low self-esteem, a negative self-concept, or "ineffectiveness" has assumed a central role in many clinically derived theories of eating disorders, e.g., (64). Constructs related to low self-esteem, especially ineffectiveness (operationalized by the EDI subscale Ineffectiveness), have been examined in many cross-sectional studies. Anorexic patients have consistently been found to exhibit lower self-esteem, a more negative self-concept, or higher levels of ineffectiveness than normal controls (5,65). The retrospective assessment of self-concept and its temporal relation to onset of the eating disorder has only been considered in one cross-sectional study: Fairburn and coworkers (63) found for the (previously) anorexic patients that negative self-evaluation prior to the onset of the eating disorder was more common than in healthy or, more specifically, psychiatric controls. Negative self-evaluation can therefore be considered a specific retrospective correlate.

Longitudinal Evidence.   Because longitudinal evidence on the role of low self-esteem or negative self-evaluation is, for the most part, based on studies with bulimia nervosa or binge-related syndromes as outcome, it cannot be classified as a risk factor for anorexia nervosa.

Perfectionism

Cross-Sectional Evidence.   From a clinical point of view it is well recognized that anorexic patients often display rigid, stereotypical, ritualistic, or perfectionistic behaviors. Most recently, these characteristics have been examined in a psychobiological light, connecting perfectionistic traits with alterations in serotonin activity in a number of cross-sectional studies. These studies found elevated scores for perfectionism in remitted anorexic and bulimic patients, even when using different measures of perfectionism, e.g., (66–68). Because none of the studies addressed premorbid perfectionism, the status of the factor perfectionism based on these studies remains a correlate.

To our knowledge, again only Fairburn et al.'s risk factor study (63) included perfectionism in their retrospective assessment of putative risk factors. They found that in (recovered) anorexic patients premorbid perfectionism was more common than in psychiatric and healthy controls. Perfectionism in these studies is therefore classified as a specific, retrospective correlate.

Longitudinal Evidence. The basis of longitudinal studies including cases of anorexia nervosa as outcome is currently too weak to classify perfectionism as a risk factor for anorexia nervosa. It therefore remains a correlate.

Athletic Competition/Participation in Weight-Related Subculture/Exercise

Members of professions that overemphasize a certain (low) weight or shape and athletes from certain sport disciplines (ballet dancers, gymnasts, wrestlers, swimmers, jockeys, etc.) were originally proposed as high-risk groups for the development of eating disorders more than 20 years ago (69). Interest in the past few years has focused primarily on the examination of eating disorder symptoms in athletes and a phenomenon called the "female athlete triad" (eating disorders, amenorrhea, osteoporosis), which a considerable number of elite athletes seem to develop, e.g., (70,71). Another major focus has been on the role of physical activity or high-level exercise in general in the development and maintenance of eating disorders (72,73).

Cross-Sectional Evidence. The few controlled studies with ballet dancers generally report that a higher percentage of dancers score in a clinically symptomatic EAT range (69,74–76) show elevations on EDI subscales (77) or on eating disorder–related symptoms and behaviors (75,77,78,86). However, rates for the full syndromes of eating disorders (anorexia and bulimia nervosa) are, when assessed, not higher than in the control groups.

The results of studies with elite athletes are less consistent. In one of the most comprehensive surveys covering six different sport disciplines, Sundgot-Borgen (79) surveyed 522 female elite athletes. 1.3% of the sample met DSM-IIIR criteria for anorexia nervosa and 8.2% for a category defined as "anorexia athletica."

More conservative results were obtained from a recent national survey of male and female student athletes (80). None of the student athletes met stringent criteria for anorexia nervosa. Using less stringent criteria, 2.85% of the females and none of the males were classified as having subclinical anorexia. However, the precedence of participation in weight-related sub-cultures to the eating disorders was not addressed in any of these studies.

Of all the studies examining the impact of physical activity or exercise in a noncompetitive context on the development of eating disorders, only one retrospectively assessed the amount of physical activity before the onset of the eating disorder. Davis et al. (81) compared a mixed eating-disordered sample of anorexic, previously anorexic, and bulimic patients with control subjects on the amount of physical activity predating the eating disorder using a structured interview. The results indicated that the eating-disordered patients were significantly more physically active than controls from ado-lescence (age 13) onward and also prior to the onset of the disorder.

On the basis of cross-sectional studies, athletic competition and parti-cipation in a competitive weight-related subculture are classified as corre-lates. However, high level of exercise is classified as a retrospective correlate.

Longitudinal Evidence. Participation in weight-related subcultures and high-level exercise have not been addressed in longitudinal studies as yet.

Other Factors

Cross-Sectional Evidence. In addition to the specific retrospective cor-relates reported above, in Fairburn ct al.'s study (63) a greater level of expo-sure to all three risk domains (personal, environmental, dieting) was found in the previously anorexic patients when compared to healthy controls but not in comparison with psychiatric controls. The exposure to the three risk domains thus seems to be a nonspecific effect.

Body dysmorphic disorder was assessed retrospectively for a period of at least 6 months prior to the onset of the eating disorder in samples of ano-rexic and bulimic patients as well as in controls. Body dysmorphic disorder (BDD) belongs to the somatoform disorder spectrum according to both ICD and DSM-IV, but similarities to OCD are also stressed by some authors. Symptoms of BDD were found to be more than three times higher in anorexic patients than in controls and were not observed at all in bulimic patients. BDD is therefore classified as a retrospective correlate of unclear specificity.

Longitudinal Evidence. Additional factors were only reported in longi-tudinal studies with primarily bulimic or binge eating disorder cases. The results will therefore be reported in the bulimia section.

Biological Risk Factors

Genetic Factors

It must be kept in mind that genes, environment, and neurobiology interact and are inseparable. The prevailing hypothesis assumes that an accumulation of various genes of small effect together with adverse environmental factors increases the risk of developing an eating disorder in those carrying the greatest genetic and environmental loading. At the moment, relevant genetic factors must be seen as *fixed markers* because they precede the onset of the eating disorder but cannot be manipulated.

Family studies provide a necessary first step in determining whether a disorder is genetic by establishing whether it clusters among biologically related individuals. These studies generally have found an increased rate of eating disorders in relatives of anorexics compared with controls. However, given that first-degree relatives share genes and environments, these studies cannot differentiate genetic versus environmental causes for family clusters. In twin studies, the contribution of additive genetic effects to liability has been estimated to be between 58% and 88% for anorexia nervosa (82–87). Even though these numbers are intriguing, the small number of studies precludes definite conclusions. In addition, in one study (88) the concordance rates of the dizygotic twins were higher than those of the monozygotic twins.

Researchers have begun directly examining genetic influences through candidate genes and linkage studies. Thus far, only a few polymorphisms have been found to be associated with anorexia nervosa. However, the literature in this area is growing rapidly, and studies are under way that include performance of genome-wide screenings in affected families [see (5)].

CNS Serotonin Activity

From a neurobiological perspective, research suggests that the (serotonin) (5-HT) system may play an important role in the pathophysiology and perhaps etiopathogenesis of eating disorders. The serotonergic system is not the only neurotransmitter system potentially implicated in the physiopathology of eating disorders but it is the most extensively studied system. Disturbances of brain serotonin activity have been described in acutely ill as well as long-term recovered patients. Research methods for the assessment of serotonin activity include neuroendocrine and behavioral responses to pharmacological challenge studies (using methyl-chlorophenylpiperazine [mcpp], fenfluramine, or tryptophan), tryptophan depletion, tryptophan availability in plasma, serotonergic parameters in platelets (^{3}H-imipramine binding, uptake of serotonin, serotonin-amplified platelet aggregation, serotonin-induced platelet calcium mobilization), and release and metabolism of serotonin in the CNS as reflected by levels of the serotonin metabolite 5-hydroxyindoleacetic acid (5-HIAA) in cerebrospinal fluid (CSF). More recently, brain imaging studies with single proton emission computed tomography (SPECT) and position emission tomography (PET) were used to characterize binding of serotonin transporters and 5-HT2A receptors (89–92). All of these studies have used a cross-sectional case-control design. Because neurobiological abnormalities cannot be assessed retrospectively, some of the studies included a *recovered study design*. The rationale in these studies is that individuals who have achieved stable remission from a disorder provide an opportunity to identify trait-related characteristics that may be risk factors for the development of the disorder. Nevertheless, it is not possible to determine whether alterations are the cause of a disorder, a reversible consequence of the disorder (which might contribute to the perpetuation of the disorder), or a "scar" caused by the abnormal behavior using this design.

In anorexia nervosa, CNS serotonergic responsiveness is substantially reduced in low-weight patients, which could be secondary to a diet-induced reduction of availability of the amino acid, tryptophan, the precursor of 5-HT, e.g., (93–98). There is some evidence that reduced brain serotonin activity persists after short-term weight recovery (92,99). In contrast, neuroendocrine responses to 5-HT-stimulating drugs have been reported to be normalized (100) and CSF concentrations of 5-HIAA even to be elevated (101) in women who were long-term weight recovered from anorexia nervosa, suggesting that hyperserotonergic function might be a trait marker in the disorder. In addition, increased CNS serotonin has been shown to be associated with obsessive-compulsive symptomatology. Obsessive personality traits frequently persist after the patient has recovered from anorexia nervosa. It has been hypothesized that increased serotonin activity might contribute to symptoms such as anxiety, perfectionism, obsessions with symmetry and exactness, and harm avoidance, which can, when coupled with psychosocial influences, make people vulnerable to developing anorexia nervosa.

Pregnancy and Perinatal Complications

Cross-Sectional Evidence.   Although associations between pregnancy and perinatal complications and schizophrenia have been reported repeatedly, e.g., (102), their association with eating disorders has received relatively little attention. Pregnancy and perinatal complications were examined in a large population-based sample of female twins (103). Information was obtained retrospectively by an interview carried out with the parents. Shorter gestational age and pregnancy complications were associated with an increased risk for anorexia nervosa. Because the risk for alcoholism, major depression, and most anxiety disorders was not significantly associated with pregnancy complications or gestational age, pregnancy complications and gestational age are classified as specific retrospective correlates of anorexia nervosa.

Cnattingius et al. (104) reported a prospectively assessed, more than three times increased risk of very preterm birth in a large case-register sample of anorexic patients. Also the risk (odds ratio, OR) of severe birth trauma (cephalhematoma) was between two- and threefold higher in anorexic patients. An elevation of these obstetrical complications was not found in a related study with patients with schizophrenia, or with affective or reactive psychosis (105). Preterm birth and birth trauma are therefore classified as specific *fixed markers* for anorexia nervosa.

Longitudinal Evidence. Pregnancy and perinatal complications have not been addressed in longitudinal studies as yet.

Pubertal Timing

Cross-Sectional Evidence. Pubertal timing effects (i.e., the age of occurrence of a pubertal event) are often confounded with pubertal status effects in cross-sectional studies limited to one age or grade. Although all girls pass through puberty, the age at which puberty begins varies considerably. An association between early pubertal timing and eating disorder symptoms or diagnosis has been observed in girls in pubertal transition as well as retrospectively after puberty completion (106,107). Whether the association between eating disorders and early sexual maturation is a function of increasing body mass index (BMI) or other aspects of puberty is not clear. Early pubertal timing as assessed in the cross-sectional studies is a nonspecific fixed marker.

Longitudinal Evidence. In none of the longitudinal studies, in which pubertal timing was addressed, did cases of anorexia nervosa emerge during the follow-up periods.

RISK FACTORS FOR BULIMIA NERVOSA

Psychosocial Risk Factors

Gender, Ethnicity, Acculturation, Age

The cross-sectional evidence for these factors has been presented in full in the anorexia nervosa section above. Their classification according to the Kraemer et al. (1) taxonomy can be summarized as follows: Female status is classifiable as a nonspecific fixed marker and non-Asian ethnicity as a fixed marker of currently unknown specificity. Furthermore, acculturation is classified as a retrospective correlate of as-yet-unknown specificity and age as a nonspecific variable risk factor.

Weight Concerns/Dieting/Negative Body Image

Cross-Sectional Evidence. Dieting has long been considered an important precursor, if not cause, of eating disorders. Clinical studies addressing the chronology of dieting and bingeing are few and the majority date back about 20 years. Onset of bulimia (i.e., onset of binge eating) has been observed in these studies to occur for the vast majority of the afflicted (73–91%) either during a period of voluntary dieting (108,109) or following weight loss (110,111). While the studies by Mitchell et al. (108) and Pyle et al. (109) remain rather vague in their description of the temporal sequence of the two behaviors, recent studies have corroborated the temporal precedence of dieting in bulimic subjects (112–114).

Experimental and laboratory-based studies on restrained eating and diet-induced binge eating yield further evidence for the relevance of this factor. One of the earliest, albeit uncontrolled, studies demonstrating the effects of prolonged dieting in a nonclinical population was reported by Keys et al. (115). Besides a variety of emotional, physical, and social changes following a period of semistarvation and average weight loss of 25%, "bingeing" was one of the behavioral changes reported, which had never been observed in the subjects prior to the experiment. In addition, so-called 'counterregulation' or behavioral disinhibition of "restrained eaters" under laboratory conditions has been regarded as an experimental analog of binge eating (116–118). Although the concepts of restrained eating and disinhibition following conditions that disrupt the dieter's restrained eating pattern (e.g., experimental preload, anxiety or stress induction, alcohol consumption) closely resemble the behavioral pattern displayed by bulimic patients, their generalizability to clinical populations has—to our knowledge—not been tested.

Taken together, the cross-sectional research provides strong evidence of the temporal sequence dieting—binge eating. Accordingly, dieting behavior can be classified as a retrospective correlate of bulimia nervosa.

Longitudinal Evidence. A factor best labeled as "weight concerns," consisting of fear of weight gain, dieting behavior, negative body image, and specific eating disorder symptoms or attitudes (e.g., bulimic behavior), has been assessed quite often in eating disorder research (12 of the total of 15 longitudinal studies). It predicted the development of eating disturbances and caseness (mixed bulimic and partial syndromes) in 9 of the 10 studies controlling for initial eating symptomatology (7,9,10,13–16,19–21). In the study by Patton et al. (13), subjects initially classified as "dieters" were found to have an almost eightfold higher risk of becoming "cases" than those initially classified as nondieters.

Weight concerns negative body image, and dieting can be classified as variable risk factors on the basis of the longitudinal studies. However, the specificity of weight concerns remains unclear, as none of the longitudinal studies included other psychiatric outcomes.

General Psychiatric Disturbance/Negative Emotionality

Cross-Sectional Evidence. Psychiatric disorders have been postulated to have a role as "primary underlying conditions" in the development of eating disorders in general (see anorexia nervosa section). However, chronology of disorder onset has only been addressed in a single cross-sectional study.

Bulik et al. (40) compared prevalence and onset of comorbid childhood anxiety disorders in anorexics, bulimics, and clinical as well as healthy controls (see anorexia nervosa section for more detail). They found the prevalence of social phobia to be highest in the bulimic group, and overanxious disorder highest in both the bulimic and anorexic groups. In regard to precedence, 94% of bulimic women with lifetime anxiety disorders reported that the onset of their anxiety disorder predated the onset of their eating disorder.

Based on logistic regressions, the authors interpret their findings as supporting the hypotheses that social phobia and overanxious disorder of childhood are nonspecific risk factors for later psychopathology (eating and affective disorders), although the association between social phobia and bulimia nervosa was particularly strong (40). Although no information was given on the rates of specific anxiety disorders preceding the eating disorders in this study, almost twice as many bulimics compared to depressed patients (53% vs. 34%) endorsed the presence of any lifetime anxiety disorder predating the onset of their further disorder.

In an attempt to explore mood- and anxiety-related prodromal symptoms of bulimia nervosa, Raffi et al. (119) found the following symptoms to be significantly more common in bulimics than controls 6 months prior to onset of the disorder: low self-esteem (see below), depressed mood, anhedonia, irritability, impaired work performance, generalized anxiety, reactivity, phobic avoidance, guilt, pessimism, and strict dieting. Because the exact sequence of the individual prodromal symptoms was not assessed, both the mood- and anxiety-related symptoms observed before the onset of the bulimia could be confounded with strict dieting. Although specificity was not tested in this study, it seems unlikely that these prodromal symptoms are specific to bulimia nervosa as they also typically occur as prodromal symptoms of depressive disorders.

Taken together, cross-sectional evidence for comorbid psychiatric disorders is limited to childhood overanxious disorder and social phobia. These disorders are therefore classified as retrospective correlates of bulimia nervosa. As the evidence for the correlate status of these disorders is limited to a single study, further studies are needed to replicate and extend these results. Prodromal mood- and anxiety-related symptoms are also classified as retrospective correlates of bulimia nervosa. However, their exact interaction with more the specific prodromal symptoms of eating disorders remains to be clarified.

Longitudinal Evidence. General psychiatric morbidity, psychopathology, and—more specifically—negative emotionality have been investigated as potential predictors of eating disturbances and disorders in seven longitudinal studies (10,13,14,16,19–21).

The change score in general psychiatric morbidity in the study by Patton et al. (13) turned out to be the only predictor of bulimia nervosa caseness. Psychiatric morbidity also was found to predict the onset of eating disorders (including partial syndromes) independent of dieting status in a further study by Patton et al. (14). Subjects in the highest psychiatric morbidity category exhibited an almost sevenfold risk of developing an eating disorder. Leon et al. (21) found negative affectivity to be the only significant (though moderate) predictor of eating disorder risk measured 3–4 years later. In four other studies (10,16,19,20), negative emotionality or psychopathology did not predict the outcome. However, two of the temperament scales (distress, fear) used in the study by Killen et al. (10) discriminated asymptomatic from symptomatic girls.

Accordingly, prior psychiatric morbidity is classified as a variable risk factor for bulimia nervosa. Although Patton et al. (13) did not address the question of specificity, longitudinal studies in other fields indicate that premorbid anxiety disorders and negative affectivity are risk factors for the development of other psychiatric conditions, including affective disorders and substance abuse (120–122). Therefore, they should be considered nonspecific risk factors.

Sexual Abuse

Cross-Sectional Evidence. Sexual abuse, especially during childhood, has been discussed as a risk factor for bulimia nervosa in many studies and reviews, e.g., (41,123). The majority of the cross-sectional studies on abuse have been conducted using *clinical* samples. Higher rates of childhood sexual abuse have been found for eating-disordered subjects (mixed anorexia and bulimia) in comparison with general-practice and nonmorbid controls (42), but not in comparison with psychiatric controls (43). Several studies addressing bulimia nervosa more specifically yielded similar results (44,46). In others no evidence of elevated rates of sexual abuse before age 16 (45) or during childhood (124) was found. In the latter study, however, higher rates of rape, sexual harassment, and molestation after age 17 were reported. In another study, significantly elevated rates of sexual abuse before age 13 were found only in bulimic patients with a comorbid borderline personality disorder (125). Only one study with a clinical sample explicitly assessed temporal precedence of abuse (46). However, in the studies by Steiger et al. (125) and Webster and Palmer (45), it seems quite likely that abuse predated eating disorder onset.

Three further studies investigating sexual abuse and bulimia nervosa were conducted using *community samples*. Dansky et al. (126) found significantly higher rates of rape, sexual molestation, aggravated assault, direct victimization, and posttraumatic stress disorder in bulimic respondents than in controls. Bulimics in a large epidemiological study were found to have experienced childhood sexual abuse approximately three times more often than comparison subjects (127). Sexual abuse was also found to be significantly more common in bulimics than in nonmorbid subjects (126). However, no difference was found between bulimics and general psychiatric patients. Though Garfinkel et al. (127) failed to report age of first sexual abuse and age of bulimia onset, the temporal sequence of abusive experiences predating eating disorder was established in the studies by Dansky et al. (126) and Welch and Fairburn (128).

Taken together, strong evidence of elevated rates of sexual abuse prior to onset of bulimia nervosa has been reported or is highly probable in five studies (two with community samples, three with clinical samples). The studies failing to address precedence also yield evidence of elevated rates of sexual abuse. No differences were found when comparing bulimics with psychiatric controls. Thus, sexual abuse is classified as a nonspecific, retrospective correlate of bulimia nervosa.

Longitudinal Evidence. The association between childhood adversities including sexual abuse and later eating- or weight-related problems has only been investigated in one longitudinal study (8). In the large community-based sample of mothers and their offspring, individuals who had experienced sexual abuse or physical neglect during childhood were at elevated risk for subsequent eating disorders and eating problems. Information on sexual abuse and physical neglect were obtained from a central registry and—for a subgroup of the sample—from maternal interviews. Sexual abuse and physical neglect are classified as nonspecific, variable risk factors on the basis of this study. However, additional prospective replication studies are needed.

Adverse Life Events

Cross-Sectional Evidence. The relationship between stressful life events and the onset of an eating disorder has been investigated in several *cross-sectional* studies with inconsistent results. Bulimic patients in the population-based study by Welch et al. (129) reported more life events in the year preceding the onset of their disorder than age-matched healthy controls (18% vs. 5% for three or more events). Adverse life events were also found to differentiate significantly between eating-disordered patients (mixed anorexic and bulimic) and healthy and psychiatric controls (51) (see anorexia section). However, bulimic patients were not found to differ significantly from normal controls regarding severe events in the studies by Troop and Treasure (47) and Schmidt et al. (48), both described above in detail, though significantly more bulimic patients had experienced a "major difficulty" and "pudicity" problems (48).

Taken together, there is some evidence that bulimic patients experience more severe life events than healthy controls. However, this appears to be the case for psychiatric patients in general. Since the reported life events predated the onset of the eating disorders in all the studies, general adverse life events are classified as nonspecific retrospective correlates.

Longitudinal Evidence. No longitudinal evidence for a relationship between adverse life events and subsequent bulimia nervosa exists to date.

BMI and Other Weight-Related Variables

Cross-Sectional Evidence. Childhood obesity, one of the many risk factors assessed retrospectively by Fairburn et al. (61), was shown to differentiate bulimic patients from psychiatric controls: approximately 40% of the bulimics vs. 13% of psychiatric and 15% of normal controls reported childhood obesity. Parental obesity was also reported more frequently by the bulimic subjects than either of the control groups. On the basis of this study, childhood and parental obesity are classified as specific retrospective correlates of bulimia nervosa.

Longitudinal Evidence. The results from longitudinal studies investigating BMI are inconsistent. In half of the studies without limitations, higher BMI or body fat was found to be predictive of eating problems (9), weight control, caseness (13), or a partial diagnosis of "binge eating" (15). In the remaining three studies without limitations, BMI or percentage of body fat at time 1 was not related to subsequent eating disturbances or caseness (10,14,19). Accordingly, higher BMI is classified as a variable risk factor. However, as the number of studies supporting versus not supporting BMI as a risk factor are equal, replication studies are needed. The specificity of BMI has not been addressed in longitudinal studies.

Early Childhood Eating and Digestive Problems

Cross-Sectional Evidence. Early childhood eating and digestive problems have not yet been investigated retrospectively in bulimic patients.

Longitudinal Evidence. Two longitudinal studies have addressed the association between early childhood eating problems and bulimia nervosa. Marchi and Cohen (12) found pica, early digestive problems, and reducing efforts to be related to later bulimic symptoms. The risk of bulimia nervosa was found to be almost seven times higher in individuals with a history of pica in early childhood. Eating problems occurring typically between ages 1 and 10 were assessed in a second longitudinal study in order to predict eating disorder diagnoses in the time span from early adolescence to young adulthood. Only eating too little was predictive of future bulimia nervosa; pica, digestive problems, not eating, not being interested in food, picky eating, and eating too slowly were not (11). The results of the longitudinal studies are inconclusive and the studies few; therefore, further research is necessary.

Family Interaction/Family Functioning/Attachment Styles

Cross-Sectional Evidence. In the majority of the cross-sectional studies on family interaction, functioning, or attachment style, bulimic (and anorexic) patients describe different aspects of their family structure as more disturbed or dysfunctional than normal controls (see anorexia section for more detail). To date, family variables have only been assessed retrospectively, for the time span prior to the onset of bulimia nervosa, in two studies.

Bulimics reported significantly more indifference, discord, lack of care, and overall adversity than anorexics and healthy controls, but did not differ from psychiatric controls (major depression) in the study by Webster and Palmer (45), which is described in detail in the anorexia section. These variables of troubled family background are therefore classified as nonspecific retrospective correlates.

In a community-based study by Fairburn et al. (61), parental variables such as high expectations, low contact, and critical comments about weight and shape by the family were found to be specifically predictive of bulimia nervosa as compared with psychiatric controls, and are therefore classified as specific retrospective correlates of bulimia nervosa.

Longitudinal Evidence. As none of the longitudinal studies assessing variables of family interaction included bulimia nervosa as an outcome, no evidence for these variables as risk factors for the disorder exists to date.

Family History/Family Psychopathology

Cross-Sectional Evidence. The majority of these studies suggest elevated rates of certain psychiatric disorders in first-degree relatives of bulimic patients: eating disorders, affective disorders, anxiety disorders, substance use disorders, and cluster B personality disorders are found more frequently among bulimics' relatives than relatives of control probands. Unfortunately, the temporal relation of the psychiatric disorders of bulimics' family members in relation to the onset of bulimia nervosa in the patient was not addressed in any of these studies.

Selected parental psychiatric disorders occurring prior to the onset of the child's bulimia nervosa were assessed retrospectively in one of the risk factor studies by Fairburn et al. (61) as part of the environmental domain risk factors. Parental depression, parental alcoholism, and parental drug abuse predating the onset of the eating disorder were significantly more common in bulimic patients than healthy controls. In addition, parental alcoholism was more common than in psychiatric controls. Based on this study, parental alcoholism is classified as a specific retrospective correlate, and parental depression and drug abuse are classified as nonspecific retrospective correlates, of bulimia nervosa.

Longitudinal Evidence. No longitudinal evidence for the role of family psychopathology as a risk factor for bulimia nervosa exists.

Low Self-Esteem/Negative Self-Concept/Ineffectiveness

Cross-Sectional Evidence. Self-esteem, self-concept, and ineffectiveness have been examined in relation to bulimia nervosa in numerous cross-sectional studies. Therein, bulimic patients have consistently been found to possess a more negative self-concept than normal controls (65,130). Self-concept deficits, as assessed in these studies, are therefore classified as correlates of bulimia nervosa.

The retrospective assessment of self-concept and its temporal relation to onset of the bulimia nervosa has been considered in two cross-sectional studies. Fairburn et al. (61) found negative self-evaluation prior to onset of eating disorder to be more common in bulimic subjects than in healthy and psychiatric controls. Low self-esteem was also reported by Raffi et al. (119) to be one of several prodromal symptoms of bulimic patients in comparison with controls. Although low self-esteem would have to be considered a highly potent retrospective correlate, the most potent prodromal symptom reported was anorexia or strict dieting. It remains unclear as to how the two prodromal symptoms were interrelated before the onset of bulimia.

Taken together, negative self-evaluation as assessed in the studies by Fairburn et al. (61) and Raffi et al. (119) can be classified as a specific retrospective correlate.

Longitudinal Evidence. Measures of self-concept have been included in four longitudinal studies (7,17,18,20). In the studies by Leon et al. (20) and Calam and Waller (19) they did not prove important in risk prediction or disordered eating. On the other hand, low self-esteem predicted elevated EAT scores 4 years later in the study by Button et al. (17). Girls in the lowest self-esteem range had an eightfold increased risk for a high EAT ($\geq$20) compared to those with high self-esteem. Similarly, Ghaderi and Scott (7) reported significantly lower self-esteem at time 1 for the incidence group that developed an eating disorder 2 years later. The EDI-Ineffectiveness subscale was included in four of the studies at baseline (9,10,20,21), but turned out to be predictive of disturbed eating patterns or caseness in only one of the multivariate analyses as part of the latent variable negative affectivity (21). However, significant differences were found in the univariate comparisons of the subsequent symptomatic and asymptomatic groups (9,10).

Based on longitudinal assessment, there seems to be a slight superiority of studies confirming the presence of a negative self-concept, low self-esteem, or higher ineffectiveness prior to the onset of an eating disorder. Exclusion of the two longitudinal studies with limitations (17,18) did not affect these results. Low self-esteem and ineffectiveness are therefore classified as variable risk factors. Based on existing studies, their specificity is unclear although it seems reasonable to assume that they are not highly specific for eating disorders. Replication studies are needed for further confirmation of risk factor status.

Perfectionism

Cross-Sectional Evidence. Elevated scores for perfectionism have been found in eating-disordered patients in a number of cross-sectional studies. The results of the studies, which warrant the classification of perfectionism as a correlate, have been presented in full in the anorexia nervosa section. However, premorbid perfectionism was not addressed in these studies. Only Fairburn et al.'s risk factor study (61) included perfectionism in their retrospective assessment of putative risk factors. Premorbid perfectionism in bulimic patients was elevated compared to healthy controls but did not differ from that of the psychiatric control group. On the basis of this study, perfectionism can be classified as a nonspecific retrospective correlate of bulimia nervosa.

Longitudinal Evidence. Perfectionism has been assessed using the corresponding EDI subscale in four longitudinal studies (9,10,20,21). In the studies by Killen et al. (9,10), perfectionism at time 1 was not found to be related to subsequent eating disturbances in multivariate analyses, but differentiated between symptomatic and asymptomatic girls at baseline in univariate comparisons (9). In both studies by Leon et al. (20,21), perfectionism did not turn out to be predictive in multivariate comparisons. No other measures of perfectionism have been employed in any of the longitudinal studies. On the basis of these results, perfectionism is classified as a correlate.

Athletic Competition/Participation in Weight-Related Subculture/Exercise

Cross-Sectional Evidence. The majority of the cross-sectional evidence for an association between athletic competition, participation in weight-related subculture, and exercise has been presented in the anorexia nervosa section above.

Results more specific to bulimia nervosa were reported in a comprehensive survey of 522 female elite athletes from six sport disciplines (79). Of the surveyed athletes, 8% met DSM-IIIR criteria for bulimia nervosa. Slightly more conservative results were obtained in a recent national survey by Johnson et al. (80), in which 1.1% of the female versus none of the male athletes met the full DSM-IV criteria for bulimia nervosa and 9.2% of the female versus 0.005% of the male athletes were classified as having subclinical bulimia. The question of temporal precedence was not addressed in these studies.

On the basis of current cross-sectional evidence, athletic competition and participation in a competitive weight-related subculture is classified as correlates of bulimia nervosa.

High level of exercise has been classified as a retrospective correlate in a mixed sample of eating-disordered patients [(81); see anorexia nervosa section]. However, there seems to be a preponderance of anorexic patients in this sample, making it unclear to what extent the results are generalizable to the diagnosis of bulimia nervosa.

Longitudinal Evidence. A longitudinal investigation of the role of athletic competition, participation in weight-related subculture, or exercise in bulimia nervosa has not yet been conducted.

Other Factors

Cross-Sectional Studies. In addition to the specific retrospective correlates reported above, Fairburn et al. (103) also found a greater level of exposure to all three assessed risk domains (personal, environmental, dieting) in bulimic patients compared with healthy controls. Exposure to the three risk domains is therefore classified as a nonspecific retrospective correlate.

Longitudinal Evidence. Girls who later turned out to be symptomatic in the study by Killen et al. (9) showed elevations on subscales of Aggressive and Unpopular in a personality inventory when compared with asymptomatic girls. In the study by Killen et al. (10), girls who developed a partial syndrome had higher 30-day prevalence of alcohol consumption. These factors thus are classified as nonspecific variable risk factors.

High use of escape–avoidance coping as well as low perceived social support were found to be prospective risk factors for subsequent eating disorders (primarily bulimia nervosa and binge eating disorder) in the study by Ghaderi and Scott (7). Accordingly, these are classified as variable risk factors but are in need of replication.

Biological Risk Factors

Genetic Factors

Similarly as in anorexia nervosa, there is an increased rate of eating disorders in bulimia nervosa relatives compared to control relatives. In twin studies, the contribution of additive genetic effects to liability to bulimia nervosa has been found to vary between 28% and 83%. The remaining variance is explained mainly by unique environmental factors. The magnitude of the contribution of shared environment is less clear, but it appears to be less prominent than of additive genetic factors (85). However, in one study (130), an equal environment assumption (EEA) violation (twin resemblance) accounted for all of the variance otherwise attributed to additive genetic effects. The EEA is central to the twin method and assumes that monozygotic and dizygotic twins are exposed to equivalent environmental influences of etiological importance. Only a small number of molecular genetic studies have been conducted for bulimia nervosa, with mostly negative results.

CNS Serotonin Activity

In bulimia nervosa, there is also considerable evidence for an impaired serotonergic responsiveness during the acute illness state, e.g., (66,132–142). Studies have shown an inverse relationship between symptom severity and measures of serotonergic responsiveness (143,144). In addition, there is evidence for an association between self-destructiveness, a history of sexual abuse, and impulsivity and reduced serotonin function (145–147). In long-term recovered patients with bulimia nervosa, 5-HIAA levels were elevated in CSF in comparison with those of controls (66). The prolactin response to fenfluramine was significantly larger than in patients with current bulimia nervosa but not compared to healthy controls (148). Moreover, recovered individuals experienced a transient return of eating disorder–related symptoms after tryptophan depletion (140). These results in recovered bulimic patients suggest that dysregulation in some CNS serotonergic pathways may persist after recovery from bulimia nervosa. Given the results in recovered patients with bulimia nervosa, it could be hypothesized that a disturbance of 5-HT activity may create vulnerability for the development of an eating disorder. However, as mentioned earlier, it cannot be ruled out that the findings related to serotonergic functions in recovered eating-disordered patients may be long-term consequences of the eating disorder rather than a premorbidly existing trait.

In addition to affecting eating behavior directly, alterations in CNS serotonin function may contribute to other psychological symptoms associated with bulimia nervosa. The diminished CNS serotonin could play a role in the high prevalence of depressive disorders in patients with bulimia nervosa. An impulsive-aggressive behavioral style, which is frequently seen in bulimic patients, may also be associated with diminished CNS serotonin function.

Taken together, the available data cannot prove whether disturbances of serotonergic function, as described above, predate the onset of eating disorder symptoms, or stem from dietary abnormalities or other changes characteristic of the disorders. Consequently, they can only be regarded as *correlates*. Studies of high-risk individuals prior to the development of an eating disorder may be clarifying.

Pregnancy and Perinatal Complications

Cross-Sectional Evidence.   In a large population-based study by Foley et al. [(103); see anorexia section], pregnancy complications were also associated with an increased risk for bulimia nervosa. Because these complications were not associated with the other psychiatric disorders they are classified as specific retrospective correlates.

Longitudinal Evidence.   Pregnancy and perinatal complications have not yet been addressed in longitudinal studies.

Pubertal Timing

Cross-Sectional Evidence.   Based on evidence from the studies by Hayward et al. (106) and Graber et al. (107), described in detail in the anorexia nervosa section above, early pubertal timing can be regarded as a nonspecific fixed marker of bulimia nervosa.

Longitudinal Evidence. Indicators of pubertal timing were also assessed in five longitudinal studies, in which neither an association with subsequent eating disturbance (9,16,19,20) nor predictive status in a structural model (21) could be found. In the study by Graber et al. (19), timing of pubertal maturation was related to eating disturbances present at study begin, with the girls in the "chronic" group evidencing earliest age of menarche. Taken together, there is no longitudinal basis for the classification of pubertal timing as a risk factor or a correlate.

RISK FACTORS FOR BINGE EATING DISORDER

Psychosocial Factors

BED is not a distinct diagnostic category like anorexia and bulimia nervosa but put part of eating disorders not otherwise specified (ED-NOS). Because the research criteria have only been put forward in the latest revision of the DSM (DSM-IV), the number of risk factor studies explicitly including the proposed BED criteria are very small. As the outcome of the longitudinal studies is often a mixture of bulimic or binge eating syndromes, it can be assumed that some of the risk factors listed in the bulimia section are also relevant for BED. Unfortunately, the majority of longitudinal studies do not permit a strict differentiation between bulimic versus binge eating–related syndromes. Therefore, only longitudinal and cross-sectional studies with explicit reliance on the research criteria for BED will be covered in this section.

Cross-Sectional Evidence. Binge eating disorder has been observed to occur predominately in females, as was also the case for anorexia and bulimia nervosa. However, the gender distribution is not quite as asymmetrical for BED: Preliminary estimates suggest a 2.5 female-to-male ratio (149). Accordingly, gender is classified as a nonspecific fixed marker for BED.

Eating disorders have generally been seen as afflictions of Caucasian females [see (29) and anorexia nervosa section]. However, though lower rates of body dissatisfaction and weight concerns have been found among African Americans, the rates of bingeing behavior are equal or elevated in comparison to Caucasians (150). African American and Caucasian ethnicity can therefore be classified as fixed markers for BED of currently unknown specificity.

Overall, only two cross-sectional studies (62,151) retrospectively assessed potential risk factors in BED patients compared to healthy controls: In the study by Fairburn et al. (62), subjects with BED reported greater levels of exposure to the following personal vulnerability factors than healthy controls: negative self-evaluation, major depression, marked conduct problems, and deliberate self-harm. With regard to environmental factors, they reported greater levels of exposure to parental criticism, high expectations, minimal affection, parental underinvolvement, and maternal low care and high overprotection. In addition, they were more likely to report sexual abuse; repeated severe physical abuse; bullying; critical comments by family about shape, weight, or eating; and teasing about shape, weight, eating, or appearance. When compared to the psychiatric controls, subjects with BED showed a higher level of exposure to the following factors: low parental contact; critical comments about shape, weight, or eating; and childhood obesity. The latter variables represent specific retrospective correlates of BED, whereas the former variables are nonspecific retrospective correlates.

Women's perception of acceptance versus rejection by their parents during childhood was the focus of the study by Dominy et al. (151). Women with BED were compared with obese and nonobese women without eating disorders on their perception of parents. BED women reported greater paternal (not maternal) neglect and rejetion than nonobese women did, while the obese non-BED women did not differ significantly from the other two groups. Perceived paternal neglect and rejection are therefore classified as *retrospective correlates*. Because no clinical control groups were included, the specificity of these correlates is not known.

Longitudinal Evidence. Two longitudinal studies (7,8) were able to identify BED cases based on the DSM-IV research criteria: Johnson et al. (8), in a large community-based sample of mothers and offspring, found that individuals who had experienced sexual abuse or physical neglect during childhood were at elevated risk for eating disorders (primarily bulimia nervosa and BED), and some eating problems during adolescence or early adulthood. Information on sexual abuse ad physical neglect had been obtained from a central registry and—for a subgroup of the sample—from maternal interviews. Sexual abuse and physical neglect in this study are classified as nonspecific, variable risk factors for BED.

Low self-esteem, high body concern, high use of escape–avoidance coping, as well as low perceived social support were found to be prospective risk factors for subsequent eating disorders in the study by Ghaderi and Scott (7). Of the 28 subjects who developed an eating disorder during follow-up, 13 were BED cases. Therefore, these factors are classified as variable risk factors.

Biological Risk Factors

Genetic Factors

There are no twin studies on BED. However, because of the low lifetime prevalence of eating disorders and the restricted power of the statistical analyses, attempts have been made to quantify the contribution of genes and environment to individual symptoms of eating disorders (e.g., binge eating) and to continuous measures of disordered eating and related attitudes (152–154). Studies with population-based twin samples suggest a genetic risk for the development of binge eating (86) with heritability estimates of 46% (155).

There are even fewer molecular genetic studies for BED than bulimia nervosa, Burnet et al. [(156), 5-HT$_{2C}$ receptor] and Ricca et al. [(157), 5-HT$_{2A}$ receptor] did not find a difference in genotype and allele frequencies between subjects with BED and controls.

CNS Serotonin Activity

At present, the possible contribution of central 5-HT dysfunction to the pathophysiology of BED has not been established. Only one study has employed a neuroendocrine challenge test with D-fenfluramine in patients with BED (144). As opposed to patients with anorexia nervosa and severe bulimia nervosa, the prolactin response was normal in BED women. Others found reduced 5-HT transporter binding in the midbrain in obese binge-eating women compared with obese control women using β-CIT SPECT (91).

As in bulimia nervosa, the satisfactory response to treatment with selective serotonin reuptake inhibitors provides indirect evidence of a possible disturbance of 5-HT transmission in these subjects. Several double-blind, placebo-controlled studies of medications that influence serotonin have been found efficacious in reducing the binge eating frequency in obese patients with BED (158–160). However, there are also studies that did not find a difference between fluoxetine and placebo in the reduction of binge eating frequency (161,162).

ADDITIONAL RISK FACTOR CHARACTERISTICS

As expected, a wide range of different indicators of *potency* for risk factors was found, depending on the methodology used to discriminate between high- and low-risk groups in the respective studies. Based on the indicators used, the potency of risk factors and retrospective correlates can be categorized as follows:

For *anorexia nervosa*, female gender and a high level of exercise are the only high-potency factors. Feeding and gastrointestinal problems, infant sleep difficulties, a high-concern parenting style, OCPD, perfectionism, and negative self-evaluation are retrospective correlates of medium potency. Sexual abuse and social support are variable risk factors of medium potency. Birth related perinatal complications and premature delivery represent fixed markers of low potency. The remaining factors are of low or unclear potency.

Factors that have been found only once and are, therefore, in need of replication are early sleeping, feeding, and gastrointestinal problems, high-concern parenting, childhood anxiety disorders, and high level of exercise.

For *bulimia nervosa*, female gender and weight concerns/dieting represent the best confirmed, most potent risk factors from longitudinal and cross-sectional studies. Sexual abuse and escape–avoidance coping are variable risk factors of medium potency; negative self-evaluation is a retrospective correlate also of medium potency. The remaining variable risk factors and retrospective correlates are of low or unclear potency. Perceived low social support, though very potent, has only been confirmed in a single sample of higher age (18–30 years) than most of the other samples. Its generalizability to early adolescence is therefore unclear.

Female gender, ethnicity, high BMI, low interoception, increased weight concerns, negative self-evaluation, and psychiatric morbidity are factors confirmed in more than one study, whereas the remaining factors are in need of replication.

SUMMARY AND CONCLUSIONS

In spite of a large number of potential risk factor studies for eating disorders, previous research is characterized by a number of limitations, which become evident when a more rigorous risk factor terminology is applied to the putative risk factors for eating disorders. The majority of so-called risk factor studies are cross-sectional, thus only allowing for the identification of correlates. However, a subset of these addressed precedence by retrospectively assessing the putative risk factor before onset of the eating disorder. Factors consistently confirmed as risk factors by longitudinal studies and as retrospective correlates and fixed markers by cross-sectional studies are gender, ethnicity, higher BMI, childhood eating problems, sexual abuse, psychiatric morbidity, low self-esteem, and weight concerns/dieting. The status of other factors (e.g., family interaction, perfectionism), frequently designated risk factors in previous reviews, could not be confirmed. The specificity of potential risk factors has only been addressed for a few retrospective correlates of anorexia and bulimia nervosa. The only well-supported high-potency factors are gender and weight concerns. Because many of the risk factors may be population specific, replication studies are needed.

Although the majority of longitudinal studies included sample sizes of several hundred subjects, the samples are still too small for consistent and meaninful risk factor detection of full syndromes of eating disorders. Given the low prevalence of eating disorders, especially of anorexia nervosa, this is not surprising. Consequently, longitudinal evidence on risk factors is much stronger for bulimia nervosa and binge-related syndromes, whereas our knowledge on risk factors for anorexia nervosa is still very limited. When attrition rates of longitudinal studies are also taken into account, one may question whether risk factor identification for full syndromes of anorexia nervosa is possible at all. Furthermore, because of the overlap of the syndromes, especially partial syndromes, previous research does not permit a valid differentiation of risk factors for bulimia nervosa versus binge eating disorder.

The majority of factors are variable risk factors, theoretically amenable to modification. No causal factors have been found, i.e., factors preceding the onset of eating disorders that change the probability of the risk of the outcome. For many of the factors (e.g., dieting, perfectionism), an experimental manipulation would seem unethical. Although randomized controlled CBT trials for bulimia nervosa can be considered a way of manipulating a variable risk factor, i.e., weight and shape concerns, the similar reductions in weight and shape concerns and dieting, achieved by such divergent treatment approaches as CBT, IPT, and pharmacotherapy, raise the question about the mechanisms of change in general.

To date, probably the most realistic way to manipulate a potential causal factor would be to target the most potent variable risk factors in a high-risk group within a preventive approach and to show that by reducing exposure to the risk factor the risk of developing the disorder can be decreased in comparison with a low-risk group. Preliminary studies (163,164) indicate that such targeted approaches may result in stronger effects than those found in previous, more universal (e.g., school-based) preventive approaches. Large-scale studies testing the causal status of variable risk factors in high-risk samples are currently under way and will help to further clarify the status of specific factors.

Finally, as pointed out above, some of the risk factors, such as maternal eating disorders, parental weight, and early feeding and gastrointestinal problems, are already present at birth or during the first years of a child's life. To manipulate these, preventive interventions would have to target parental attitudes and behaviors. To our knowledge, none of the prevention programs to date have focused on or included parents in order to reduce the risk for their children. However, the identification of risk factors during different developmental periods could result in differential recommendations for preventive intervention in the future.

REFERENCES

1. Kraemer HC, Kazdin AE, Offord DR, Kessler RC, Jensen PS, Kupfer DJ. Coming to terms with the terms of risk. Arch Gen Psychiatry 1997; 54:337–343.

2. Kazdin AE, Kraemer HC, Kessler RC, Kupfer DJ, Offord DR. Contributions of risk factor research to developmental psychopathology. Clin Psychol Rev 1997; 17:375–406.
3. Kazdin AE. Research Designs in Clinical Psychology. 3d ed. Boston: Allyn and Bacon, 1998.
4. Rutter M. Beyond longitudinal data: causes, consequences, changes, and continuity. J Consult Clin Psychol 1994; 62:928–940.
5. Jacobi C, Hayward C, de Zwaan M, Kraemer H, Agras WS. Coming to terms with risk factors for eating disorders: application of risk terminology and suggestions for a general taxonomy. Psychol Bull. In press.
6. Kraemer HC, Kazdin AE, Offord DR, Kessler RC, Jensen PS, Kupfer DJ. Measuring the potency of risk factors for clinical or policy significance. Psychol Meth 1999; 4:257–271.
7. Ghaderi A, Scott B. Prevalence, incidence and prospective risk factors for eating disorders. Acta Psychiatrica Scand 2001; 104:122–130.
8. Johnson JG, Cohen P, Kasen S, Brook JS. Childhood adversities associated with risk for eating disorders or weight problems during adolescence or early adulthood. Am J Psychiatry 2002; 159:394–400.
9. Killen JD, Taylor CB, Hayward C, Wilson DM, Haydel KF, Hammer LD, Simmonds B, Robinson TN, Litt I, Varady A, Kraemer H. Pursuit of thinness and onset of eating disorder symptoms in a community sample of adolescent girls: a three year prospective analysis. Int J Eat Disord 1994; 16:227–238.
10. Killen JD, Taylor CB, Hayward C, Haydel KF, Wilson DM, Hammer LD, Kraemer HC, Blair-Greiner A, Strachowski D. Weight concerns influence the development of eating disorders: a 4-year prospective study. J Consul Clin Psychol 1996; 64:936–940.
11. Kotler LA, Cohen P, Davis M, Pine DS, Walsh BT. Longitudinal relationships between childhood, adolescent, and adult eating disorders. J Am Acad Child Adol Psychiatry 2001; 40:1424–1440.
12. Marchi M, Cohen P. Early childhood eating behaviors and adolescent eating disorders. J Am Acad Child Adol Psychiatry 1990; 29:112–117.
13. Patton GC, Johnson-Sabine E, Wood K, Mann AH, Wakeling A. Psychol Med 1990; 20:383–394.
14. Patton GC, Selzer R, Coffey C, Carlin JB, Wolfe R. Onset of adolescent eating disorders: population based cohort study over 3 years. Br Med J 1999; 318:765–768.
15. Vollrath M, Koch R, Angst J. Binge eating and weight concerns among young adults. Results from the Zurich Cohort Study. B J Psychiatry 1992; 160:498–503.
16. Attie I, Brooks-Gunn J. Development of eating problems in adolescent girls: a longitudinal study. Dev Psychol 1989; 25:70–79.
17. Button EJ, Sonuga-Barke EJS, Davies J, Thompson M. A prospective study of self esteem in the prediction of eating problems in adolescent schoolgirls: questionnaire findings. Br J Clin Psychol 1996; 35:193–203.
18. Calam R, Waller G. Are eating and psychosocial characteristics in early teen-

age years useful predictors of eating characteristics in early adulthood? A 7-year longitudinal study. Int J Eat Disord 1998; 24:351–362.

19. Graber JA, Brooks-Gunn J, Paikoff RL, Warren MP. Prediction of eating problems: an 8-year study of adolescent girls. Dev Psychol 1994; 30:823–834.

20. Leon GR, Fulkerson JA, Perry CL, Early-Zald MB. Prospective analysis of personality and behavioral influences in the later development of disordered eating. J Abnormal Psychol 1995; 104:140–149.

21. Leon GR, Fulkerson JA, Perry CL, Keel PK, Klump KL. Three to four year prospective evaluation of personality and behavioral risk factors for later disordered eating in adolescent girls and boys. J Youth Adol 1999; 28:181–196.

22. Lewinsohn PM, Hops H, Roberts RE, Seeley JR, Andrews JA. Adolescent psychopathology: I. Prevalence and incidence of depression and other DSM-III-R disorders in high school students. J Abnormal Psychol 1993; 102:133–144.

23. Nielsen S. The epidemiology of anorexia nervosa in Denmark from 1973 to 1987: a nationwide register study of psychiatric admission. Acta Psychiatrica Scand 1990; 81:507–514.

24. Schotte DE, Stunkard AJ. Bulimia vs. bulimic behaviors on a college campus. JA 1987; 258:1213–1215.

25. Whitaker AH, Johnson J, Shaffer D, Rapoport JL, Kalikow K, Walsh BT, Davis M, Braimann S, Dolinsky A. Uncommon troubles in young people: prevalence estimates of selected psychiatric disorders in a nonreferred adolescent population. Arch Gen Psychiatry 1990; 47:487–496.

26. Hsu LKG. Epidemiology of the eating disorders. Psychiatric Clin North Am 1996; 19:681–700.

27. American Psychiatric Association. Diagnostic and Statistical Manual of Mental Disorders. 4th ed. Washington, DC, 1994.

28. Blazer DG, Kessler RC, McGonagle KA, Swartz MS. The prevalence and distribution of major depression in a national community sample: the National Comorbidity Survey. Am J Psychiatry 1994; 151:979–986.

29. Striegel Moore R, Smolak L. The role of race in the development of eating disorders. In: Smolak L, Levine MP, Striegel-Moore R, eds. The Develomental Psychopathology of Eating Disorders. Mahwah, NJ: Lawrence Erlbaum Associates, 1996:259–284.

30. Crago M, Shisslak CM, Estes LS. Eating disturbances among American minority groups: a review. Int J Eat Disord 1996; 19:239–248.

31. Chen CN, Wong J, Lee N, Chan-Ho MW, Lau JT, Fung M. The Shatin Community mental health survey in Hong Kong. II. Major findings. Arch Gen Psychiatry 1993; 50:125–133.

32. Ohzeki T, Hanaki K, Motozumi H, Ishitani N, Matsuda-Ohtahara H, Sunaguchi M, Shiraki K. Prevalence of obesity, leanness and anorexia nervosa in Japanese boys and girls aged 12–14 years. Ann Nutr Metab 1990; 34:208–212.

33. Davis C, Katzman MA. Perfection as acculturation: psychological correlates

of eating problems in Chinese male and female students living in the United States. Int J Eat Disord 1999; 25:65–70.

34. Gowen LK, Hayward C, Killen JD, Robinson TN, Taylor CB. Acculturation and eating disorder symptoms in adolescent girls. J Res Adol 1999; 9:67–83.

35. Hooper MSH, Garner DM. Application of the eating disorders inventory to a sample of black, white and mixed race schoolgirls in Zimbabwe. Int J Eat Disord 1986; 5:161–168.

36. Woodside DB, Garfinkel P. Age of onset in eating disorders. Int J Eat Disord 1992; 12:31–36.

37. Mitchell JE, Specker SM, de Zwaan M. Comorbidity and medical complications of bulimia nervosa. J Clin Psychiatry 1991; 52(Suppl 10):13–20.

38. Wonderlich SA, Mitchell JE. Eating disorders and comorbidity: Empirical, conceptual, and clinical implications. Psychopharmacol Bull 1997; 33:381–390.

39. Rastam M. Anorexia nervosa in 51 Swedish adolescents: premorbid problems and comorbidity. J Am Acad Child Adol Psychiatry 1992; 31:819–829.

40. Bulik CM, Sullivan PF, Fear JL, Joyce PR. Eating disorders and antecedent anxiety disorders: a controlled study. Acta Psychiatrica Scand 1997; 96:101–107.

41. Pope HG, Hudson JI. Is childhood sexual abuse a risk factor for bulimia nervosa? Am J Psychiatry 1992; 149:455–463.

42. Brown L, Russell J, Thornton C, Dunn S. Experiences of physical and sexual abuse in Australian general practice attenders and an eating disordered population. Aust N Z J Psychiatry 1997; 31:398–404.

43. Folsom V, Krahn D, Nairn K, Gold L, Demitrack MA, Silk KR. The impact of sexual and physical abuse on eating disordered and psychiatric symptoms: a comparison of eating disordered and psychiatric inpatients. Int J Eat Disord 1993; 13:249–257.

44. Steiger H, Zanko M. Sexual traumata among eating-disordered, psychiatric, and normal female groups. J Interpers Viol 1990; 5:74–86.

45. Webster JJ, Palmer RL. The childhood and family background of women with clinical eating disorders: a comparison with women with major depression and women without psychiatric disorder. Psychol Med 2000; 30:53–60.

46. Vize CM, Cooper PJ. Sexual abuse in patients with eating disorder, patients with depression and normal controls. A comparative study. Br J Psychiatry 1995; 167:80–85.

47. Troop NA, Treasure JL. Psychosocial factors in the onset of eating disorders: responses to life events and difficulties. Br J Med Psychol 1997; 70:373–385.

48. Schmidt U, Tiller J, Blanchard M, Andrews B, Treasure J. Is there a specific trauma precipitating anorexia nervosa? Psychol Med 1997; 27:523–530.

49. Rastam M, Gillberg C. Background factors in anorexia nervosa. A controlled study of 51 teenage cases including a population sample. Eur Child Adol Psychiatry 1992; 1:54–65.

50. Horesh N, Apter A, Lepkifker E, Ratzoni G, Weizman R, Tyrano S. Life events and severe anorexia nervosa in adolescence. Acta Psychiatrica Scand 1995; 91:5–9.

51. Horesh N, Apter A, Ishai J, Danziger Y, Miculincer M, Stein D, Lepkifker E,

Minouni M. Abnormal psychosocial situations and eating disorders in adolescence. J Am Acad Child Adol Psychiatry 1996; 35:921–927.

52. Gowers SG, North CD, Byram V. Life event precipitants of adolescent anorexia nervosa. J Child Psychol Psychiatry 1996; 37:469–477.
53. Minuchin S, Rosman BL, Baker L. Psychosomatic Families: Anorexia Nervosa in Context. Cambridge, MA: Harvard University Press, 1978.
54. Bruch H. Eating Disorders: Obesity, Anorexia Nervosa, and the Person Within. New York: Basic Books, 1973.
55. Cole-Detke H, Kobak R. Attachment processes in eating disorder and depression. J Consul Clin Psychol 1996; 64:282–290.
56. Friedmann MA, Wilfley DE, Welch RR, Kunce JT. Self-directed hostility and family functioning in normal-weight bulimics and overweight binge eaters. Addict Behav 1997; 22:367–375.
57. McNamara K, Loveman C. Differences in family functioning among bulimics, repeat dieters, and nondieters. J Clin Psychol 1990; 46:518–523.
58. Shisslak CM, McKeon RT, Crago M. Family dysfunction in normal weight bulimic and bulimic anorexic families. J Clin Psychol 1990; 46:185–189.
59. Strober M, Humphrey LL. Familial contributions to the etiology and course of anorexia nervosa and bulimia. J Consult Clin Psychol 1987; 55:654–659.
60. Shoebridge P, Gowers SG. Parental high concern and adolescent-onset anorexia nervosa. Br J Psychiatry 2000; 176:132–137.
61. Fairburn CG, Welch SL, Doll HA, Davies BA, O'Connor ME. Risk factors for bulimia nervosa. A community-based case-control study. Arch Gen Psychiatry 1997; 54:509–517.
62. Fairburn CG, Doll HA, Welch SL, Hay PJ, Davies BA, O'Connor ME. Risk factors for binge-eating disorder: a community-based case-control study. Arch Gen Psychiatry 1998; 55:425–432.
63. Fairburn CG, Cooper Z, Doll HA, Welch SL. Risk factors for anorexia nervosa. Three integrated case-control comparisons. Arch Gen Psychiatry 1999; 56:468–476.
64. Bruch H. Perceptual and conceptual disturbances in anorexia nervosa. Psychosom Med 1962; 14(2):187–194.
65. Jacobi C. Zur Spezifität und Veränderbarkeit von Beeinträchtigungen des Selbstkonzepts bei Essstörungen. Regensburg: S. Roderer Verlag, 1999.
66. Kaye WH, Greeno CG, Moss H, Fernstrom J, Fernstrom M, Lilenfeld LR, Weltzin TE, Mann JJ. Alterations in serotonin activity and psychiatric symptoms after recovery from bulimia nervosa. Arch Gen Psychiatry 1998; 55:927–935.
67. Srinivasagam NM, Kaye WH, Plotnicov KH, Greeno C, Weltzin TE, Rao R. Persistent perfectionism, symmetry, and exactness after long-term recovery from anorexia nervosa. Am J Psychiatry 1995; 152:1630–1634.
68. Bastiani AM, Rao R, Weltzin T, Kaye WH. Perfectionism in anorexia nervosa. Int J Eat Disord 1995; 17:147–152.
69. Garner DM, Garfinkel PE. Sociocultural factors in anorexia nervosa. Lancet 1978; 2:674.
70. Brownell KD. Eating disorders in athletes. In: Brownell KD, Fairburn CG,

eds. Eating Disorders and Obesity. A Comprehensive Handbook. New York: Guilford Press, 1995:191–196.

71. Putukian M. The female athlete triad. Clin Sports Med 1998; 17:675–696.
72. Davis C, Fox J, Cowles M, Hastings P, Schwass K. The functional role of exercise in the development of weight and diet concerns in women. J Psychosom Res 1990; 34:563–574.
73. Davis C, Katzman DK, Kaptein S, Kirsh C, Brewer H, Kalmbach K, Olmstedt MP, Woodside DB, Kaplan AS. The prevalence of high-level exercise in the eating disorders: etiological implications. Comprehen Psychiatry 1997; 38:321–326.
74. Joseph A, Wood IK, Goldberg SC. Determining populations at risk for developing anorexia nervosa based on selection of college major. Psychiatry Res 1982; 7:53–58.
75. Abraham S. Eating and weight controlling behaviors of young ballet dancers. Psychopathology 1996a; 29:218–222.
76. Abraham S. Chracteristics of eating disorders among young ballet dancers. Psychopathology 1996b; 29:223–229.
77. Kurtzman FD, Yager J, Landsverk J, Wiesmeier E, Bodurka DC. Eating disorders among selected female student populations at UCLA. J Am Diet Assoc 1989; 89:45–53.
78. Braistedt JR, Mellin L, Gong EJ, Irwin CE Jr. The adolescent ballet dancer. Nutritional practices and characteristics associated with anorexia nervosa. J Adol Health Care 1985; 6:365–371.
79. Sundgot-Borgen J. Risk and trigger factors for the development of eating disorders in female elite athletes. Med Sci Sports Exercise 1994; 26:414–419.
80. Johnson C, Powers PS, Dick R. Athletes and eating disorders: the National Collegiate Athletic Association study. Int J Eat Disord 1999; 26:179–188.
81. Davis C, Kennedy SH, Ravelski E, Dionne M. The role of physical activity in the development and maintenance of eating disorders. Psychol Med 1994; 24:957–967.
82. Holland AJ, Hall A, Murray R, Russell GFM, Crisp AH. Anorexia nervosa: a study of 34 twin pairs and one set of triplets. Br J Psychiatry 1984; 145:414–419.
83. Holland AJ, Sicotte N, Treasure J. Anorexia nervosa: evidence for a genetic basis. J Psychosom Res 1988; 32:561–571.
84. Treasure J, Holland A. Genetic vulnerability to eating disorders: evidence from twin and family studies. In: Remschmidt H, Schmidt MH, eds. Child and Youth Psychiatry: European Perspectives. New York: Hogrefe and Huber, 1989:59–68.
85. Bulik CM, Sullivan PF, Wade TD, Kendler KS. Twin studies of eating disorders: a review. Int J Eat Disord 2000; 27:1–20.
86. Wade TD, Bulik CM, Neale M, Kendler KS. Anorexia nervosa and major depression: Shared genetic and environmental risk factors. Am J Psychiatry 2000; 157:469–471.
87. Klump KL, Miller KB, Keel PK, McGue M, Iacono WG. Genetic and

environmental influences on anoexia nervosa syndromes in a population-based twin sample. Psychol Med 2001; 31:737–740.

88. Walters EE, Kendler KS. Anorexia nervosa and anorexic-like syndromes in a population-based female twin sample. Am J Psychiatry 1995; 152:64–71.

89. Kaye WH, Frank GKW, Meltzer CC, Price JC, McConaha CW, Crossan PJ, Klump KL, Rhodes L. Altered serotonin 2A receptor activity in women who have recovered from bulimia nervosa. Am J Psychiatry 2001; 158:1151–1154.

90. Tauscher J, Pirker W, Willeit M, de Zwaan M, Bailer U, Neumeister A, Asenbaum S, Lennkh C, Praschak-Rieder N, Brücke T, Kasper S. $[^{123}I]$-β-CIT and single photon emission computed tomography reveal reduced brain serotonin transporter availability in bulimia nervosa. Biol Psychiatry 2001; 49:326–332.

91. Kuikka JT, Tammela L, Karhunen L, Rissanen A, Bergstroem KA, Naukkarinen H, Vanninen E, Karhu J, Lappalainen R, Repo-Tiihonen E, Tiihonen J, Uusitupa M. Reduced serotonin transporter binding in binge eating women. Psychopharmacology 2001; 155:310–314.

92. Frank GK, Kaye WH, Meltzer CC, Price JC, Greer P, McConaha C, Skovira K. Reduced 5-HT2A receptor binding after recovery from anorexia nervosa. Biol Psychiatry 2002; 52:896–906.

93. Brewerton TD, Jimerson DC. Studies of serotonin function in anorexia nervosa. Psychiatry Res 1996; 62:31–42.

94. Hadigan CM, Walsh BT, Buttinger C, Hollander E. Behavioural and neuroendocrine responses to meta-CPP in anorexia nervosa. Biol Psychiatry 1995; 37:504–511.

95. Kaye WH, Ebert MH, Raleigh M, Lake R. Abnormalities in CNS monoamine metabolism in anorexia nervosa. Arch Gen Psychiatry 1984; 41:350–355.

96. Kaye WH, Gwirtsman HE, George DT, Jimerson DC, Ebert MH. CSF 5-HIAA concentrations in anorexia nervosa: reduced values in underweight subjects normalise after weight restoration. Biol Psychiatry 1988; 23:102–105.

97. Monteleone P, Brambilla F, Bortolotti F, La Rocca A, Maj M. Prolactin response to d fenfluramine is blunted in people with anorexia nervosa. B J Psychiatry 1998b; 172:438–442.

98. Ward A, Brown N, Lightman S, Campbell IC, Treasure J. Neuroendocrine, appetitive and behavioural responses to d-fenfluramine in women recovered from anorexia nervosa. Br J Psychiatry 1998; 172:351–358.

99. Frank GK, Kaye WH, Weltzin TE, Perel J, Moss H, McConaha C, Pollice C. Altered response to meta-chlorophenylpiperazine in anorexia nervosa: support for a persistent alteration of serotonin activity after short-term weight restoration. Int J Eat Disord 2001; 30:57–68.

100. O'Dwyer AM, Lucey JV, Russell GMF. Serotonin activity in anorexia nervosa after long-term weight restoration: response to D-fenfluramine challenge. Psychol Med 1996; 26:353–359.

101. Kaye WH, Gwirtsman, El H, George DT, Ebert MH. Altered serotonin activity in anorexia nervosa after long-term weight restoration. Does elevated cerebrospinal fluid 5-hydroxyindoleacetic acid level correlate with rigid and obsessive behavior? Arch Gen Psychiatry 1991; 48:556–562.

102. Geddes JR, Lawrie SM. Obstetric complications and schizophrenia: a meta-analysis. Br J Psychiatry 1995; 167:86–93.
103. Foley DL, Thacker LR, Aggen SH, Neale MC, Kendler KS. Pregnancy and perinatal complications associated with risks for common psychiatric disorders in a population-based sample of female twins. Am J Med Genet 2001; 105:426–431.
104. Cnattingius S, Hultman CM, Dahl M, Sparén P. Very preterm birth, birth trauma, and the risk of anorexia nervosa among girls. Arch Gen Psychiatry 1999; 56:634–638.
105. Hultman CM, Sparén P, Takei N, Murray RM, Cnattingius S. Prenatal and perinatal risk factors for schizophrenia, affective psychosis, and reactive psychosis of an early onset: case control study. Br Med J 1999; 318:421–426.
106. Hayward C, Killen JD, Wilson DM, Hammer LD, Litt IF, Kraemer HC, Haydel F, Varady A, Taylor CB. Psychiatric risk associated with early puberty in adolescent girls. J Am Acad Child Adol Psychiatry 1997; 36:255–262.
107. Graber JA, Lewinsohn PM, Seeley JR, Brooks-Gunn J. Is psychopathology associated with the timing of pubertal development? J Am Acad Child Adol Psychiatry 1997; 36:1768–1776.
108. Mitchell JE, Hatsukami D, Pyle RL, Eckert ED. The bulimia syndrome: course of the illness and associated problems. Comprehens Psychiatry 1986; 27:165–170.
109. Pyle RL, Mitchell MD, Eckert ED. Bulimia: a report of 34 cases. J Clin Psychiatry 1981; 42:60–64.
110. Russell GF. Bulimia nervosa: an ominous variant of anorexia nervosa. Psychol Med 1979; 9:429–448.
111. Garfinkel, Modolfsky, Garner. The heterogeneity of anorexia nervosa: Bulimia as a distinct subgroup. Arch Gen Psychiatry 1980; 37:1036–1040.
112. Brewerton TD, Dansky BS, Kilpatrick DG, O'Neil PM. Which comes first in the pathogenensis of bulimia nervosa, dieting or bingeing? Int J Eat Disord 2000; 28:259–264.
113. Mussell MP, Mitchell JE, Fenna CJ, Crosby RD, Miller JP, Hoberman HM. A comparison of onset of binge eating versus dieting in the development of bulimia nervosa. Int J Eat Disord 1997; 21:353–360.
114. Haiman C, Devlin MJ. Binge eating before the onset of dieting: A distinct subgroup of bulimia nervosa? Int J Eat Disord 1999; 25:151–157.
115. Keys A, Brozek J, Hentschel A, Mickelsen O, Taylor HL. The Biology of Human Starvation. Minneapolis: University of Minnesota Press, 1950.
116. Polivy J, Herman PC. Dieting and bingeing. A causal analysis. Am Psychol 1985; 40:193–201.
117. Ruderman AJ. Dietary restraint: a theoretical and empirical review. Psychol Bull 1986; 99:247–262.
118. Tuschl RJ. From dietary restraint to binge eating: some theoretical considerations. Appetite 1990; 14:105–109.
119. Raffi AR, Rondini M, Grandi S, Fava GA. Life events and prodromal symptoms in bulimia nervosa. Psychol Med 2000; 30:727–731.

120. Hayward C, Killen JD, Kraemer HC, Taylor CB. Predictors of panic attacks in adolescents. J Am Acad Child Adol Psychiatry 2000; 39:207–214.
121. Ingram RE, Price JM, Eds. Vulnerability to Psychopathology. New York: Guildford Press, 2000.
122. Pine DS, Cohen P, Gurley D, Brook J, Ma Y. The risk for early adulthood anxiety and depressive disorders in adolescents with anxiety and depressive disorders. Arch Gen Psychiatry 1998; 55:56–64.
123. Wonderlich SA, Brewerton TD, Jocic Z, Dansky B, Abbott DW. Relationship of childhood sexual abuse and eating disorders. J Am Academy of Child and Adolescent Psychiatry 1997; 36:1107–1115.
124. Casper RC, Lubomirsky S. Individual psychopathology relative to reports of unwanted sexual experiences as predictor of a bulimic eating pattern. Int J Eat Disord 1997; 21:229–236.
125. Steiger H, Léonard S, Ng Ying Kin NMK, Ladouceur C, Ramdoyal D, Young SN. Childhood abuse and platelet tritiated-paroxetine binding in bulimia nervosa: implications of borderline personality disorder. J Clin Psychiatry 2000; 61:428–435.
126. Dansky BS, Brewerton TD, Kilpatrick DG, O'Neal PM. The National women's study: Relationship of victimization and posttraumatic stress disorder to bulimia nervosa. Int J Eat Disord 1997; 21:213–228.
127. Garfinkel PE, Lin E, Goering P, Spegg C, Goldbloom DS, Kennedy S, Kaplan AS, Woodside DB. Bulimia nervosa in a Canadian community sample: prevalence and comparison of subgroups. Am J Psychiatry 1995; 152:1052–1058.
128. Welch SL, Fairburn CG. Sexual abuse and bulimia nervosa: three integrated case-control comparisons. Am J Psychiatry 1994; 151:402–407.
129. Welch SL, Doll HA, Fairburn CG. Life events and the onset of bulimia nervosa: A controlled study. Psychol Med 1997; 27:515–522.
130. Jacobi C, Paul Th, de Zwaan M, Nutzinger DO, Dahme B. Specificity of self-concept disturbances in eating disorders. Int J Eat Disord. In press.
131. Hettema JM, Neale MC, Kendler KS. Physical similarity and the equal-environment assumption in twin studies of psychiatric disorders. Behav Gene 1995; 25:327–335.
132. Brewerton TD, Mueller EA, Lesem MD, Brandt HA, Quearry B, George DT, Murphy DL, Jimerson DC. Neuroendocrine responses to m-chlorophenylpiperazine and l-tryptophan in bulimia. Arch Gen Psychiatry 1992; 49:852–861.
133. Goldbloom DS, Garfinkel PE, Katz R, Brown G. The hormonal response to intravenous 5-hydroxytryptophan in bulimia nervosa. Psychosom Med 1990; 52:225–226.
134. Jimerson DC, Wolfe BE, Metzger ED, Finkelstein DM, Cooper TB, Levine JM. Decreased serotonin function in bulimia nervosa. Arch Gen Psychiatry 1997; 54:529–534.
135. Kaye WH, Gendall KA, Fernstrom MH, Fernstrom JD, McConaha CW, Weltzin TE. Effects of acute tryptophan depletion on mood in bulimia nervosa. Biol Psychiatry 2000; 4:151–157.
136. Levitan RD, Kaplan AS, Joffe RT, Levitt AJ, Brown GM. Hormonal and

subjective responses to intravenous meta-Chlorphenylpiperazine in bulimia nervosa. Arch Gen Psychiatry 1997; 54:521–527.

137. McBride PA, Anderson GM, Khait VD, Sunday SR, Halmi KA. Serotonergic responsivity in eating disorders. Psychopharmacol Bull 1991; 27:365–372.

138. Monteleone P, Brambilla F, Bortolotti F, Ferraro C, Maj M. Plasma prolactin response to D-fenfluramine is blunted in bulimic patients with frequent binge episodes. Psychol Med 1998a; 28:975–983.

139. Oldman A, Walsh A, Salkovskis P, Fairburn CG, Cowen PJ. Biochemical and behavioural effects of acute tryptophan depletion in abstinent bulimic sub jects: a pilot study. Psychol Med 1995; 25:995–1001.

140. Smith KA, Fairburn CG, Cowen PJ. Symptomatic relapse in bulimia nervosa following acute tryptophan depletion. Arch Gen Psychiatry 1999; 56:171–176.

141. Weltzin TE, Fernstrom MH, Fernstrom JD, Neuberger SK, Kaye WH. Acute tryptophan depletion and increased food intake and irritability in bulimia nervosa. Am J Psychiatry 1995; 152:1668–1671.

142. Weltzin TE, Fernstrom JD, McConaha C, Kaye WH. Acute tryptophan depletion in bulima: effects on large neutral amino acids. Biol Psychiatry 1994; 35: 388–397.

143. Jimerson DC, Lesem MD, Kaye WH, Brewerton TD. Low serotonin and dopamine metabolite concentration in cerebrospinal fluid from bulimic patients with frequent binge episodes. Arch Gen Psychiatry 1992; 49:132–138.

144. Monteleone P, Brambilla F, Bortolotti F, Maj M. Serotonergic dysfunction across the eating disorders: relationship to eating behaviour, nutritional status and general psychopathology. Psychol Med 2000; 30:1099–1110.

145. Steiger H, Gauvin L, Israel M, Koerner N, Ng Ying Kin NMK, Paris J, Young SN. Association of serotonin and cortisol indices with childhood abuse in bulimia nervosa. Arch Gen Psychiatry 2001a; 58:837–843.

146. Steiger H, Koerner N, Engelberg MJ, Israel M, Ng Ying Kin NMK, Young SN. Self-destructiveness and scrotonin function in bulimia nervosa. Psychiatry Res 2001b; 103:15–26.

147. Steiger H, Young SN, Ng Ying Kin NMK, Koerner N, Israel M, Lageix P, Paris J. Implications of impulsive and affective symptoms for serotonin function in bulimia nervosa. Psychol Med 2001c; 31:85–95.

148. Wolfe BE, Metzger ED, Levine JM, Finkelstein DM, Cooper TB, Jimerson DC. Serotonin function following remission from bulimia nervosa. Neuropsychopharmacology 2000; 22:257–263.

149. Spitzer RL, Devlin M, Walsh BT, Hasin D, Wing R, Marcus M, Stunkard A, Wadden T, Yanovski S, Agras S, Mitchell J, Nonas C. Binge-eating disorder: A multisite field trial of the diagnostic criteria. Int J Eat Disord 1992; 11:191–203.

150. Striegel-Moore RH, Schreiber GB, Lo A, Crawford P, Obarzanek E, Roding J. Eating disorder symptoms in a cohort of 11 to 16-year-old black and white girls: The NHLBI growth and health study. Int J Eat Disord 2000; 27:49–66.

151. Dominy NL, Johnson WB, Koch C. Perception of parental acceptance in women with binge-eating disorder. J Psychol 2000; 134:23–36.

152. Rutherford J, McGuffin P, Katz RJ, Murray RM. Genetic influences on eating attitudes in a normal female twin population. Psychol Med 1993; 23:425–436.
153. Klump KL, McGue M, Iacono WG. Age differences in genetic and environmental influences on eating attitudes and behaviors in preadolescent and adolescent female twins. Journal of Abnormal Psychology 2000; 109:239–251.
154. Wade T, Martin NG, Tiggemann M. Genetic and environmental risk factors for the weight and shape concerns characteristic of bulimia nervosa. Psychological Medicine 1998; 28:761–771.
155. Sullivan PF, Bulik CM, Kendler KS. Genetic epidemiology of binging and vomiting. British Journal of Psychiatry 1998; 173:75–79.
156. Burnet PWJ, Smith KA, Cowen PJ, Harrison PJ. Allelic variation of the 5-HT$_{2C}$ receptor in bulimia nervosa and binge-eating disorder. Psychiatric Genetics 1999; 9:101–104.
157. Ricca V, Nacmias B, Cellini E, Di Bernardo M, Rotella CM, Sorbi S. 5-HT$_{2A}$ receptor gene polymorphism and eating disorders. Neuroscience Letters 2002; 323:105–108.
158. Stunkard A, Berkowitz R, Tanrikut C, Reiss E, Young L. d-Fenfluramine treatment of binge-eating disorder. Am J Psychiatry 1996; 153:1445–1449.
159. Hudson JI, McElroy SL, Raymond NC, Crow S, Keck PE, Carter WP, Mitchell JE, Strakowski SM, Pope HG, Coleman B, Jonas JM. Fluvoxamine in the treatment of binge-eating disorder. Am J Psychiatry 1998; 155:1756–1762.
160. McElroy SL, Casato LS, Nelson EB, Lake KA, Soutullo CA, Keck PE Jr, Hudson JI. Placebo-controlled trial of sertraline in the treatment of binge eating disorder. Am J Psychiatry 2000; 157:1004–1006.
161. Grilo CM, Masheb RM, Heninger G, Wilson GT. Psychotherapy and medication for binge eating disorder, Abstract 095. International Conference on Eating Disorders, Boston, April 25–28, 2002.
162. Devlin M. Psychotherapy and medication for binge eating disorder, Abstract Plenary Session. International Conference on Eating Disorders, Boston, April 25–28, 2002.
163. Taylor CB, Altman T. Priorities in prevention research for eating disorders. Psychopharmacol Bull 1997; 33:413–417.
164. Winzelberg AJ, Eppstein D, Eldredge KL, Wilfley D, Dasmahapatra R, Dev P, Taylor CB. Effectiveness of an Internet-based program for reducing risk factors for eating disorders. J Consult Clin Psychol 2000; 68:346–350.

7

Role of Genetics in Anorexia Nervosa, Bulimia Nervosa, and Binge Eating Disorder

Cynthia M. Bulik
University of North Carolina
Chapel Hill, North Carolina, U.S.A.

THE BURDEN OF PLAUSIBILITY

Research on the etiology of eating disorders has lagged behind other areas of psychiatry, in part due to the imminent plausibility of sociocultural theories about the illness. Perhaps more than any other psychiatric disorder, social explanations that focus on Western societies' drive for thinness and beauty ideals as motivators for dieting and symbols of control provide a highly probable explanation for why young girls engage in unhealthy weight loss practices. The face validity of these explanations has inhibited our progress due to a burden of plausibility. The sheer convenient believability of sociocultural explanations has influenced research directions and hindered recognition of the seriousness of eating disorders. The perception that anorexia nervosa (AN) and bulimia nervosa (BN) are volitional disorders has obscured the facts regarding morbidity, comorbidity, and mortality.

The tide is turning. Over the past decade there has been a concentrated effort to advance our understanding of the influence of genes and environment on eating disorders that has resulted in a number of centers conducting highly sophisticated family, twin, and genetic studies. The mosaic of findings has pointed us toward the conclusion that genetic effects play a moderate to substantial role in liability to AN and BN. Less is known about the role of genetics in binge eating disorder (BED), although results are not far behind. The consistency of these findings across centers warrants a recommendation that all practitioners in the field consider developing at least a passing familiarity with their meaning and their implications for etiology, prevention, and management of eating disorders.

This chapter reviews the value and methods associated with family and twin studies, current findings relevant to eating disorders, and implications for prevention and clinical practice.

ROLE OF GENETICS IN ANOREXIA NERVOSA, BULIMIA NERVOSA, AND BINGE EATING DISORDER

Methods of Genetic Epidemiology: Family, Twin, and Adoption Studies

There are three major research designs in genetic epidemiology that allow for the unraveling of the relative contribution of genes and environment to the etiology of complex behavioral traits or disorders.

Family Studies

The first step is to determine whether a trait or disorder runs in families. This question can be addressed by the standard family study, which determines whether there is a significantly greater lifetime risk of eating disorders in biological relatives of individuals who have an eating disorder in comparison to relatives of individuals without eating disorders. If risk to relatives is not increased, then the probability of the disorder being influenced by genetic factors is low. Family studies are limited in that they cannot tell you the extent to which the familial aggregation is due to genes and to what extent it is due to environment.

Adoption Studies

Two additional designs are possible that enable the disentangling of genetic and environmental effects: adoption and twin designs. In an adoption paradigm, one compares the degree of similarity between an adoptee and his or her biological versus adoptive parents. A greater similarity to biological parents suggests genetic effects whereas greater similarity to adoptive parents suggests environmental effects. Although adoption studies are statistically powerful, adoption is rare and many of the assumptions of the method are often not met (e.g., random placement). Moreover, when studying relatively rare conditions such as eating disorders, the prevalence of the disorders is often too low to allow meaningful conclusions to be drawn from adoption studies.

Twin Studies

Twin studies are often the only practical design for teasing out the relative contributions of genetic and environmental factors to complex traits. Monozygotic (MZ) twins emerge from two genetically identical embryos. Therefore, any differences between MZ twins provides strong evidence for the role of environmental influences (1, pp. 171–172). Dizygotic (DZ) twins result from the fertilization of two ova by different spermatozoa. DZ twins are no more similar genetically than nontwin siblings and share—on average—half of their genes identical by descent. Thus, differences between DZ twins can result from genetic and/or environmental effects.

The classical twin study uses the similarities and differences between MZ and DZ twin pairs to quantify and qualify genetic and environmental causes for a particular trait. Using structural equation modeling techniques, one is able to parse liability to a trait into three sources of variability: additive genetic effects (a^2), common or shared environmental effects (c^2), and unique environmental effects (e^2).

Additive Genetic Effects (abbreviation "A"). Additive genetic effects result from the cumulative impact of many individual genes each of small effect. The presence of A is inferred when the correlation between MZ twins is greater than the correlation between DZ twins. For example, the correlation between MZ twins for Body Dissatisfaction from the Eating Disorders Inventory was 0.60 for MZ twins and 0.13 for DZ twins in a study conducted by Klump et al. (2). The fact that the MZ twin correlation was more than twice the DZ correlation suggests that genes affect Body Dissatisfaction as measured by the EDI *in this sample*.

Common Environmental Effects (abbreviation "C"). Common environmental effects result from etiological influences to which both members of a twin pair are exposed regardless of zygosity. Thus, common environmental effects contribute equally to the correlation between MZ and between DZ twins. For example, if the correlation for body dissatisfaction had been 0.61 for MZ and 0.61 for DZ twins, then we would infer that common environment was influencing the trait.

Individual-Specific Environmental Effects (abbreviation "E"). The second type of environmental effect results from etiological influences to which one member of a twin pair is exposed but not the other. Thus, individual-specific environmental effects contribute to differences between members of a twin pair and decrease the magnitude of the correlation between both MZ and DZ twin pairs. In the simplest case, if the correlation between both MZ and DZ is 0, then the trait is entirely determined by individual-specific environmental effects. Examples include one member of a twin pair being exposed to a traumatic experience not shared with the cotwin.

More sophisticated analyses allow one to quantify the relative contributions of A, C, and E. The proportion of variance due to A (additive genetic effects) is a^2 (also known as "heritability"). The proportion of variance due to C is c^2 and the proportion due to E is e^2. The value of e^2 also incorporates measurement error. Finally, a^2, c^2, and e^2 must add up to the total variance of 1.

What Is Heritability? What Isn't Heritability?

The methodology and terminology of twin studies can easily lead to misinterpretation. Heritability estimates are often quoted with little understanding of their meaning or of their limitations.

Allison and Faith (3) discuss a number of ways in which the concept of heritability can be misinterpreted. For example, hypothesize for a moment that a researcher reports in a scientific paper that the heritability of BN is 83% with a 95% confidence interval of 49–100%. Normally, the media are very interested in such findings. Unfortunately, in their attempt to interpret the findings they often lead readers astray. Here are a couple of errant headlines that highlight common misinterpretations.

1. Researchers say 83% of the reason people develop bulimia is genetic.
2. Research says 83% of bulimia cases are caused by genes.
3. If you have the bulimia gene, there's an 83% chance you'll develop bulimia.

Each of these grossly misrepresents what the heritability estimate tells us.

Even more challenging is helping patients incorporate this information into their schema regarding the causes of their illness. The two concepts that are keyto understanding heritability are confidence intervals and variability in liability. Even though the research may come up with a point estimate like 83% heritable, it is critical to pay attention to the confidence interval that bounds the estimate. So it is more accurate to say that between 49% and 100% of the variance in liability to BN is due to genetic effects. The second part of the equation is variance. We all vary in terms of our risk for developing BN. What these results are saying is that genes play a role in determining the extent to which an individual is likely to develop BN (or whatever the relevant trait may be).

Another critical point is that there is not one *true* heritability estimate for any given trait or disorder. It is inaccurate to say "The heritability of bulimia nervosa is 83%." Heritability is a statistic that varies across populations and across time. Kendler and Pedersen (4) illustrated beautifully how heritability estimates can change for a trait over time. They explored the pattern of twin resemblance for regular tobacco use in a population-based sample of Swedish twins. Results for males suggested both genetic and rearing–environmental effects, which, in the best-fit biometrical model, accounted for 61% and 20% of the variance in liability to regular tobacco use, respectively. For women, the pattern differed by birth cohort. In women born before 1925, rates of regular tobacco use were low and twin resemblance was influenced primarily by environmental factors. In later cohorts, rates of regular tobacco use in women increased substantially and heritability estimates were on par with those seen in men (63%). Thus, the genetic influences were only detectable in females once social constraints on female tobacco use were relaxed and smoking became more prevalent.

Family and Twin Studies of Eating Disorders

Family Studies of Eating Disorders

There are now a series of large, well-controlled family studies of eating disorders. The vast majority of controlled family studies (5–10) have found a significantly greater lifetime prevalence of eating disorders among relatives of eating-disordered individuals in comparison to relatives of controls. The relative risk of anorexia in first-degree family members of individuals with anorexia has been reported to be 11.3 (10). That means that relatives of individuals with AN are 11.3 times more likely to have an AN than relatives of controls. For BN, the relative risk in female relatives of probands with BN was reported to be 4.4 (10). Moreover, several studies have found increased rates of both AN and BN, and eating disorder not otherwise specified (ED-NOS) (i.e., coaggregation) in relatives of individuals with AN as well as individuals with BN, compared to rates among relatives of controls (5–10), suggesting that the various eating disorders share transmissible risk factors. Moreover, relatives of individuals with AN and BN have also been found to have a significantly increased rate of subthreshold eating disorders compared to relatives of controls (9,10), suggesting that the eating disorders do not "breed true" but are expressed in families as a broad spectrum of eating-related pathology. Anorexia may have a slightly stronger tendency to aggregate specifically in families; Woodside et al. (11) reported a tendency for anorexia to cluster more in families of probands with anorexia than in probands with bulimia, possibly suggesting some specificity of clustering for anorexia.

Much less is known about the familiality of BED. Brody et al. (12) noted that binge eating is more commonly reported in family members of individuals with BED than in family members of individuals without BED. A small study by Fowler and Bulik (13) found that the percentage of BED individuals who reported at least one first-degree relative with BED (60%) was significantly higher than for those without BED (5%), providing preliminary evidence for the familiality of the disorder.

In summary, family study data reveal an elevation in the lifetime prevalence of eating disorders among the relatives of people with eating disorders. In addition, the coaggregation in families of persons with AN, BN, or milder eating disturbances suggests shared etiological factors across these conditions. Large controlled family studies of BED have yet to be conducted, although preliminary evidence suggests that BED is familial as well. Such studies are important as the demonstration of familiality and the determination of the causes of that familiality have the potential to play a critical role in the ongoing debate of whether BED should emerge as a free-standing eating disorders diagnosis or is best subsumed under another existing condition—the current psychiatric nosology (14–16).

Twin Studies of Eating Disorders.

Given that there have been no adoption studies of eating disorders, we have had to rely on twin studies to separate out the effects of genes and environment on the observed familial aggregation of these traits.

The Equal Environment Assumption

One of the key assumptions underlying twin studies is the equal environment assumption (EEA), which posits that MZ and DZ twins are equally correlated for their exposure to environmental influences that are of etiological relevance to the trait under study (1). In other words, this means that MZ twins are no more likely to have received similar exposure to an environmental factor that may play a causal role in eating disorders than DZ twins. It is well known (and commonly observed by the casual observer) that the environments shared by MZ twins are often more similar than the environments shared by DZ twins. This could include common environments such as sharing a bedroom or dressing alike. Although this suggests a more correlated environment in MZ than DZ twins, the relevant point is that this dimension is not one that is assumed to be of etiological relevance to eating disorders. There are no extant data to suggest that being dressed like one's twin or sharing a bedroom increases one's risk of developing an eating disorder. Violations of the EEA are critical only when the violation occurs in domains that are relevant to the etiology of the trait. Such an example might be if mothers of MZ twins were more likely to put both twins on a diet than mothers of DZ twins.

If the EEA is violated, then the greater resemblance of MZ twins in comparison to DZ twins could actually be due to environmental factors. A violation of the EEA does not necessarily invalidate the results of a twin study but may influence the magnitude of the estimated genetic and environmental components. Studies of the EEA with regard to eating disorders suggest that this assumption has not been violated in twin studies (17–20).

There is more work to be done in validating the EEA in eating disorders research. Many of the existing evaluations of the EEA focus on very global environments. No tests of the EEA have yet been performed that probe into specific environmental factors that may be of etiological relevance to AN and BN (e.g., codieting with your twin, joining activities that promote dieting).

Twin Studies of Anorexia Nervosa

Isolated case reports of MZ twins concordant for AN have appeared sporadically in the literature (21–24). The first systematic study of clinically ascertained twins with AN found that concordance for MZ twins was substantially greater than for DZ twins (25–27). Reanalysis of these data (assuming a population prevalence of AN of 0.75%) revealed evidence of familial aggregation with parameter estimates of 88% for a^2, 0 for c^2, and 12% for e^2. This reanalysis suggested the role of additive genetic effects and some unique environmental effects with no contribution from common environment.

Twin studies of AN have been difficult to conduct due to the low prevalence of the disorder. Because of the relative rarity, each of these studies has had to adopt some strategy to boost statistical power either by broadening the criteria for anorexia nervosa (28), basing the study on a large sample but simply relying on self-report diagnosis of anorexia (29), or exploring the heritability of anorexia in the context of a bivariate twin study paired with a higher prevalence condition such as major depression (30). Although scientifically defensible, having to adopt these strategies underscores the difficulties of conducting sufficiently powered twin studies with rare complex traits.

Reviewing these studies briefly, Wade et al. (30) derived heritability estimates for AN in the context of studying the nature of the comorbid relationship between AN and major depression. The heritability of AN was estimated to be 58%, although the authors could not rule out a contribution of shared environment to the liability to AN due to limited statistical power. Kortegaard et al. (29) conducted a twin study on 34,142 Danish twins based on self-reported diagnosis of AN. They reported heritability estimates of 0.48 and 0.52 for narrow and broad definitions of AN, with no influence of common environment. Finally, Klump et al. (28) estimated the heritability of broadly defined AN to be 0.74 in 17-year-old female twins with the remaining variance accounted for by individual-specific environmental effects.

On balance, we can conclude from family studies (see 31 for a review) that AN is familial and at least preliminarily from twin studies that the familiality appears to be due primarily to additive genetic effects. Before that can be stated with confidence, we will require larger population-based studies or pooling of data across existing twin samples.

Twin Studies of Bulimia Nervosa

Twin studies of BN have been more successful than those of AN given the higher population prevalence of the disorder. Similar to AN, hints of genetic effects on bulimia first begin to emerge with reports of concordant MZ twins in the literature (32). Case series of twins with BN revealed consistently greater concordance for BN in MZ than DZ twin pairs (27,33,34). Pooling data from these case series for twin modeling and assuming a population prevalence of BN of 2.5% revealed evidence of familial aggregation with 47% of the variance accounted for by additive genetic effects, 30% by common environmental effects, and 23% by unique environmental effects. However, the sample sizes were small and the estimates imprecise.

Population-based studies of BN have been conducted in the United States (35,36), Australia (37,38), and via self-report diagnoses in Denmark (29). The studies that have estimated the heritability of BN based on a single occasion of measurement suggest a moderate contribution of additive genetic effects (point estimates ranging from 0.31 to 0.54 with confidence intervals ranging from 0 to 0.86), a negligible contribution of shared environmental effects, and a more substantial contribution of unique environmental effects to liability to BN (29,35,36,38). Despite the higher prevalence of bulimia these studies still had limited statistical power as reflected in the broad confidence intervals (36).

One approach to enhancing statistical power is to incorporate more than one wave of measurement into the twin model. Two studies have successfully employed this approach (36,38). This model (called the measurement twin model) controls for unreliability of diagnosis, increases power to detect both a^2 and c^2, and provides the most reliable information regarding the nature and magnitude of genetic and environmental contributions to latent liability to BN. The results of these two measurement model studies reveal a markedly greater contribution of additive genetic effects to the liability to BN (59% and 83%, respectively), a negligible contribution of shared environment (0 in both studies), and a moderate contribution of unique environmental effects (41% and 17%). It is critical to note that these two studies had greater power to detect both c^2 and a^2. In these studies, the point estimates of a^2 were higher and the confidence intervals suggested a substantial contribution of a^2. The point estimates of c^2 were quite low, but the confidence intervals allowed for the possibility of some contribution of shared environment. In both studies the confidence intervals for the a^2 estimates and the c^2 estimates were nonoverlapping. Thus, by controlling for measurement error and increasing statistical power, it appears that the contribution of additive genetic effects to liability to BN is more substantive than the contribution of common environment.

In summary, from twin and family studies, we can conclude that BN is familial and that there appears to be a moderate to substantial contribution made by genetic factors and unique environmental factors to liability to the disorder. The contribution of shared environment is less certain but appears to be less prominent than the effect of genes and of unique environment. A reasonable next step for twin studies is to determine the precise nature of the unique environmental effects that increase risk for developing BN.

Twin Studies of Binge Eating Disorder

As many of the twin registries were established prior to the emergence of BED as a disorder requiring further investigation in the literature. Much of the existing interview and self-report screenings did not include questions that enable a diagnosis of BED. Two more recent waves of data collection are currently underway which will allow us to address the heritability of BED (39,40). In the meantime, some information regarding the heritability of the symptom of binge eating is available.

Sullivan et al. (20) explored genetic and environmental contributions to the symptoms of objective binge eating and self-induced vomiting by incorporating both behaviors into a bivariate twin model. The prevalences of each of these individual symptoms were higher than prevalences for the full syndrome of BN. Therefore, the power to detect a^2 and c^2 was greater as reflected in the narrower confidence intervals. Two findings from this study are relevant to BED. The association between having ever binged (23.6%) and having ever induced vomiting (4.8%) was very strong [odds ratio (OR) = 8.78, $p \ll 0.00001$]. The best-fitting model indicated that lifetime bingeing and vomiting were both heritable (46% and 72%) and influenced by individual-specific environmental factors (54% and 28%). The overlap between the genetic ($r_a = 0.74$) and individual-specific environmental factors ($r_e = 0.48$) for the two traits was substantial but less than unity. So, what this study tells us that is relevant to BED is first that binge eating as a symptoms is itself heritable, and although the genetic and environmental correlations between binge eating and vomiting are substantial, they are not complete. That is, although there appear to be genetic and environmental factors that influence both binge eating and vomiting, there are also genetic and environmental factors that uniquely influence these symptoms (i.e., they are not perfectly correlated).

USING TWIN STUDIES TO EXPLORE THE RELATION BETWEEN ANOREXIA AND BULIMIA NERVOSA

AN and BN are probably neither completely independent nor completely overlapping conditions. Despite the frequency with which these disorders occur both concurrently and sequentially, we know little about the pattern and predictors of the observed comorbidity. A number studies of the outcome of anorexia have been conducted that specifically address the percentage of patients who have developed BN at the time of follow-up assessment (41–48).

The duration of follow-up intervals ranged from 4 to 22 years, and the percentage of individuals at follow-up who met diagnostic criteria for DSM-III bulimia or DSM-IIIR BN ranged from 8% to 41%. Across studies, the percentage of individuals with BN tended to be greater the longer the follow-up interval. In a pilot study with a very long observation period of 22 years, Hsu et al. (44) reported that 19% of women with AN met criteria for BN at follow-up. In addition to frank diagnoses of BN, 14–36% of women in these studies met criteria for ED-NOS (42,43,45,46) which includes women with bulimic symptoms of insufficient frequency or duration to qualify for a diagnosis of BN. Further evidence for the relation between AN and BN is reflected in the fact that a significant minority (22–37%) of women with BN in clinical samples report a history of AN [(49–54), for example]. Finally, cross-sectional investigations identify a range of symptom combinations ranging from the restricting subtype of anorexia, the mixed clinical picture of anorexia and bulimia, current bulimia with a history of anorexia, and bulimia with no history of anorexia (49,55).

The above clinical studies are all subject to referral bias, which could conceivably inflate the observed frequency with which anorexia and bulimia co-occur either concurrently or sequentially. Arguing against this, however, epidemiological studies of nonclinical populations indicate an elevated odds ratio between anorexia and bulimia (OR = 8.2) (35,56). To date, no twin study has had sufficient power to explore the extent to which genetic and

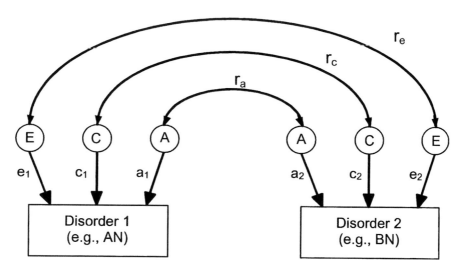

FIGURE 1 Bivariate twin model exploring the nature of the genetic and environmental relation between anorexia (AN) and bulimia nervosa (BN).

environmental factors that contribute to liability to anorexia and bulimia are shared.

Bivariate twin analysis is able to decompose the covariance between two disorders. A bivariate twin model (Fig. 1) decomposes the observed correlation between two disorders into the part due to additive genes, familial environment, and unique environmental influences. These are potentially powerful tools because the degree to which two disorders share genetic or environmental risk factors can have important implications for nosology. This key analysis has not been accomplished in existing population-based studies of twins due to lack of statistical power. By addressing this question in a larger sample, we would be able to address a critical question in the field, namely, what is the nature of the relation between anorexia and bulimia nervosa?

WHY DO WE NOT DETECT COMMON ENVIRONMENTAL EFFECTS IN TWIN STUDIES OF EATING DISORDERS?

One of the most frequently asked questions is to explain the relative infrequency with which common environment has been found to contribute to etiology of AN and BN (57). To understand this it is important to approach the question both methodologically (why is it hard to detect shared environment in twin studies?) and definitionally (what is shared environment and how does it differ from unique environment or from what is commonly termed family environment?).

If we approach the methodological issues first, a quick glance at the point estimates suggests that there is minimal contribution of shared environment in most of the twin studies of eating disorders. As noted above, without the confidence intervals the point estimates can be misleading. In all of the studies reviewed above, the confidence intervals do not eliminate the possibility of a contribution of c^2 to the etiology of eating disorders. However, they do suggest that the contribution of shared environment is substantially less than the contribution of genes.

Second, is possible that "common" or "shared" environment truly does not influence risk of eating disorders and that our results simply reflect reality. Saying that common environment does not influence a trait is *not* equivalent to saying that "family environment" has no influence on risk for the trait. What we casually refer to as "family environment" is composed of factors that qualify both as common environment and as unique environmental features (58), and research strongly suggests that children raised in the same families experience surprisingly different environments (59).

For example, let's assume for a moment that maternal dieting is an environmental factor (although we will illustrate later that this may be a fallacious assumption). Since both members of a twin pair are exposed to maternal dieting, we could conceptualize this as a shared environmental factor. Although the shared component is that both twins were exposed to this behavior, the exposure may be uniquely experienced by each twin. Whereas one twin might climb on board and adopt the behavior herself to try to lose weight and boost her own self-esteem, the other twin might recognize the futility and vow never to become so ruled by her weight and appearance. Thus, what appeared to be a common environmental experience actually exerted more influence through its unique environmental effects.

In addition, the relative absence of shared environmental effects does not mean that the environment does not impact on liability to eating disorders at all. Indeed, all studies have found that a substantial portion of the variance resulted from nonshared environmental factors (57). These unique environmental factors simply appear to be more etiologically relevant than the shared ones.

Also, several observational and self-report studies have found differences between the family environment of women with eating disorders and controls (60–65). The problem with these family environment designs is that they cannot take into account the presence of gene–environment correlations. Many of the variables that are assumed to be "environmental" may be influenced or elicited by features of either the child or the parent that are genetically mediated.

Genotype–environment correlation arises when the exposure to positive or negative environmental influences is not randomly distributed with respect to genetic differences. For example, girls who are genetically more prone to drive for thinness may evoke more intrusive comments about eating and dieting from their parents (evocative gene–environment correlation) and actively seek peers or activities that reinforce their drive to lose weight, such as, ballet or gymnastics (active gene–environment correlation). Another type of gene–environment correlation ("passive" correlation) reflects the fact that children receive genotypes that are correlated with their family environment. This type of gene–environment correlation reflects that one receives one's genes from the same individuals who create one's environment. Moreover, the environment that they create for you is in part determined by their genotype. Concretely, one can imagine a mother with a history of an eating disorder who still has lingering concerns about her own weight who has passed on this genetic predisposition to her daughter. In addition, she contributes to an environment in the household that is highly weight focused by only buying low-fat foods, watching her daughter's caloric intake, and often commenting about the size and shape of her own body. Thus, the daughter is not only dealing with the impact of her inherited genotype; she is also being raised in an environment that may facilitate the expression of that genetic predisposition.

Last, shared environmental factors may be important to the etiology of eating disorders but may only exert their influence in concert with an individual's genetic makeup. Thus, the independent main effect of shared environmental factors may be small, but their effects via one of several types of gene x–environment interactions might be profound (66).

IMPLICATIONS OF FAMILY AND TWIN FOR PREVENTION AND CLINICAL PRACTICE

The upsurge in family, twin, and genetic research has generated enormous interest in patient advocacy and family groups. In many ways these findings have assisted in legitimizing the disorders and have helped to erase an existing prejudice that somehow individuals with eating disorders "choose" to have AN or BN. Results from twin studies underscore that these disorders are no less influenced by genes than major psychiatric disorders such as bipolar disorder and schizophrenia, which are comfortably viewed as biologically mediated in most spheres.

One potential pitfall to be avoided in clinical practice is interpreting these results as genetic determinism. When describing the genetic research to patients and families it is imperative to underscore that the presence of a genetic predisposition in no way guarantees expression of the trait. One way of empowering families over their genotypes is to reframe the concept of gene–environment correlation in a positive light. Some parents develop guilty and powerless feelings about having passed on genes that might increase risk for eating disorders in their children. By emphasizing the fact that they have the ability to influence environment and that environment can serve a protective function as well as an evocative function, parents can begin to see that although there is nothing they can do to alter the passing down of DNA, they can alter environments that influence the likelihood of genes being expressed.

Another important ramification of family and twin studies concerns prevention. Our global efforts at preventing eating disorders have been unimpressive and in some cases have caused more problems than they prevented. Combined, the results of family and twin studies confirm that offspring of women with anorexia and bulimia constitute a high-risk group for eating disorders. Targeted prevention programs could be tested that intervene at several different points along the continuum. The earliest intervention point could focus on enhanced prenatal and postnatal care for women with current or even historical eating disorders. These efforts would focus on healthy and adequate nutrition during pregnancy, dealing with issues that arise as body size increases with pregnancy, developing healthy feeding and parenting styles after birth, and having realistic postdelivery expectations about the resumption of normal body weight (67).

A second preventive option would be to develop programs for mothers with eating disorders or food and weight issues to help them develop tools to model healthy eating behaviors and healthy body esteem and self-esteem to their daughters (and sons). As noted above, although at this stage little can be done to alter the transmission of susceptibility genes to offspring of women and men with eating disorders, we can assist in modifying the environments that these individuals create that may contribute to the expression of those genetic predispositions.

A third preventive option could focus on the offspring themselves. In much the same manner that children of alcoholics are encouraged to delay the onset of alcohol consumption, offspring of individuals with eating disorders could be provided with assistance to avoid the pitfalls of dieting, for developing non-body-centered self-esteem, and other ways to prevent the development of eating disorders.

CONCLUSIONS

We have been aware for decades that family and society influence risk for eating disorders. We have been less clear on how they exert their influence. Family and twin studies have helped us understand the nontrivial role of genes in influencing risk. Somewhat paradoxically, given recent advances in technology, the study of genes has become more tractable and practical than the study of environments. All of the twin studies to date have shown that nonshared environment significantly influences liability to eating disorders (57). We should not abandon research on environment simply because our tools to explore the human genome have become more practical. The environment is amazingly complex and no doubt exerts its influence in myriad often idiosyncratic ways. Nonetheless, a complete understanding of pathways of risk to eating disorders will necessarily require further research designed to identify both the specific genes that influence risk and the specific environmental factors that evoke and inhibit expression of those genes.

REFERENCES

1. Plomin R, DeFries JC, McClearn GE, Rutter M. Behavioral Genetics. 3d ed. New York: W.H. Freeman & Co, 1994.
2. Klump KL, McGue M, Iacono WG. Genetic relationships between personality and eating attitudes and behaviors. J Abnorm Psychol 2002; 111:380–389.
3. Allison D, Faith M. Genetic and environmental influences on human body weight: implications for the behavior therapist. Nutrition Today 2000; 35:18–21.
4. Kendler KS, Thornton LM, Pedersen NL. Tobacco consumption in Swedish

twins reared apart and reared together. Arch Gen Psychiatry 2000; 57(9):886–892.

5. Gershon E, Schreiber J, Hamovit J, Dibble E, Kaye W, Nurnberger J, Anersen A, Ebert M. Anorexia nervosa and major affective disorders associated in families: a preliminary report. In: Guze SB, Earls FJ, Barrett JE, eds. Childhood Psychopathology and Development. New York: Raven Press, 1983:279–284.

6. Hudson JI, Pope HG, Jonas JM, Yurgelun-Todd D, Frankenburg FR. A controlled family history study of bulimia. Psychol Med 1987; 17:883–890.

7. Kassett J, Gershon E, Maxwell M, Guroff J, Kazuba D, Smith A, Brandt H, Jimerson D. Psychiatric disorders in the first-degree relatives of probands with bulimia nervosa. Am J Psychiatry 1989; 146:1468–1471.

8. Strober M, Lampert C, Morrell W, Burroughs J, Jacobs C. A controlled family study of anorexia nervosa: evidence of familial aggregation and lack of shared transmission with affective disorders. Int J Eating Disord 1990; 9:239–253.

9. Lilenfeld L, Kaye W, Greeno C, Merikangas K, Plotnikov K, Pollice C, Rao R, Strober M, Bulik C, Nagy L. A controlled family study of restricting anorexia and bulimia nervosa: comorbidity in probands and disorders in first-degree relatives. Arch Gen Psychiatry 1998; 55:603 610.

10. Strober M, Freeman R, Lampert C, Diamond J, Kaye W. Controlled family study of anorexia nervosa and bulimia nervosa: evidence of shared liability and transmission of partial syndromes. Am J Psychiatry 2000; 157:393–401.

11. Woodside D, Field LL, Garfinkel P, Heinmaa M. Specificity of eating disorders diagnoses in families of probands with anorexia nervosa and bulimia nervosa. Comp Psychiatry 1998; 39:261–264.

12. Brody ML, Walsh BT, Devlin MJ. Binge eating disorder: reliability and validity of a new diagnostic category. J Consult Clin Psychol 1994; 62(2):381–386.

13. Fowler S, Bulik C. Family environment and psychiatric history in women with binge eating disorder and obese controls. Behav Change 1997; 14:106–112.

14. Kendell RE. Clinical validity. Br J Psychiatry 1989; 19:45–55.

15. Kendler KS. Toward a scientific psychiatric nosology. Arch Gen Psychiatry 1990; 47:969–973.

16. Robins E, Guze SB. Establishment of diagnostic validity in psychiatric illness: its application to schizophrenia. Am J Psychiatry 1970; 126:107–111.

17. Klump KL, Holly A, Iacono WG, McGue M, Willson LE. Physical similarity and twin resemblance for eating attitudes and behaviors: a test of the equal environments assumption. Behav Genet 2000; 30(1):51–58.

18. Bulik C, Sullivan P, Wade T, Kendler K. Twin studies of eating disorders: a review. Int J Eat Disord 2000; 27:1–20.

19. Kendler KS, Neale MC, Kessler RC, Heath AC, Eaves LJ. A test of the equal environment assumption in twin studies of psychiatric illness. Behav Genet 1993; 23:21–27.

20. Sullivan PF, Bulik CM, Kendler KS. The genetic epidemiology of binging and vomiting. Br J Psychiatry 1998; 173:75–79.

21. Askevold F, Heiberg A. Anorexia nervosa: two cases in discordant MZ twins. Psychother Psychosom 1979; 32:223–228.

22. Suematsu H, Kuboki T, Ogata E. Anorexia nervosa in monozygotic twins. Psychother Psychosom 1986; 45:46–50.
23. Vandereycken W, Pierloot R. Anorexia nervosa in twins. Psychother Psychosom 1981; 35:55–63.
24. Nowlin N. Anorexia nervosa in twins: case report and review. J Clin Psychiatry 1983; 44:101–105.
25. Holland AJ, Hall A, Murray R, Russell GFM, Crisp AH. Anorexia nervosa: a study of 34 twin pairs and one set of triplets. Br J Psychiatry 1984; 145:414–419.
26. Holland AJ, Sicotte N, Treasure J. Anorexia nervosa: evidence for a genetic basis. J Psychosom Res 1988; 32(6):561–571.
27. Treasure J, Holland A. Genetic vulnerability to eating disorders: evidence from twin and family studies. In: Remschmidt H, Schmidt M, eds. Child and Youth Psychiatry: European Perspectives. New York: Hogrefe & Huber, 1989:59–68.
28. Klump KL, Miller KB, Keel PK, McGue M, Iacono WG. Genetic and environmental influences on anorexia nervosa syndromes in a population-based twin sample. Psychol Med 2001; 81(4):737–740.
29. Kortegaard LS, Hoerder K, Joergensen J, Gillberg C, Kyvik KO. A preliminary population-based twin study of self-reported eating disorder. Psychol Med 2001; 31:361–365.
30. Wade TD, Bulik CM, Neale M, Kendler KS. Anorexia nervosa and major depression: shared genetic and environmental risk factors. Am J Psychiatry 2000; 157:469–471.
31. Lilenfeld L, Kaye W, Strober M. Genetics and family studies of anorexia nervosa and bulimia nervosa. In: Balliere's Clinical Psychiatry, 1997:177–197.
32. Kaminer Y, Feingold M, Lyons K. Bulimia in a pair of monozygotic twins. J Nerv Ment Dis 1988; 176:246–248.
33. Fichter MM, Noegel R. Concordance for bulimia nervosa in twins. Int J Eat Disord 1990; 9:255–263.
34. Hsu GLK, Chesler BE, Santhouse R. Bulimia Nervosa in eleven sets of twins: a clinical report. Int J Eat Disord 1990; 9:275–282.
35. Kendler KS, MacLean C, Neale MC, Kessler RC, Heath AC, Eaves LJ. The genetic epidemiology of bulimia nervosa. Am J Psychiatry 1991; 148:1627–1637.
36. Bulik CM, Sullivan PF, Kendler KS. Heritability of binge-eating and broadly defined bulimia nervosa. Biol Psychiatry 1998; 44(12):1210–1218.
37. Wade T, Neale MC, Lake RIE, Martin NG. A genetic analysis of the eating and attitudes associated with bulimia nervosa: dealing with the problem of ascertainment. Behav Genet 1999; 29:1–10.
38. Wade TD, Martin N, Neale M, Tiggemann M, Trealor S, Heath A, Bucholz K, Madden P. The structure of genetic and environmental risk factors for three measures of disordered eating characteristic of bulimia nervosa. Psychol Med 1999; 29:925–934.
39. Anderson C, Bulik CM. A twin study of binge-eating disorder (in preparation).
40. Reichborn-Kjennerud T, Tambs K, Harris JR, Bulik CM. Gender differences in binge-eating in the absence of compensatory behaviors.
41. Eckert ED, Halmi KA, Marchi P, Grove W, Crosby R. Ten-year follow-up of

anorexia nervosa: clinical course and outcome. Psychol Med 1995; 25:143–156.

42. Gillberg IC, Rastam M, Gillberg C. Anorexia nervosa outcome: six-year controlled longitudinal study of 51 cases including a population cohort. J Am Acad Child Adol Psychiatry 1994; 33:729–739.

43. Herpertz-Dahlman B, Wewetzer C, Schulz E, Remschmidt H. Course and outcome in adolescent anorexia nervosa. Int J Eat Disord 1996; 19:335–345.

44. Hsu G, Crisp A, Callender J. Psychiatric diagnoses in recovered and unrecovered anorectics 22 years after onset of illness: a pilot study. Comp Psychiatry 1992; 33:123–127.

45. Schork EJ, Eckert ED, Halmi KA. The relationship between psychopathology, eating disorder diagnosis, and clinical outcome at 10-year follow-up in anorexia nervosa. Comp Psychiatry 1994; 35:113–123.

46. Smith C, Feldman S, Nasserbakht A, Steiner H. Psychological characteristics and DSM-III-R diagnoses at 6-year follow-up of adolescent anorexia nervosa. J Am Acad Child Adol Psychiatry 1993; 32:1237–1245.

47. van der Ham T, van Strien D, van Engeland H. A four-year prospective follow-up study of 49 eating-disordered adolescents: differences in course of illness. Acta Psych Scand 1994; 90:229–235.

48. Zipfel S, Lowe B, Reas DL, Deter HC, Herzog W. Long-term prognosis in anorexia nervosa: lessons from a 21-year follow-up study. Lancet 2000; 355(9205):721–722.

49. Braun DL, Sunday SR, Halmi KA. Psychiatric comorbidity in patients with eating disorders. Psychol Med 1994; 24:859–867.

50. Fairburn CG, Cooper PJ. The clinical features of bulimia nervosa. Br J Psychiatry 1984; 144:238–246.

51. Pyle RL, Mitchell JE, Eckert ED. Bulimia: a report of 34 cases. J Clin Psychiatry 1981; 42:60–64.

52. Russell GFM. Bulimia nervosa: an ominous variant of anorexia nervosa. Psychol Med 1979; 9:429–448.

53. Schmidt U, Keilen M, Tiller J, Treasure J. Clinical symptomatology and etiological factors in obese and normal weight bulimic patients: a retrospective case-control study. J Nerv Ment Dis 1993; 181:200–202.

54. Sullivan PF, Bulik CM, Carter FA, Gendall KA, Joyce PR. The significance of a prior history of anorexia in bulimia nervosa. Int J Eat Disord 1996; 20:253–261.

55. Herzog DB, Keller MM, Sacks NR, Yeh CJ, Lavori PW. Psychiatric comorbidity in treatment-seeking anorexics and bulimics. J Am Acad Child Adol Psychiatry 1992; 31:810–818.

56. Walters EE, Kendler KS. Anorexia nervosa and anorexic-like syndromes in a population-based female twin sample. Am J Psychiatry 1995; 152:64–71.

57. Klump KL, Wonderlich S, Lehoux P, Lilenfeld LR, Bulik CM. Does environment matter? A review of nonshared environment and eating disorders. Int J Eat Disord 2002; 31(2):118–135.

58. Silberg JL, Erickson MT, Meyer JM, Eaves LJ, Rutter ML, Hewitt JK. The

application of structural equation modeling to maternal ratings of twins' behavioral and emotional problems [published erratum appears in J Consult Clin Psychol 1994 Dec; 62(6):1234]. J Consult Clin Psychol 1994; 62(3):510–521.

59. Dunn J, Plomin R. Separate Lives: Why Siblings Are So Different. New York: Basic Books, 1990.

60. Fallon BA, Sadik MSW, Saoud JB, Garfinkel RS. Childhood abuse, family environment, and outcome in bulimia nervosa. J Clin Psychiatry 1994; 55(10):424–428.

61. Humphrey LL, Apple RF, Kirschenbaum DN. Differentiating bulimic-anorexic from normal families using interpersonal and behavioral observational systems. J Consult Clin Psychol 1986; 54(2):190–195.

62. Humphrey L. Family relations in bulimic-anorexia and nondistressed families. Int J Eat Disord 1986; 5:223–232.

63. Wonderlich S. Relationship of family and personality factors in bulimia. In: Crowther J, Tennenbaum D, Hobfall S, Parvis S, eds. The Etiology of Bulimia Nervosa: The Individual and Familial Context. Washington, D.C.: Hemisphere Publishers, 1992:103–126.

64. Woodside D, Shekter-Wolfson L, Garfinkel P, Olmsted M, Kaplan A, Maddocks S. Family interactions in bulimia nervosa: I. Study design, comparisons to established population norms, and changes over the course of an intensive day hospital treatment program. Int J Eat Disord 1995; 17:105–115.

65. Woodside D, Shekter-Wolfson L, Garfinkel P, Olmsted M. Family interactions in bulimia nervosa II: complex intrafamily comparisons and clinical significance. Int J Eat Disord 1995; 17:117–126.

66. Kendler KS, Eaves LJ. Models for the joint effect of genotype and environment on liability to psychiatric illness. Am J Psychiatry 1986; 143:279–289.

67. Mitchell-Gieleghem A, Mittelstaedt ME, Bulik CM. Eating disorders and childbearing: concealment and consequences. Birth 2002; 29(3):182–191.

8

Psychiatric Comorbidity Associated with Anorexia Nervosa, Bulimia Nervosa, and Binge Eating Disorder

Lisa Rachelle Riso Lilenfeld
Georgia State University
Atlanta, Georgia, U.S.A.

OVERVIEW

The term "comorbidity" was introduced in the medical literature by Feinstein (1) to refer to patients with two co-occurring diseases. In recent years, this concept has become well known in the field of psychiatry. Extensive comorbidity has been documented among a number of psychiatric disorders, not the least of which are eating disorders. Such comorbidity has several important clinical and research implications, as reviewed by Klein and Riso (2). First, the presence of comorbid disorders may affect the course and treatment response of the primary disorder. Second, comorbidity can make it unclear as to whether associations between the primary disorder and other variables are true associations or instead correlations with a comorbid condition. Third, a great degree of comorbidity may lead to reevaluation of the validity of a diagnostic category. That is, it may suggest an alternative diagnostic grouping. Fourth, high rates of comorbidity may provide important information regarding the etiology of the primary disorder, as well as the comorbid disorders.

Klein and Riso (2) provide an in-depth review of the many reasons for which comorbidity may exist. A brief overview of those most relevant to the field of eating disorders will be provided here. The first, possibly least interesting, but important reason for comorbidity that is often overlooked is simply chance. Two disorders with high prevalences will co-occur within individuals simply on the basis of chance due to base rates. While anorexia nervosa is a relatively uncommon disorder with a lifetime prevalence rate of approximately 0.5–1.0% among young females, bulimia nervosa and binge eating disorder are more common with lifetime prevalence estimates of approximately 1–3% and 3%, respectively, among this population (3). A second reason comorbidity may be observed is sampling bias, often referred to as "Berkson's bias" (4). This is particularly relevant in the field of psychiatry, where studies using clinical populations can produce high estimates of comorbidity. This occurs because individuals with multiple disorders are more likely to seek treatment than individuals with one disorder. This bias has often led to higher comorbidity estimates in studies where eating disorder subjects are recruited from treatment centers as opposed to studies in which subjects are recruited from the community. A third reason for comorbidity is population stratification. That is, each of two disorders may be associated with distinct risk factors. If both sets of risk factors happen to have an increased prevalence in the same subgroup of the population (e.g., as has been proposed for bulimia nervosa and substance abuse), the rate of comorbidity is higher than that expected by chance for the population as a whole. A fourth reason is overlapping diagnostic criteria. For example, one of the criteria for borderline personality disorder is potentially dangerous impulsive behavior, among which binge eating is listed. Thus, someone with this symptom would simultaneously partially meet one criterion for borderline personality disorder, as well as for bulimia nervosa or binge eating disorder, obviously increasing the likelihood of comorbidity of the personality disorder and eating disorder. A fifth reason for comorbidity is known as "multiformity," referring to the fact that disorders may assume multiple heterogeneous forms. For instance, the comorbid disorder might be an alternative manifestation of the target disorder. For instance, some have suggested that anorexia nervosa and obsessive-compulsive disorder (OCD) may be alternate forms of the same underlying pathology (5).

The last two reasons for comorbidity, which the majority of eating disorder comorbidity studies have focused on, are among the more interesting. First, one disorder may be a risk factor for another. For instance, it has been suggested that anxiety disorders may be a risk factor for eating disorders (6). The final reason for comorbidity to be reviewed here is overlapping etiological processes. That is, there may be overlapping risk factors that contribute to "pure" forms of each disorder. Thus, the two disorders can appear in their pure forms as well as comorbidly. For instance, low self-esteem and perfectionism may be risk factors for both depression and eating disorders, which would contribute to their co-occurrence. In addition, depression and eating disorders each have their own set of unique risk factors, leading to these disorders often appearing without the other.

As mentioned at the outset of this chapter, the different reasons for comorbidity among eating disorders and other psychiatric disorders are important from both a basic science and clinical perspective. Patterns of comorbidity may help us further refine our diagnostic categories, which have continued to evolve; however, there is general agreement that such categories are in need of further refinement (7). Comorbidity patterns may help to identify taxons, i.e., naturally occurring categories that exist in the world (8), such that our diagnostic system would reflect true relationships among different forms of psychopathology.

Clinically, as much as comorbidity patterns may lead to a better understanding of underlying etiological processes, this may help in our conceptualization model of eating disorders, which may in turn lead to more effective treatment aimed at these etiological factors. Alternatively, or additionally, understanding comorbidity patterns may lead to better identification of risk factors, which may ultimately aid in prevention. At the very least, clinicians who treat eating-disordered patients must be well versed in the most commonly observed comorbid psychiatric disorders in this population, as these disorders should often be a focus of treatment, either separately (as suggested by some in the case of comorbid substance abuse) or in conjunction with the eating disorder treatment (as suggested in the case of comorbid depression). Thus, clinicians must be sure to conduct a thorough psychiatric assessment focused on eating disorder symptoms, as well as comorbid conditions, particularly major depressive disorder, all anxiety disorders, substance use disorders, and cluster B and C personality disorders. Onset patterns, i.e., whether the eating disorder preceded the comorbid disorder(s), may also be relevant to treatment.

The remainder of the chapter is devoted to reviewing comorbidity among anorexia nervosa, bulimia nervosa, and binge eating disorder, beginning with an emphasis on general differences between subtypes in a diagnostic category.

EATING DISORDER SUBTYPES

Anorexia Nervosa

The two DSM-IV diagnostic subtypes of anorexia nervosa, restricting type and bingeing-purging type, display somewhat different patterns of comorbidity. Both subtypes share the same core symptoms (refusal to maintain a minimally normal body weight, intense fear of weight gain, body image disturbance, and amenorrhea in postmenarcheal females). The key difference between the two subtypes is that weight loss is accomplished primarily through dieting, fasting, or excessive exercise in restricting-type anorexia nervosa, without any regular binge eating or purging. In the bingeing-purging type, the individual regularly engages in bingeing and/or purging, so that weight loss may be accomplished through misuse of laxative, diuretics, or enemas, in addition to the methods used in the restricting type.

While some comorbid disorders are common among both types of anorexia nervosa, such as depression and anxiety disorders, other comorbid disorders are found to be associated primarily with the bingeing–purging form of anorexia nervosa, such as substance use disorders. In fact, in many ways, patterns of comorbidity for bingeing-purging anorexia nervosa more closely resemble comorbid patterns for bulimia nervosa than they do for restricting-type anorexia nervosa. Specific comorbidity findings are reviewed in the following section.

Bulimia Nervosa

The two DSM-IV diagnostic subtypes of bulimia nervosa are purging type and nonpurging type. Both share the same core symptoms of binge eating, inappropriate compensatory methods to prevent weight gain, and self-evaluation being unduly influenced by body shape and weight. What distinguishes the subtypes is the compensatory methods used. Purging-type bulimia nervosa involves regular use of self-induced vomiting or misuse of laxatives, diuretics, or enemas. Those with nonpurging-type bulimia nervosa use fasting or exercise, but not vomiting, laxatives, diuretics, or enemas, as compensatory methods to prevent weight gain. Bulimic patients may also use diet pills (e.g., stimulants) to prevent weight gain, although the DSM-IV does not specify this type of compensatory strategy in either subtype definition. If none of the other purging methods are used, then a patient who abuses diet pills as their compensatory strategy of choice is usually classified as having nonpurging-type bulimia nervosa.

Nearly all comorbidity studies of bulimia nervosa have been conducted with individuals who have the purging subtype. Patterns of comorbidity among this subtype of bulimia nervosa often resemble patterns seen with the bingeing–purging subtype of anorexia nervosa. Both disorders share the symptoms of binge eating and purging (though it may be one or the other rather than both in bingeing–purging anorexia nervosa). Thus, it may be this (these) particular symptom(s) that are critical in accounting for the observed comorbidity.

Binge Eating Disorder

As binge eating disorder was only recently defined and included as an example of Eating Disorder-Not Otherwise Specified (ED-NOS) in the DSM-IV, many fewer studies of comorbidity have been conducted than such studies of anorexia nervosa and the purging type of bulimia nervosa. However, comorbidity patterns have recently begun to emerge and may help us to better understand how this disorder may share important features with, as well as be distinguished from, the more well-known eating disorders. Understanding comorbidity of binge eating disorder may not only help our treatment of the condition but may help further refine this diagnostic category, which has been a subject of great debate since its inclusion in the appendix of the DSM-IV as "warranting further study." Thus, refinement of this disorder, specifically regarding the decision as to whether it warrants its own diagnostic category, may be greatly aided by comorbidity data.

PSYCHIATRIC COMORBIDITY

It is well recognized that both anorexia nervosa and bulimia nervosa are often accompanied by other psychiatric symptoms and syndromes, in particular depression, anxiety disorders and substance use disorders. Of great importance in recognizing and studying comorbidity and eating disorders is that these comorbidities are likely substantially exaggerated by malnutrition and pathological eating behaviors (9). Thus, one must always question whether the apparent comorbid presentation of mood disturbance or high anxiety is a function of the physiological consequences of the eating disorder itself. Even if the comorbid disorder predates the eating disorder, it is possible that the mood or anxiety pathology is exacerbated by, if not caused by, the consequences of starvation in the case of anorexia nervosa or erratic consummatory behaviors in the case of bulimia nervosa. In some patients, it is clear that the comorbidity antedates weight loss or disordered eating, or persists after weight recovery or abstinence from bingeing and purging (10–12), suggesting that the comorbid problems may not simply be sequalae of malnutrition or pathological eating behavior. Whether such comorbid pathology enhances vulnerability to the development of eating disorders remains uncertain.

In the absence of high-risk paradigms, unraveling the precise nature of the mechanisms underlying eating disorder comorbidities is a formidable task. Family studies, in which patterns of comorbidity in relatives are assessed, are probably the single most useful means of testing alternative models of comorbidity (2). Several recent family studies (13–15) have shed light on comorbid disorders that may share a common familial vulnerability with eating disorders and will be briefly reviewed. The three areas of comorbid psychopathology of greatest relevance to eating disorders are mood disorders, anxiety disorders, and substance use disorders, all to be reviewed below with regard to what we know about comorbidities of each with anorexia nervosa, bulimia nervosa, and binge eating disorder. In addition, impulse control disorders, schizophrenia and other psychotic disorders, dissociative disorders, somatoform disorders, as well as attention deficit-hyperactivity disorder (ADHD) and disruptive behavior disorders will also be briefly covered.

Mood Disorders

It is well known that individuals with eating disorders often have symptoms of depression. While the reasons for this frequent comorbidity has been a subject of debate, the frequent presence of comorbid depression among individuals with eating disorders has not.

As previously reviewed, there are many potential reasons for comorbidity. First, one must ask whether the rate of depression among people with eating disorders exceeds that expected by a chance association of these potentially independent disorders. The nature of the population under study will have a great effect on the answer to this question. That is, rates of depression among those with eating disorders recruited from a clinic or other treatment sample will nearly always be significantly higher than rates of depression among a community sample of individuals with eating disorders. Most comorbidity studies have been conducted with samples of convenience (i.e., treatment samples) and are thus subject to referral bias, which results in an increased rate of comorbid depression observed. This is likely to occur because people with more than one disorder are more likely to seek treatment (i.e., Berkson's bias). In general, a clinical sample is likely to be more disturbed than an epidemiological sample. Nonetheless, depression comorbidity rates among a clinical sample may be of greatest interest to clinicians, as these are the patients they are most likely to encounter! Thus, comorbidity studies using clinical samples may be of greatest relevance to clinicians treating patients with eating disorders, though it is important to keep in mind that this is just a subset of the larger population of individuals with eating disorders. So, the reasons for such comorbidity remain uncertain and are likely related to sampling.

It is agreed that the presence of depressive comorbidity is very common, but just how common? With the aforementioned in mind, rates of comorbid depression among individuals with eating disorders have been found to vary markedly, again likely due to referral biases. Rates among clinical samples have nearly always been significantly higher than rates observed in nonpsychiatric control subjects. In addition, elevated rates of depressive disorders, particularly major depressive disorder, have been observed among all types of eating disorders. Lifetime rates of major depression appear to be relatively equally distributed across eating disorder subtypes, though there is some suggestion that bingeing–purging anorexic and purging bulimic patients have higher rates of depression than restricting-type anorexic patients (16). It is generally accepted that at least half of treatment-seeking individuals with anorexia or bulimia nervosa will meet lifetime criteria for a depressive disorder, with rates ranging from 24% to 88% (17–25).

Rates of dysthymic disorder have not been consistently gathered in the same way that those of major depressive disorder have, though existing data suggest that this comorbid condition may also be elevated among those with bulimia nervosa (26). In contrast to unipolar mood disorders, bipolar mood disorders appear to be relatively uncommon among this population.

Seasonal affective disorder (SAD) has received quite a bit of attention in the eating disorders field in the past decade. This is because a growing body of research suggests seasonal variations in mood patterns and eating behaviors among patients with eating disorders, particularly those with bulimia nervosa. Patients diagnosed with SAD often demonstrate dysfunctional eating behaviors similar to those found in bulimic patients. In fact, both disorders are characterized by disturbances in eating, appetite, weight, mood, sleep, and energy. Research conducted primarily in North America has estimated the comorbidity rates of winter SAD to range between 27% and 42%, with lower percentages in other seasons (27–30), based on the Seasonal Pattern Assessment Questionnaire. While higher global seasonality scores have been reported among those with various types of eating disorders compared to control subjects (31), most studies have found that individuals with bulimia nervosa specifically are most heavily influenced by seasonality (27,30,32,33). In general, patients with anorexia nervosa show less seasonal mood and weight variation (32). Although most of the research has been concentrated in North America, a Japanese study also cited the greatest seasonal changes in bulimic patients specifically, albeit less seasonal variation in mood and eating behavior than that found in North American patients (33). Neurochemical dysregulation, such as serotonin dysfunction, has been proposed as a possible link between these two disorders (e.g., 34). Phototherapy has been demonstrated to be effective in decreasing depressive and bulimic symptoms for some patients with SAD and bulimia nervosa (35–37).

Some have proposed that depression and eating disorders share a similar underlying diathesis, which may account for their frequent comorbidity (e.g., 38). However, other family and twin study data refute the shared diathesis hypothesis (14,39–41) and suggest that eating disorders are not simply an alternate form of depressive disorder.

Indeed, there has been considerable controversy regarding the direction of the association between depression and eating disorders. In an attempt to unravel the nature of the association, several retrospective studies have found that a significant proportion of individuals have depressive symptoms before the onset of their eating disorder (19,21,25,42). However, a more recent review of this literature suggests that it is more common for the eating disorder to precede the onset of the depressive disorder (43). If this is the case, we must remember the potential role of starvation and erratic consummatory patterns in producing secondary depressive symptoms (9). Thus, in some cases, it is likely that the primary eating disorder may in fact produce, or at least exaggerate, the observed depressive symptomatology.

The role of starvation is of such great clinical importance when treating an eating-disordered patient that the patient should be informed of the likelihood that her mood may improve with weight restoration and resumption of normal eating patterns. It is a good idea to review the details of the landmark Keys et al. (9) semistarvation study with the patient, so that she may appreciate the nature of her mood symptoms as at least partly due to the consequences of her disordered eating patterns.

The treating clinician might summarize the following for the patient: In the 1940s, Ancel Keys and colleagues at the University of Minnesota conducted a landmark study of the effects of semistarvation among healthy young men who were "conscientious objectors" to World War II. These men were carefully screened at the beginning of the study to ensure that they were extremely physically and psychologically healthy. It was discovered that after an imposed period of semistarvation and a loss of body weight comparable to that observed among individuals with anorexia nervosa, these previously healthy young men began to experience numerous disturbing physical and psychological symptoms that had not been present before their weight loss. These psychological and behavioral symptoms included depressed mood, anxiety, ruminative thoughts about food, hoarding, and other unusual food rituals. Thus, the point to emphasize to one's depressed anorexic patient is that the restriction of food and resulting weight loss itself caused such problems in these previously healthy individuals. Weight restoration was subsequently found to reverse these symptoms in most subjects. This is an important point to make to the depressed anorexic patient because, although there is no guarantee, particularly if the patient evidenced premorbid depression, it is still likely that her mood will improve with weight restoration. This same point may be made to the patient with bulimia nervosa, as it is quite likely that the erratic eating patterns inherent in this disorder may cause, or at least exacerbate, similar mood problems. In addition, the bulimic patient, though usually at normal body weight, may in fact be below her expected weight due to food restriction that is commonly observed between bulimic episodes (44). Thus, the same process may apply and should be explained to these patients as well.

All of the previously reviewed mood disorder comorbidity research has been conducted with anorexic or bulimic individuals. Recent studies of individuals with binge eating disorder similarly suggest elevated rates of depressive disorders, but not bipolar mood disorders. Comparable to that observed among treatment-seeking patients with anorexia nervosa and bulimia nervosa, approximately 50% of binge eating disorder patients have been found to have a lifetime history of major depressive disorder and high levels of depressive symptomatology (45–47). In addition, women with binge eating disorder from a non-treatment-seeking sample evidenced similarly elevated rates of major depression compared to control subjects (48).

Although it is more common for people to lose weight during depressive episodes, there is evidence that obese individuals may instead be especially likely to gain weight while depressed. Results from a large epidemiological study of female twins suggests the existence of three clinically significant depressive syndromes, one of which was labeled "atypical depression" (49). This type of depression was characterized by increased eating, hypersomnia, and a proclivity to obesity, which describes the usual presentation seen in binge eating disorder patients. Recent evidence has suggested that this pattern of depression may be familial (49).

As is the case for anorexia and bulimia nervosa, the causal relationship between binge eating disorder and depression is unclear. The Kendler et al. (49) twin study suggests the possibility of a familial tendency toward depression, which is accompanied by overeating and obesity. However, it is important to recognize that both obesity and binge eating may contribute to depressive symptomatology. Onset of binge eating disorder more often appears to predate that of major depressive disorder (50), similar to the onset pattern found with other eating disorders (43). Because obesity is associated with stigmatization in our society, the effects of coping with such prejudice may be depressogenic. Furthermore, the sense of feeling out of control over eating is extremely aversive, and may cause or exacerbate depressive symptoms. In fact, severity of depression among individuals with binge eating disorder has been found to be strongly associated with the frequency of binge eating (51).

Anxiety Disorders

As with mood disorders, most comorbidity studies of anxiety disorders and eating disorders have been conducted with anorexia and bulimia nervosa rather than binge eating disorder, so these findings will be reviewed first. Also similar to that found with mood disorders, lifetime prevalence rates of anxiety disorders vary markedly across studies. Rates of any anxiety disorder have ranged from 23% to 66% among anorexic and 25% to 75% among bulimic individuals (22,23,25,38,42,52–62).

When subtypes of anorexic and bulimic subjects are examined, similar to findings with depression, bulimic symptomatology appears to be more predictive of anxiety disorder comorbidity. Specifically, bulimic individuals have been found to have significantly higher lifetime rates of comorbid anxiety disorders than restricting-type anorexic subjects, whereas anorexic subjects with bulimic symptomatology (i.e., bingeing-purging anorexia nervosa) appear to fall in between the two groups (16).

Two of the specific anxiety disorders that are among the most common in their co-occurrence with both anorexia and bulimia nervosa are social phobia and OCD. Lifetime prevalence rates among clinical samples of patients with anorexia nervosa range from 24% to 55% for social phobia and from 10% to 66% for OCD (14,16,52,63,64). Lifetime prevalence rates among clinical samples of patients with bulimia nervosa range from 17% to 59% for social phobia and from 3% to 43% for OCD (14,16,25,38,52,55,63–65). Two studies of bulimic individuals from the community found a lifetime prevalence rate of 42% to 46% for social phobia and one found a rate of 9% for OCD (24,61).

In making a comorbid diagnosis of social phobia in an eating-disordered patient, it is important to assess whether the patient's social fears are limited to eating behavior alone, as this is not at all uncommon among anorexic individuals in particular. If the fear of humiliation or embarrassment and avoidance is not specific to food and food-related cues, then an additional diagnosis of social phobia may be considered. There has not been much focus on the potential reasons for this comorbidity in the eating disorders literature. The fact that social phobia has among the highest anxiety disorder comorbidity rates in an eating-disordered population may simply be a function of the fact that it is the most common anxiety disorder in the general population as well. Thus far, no twin or family study data have suggested a meaningful etiological link between anorexia or bulimia nervosa and social phobia.

In contrast, much has been written about a potentially meaningful relationship between eating disorders, particularly anorexia nervosa, and OCD. Similar to determining whether a comorbid diagnosis of social phobia is warranted, in this case it is important for the clinician to evaluate whether the content of the obsessions and/or compulsions is restricted to food, eating, or weight concerns. It is very common for anorexic patients to engage in eating rituals, such as chewing one's food a specific number of times or cutting food into a specific number of pieces. It is also common for anorexic and bulimic patients to be preoccupied with thoughts and images about eating and weight loss. Before making a comorbid diagnosis of OCD, it is important to ensure that the "obsessions" and "compulsions" are not restricted to these areas of focus.

Indeed, many anorexic and bulimic patients have additional preoccupations and rituals that warrant a comorbid diagnosis of OCD. Some have suggested that anorexia nervosa is an etiologically similar variant of OCD (e.g., 5) and may best be considered on the obsessive-compulsive spectrum of illness. While this fits with our clinical experience of frequently obsessive and ritualistic anorexic patients, it is not supported by empirical data. Indeed, several family studies of anorexic and bulimic individuals have found elevated rates of OCD among their relatives (14,15,22,66), which initially seemed suggestive of a potentially shared etiology. However, closer examination of the patterns of cosegregation of OCD and eating disorders suggests that these two disorders are actually independently transmitted in families (14,15). That is, OCD has been found to be elevated primarily among the relatives of those eating-disordered individuals who themselves have OCD. Thus, although OCD and eating disorders frequently co-occur within individuals and within families, there is no evidence of a shared etiological factor from family study data. However, recent research suggests the possibility that OCD and anorexia nervosa may both be linked to a polymorphism of the $5\text{-}HT_{2a}$ receptor (67–72), although some studies have not supported this association for either or both disorders (73,74).

In addition to OCD and social phobia, post-traumatic stress disorder (PTSD) is an anxiety disorder of great importance to consider in individuals with eating disorders because it coexists specifically with binge eating problems so frequently. Lifetime prevalence rates of PTSD among bulimic individuals have been found to range from 11% to 52% (14,75–77). Most notably, the National Women's Study, a very large and representative epidemiological sample, yielded lifetime prevalence rates of 37% among women with bulimia nervosa and 22% among women with binge eating disorder (77). Elevated rates of both sexual and aggravated assault among women with bulimia nervosa suggests that victimization may contribute to the development of and/or maintenance of bulimia nervosa. Others have concluded that while PTSD is a common and important clinical variable among women with eating disorders, it may not be directly related to the eating disorder per se but rather to the comorbid depressive, anxiety, and dissociative symptoms that often coexist with an eating disorder (76).

The suggestion that there may be a meaningful etiological relationship between anxiety disorders and eating disorders remains. Because anxiety disorders often precede the development of the eating disorder (25,78), it has been suggested that anxiety disorders may serve as a risk factor for the development of anorexia nervosa or bulimia nervosa. We are currently awaiting more data to confirm or refute this hypothesis.

Anxiety disorder comorbidity appears to be more clearly linked with anorexia nervosa and bulimia nervosa than binge eating disorder. Lifetime prevalence rates of any anxiety disorder in obese binge eaters have ranged from 9% to 46% (45,47,48,79–81). Only one of these studies (45) has found significantly increased rates of anxiety disorders among obese binge eaters compared to obese nonbinge eaters. One issue to consider in reviewing these findings is that the diagnostic criteria used for binge eating in some earlier studies was not DSM-IV binge eating disorder. However, again, all but one study (45) that did use the current definition of binge eating disorder found no significant group differences in lifetime rates of anxiety disorders. All of these studies utilized treatment-seeking samples. One recent comorbidity study of a non-treatment-seeking community sample of binge eating disorder individuals likewise suggests no significantly elevated rates of any anxiety disorders compared with non-eating-disordered overweight women from the community (48). The one important exception to these findings is the National Women's Study, which found PTSD to occur at a rate of 22% among women with binge eating disorder in the community (77).

At present, we can conclude that anxiety disorders are common among anorexic and bulimic patients, though we know less about those individuals with anorexia nervosa and bulimia nervosa in the community. Thus far, the common co-occurrence does not seem to be due to a shared etiologic factor between eating disorders and anxiety disorders, though more family and twin study research would aid in making a firmer conclusion. Individuals with binge eating disorder, including both treatment-seeking as well as community samples, do not appear to have similarly elevated rates of anxiety disorders, with the possible exception of PTSD. However, many fewer studies of binge eating disorder have been conducted compared to anorexia nervosa and bulimia nervosa.

Substance Use Disorders

Substance use disorders are the type of comorbidity where distinguishing between anorexia nervosa and bulimia nervosa is most critical. Individuals with bulimic symptomatology in the form of bulimia nervosa or the bingeing–purging type of anorexia nervosa, have elevated rates of substance use disorders (23,58,82), whereas those with restricting-type anorexia nervosa do not (23,58). Since 1977, more than 50 studies have examined the relationship between bulimic symptomatology and substance use disorders (83–85). In a review of clinical samples of bulimic individuals, Holderness et al. (83)

estimated that 23% had alcohol abuse or dependence. Interestingly, one recent prospective longitudinal study (86) found that anorexic women with bulimic symptomatology were nearly seven times more likely to develop substance use disorders than those with restricting-type anorexia nervosa.

Questions of a potentially shared vulnerability between bulimia nervosa and substance use disorders have been raised, similar to the question regarding the nature of the relationship between anorexia nervosa and OCD, for similar reasons. First, rates of comorbidity are high. That is, a higher proportion of bulimic individuals have a comorbid substance use disorder than would be expected by chance. Second, there is overlap in the clinical presentation, at least among a subset of eating-disordered individuals. Some have written about "multi-impulsive bulimia" (87,88), characterized by multiple impulsive behaviors, such as binge eating, substance abuse, shoplifting, promiscuity, and reckless driving (reviewed below). Many have theorized that this shared impulsivity between bulimia nervosa and substance use disorders may account for the frequently observed comorbidity. Third, there are elevated rates of substance use disorders among the relatives of bulimic individuals (13,89–91). Again, this may be suggestive of a potentially shared etiology. However, closer examination of the patterns of cosegregation of bulimia nervosa and substance use disorders suggests that these two disorders are actually independently transmitted in families (13,15), similar to what has been concluded about the relationship between eating disorders and OCD. This conclusion comes from the finding that substance use disorders are elevated primarily among the relatives of those bulimic individuals who themselves have a substance use disorder. Additional findings supporting this conclusion come from examining rates and patterns of eating disorders among family members of alcohol-dependent individuals (92). Finally, these family study findings converge with multivariate genetic modeling of the large population-based twin study database investigated by Kendler and colleagues (41), in which it was found that bulimia nervosa and alcoholism were attributable to distinct genetic factors.

Thus, although substance use disorders and bulimia nervosa frequently co-occur within individuals and within families, there is no evidence of a shared etiological factor from these family study data. Interestingly, however, data from a large national, representative, epidemiological sample of women suggest that comorbid PTSD may be one explanation for why alcohol abuse so commonly coexists with bulimia nervosa (93).

As has been true for mood and anxiety disorders, while there is a substantial literature demonstrating elevated rates of substance use disorders in women with bulimia nervosa (83) and the relatives of substance-abusing bulimics, much less is known about substance use disorders in binge eating disorder patients and their families. Lifetime rates of any substance use disorder have ranged from 8% to 33% in studies of individuals with DSM-IV binge eating disorder (45,47,48,81,94,95). All but one (81) of these studies found no increased rates among the binge eating disorder group compared to a control group. The first of these studies (45) found no increased rate of substance abuse among obese binge eating–disordered patients themselves but, interestingly, did find an elevated rate of substance abuse in the family members of obese binge eating–disordered subjects compared to those of obese non–binge eating–disordered subjects. Likewise, more recent studies of a non-treatment-seeking sample (48), as well as a treatment sample compared to a general psychiatric control group (95), found no evidence of increased rates of substance use disorders among binge eating–disordered individuals. Thus, most of the modest existing literature suggests no elevated rates of substance use disorders among binge eating–disordered individuals compared to control groups.

In summary, many bulimic and bingeing–purging anorexic patients experience alcohol and/or drug problems, sometimes simultaneously. As a result, eating disorders have often been viewed as a form of addiction. The addiction model of eating disorders is illustrated by the 12-step approach of Overeaters Anonymous and similar treatment programs. One assumption of this treatment approach is that some people are biologically vulnerable to certain foods (e.g., sugar) that can cause chemical dependence; thus, abstinence from these foods is required. A second assumption is that an eating disorder is a lifelong illness that can be managed but never truly eliminated. However, most empirical research does not support these assumptions as they apply to eating disorders and, thus, does not support the notion of eating disorders as a form of addiction like alcoholism (96). More research is needed to understand the reasons behind the co-occurrence of bulimic disorders and substance use disorders, as well as the reasons for the lack of apparent relationship between binge eating disorder and substance use disorders. A final interesting area of future research is the possibility of a protective function against substance use disorders served by restricting-type anorexia nervosa.

Impulse Control Disorders

As previously mentioned, some researchers have described a condition called "multi-impulsive bulimia" (87,88), characterized by multiple impulsive behaviors, such as binge eating, substance abuse, shoplifting, promiscuity, and reckless driving. Indeed, much has been written about impulsivity in women with eating disorders, particularly bulimia nervosa (e.g., 97). It has been suggested by numerous investigators that decreased serotonin functioning may account for such impulsive behavior. In addition to bingeing and purging behavior, a subset of these patients also engage in intentional self-injury (e.g., 98,99). In contrast, there are very few reports of comorbid DSM-IV impulse control disorders, such as intermittent explosive disorder, kleptomania, pyromania, pathological gambling, and trichotillomania, with a few exceptions where shoplifting and other theft were reported in clinical samples (100, 101).

Thus, impulse control problems most typically take the form of substance abuse and self-injury among individuals with eating disorders, specifically those with bulimic symptomatology. Of greatest clinical relevance, such impulsive behaviors are associated with poor long-term prognosis among those with bulimic symptomatology (i.e., bulimia nervosa or bingeing–purging anorexia nervosa), even following treatment (102,103).

Schizophrenia and Other Psychotic Disorders

Investigations of comorbidity between psychotic disorders and eating disorders has primarily focused on anorexia nervosa. Indeed, the delusional nature of the body distortion and fear of fatness among clearly underweight and sometimes emaciated individuals is noteworthy. The general consensus is that in most cases where psychotic symptoms are present, they are likely to be secondary to the eating disorder (e.g., as a result of malnutrition; 9) or secondary to another comorbid disorder rather than a primary psychotic illness. A systematic study of 130 consecutive eating disorder inpatients found that 17 displayed psychotic symptoms (104). Nearly all of these patients' psychotic symptoms occurred in the context of a primary mood disorder. No cases of schizophrenia or organic psychosis were identified. Thus, the psychotic symptoms in each case were attributable to a psychiatric disorder other than the eating disorder, nearly always a mood disorder.

A few early reports describe several patients with both anorexia nervosa and schizophrenia (105,106). However, further examination of these cases suggests that many of these patients actually had major depression with psychotic features rather than schizophrenia (104). Thus, a diagnosis of major mood disorder should be considered likely in any eating disorder patient who displays psychotic symptoms.

It has been suggested that there may be a link between psychosis and eating disorders via the 5-HT_{1c} receptor (107). Likewise, antipsychotic medications, such as olanzapine and risperidone, are now often used in the management of anorexia nervosa, even for patients without clear psychosis, in order to target the delusional nature of body image distortions (108,109). Substantial weight gain is an obvious side effect with interesting implications for the management of a disorder whose hallmark symptom is an intense fear of fatness.

Dissociative Disorders

Nearly all studies of dissociative pathology and eating disorders have examined dissociation as a continuous variable (110–112), as opposed to diagnosable dissociative disorders. Specifically, the Dissociative Experiences Scale (113) is the most commonly used measure for this purpose. Interestingly, however, Waller and colleagues (114) successfully created a more effective categorical measure of dissociation from this dimensional assessment instrument and used it to classify eating disorder patients as "high" or "low" dissociators. Dissociation has been demonstrated particularly among patients with a history of trauma (e.g., 115), self-mutilation (e.g., 116,117), and those who have a psychiatric disorder that involves impulsive behaviors, such as substance abuse and bulimia nervosa (118). It is thought that these behaviors serve the function of allowing the individual to escape from an awareness of intolerable emotional states (119,120). Among eating disorder populations, anorexic patients with bingeing and purging symptomatology and bulimic patients demonstrate the most pathological level of dissociation (118,121).

Somatoform Disorders

Very little empirical research on somatoform and eating disorder comorbidity has been conducted. However, "somatoform dissociation" has been assessed with the Somatoform Dissociation Questionnaire and has been found to be characteristic of patients with dissociative disorders and a core feature in many patients with somatoform disorders, as well as in some patients with eating disorders (122,123). Examples of somatoform dissociation include motor inhibitions and analgesia. It is not surprising that these symptoms are strongly associated with a history of trauma (122).

ADHD and Disruptive Behavior Disorders of Childhood

Little research on these childhood disorders has been conducted in the field of eating disorders. ADHD and disruptive behavior disorders of childhood are considered to be virtually nonexistent among individuals with restricting-type anorexia nervosa, as these individuals instead report having been well behaved, perfectionists, and having excelled in school, all of which are corroborated by family member reports. Some individuals with bulimia nervosa likewise have similar childhood histories. However, some report disruptive disorders of childhood to predate their eating disorder. These are typically individuals who would be classified as having multi-impulsive bulimia. There has been some suggestion that eating might help fulfill the need for high stimulation among individuals with ADHD, decrease agitation, or satisfy a need for control (124). While some recommend screening for ADHD in bulimic and binge eating disorder populations because of the presence of poor self-control and impulsivity in this population, there is little empirical evidence to support the suggested comorbid link.

Interestingly, there is one report of oppositional defiant disorder occurring at elevated rates in adolescents with eating disorders where bingeing and purging symptoms are present (125). In addition, there is one report of an association between eating-disordered behavior and aggressive conduct in adolescent girls (126). Conduct disorder per se was not assessed, but these authors examined a continuous measure of conduct disorder–like symptoms, including robbery and aggravated battery. They found that the odds of involvement in aggressive behavior was significantly higher among those adolescent girls endorsing eating disturbances, including not only bingeing and purging behavior, but also food restriction. This finding contrasts with the typical clinical description of the average eating-disordered adolescent who is usually described as passive, compliant, and rarely aggressive (e.g., 105). Thus, there is little empirical research on disruptive behavior disorders in this population, but there are several reports suggestive of an association between eating disturbance and aggressive behavior during adolescence.

SUMMARY

There are many reasons for the coexistence of two disorders. Reasons for the comorbidity of eating disorders and other psychiatric disorders is under study and much remains to be learned. We know that among clinical samples, elevated rates of depressive disorders, particularly major depressive disorder, have been observed among individuals with all types of eating disorders. In addition, elevated rates of anxiety disorders, particularly social phobia and OCD, have been found among individuals with anorexia nervosa and bulimia nervosa, but not binge eating disorder. Substance use disorders are common among individuals with bulimic symptomatology, in the form of bulimia nervosa or bingeing–purging anorexia nervosa, but not binge eating disorder.

It is important to remember that most comorbidity studies have been conducted with samples of convenience (i.e., treatment samples) and thus are subject to referral bias, which will usually result in higher comorbidity rates than would be found in a community sample. This is likely to occur because people with more than one disorder are more likely to seek treatment (i.e., Berkson's bias). Thus, in general, a clinical sample is likely to be more disturbed than an epidemiological sample.

Finally, it is also important to remember that the comorbidity observed with eating disorders (especially depressive and anxiety disorders) may be created, or at least exacerbated, by malnutrition and pathological eating behaviors. The extent to which such comorbid pathology actually increases the risk of developing an eating disorder remains the focus of ongoing research.

REFERENCES

1. Feinstein AR. The pre-therapeutic classification of co-morbidity in chronic disease. J Chron Dis 1970; 23:455–468.
2. Klein DN, Riso LP. Psychiatric disorders: problems of boundaries and comorbidity. In: Costello CG, ed. Basic Issues in Psychopathology. New York: Guilford, 1993:19–66.
3. American Psychiatric Association. Diagnostic and statistical manual of mental disorders. 4th ed. Washington, D.C., 1994.
4. Berkson J. Limitations of the application of fourfold table analysis to hospital data. Biometrics 1946; 2:47–53.
5. Rothenberg A. Eating disorder as a modern obsessive-compulsive syndrome. Psychiatry 1986; 49:45–52.
6. Fahy TA, Osacar A, Marks I. History of eating disorders in female patients with obsessive-compulsive disorder. Int J Eat Disord 1993; 14:439–443.
7. Westen D. Unresolved issues in the classification, diagnosis, and comorbidity of eating disorders. In: Maj M, Halmi K, Lopez-Ibor JJ, Sartorius N. eds. World Psychiatric Association: Evidence and Experience in Psychiatry. Vol. 6. Eating Disorders, New York: John Wiley and Sons, 2003:34–37.
8. Gleaves DH, Lowe MR, Snow AC. Continuity and discontinuity models of bulimia nervosa: a taxometric investigation. J Abnorm Psychol 2000; 109:56–68.
9. Keys A, Brozek J, Henschel A, Mickelsen O, Taylor HL. The Biology of Human Starvation. Minneapolis: University of Minnesota Press, 1950.
10. Strober M. Personality and symptomatological features in young, nonchronic anorexia nervosa patients. J Psychosom Res 1980; 24:353–359.
11. Srinivasagan NM, Plotnicov KH, Greeno C, Weltzin TE, Rao R, Kaye WH. Persistent perfectionism, symmetry, and exactness in anorexia nervosa after long-term recovery. Am J Psychiatry 1995; 152:1630–1634.
12. Pollice CP, Kaye WH, Greeno CG, Weltzin TE. Relationship of depression, anxiety, and obsessionality to state of illness in anorexia nervosa. Int J Eat Disord 1997; 21:367–376.
13. Kaye WH, Lilenfeld LR, Plotnicov K, Merikangas KR, Nagy L, Strober M, Bulik CM, Moss H, Greeno CG. Bulimia nervosa and substance dependence. Alcohol Clin Exp Res 1996; 20:878–881.
14. Lilenfeld LR, Kaye WH, Greeno CG, Merikangas KR, Plotnicov K, Pollice C, Rao R, Strober M, Bulik CM, Nagy L. A controlled family study of anorexia nervosa and bulimia nervosa: psychiatric disorders in first-degree relatives and effects of proband comorbidity. Arch Gen Psychiatry 1998; 55:603–610.

15. M. Strober. Unpublished data, 2000.

16. Laessle RG, Wittchen HU, Fichter MM, Pirke KM. The significance of sub-groups of bulimia and anorexia nervosa: lifetime frequency of psychiatric disorders. Int J Eat Disord 1989; 8:569–574.

17. Hatsukami D, Eckert E, Marchi P, Sampugnaro V, Apple R, Cohen J. Affective disorders and substance abuse in women with bulimia. Psychol Med 1984; 14:701–704.

18. Herzog DB. Are anorexic and bulimic patients depressed? Am J Psychiatry 1984; 141:1594–1597.

19. Hudson JI, Pope HG, Jonas JM, Yurgelun-Todd D. Phenomenologic relationship of eating disorders to major affective disorder. Psychiatry Res 1983; 9:345–354.

20. Herzog DB. Bulimia in the adolescent. Am J Dis Child 1982; 136:985–989.

21. Walsh BT, Roose SP, Glassman AH, Glades MA, Sadik C. Depression and bulimia. Psychosom Med 1985; 47:123–131.

22. Halmi KA, Eckert E, Marchi P, Sampugnaro V, Apple R, Cohen J. Comorbidity of psychiatric diagnoses in anorexia nervosa. Arch Gen Psychiatry 1991; 48:712–718.

23. Herzog D, Keller M, Sacks N, Yeh C, Lavori P. Psychiatric comorbidity in treatment seeking anorexics and bulimics. J Am Acad Child Adol Psychiatry 1992; 31:810–818.

24. Bushnell JA, Wells JE, McKenzie JM, Hornblow AR, Oakley-Browne MA, Joyce PR. Bulimia comorbidity in the general population and in the clinic. Psychol Med 1994; 24:605–611.

25. Brewerton TD, Lydiard RB, Herzog DB, Brotman AW, O'Neil PM, Ballenger JC. Comorbidity of axis I psychiatric disorders in bulimia nervosa. J Clin Psychiatry 1995; 56:77–80.

26. Gwirtsman HE, Roy-Byrne P, Yager J, Gerner RH. Neuroendocrine abnormalities in bulimia. Am J Psychiatry 1983; 140:559–563.

27. Blouin A, Blouin J, Aubin P, Carter J, Goldstein C, Boyer H, Perez E. Seasonal patterns of bulimia nervosa. Am J Psychiatry 1992; 149:73–81.

28. Ghadirian AM, Marini N, Jabalpurwala S, Steiger H. Seasonal mood patterns in eating disorders. Gen Hosp Psychiatry 1999; 21:354–359.

29. Lam RW, Solymon L, Tompkins A. Seasonal mood symptoms in bulimia nervosa and seasonal affective disorder. Compr Psychiatry 1991; 32:552–558.

30. Lam RW, Golner EM, Grewal A. Seasonality of symptoms in anorexia and bulimia nervosa. Int J Eat Disord 1996; 19:35–44.

31. Brewerton TD, Krahn DD, Hardin TA, Wehr TA, Rosenthal NE. Findings from the Seasonal Pattern Assessment Questionnaire in patients with eating disorders and control subjects: effects of diagnosis and location. Psychiatry Res 1994; 52:71–84.

32. Fornari VM, Braun DL, Sunday SR, et al. Seasonal patterns in eating disorder subgroups. Compr Psychiatry 1994; 35:450–456.

33. Yamatsuji M, Yamashita T, Arii I, Taga C, Tatara N, Fukui K. Seasonal variations in eating disorder subtypes in Japan. Int J Eat Disord 2003; 33:71–77.

34. Brewerton TD, Brandt HA, Lesem MD, Murphy DL, Jimerson DC. Serotonin in eating disorders. In: Coccaro EF, Murphy DL, eds. Serotonin in Major Psychiatric Disorders. Spiefel D, ed. Progress in Psychiatry Monograph Series. Washington, DC: American Psychiatric Press, 1990:153–184.

35. Lam RW, Lee SK, Tam EM, Grewal A, Yatham LN. An open trial of light therapy for women with seasonal affective disorder and comorbid bulimia nervosa. J Clin Psychiatry 2001; 62:164–168.

36. Braun DL, Sunday SR, Fornari VM, Halmi KA. Bright light therapy decreases winter binge frequency in women with bulimia nervosa: a double-blind, placebo-controlled study. Compr Psychiatry 1999; 40:442–448.

37. Blouin AG, Blouin JH, Iversen H, Carter J, Goldstein C, Goldfield G, Perez E. Light therapy in bulimia nervosa: a double-blind placebo-controlled study. Psychiatry Res 1996; 60:1–9.

38. Hudson JI, Pope HG, Yurgelun-Todd D, Jonas JM, Frankenburg FR. A controlled study of lifetime prevalence of affective and other psychiatric disorders in bulimic outpatients. Am J Psychiatry 1987; 144:1283–1287.

39. Strober M, Lampert C, Morrell W, Burroughs J, Jacobs C. A controlled family study of anorexia nervosa: evidence of familial aggregation and lack of shared transmission with affective disorders. Int J Eat Disord 1990; 9:239–253.

40. Biederman J, Rivinus T, Kemper K, Hamilton D, MacFayden J, Harmatz J. Depressive disorders in relatives of anorexia nervosa patients with and without a current episode of nonbipolar major depression. Am J Psychiatry 1985; 142:1495–1496.

41. Kendler KS, Walters EE, Neale MC, Kessler RC, Heath AC, Eaves LJ. The structure of the genetic and environmental risk factors for six major psychiatric disorders in women. Arch Gen Psychiatry 1995; 52:374–383.

42. Piran N, Kennedy S, Garfinkel PE, Owens M. Affective disturbance in eating disorders. J Nerv Ment Dis 1985; 173:395–400.

43. Cooper PJ. Eating disorders and their relationship to mood and anxiety disorders. In: Brownell KD, Fairburn CG, eds. Eating Disorders and Obesity: A Comprehensive Handbook. New York: Guilford Press, 1995:159–164.

44. Vitousek K, Manke F. Personality variables and disorders in anorexia nervosa and bulimia nervosa. J Abnorm Psychol 1994; 103:137–147.

45. Yanovski SZ, Nelson JE, Dubbert BK, Spitzer RL. Association of binge eating disorder and psychiatric comorbidity in the obese. Am J Psychiatry 1993; 150:1472–1479.

46. Marcus MD, Wing RR, Ewing L, Kern E, Gooding W, McDermott M. Psychiatric disorders among obese binge eaters. Int J Eat Disord 1990; 9:69–77.

47. Specker S, de Zwaan M, Raymond N, Mitchell J. Psychopathology in subgroups of obese women with and without binge eating disorder. Compr Psychiatry 1994; 35:185–190.

48. Telch CF, Stice E. Psychiatric comorbidity in women with binge eating disorder: prevalence rates from a non-treatment-seeking sample. J Consult Clin Psychol 1998; 66:768–776.

49. Kendler KS, Eaves LJ, Walters EE, Neale MC, Heath AC, Kessler RC. The

identification and validation of distinct depressive syndromes in a population-based sample of female twins. Arch Gen Psychiatry 1996; 53:391–399.

50. Mussell MP, Mitchell JE, Weller CL, Raymond NC, Crow SJ, Crosby RD. Onset of binge eating, dieting, obesity, and mood disorders among subjects seeking treatment for binge eating disorder. Int J Eat Disord 1995; 17:395–401.

51. Smith DE, Marcus MD, Lewis C, Fitzgibbon M, Schreiner P. Prevalence of binge eating disorder, obesity and depression in a biracial cohort of young adults. Ann Behav Med 1998; 20:227–232.

52. Fornari V, Kaplan M, Sandberg DE, Mathews M, Skolnick N, Katz JL. Depressive and anxiety disorders in anorexia nervosa and bulimia nervosa. Int J Eat Disord 1992; 12:21–29.

53. Laessle RG, Kittl S, Fichter MM, Wittchen H, Pirke KM. Major affective disorder in anorexia nervosa and bulimia: a descriptive diagnostic study. Br J Psychiatry 1987; 151:785–789.

54. Toner BB, Garfinkel PE, Garner DM. Affective and anxiety disorders in the long-term follow-up of anorexia nervosa. Int J Psychiatry Med 1988; 18:357–364.

55. Schwalberg MD, Barlow DH, Alger SA, Howard LJ. Comparison of bulimics, obese binge eaters, social phobics, and individuals with panic disorder on comorbidity across DSM-III-R anxiety disorders. J Abnorm Psychol 1992; 101:675–681.

56. Smith C, Feldman SS, Nasserbakht A, Steiner H. Psychological characteristics and DSM-III-R diagnoses at 6-year follow-up of adolescent anorexia nervosa. J Am Acad Child Adol Psychiatry 1993; 32:1237–1245.

57. Bossert-Zaudig S, Zaudig M, Junker M, Wiegand M, Krieg JC. Psychiatric comorbidity of bulimia nervosa inpatients: relationship to clinical variables and treatment outcome. Eur Psychiatry 1993; 8:15–23.

58. Braun DL, Sunday S, Halmi KA. Psychiatric comorbidity in patients with eating disorders. Psychol Med 1994; 24:859–867.

59. Deep AL, Nagy LM, Weltzin TE, Rao R, Kaye WH. Premorbid onset of psychopathology in long-term recovered anorexia nervosa. Int J Eat Disord 1995; 17:291–297.

60. Thiel A, Broocks A, Ohlmeier M, Jacoby GE, Schussler G. Obsessive-compulsive disorder among patients with anorexia nervosa and bulimia nervosa. Am J Psychiatry 1995; 152:72–75.

61. Garfinkel PE, Lin E, Goering P, Speff C, Goldbloom DS, Kennedy S, Kaplan AS, Woodside DB. Bulimia nervosa in a Canadian community sample: prevalence and comparison of subgroups. Am J Psychiatry 1995; 152:1052–1058.

62. Keck PE Jr, Pope HG Jr, Hudson JI, McElroy SL, Yurgelun-Todd D, Hundert EM. A controlled study of phenomenology and family history in outpatients with bulimia nervosa. Compr Psychiatry 1990; 31:275–283.

63. Thornton C, Russell J. Obsessive compulsive comorbidity in the dieting disorders. Int J Eat Disord 1997; 21:83–87.

64. Godart NT, Flament MF, Lecrubier Y, Jeammet P. Anxiety disorders in ano-

rexia nervosa and bulimia nervosa: comorbidity and chronology of appearance. Eur Psychiatry 2000; 15:38–45.

65. Powers PS, Coovert DL, Brightwell DR, Stevens BA. Other psychiatric disorders among bulimic patients. Compr Psychiatry 1988; 29:503–508.
66. Pasquale L, Sciuto G, Cocchi S, Ronshi P, Billodi L. A family study of obsessive compulsive, eating, and mood disorders. Eur Psychiatry 1994; 9:33–38.
67. Collier DA, Arranz MJ, Li T, Mupita D, Brown N, Treasure J. Association between 5-HT$_{2A}$ gene promoter polymorphism and anorexia nervosa. Lancet 1994; 350:412.
68. Hinney A, Ziegler A, Nothen MM, Remschmidt H, Hebebrand J. 5-HT$_{2A}$ receptor gene polymorphisms, anorexia nervosa, and obesity. Lancet 1997; 350: 1324–1325.
69. Enoch MA, Kaye WH, Rotondo A, Greenberg BD, Murphy DL, Goldman D. 5-HT$_{2A}$ promoter polymorphism -1438G/A, anorexia nervosa, and obsessive-compulsive disorder. Lancet 1998; 351:1785–1786.
70. Sorbi S, Nacmias B, Tedde A, Ricca V, Mezzani B, Rotella CM. 5-HT$_{2A}$ promoter polymorphism in anorexia nervosa. Lancet 1998; 351:1785.
71. Nacmias B, Ricca V, Tedde A, Mezzani B, Rotella CM, Sorbi S. 5-HT$_{2A}$ receptor gene polymorphisms in anorexia nervosa and bulimia nervosa. Neurosci Lett 1999; 277:134–136.
72. Nishiguchi N, Matsushita S, Suzuki K, Muryama M, Shirakawa O, Higuchi S. Association between 5HT$_{2A}$ receptor gene promoter region polymorphism and eating disorders in Japanese patients. Biol Psychiatry 2001; 50:123–128.
73. Ziegler A, Hebebrand J, Gorg T, Rosenkranz K, Fichter MM, Herpertz-Dahlmann B, Remschmidt H, Hinney A. Further lack of association between the 5-HT$_{2A}$ gene promoter polymorphism and susceptibility to eating disorders and a meta-analysis pertaining to anorexia nervosa. Mol Psychiatry 1999; 4: 410–412.
74. Karwautz A, Rabe-Hesketh S, Hu X, Zhao J, Sham P, Collier DA, Treasure JL. Individual-specific risk factors for anorexia nervosa: a pilot study using a discordant sister-pair design. Psychol Med 2001; 31:317–329.
75. Turnbull SJ, Troop NA, Treasure JL. The prevalence of post-traumatic stress disorder and its relation to childhood adversity in subjects with eating disorders. Eur Eating Dis Rev 1997; 5:270–277.
76. Gleaves DH, Eberenz KP, May MC. Scope and significance of posttraumatic symptomatology among women hospitalized for an eating disorder. Int J Eat Disord 1998; 24:147–156.
77. Dansky BS, Brewerton TD, Kirkpatrick DG, O'Neil PM. The National Women's Study: relationship victimization and posttraumatic stress disorder to bulimia nervosa. Int J Eat Disord 1997; 21:213–228.
78. Bulik CM, Sullivan PF, Fear JL, Joyce PR. Eating disorders and antecedent anxiety disorders: a controlled study. Acta Psychiatr Scand 1997; 96:101–107.
79. Hudson JI, Pope HG Jr, Yurgelun-Todd D. Bulimia and major affective disorder: experience with 105 patients. Psychiatr Psychobiol 1988; 3:37–47.
80. de Zwaan M, Nutzinger DO, Schoenbeck G. Binge eating in overweight women. Compr Psychiatry 1992; 33:256–261.

81. Mussell MP, Mitchell JE, de Zwaan M, Crosby RD, Seim HC, Crow SJ. Clinical characteristics associated with binge eating in obese females: a descriptive study. Int J Obes Relat Metab Disorders 1996; 20:324–331.

82. Bulik CM, Sullivan PF, Epstein LH, McKee M, Kaye WH, Dahl RE, Weltzin TE. Drug use in women with anorexia and bulimia nervosa. Int J Eat Disord 1992; 11:213–225.

83. Holderness CC, Brooks-Gunn J, Warren WP. Co-morbidity of eating disorders and substance abuse. Int J Eat Disord 1994; 16:1–34.

84. Krahn DD. The relationship of eating disorders and substance abuse. J Subst Abuse 1991; 3:239–253.

85. Wilson GT. The addiction model of eating disorders: a critical analysis. Adv Behav Res Ther 1991; 13:27–72.

86. Strober M, Freeman R, Bower S, Rigali J. Binge eating in anorexia nervosa predicts later onset of substance use disorder: a ten-year prospective, longitudinal follow-up of 96 adolescents. J Youth Adol 1996; 25:519–532.

87. Lacey J, Evans C. The impulsivist: a multi-impulsive personality disorder. Br J Addict 1986; 81:641–649.

88. Fichter MM, Quadflieg N, Rief W. Course of multi-impulsive bulimia. Psychol Med 1994; 24:591–604.

89. Lilenfeld LR, Kaye WH, Greeno CG, Merikangas KR, Plotnicov K, Pollice C, Rao R, Strober M, Bulik CM, Nagy L. Psychiatric disorders in women with bulimia nervosa and their first-degree relatives. Int J Eat Disord 1997; 22:253–264.

90. Bulik CM. Family histories of bulimic women with and without comorbid alcohol abuse or dependence. Am J Psychiatry 1991; 148:1267–1268.

91. Mitchell JE, Hatsukami D, Pyle R, Eckert E. Bulimia with and without a family history of drug abuse. Addict Behav 1988; 12:245–251.

92. Schuckit MA, Tipp JE, Anthenelli RM, Bucholz KK, Hesselbrock VM, Nurnberger JI. Anorexia nervosa and bulimia nervosa in alcohol-dependent men and women and their relatives. Am J Psychiatry 1996; 153:74–82.

93. Dansky BS, Brewerton TD, Kilpatrick DG. Comorbidity of bulimia nervosa and alcohol use disorders: results from the National Women's Study. Int J Eat Disord 2000; 27:180–190.

94. Brody MJ, Walsh BT, Devlin MJ. Binge eating disorder: reliability and validity of a new diagnostic category. J Consult Clin Psychol 1994; 62:381–386.

95. Wilfley DE, Friedman MA, Dounchis JZ, Stein RI, Welch RR, Ball SA. Comorbid psychopathology in binge eating disorder: relation to eating disorder severity at baseline and following treatment. J Consult Clin Psychol 2000; 68: 641–649.

96. Wilson GT. Eating disorders and addictive disorders. In: Brownell KD, Fairburn CG, eds. Eating Disorders and Obesity: A Comprehensive Handbook. New York: Guilford Press, 1995:165–170.

97. Steiger H, Lehoux PM, Gauvin L. Impulsivity, dietary control and the urge to binge in bulimic syndromes. Int J Eat Disord 1999; 26:261–274.

98. Favaro A, Santonastaso P. Impulsive and compulsive self-injurious behavior in bulimia nervosa: prevalence and psychological correlates. J Nerv Ment Dis 1998; 186:157–165.

99. Lledo EP, Waller G. Bulimic psychopathology and impulsive behaviors among nonclinical women. Int J Eat Disord 2001; 29:71–75.

100. Bridgeman J, Slade PD. Shoplifting and eating disorders: a psychological medical-legal perspective. Eur Eat Dis Rev 1996; 4:133–148.

101. Penas-Lledo E, Vaz FJ, Ramos MI, Waller G. Impulsive behaviors in bulimic patients: relation to general psychopathology. Int J Eat Disord 2002; 32:98–102.

102. Agras WS, Crow SJ, Halmi KA, Mitchell JE, Wilson GT, Kraemer HC. Outcome predictors for the cognitive behavior treatment of bulimia nervosa: data from a multisite study. Am J Psychiatry 2000; 157:1302–1308.

103. Sohlberg S, Norring C, Holmgren S, Rosmark B. Impulsivity and long-term prognosis of psychiatric patients with anorexia nervosa/bulimia nervosa. J Nerv Ment Dis 1989; 177:249–258.

104. Hudson JI, Pope HG Jr, Jonas JM. Psychosis in anorexia nervosa and bulimia. Br J Psychiatry 1984; 145:420–423.

105. Bruch H. Eating Disorders: Obesity, Anorexia Nervosa and the Person Within. New York: Basic Books, 1973.

106. Hsu LKG, Meltzer ES, Crisp AH. Schizophrenia and anorexia nervosa. J Nerv Ment Dis 1981; 169:273–276.

107. Salmon G. Atypical anorexia nervosa and schizophrenia: are they linked by the 5-HT$_{1c}$ receptor? Eur Eat Disord Rev 1996; 4:189–194.

108. Lavia MC, Gray N, Kaye WH. Case reports of olanzapine treatment of anorexia nervosa. Int J Eat Disord 2000; 27:363–366.

109. Newman-Toker J. Risperidone in anorexia nervosa. J Am Acad Child Adol Psychiatry 2000; 39:941–942.

110. Everill JT, Waller G, MacDonald W. Dissociation in bulimic and non-eating disordered women. Int J Eat Disord 1995; 17:127–134.

111. Everill JT, Waller G. Dissociation and bulimia: research and theory. Eur Eat Dis Rev 1995; 3:129–147.

112. Vanderlinden J, Vandereycken W, van Dyck R, Vertommen H. Dissociative experiences and trauma in eating disorders. Int J Eat Disord 1993; 13:187–193.

113. Carlson EB, Putnam FW. An update on the dissociative experiences scale. Dissociation 1993; 6:16–27.

114. Waller NG, Putnma FW, Carlson EB. Types of dissociation and dissociative types: a taxometric analysis of dissociative experiences. Psychol Measures 1996; 1:300–321.

115. van der Kolk BA, Pelcovitz D, Roth S, Mandel FS, McFarlane A, Herman JL. Dissociation, somatization, and affect dysregulation: the complexity of adaptation to trauma. Am J Psychiatry 1996; 153:83–93.

116. Shearer SL. Dissociative phenomena in women with borderline personality disorder. Am J Psychiatry 1994; 151:1324–1328.

117. Brodsky BS, Cloitre M, Dulit RA. Relationship of dissociation to self mutilation and childhood abuse in borderline personality disorder. Am J Psychiatry 1995; 152:1788–1792.

118. Waller G, Ohanian V, Meyer C, Everill J, Rouse H. The utility of dimensional

and categorical approaches to understanding dissociation in the eating disorders. Br J Clin Psychol 2001; 40:387–397.

119. Baumeister R, Heatherton T, Tice D. Losing Control: How and Why People Fail at Self-Regulation. London: Academic Press, 1994.
120. Suycmoto KL. The functions of self-mutilation. Clin Psychol Rev 1998; 18:531–554.
121. Nagata T, Kiriike N, Iketani T, Kawarada Y, Tanaka H. History of childhood sexual or physical abuse in Japanese patients with eating disorders: relationship with dissociation and impulsive behaviors. Psychol Med 1999; 29:935–942.
122. Nijenhuis ERS. Somatoform dissociation: major symptoms of dissociative disorders. J Trauma Dissoc 2000; 1:7–32.
123. Zerbe KJ, Giorgio C. Whose body is it anyway? Understanding and treating psychosomatic aspects of eating disorders. Rev Psychoanal Meth Res Clin Exp 1999; 6:13–32.
124. Fleming J, Levy L. Eating disorders in women with AD/HD. In: Quinn P, Nadeau K, eds. Gender Issues and AD/HD: Research, Diagnosis, and Treatment. Silver Spring, MD: Advantage Books, 2002.
125. Geist R, Davis R, Heinmaa M. Binge/purge symptoms and comorbidity in adolescents with eating disorders. Can J Psychiatry 1998; 43:507–512.
126. Thompson KM, Wonderlich SA, Crosby RD, Mitchell JE. The neglected link between eating disturbances and aggressive behavior in girls. J Am Acad Child Adol Psychiatry 1999; 38:1277–1284.

9

Personality Traits and Disorders Associated with Anorexia Nervosa, Bulimia Nervosa, and Binge Eating Disorder

Howard Steiger and Kenneth R. Bruce
Douglas Hospital and McGill University
Montreal, Quebec, Canada

In 1689, Thomas Morton reported two cases of anorexia nervosa (AN): one involving a "sad and anxious" girl who "poured over books," another involving a young boy prone to "studying too hard" (1). With these reports, Morton not only introduced AN to the medical literature; he introduced the concept that AN frequently co-occurs with perfectionistic or compulsive personality traits. Likewise, 19th century observations on bulimia nervosa (BN) documented instability of mood and behavior (2). All of this says that there is a history behind the association between eating disorders (EDs) and problematic personality tendencies.

The connection may not be new, but many questions remain: Is there an ED-prone personality type? Do AN and BN coincide with different personality characteristics? Do EDs always involve personality problems? In this chapter, we study personality traits and disorders in AN, BN, and binge eating disorder (BED). We examine the coaggregation of eating symptoms with personality trait variations and evidence that such co-occurrence involves shared developmental, familial, neurobiological, and hereditary pathways. We also discuss the bearing of personality pathology, in the EDs, for clinical typology, treatment needs, and prognosis.

EATING AND PERSONALITY PATHOLOGIES

Personality "traits" refer to enduring patterns of perception, thought, and feeling. Traits are presumed to exist on a continuum (from absent to strongly present) and are believed to structure feelings, actions, and reactions in predictable ways across situations (3). For example, someone who regularly worries about things going wrong might be said to display "trait anxiety." Personality "disorders" (PDs) also represent stable (or frequently recurring) patterns of inner experience and behavior. However, they imply more pervasive anomalies that adversely and profoundly affect thought, mood, behavior, and social functioning (3). PDs are conceived to be categorical (i.e., present or absent) and to involve a systematic convergence of tendencies (e.g., mood lability, impulsivity, and interpersonal instability).

Personality Traits in the EDs

The first formal psychometric studies on the EDs were published in the mid-1970s. These reports (on AN, at the time) led to emphasis on various traits—obsessionality, social anxiety, introversion, "neuroticism," and depression. These same reports introduced a distinction between an ED subtype characterized solely by restriction of food intake (the "restricters") and variants implicating binge eating and purging (the "bingers–purgers"). AN, restricting subtype (AN-R) was associated with a "conforming, obsessional, and emotionally and socially reserved" personality stereotype, whereas AN/binge–purge subtype (AN-BP) was linked with a more dramatic psychopathology, with an "impulsive, antisocial, or externalizing" flavor (4). Later studies on BN broadened the boundaries of a hypothetical association between binge eating and impulsive/erratic characteristics (5)—and the stage was set for belief in a systematic distinction, as to associated personality characteristics, between "restrictive" ED variants (i.e., AN-R) and "binger–purger" variants (exemplified by BN or AN-BP).

   Although fit proves to be imperfect, contemporary studies generally corroborate the "restricter/binger difference" concept: With the Multidimensional Personality Questionnaire, Casper and colleagues (6) found greater self-control, conscientiousness, and emotional inhibition in AN-R than in BN or AN-BP. Norman and colleagues (7), using the Millon Clinical Multiaxial Inventory, found Avoidant personality traits to predominate in AN-R, and Histrionic traits in BN or AN-BP. Partially "echoing" such tendencies, studies applying the Tridimensional Personality Questionnaire (TPQ) have reported normal-weight bulimics to display elevated novelty seeking relative to restricter anorexics (8,9). However, results on TPQ dimensions of Harm Avoidance and Reward Dependence have not lent themselves to simple interpretation within a restricter/binger difference framework. Using a comparable scale, the Temperament and Character Inventory (TCI), Diaz-Marsa and colleagues (10) found anorexic patients to have stronger loadings on a measure of persistence (largely "compulsive" personality) than bulimics, whereas bulimics showed more impulsivity. Finally, bingers have been reported to display more ideational disturbances and more anger than restricters on the Minnesota Multiphasic Personality Inventory 2 (MMPI-2) (11). The preceding supports belief in a systematic coaggregation (at a group level) between AN-R and perfectionistic, approval seeking, or compulsive traits, on the one hand, and between binger–purger ED variants (AN-BP and BN) and impulsivity, emotionality, or risk taking on the other. However, a caveat is needed: "Average" traits in diagnostic subgroups risk obscuring meaningful within-subtype heterogeneities. We address the issue of within-subtype heterogeneity in a later section.

Specific Traits

A. Perfectionism. A hypothetical link between AN and perfectionism seems to be well-supported empirically, with restricter and binger–purger anorexics both producing higher self-rated perfectionism scores than healthy controls (12,13) Recent findings suggest that a connection with perfectionism may extend to BN (14) and to BED (15). However, any such link may be stronger for BN than for BED (16). Perfectionism appears to exist premorbidly in ED sufferers (17) and in AN sufferers after long-term weight recovery (13), and furthermore to be common in relatives of those who develop an ED (14,18). While such findings all support the speculation that perfectionism may be a risk factor for ED development, specificity of the association with EDs (versus other forms of maladjustment) still needs to be established.

B. Impulsivity. Findings suggest remarkable capacities for nonreflectiveness or behavioral impulsivity in "bingers–purgers." Self-report scales show that bulimic individuals often fail to consider consequences of their actions and often act on impulse (19). Furthermore, various studies report bulimics to show prominent parasuicidality or self-mutilation: Mitchell and colleagues (20) estimated that about 20% of their bulimic cohort showed repeated suicidal gestures, self-mutilation, or other forms of self-destructive impulsivity. Likewise, Newton and colleagues (21) found almost half of a cohort of normal-weight bulimics to engage in combinations of substance abuse, drug overdoses, suicidal gestures, self-mutilation, sexual disinhibition, or shoplifting. A similar report, based on semistructured interviewing techniques, showed nearly 40% of bulimic individuals to display multiple forms of destructive impulsivity (22). Combined characteristics of suicidality, self-aggression, shoplifting, substance abuse, and sexual promiscuity compose the features of what Hubert Lacey and his colleagues (23) some years ago dubbed "multi-impulsive" bulimia—a subtype of BN in which binge eating represented only one instance of pervasive dysregulation of impulse controls. The general propensity toward impulsivity may extend, it appears, to "binger" populations in general. For example, studies have supported the idea that binge–purge AN has a more complicated clinical course, with greater risk for suicide than restricting AN (24). Similarly, a study of 495 eating-disordered outpatients by Favaro and Santonastaso (25) indicated that 13% reported a past suicide attempt and 29% reported current suicidal ideation, with suicidality being more prevalent among binge–purge anorexics and purging bulimics than other ED subtypes. This study also linked suicidal acts to a history of sexual abuse (a theme to which we return below). Extending the putative link between binge eating and self-destructiveness even further, Paul and his group (26) assessed self-injuriousness in women with AN, BN, or BED, and found lifetime rates to be elevated in both BED and BN (at 35.8% and 34.3%, respectively).

The idea that binge eating syndromes are linked to behavioral impulsivity or response inhibition may hold as a generalization. However, potentially important heterogeneities emerge among "binger" patients (5,27–31)— with a sizable proportion of cases found to display the perfectionistic or compulsive tendencies that have been typically associated with restricting-type AN. Such variations have led some theorists to postulate the existence of distinct "binger" subtypes, with distinct etiological paths (5,23,30,31). The idea here is that in only some bulimics is binge eating driven by a pervasive "dysregulatory pathology" (affecting mood and impulse regulation). In others, binge eating is thought to have a more circumscribed etiology. We elaborate on this point in "Within-Subtype Heterogeneity as to Personality Features" (to follow).

Personallty Disorders in the EDs

Details on the link between eating and personality disorders are provided in several excellent, comprehensive reviews (4,5,27–29). Consequently, in the present context, we enumerate broad, empirically supported generalizations:

1. PDs are undoubtedly more common in anorexic and bulimic women than in healthy comparison cases. Estimated PD prevalences in eating-disordered samples vary from roughly 20% to nearly 100%, with most commonly cited figures occupying the 50–75% range. Corroborating this point, a recent meta-analytical review of findings from 28 available studies finds 58% of women with an ED to have a PD, compared to 28% of comparison women (29).
2. Restrictive AN is associated mainly with DSM Cluster C ("Anxious–Fearful") PD subtypes, typified by anxiousness, orderliness, and preference for control. More rarely, AN-R coincides with Cluster A ("Odd–Eccentric") PDs (e.g., Schizoid PD)— having a particularly stilted quality, but still characterized by

inhibition and restricted emotionality. The PD subtype reported to occur most frequently in AN-R is Obsessive-Compulsive PD (with Avoidant and Dependent PDs also sometimes named as modal diagnoses).

3. Binger–purger variants show greater heterogeneity as to comorbid PD variations. If present, PDs will often occupy the DSM Cluster B ("Dramatic–Erratic") spectrum (i.e., Borderline, Histrionic, and Narcissistic PDs), in which attention and sensation seeking, and mood lability, excitability, and impulsivity are prominent. However, suggesting that there is no simple dichotomy as to personality traits across restricter and binger ED subtypes, and no overly direct connection between binge eating potentials and "dysregulation" (as a trait), bingers–purgers are noted to display PDs of the Cluster C ("Anxious–Fearful") type about as frequently as those of the Cluster B ("Dramatic–Erratic") type. Heterogeneous personality profiles associated with the binge–purge syndromes have, again, been taken to imply that these syndromes may have heterogeneous etiological paths (see "Within-Subtype Heterogeneity as to Personality Features").

4. Borderline personality disorder (BPD) is a particularly malignant Dramatic–Erratic variant, characterized by massive dysregulation of affects and impulse controls, chaotic interpersonal functioning, and repeated parasuicidality. Modal figures suggest that BPD, or an apparent "borderline-spectrum" personality (in which self-destructive impulsivity and parasuicidality are prominent), may be present in up to a one-third of bingers–purgers. Although rare in AN-R, BPD is apparently common in AN-BP.

5. Patterns of PD comorbidity in BED resemble those obtained in BN: Accumulating evidence suggests a general propensity towards personality pathology, possibility of special affinity with Cluster B ("Dramatic–Erratic") PD subtypes (32), but nonnegligible presence of Cluster C ("Anxious–Fearful") PDs (33,34).

State–Trait Debate

Since malnutrition can adversely affect personality functioning (35), apparent personality problems seen in ED sufferers could be attributed to "state" sequelae of an active ED. Consistent with this, various findings show EDs to exacerbate features with a "characterological coloring" (36,37). However, in counterpoint, retrospective findings often suggest that personality problems predate ED onset in ED sufferers. Råstam (38) estimated that 67% of a group of 51 adolescent anorexics had a PD prior to ED onset, the most common of which (in 35% of cases) was obsessive-compulsive PD. Similarly, Nagata and colleagues estimated that parasuicidality predated onset of eating symptoms in 80% of ED patients showing such self-destructiveness (39). Suggesting a similar independence of personality pathology from ED sequelae, many findings indicate personality problems to be relatively persistent in recovered (or recovering) ED sufferers. One study reports 26% of recovered anorexics or bulimics to show an ongoing PD——more often a Dramatic–Erratic Cluster PD in the case of BN (40). Others report persistence of obsessions, compulsions, social interaction problems (41), and perfectionism (42) in AN, even years after weight recovery.

PUTATIVE SUBSTRATES FOR AN EATING– AND PERSONALITY–PATHOLOGY "INTERFACE"

In the following sections, we explore psychosocial and psychobiological factors that may contribute to convergence of eating and personality disturbances.

Family/Developmental Characteristics

Given systematic coaggregation of personality traits with ED subtypes, data associating family interaction patterns with eating and personality problems present various explicative potentials. On the personality side of this question, some principled connections emerge: There have been inconsistent indications of a link between obsessive-compulsive personality traits and familial overinvolvement or overcontrol (43), and between impulsive (or borderline) personality traits and parental neglect, hostility, or inconsistency (44).

In light of the preceding, data on family interaction patterns in ED subtypes become suggestive. Studies on anorexic restricters and their relatives have often corroborated concepts of enmeshment, overprotection, and emotional constraint. In contrast, studies have associated binge–purge syndromes with relatively more overt familial discord, disengagement, and hostility (31, 45). Data on family interaction patterns in BED are inconclusive but suggest comparable family interactions to those found in BN. For example, Hodges and her colleagues (46) found BED women to describe their families as less cohesive, expressive, and independent, and more conflictual and controlling, than did normal-control women. Reiterating this notion, Tachi (47), working in Japan, found women with BN and BED to perceive their families as being relatively disengaged. Similarly, obese women with BED have been found to report more paternal rejection than do obese women without BED (48).

Several research groups have noted severity of family dysfunction to correspond much more closely to severity of personality pathology in eating-disordered individuals than to severity of eating symptoms (49,50). This raises doubts about the extent to which family interaction patterns may be specific to ED development—and the possibility that systematic convergences between family interaction patterns and ED subtypes might reflect indirect (personality-mediated) effects of family–environment variables acting on eating-related-symptom development. For example, familial disturbances might heighten explosiveness or impulsivity, and indirectly amplify impulse-driven ED behaviors (like frequent vomiting).

Childhood Abuse

EDs, personality pathology, and especially BPD have all been associated with childhood abuse or neglect. Studies suggest, for example, that more than 50% of individuals suffering from BPD (51,52) and roughly 30% of those suffering from an ED (53,54) have experienced childhood sexual abuse. Childhood abuse experiences therefore represent one possible area of commonality underlying convergence of eating and personality disturbances. However, assessment of this possibility asks that various findings be properly considered:

1. Clinical studies have associated childhood abuse preferentially with bulimic (rather than restrictive) forms of EDs (55,56). Corroborating this view, survivors of childhood abuse report higher frequencies of BN than of AN (57). In addition, studies in nonclinical, community samples suggest a selective association between victimization experiences and bulimic symptoms (58).
2. Studies in samples of clinical EDs generally show childhood abuse to covary more directly with personality variables (impulsivity, dissociation, interpersonal problems, etc.) than with eating-related symptom variables. We cite a few illustrative examples: One study of 133 eating-disordered women showed those reporting childhood abuse to display elevated personality pathology but not more severe eating symptoms (58). Another showed bulimics with a history of sexual or physical abuse to have more posttraumatic symptoms and more substance dependence, but not more eating symptoms (40). Several studies by our group are pertinent. One showed a systematic association between childhood sexual or physical abuse and likelihood of comorbid BPD, with no corresponding elevation in eating-related symptom severity (59). A second showed childhood abuse (sexual or physical) to predict more self-injuriousness, posttraumatic stress disorders, and (nonsignificantly) more BPD in bulimic women (60). A third indicated an association between severity of sexual and physical trauma and severity of specific pathological personality characteristics, such as submissiveness (61). Bearing closely on this question, Wonderlich and colleagues documented findings suggesting that abuse may moderate eating-related

symptom severity indirectly, through exaggeration of tendencies such as impulsivity (62).

Although it is premature to draw firm conclusions, preliminary observations have suggested that sexual abuse may be less prevalent in BED than in BN. For example, Yanovski and colleagues (32) did not find sexual abuse to be more common in obese BED participants than in obese participants without BED. Providing an apparent parallel, a telephone survey of 3006 women linked history of forcible assault or rape to BN more than to BED or non-eating-disordered status (57).

Neurobiology of Eating and Personality Disturbances

As a general rule, studies on the neurobiology of eating behavior indicate that reducing brain serotonin (5-hydroxytryptamine, 5-HT) activity disinhibits eating, whereas increasing 5-HT neurotransmission results in reduced eating (63). In this light, it is intriguing to note that studies of the 5-HT system in ED patients have associated BN and AN-BP with reduced activity of the 5-HT system, while AN-restrictive subtype has been associated with the converse (63,64). An obvious conjecture is that binge eating symptoms correspond to reductions in 5-HT neurotransmission, whereas restrictive symptoms implicate increases.

In light of the preceding, it is intriguing that findings indicate 5-HT status to covary along with ED-relevant personality trait variations as follows: The literature indicates "impulsive" populations in general (suicide completers, fire setters, violent offenders, individuals with BPD) to often display decreased 5-HT activity (65). In contrast, anxious and compulsive populations, at least inconsistently, display increased 5-HT tone. Such data have supported the proposal that "impulsive" and "compulsive" traits may occupy opposite poles of a continuum of 5-HT hypo- to hyperactivity (66). If so, neurobiological correlates of personality traits—like impulsivity and compulsivity—could underlie the association of bulimic ED variants with decreased 5-HT tone and of restrictive ED variants with increased 5-HT. In turn, 5-HT mechanisms might act as neurobiological "bridge" between impulsive personality traits and binge-eating tendencies, and between compulsive traits and dietary overcontrol.

Several studies in ED sufferers are consistent with just such personality-mediated variations of 5-HT activity. One series, in BN, links impulsivity (or disinhibition) with alterations in 5-HT activity, showing (a) reduced neuroendocrine response after administration of a 5-HT agonist in self-reportedly hostile (67) or self-mutilative (68) bulimics; (b) lower platelet monoamine oxiydase (MAO) concentrations (a proxy for level of 5-HT activity) in bulimics reporting impulsivity or borderline traits (69); (c) lower platelet paroxetine binding in bulimics reporting greater "nonplanning" impulsivity

(70). In addition, we have recently documented unusually high baseline pro-lactin and elevated density of platelet 5-HT reuptake sites in highly compul-sive bulimics (71). Together, such findings suggest that 5-HT alterations in the EDs might reflect different personality tendencies in different segments of the eating-disordered population. In other words, there may be serotonergic mediation of affinities observed between ED subtypes and personality trait variations.

We add that we have recently found childhood abuse (in bulimics and, to a lesser extent, in nonbulimics) to predict (a) blunted prolactin reponses to a 5-HT agonist and (b) abnormally low basal plasma cortisol concentrations (60). Such findings associate childhood abuse with alterations in adult brain function of a type that could (in theory) impact adversely on impulse controls, stress responses, and satiety. In other words, abuse-linked neurobiological alterations could contribute to ED vulnerability and to various aspects of ED phenomenology.

Genetics

Findings on the molecular genetics of eating and personality disorders are in a nascent state. Nonetheless, preliminary findings may help inform our study of the convergence of ED subtypes and personality trait variations. In BN, data have pointed to gene variations that may be simultaneously linked to binge eating and impulsive potentials. For example, Nishiguchi and colleagues (72) reported a link, in a heterogeneous anorexic–bulimic sample, between a polymorphism in the 5-HT_{2A} receptor gene and the presence of (a) disinhib-ited eating and (b) traits (largely impulsivity). In a related vein, Devlin and colleagues linked drive for thinness and obsessionality, in 196 patients with AN-restrictive subtype, to specific gene loci (73). Such findings raise the intriguing specter that genetic factors may be substrates of a link between bulimic eating tendencies and an "impulsive/behaviorally dysregulated" phe-notype—and between restrictive eating patterns and compulsive personality characteristics.

CLINICAL IMPLICATIONS OF PERSONALITY PATHOLOGY

Symptoms

Intuitively, personality pathology might be though to confer risk for more severe eating symptomatology. However, empirical treatments provide limited support for this idea. (Here we see the first of several instances of apparent independence between eating and personality pathologies.) Johnson and his colleagues (74) compared patients with and without self-reported BPD features. Borderlines differed from nonborderlines in showing greater depression, self-mutilation, drug abuse, and history of sexual abuse, but not greater binge/purge frequencies or other eating-specific symptoms. In a similar study, Wonderlich and Swift (75) examined clinical profiles in 75 eating-disordered women, divided (according to structured interviews) into those with and without BPD. Borderline patients displayed more suicidality, depression, anxiety, and self-mutilation than did their nonborderline counterparts. However, except for more frequent vomiting, borderline patients displayed negligibly more severe eating symptoms. Our group conducted a similar multidimensional evaluation, rating eating and general psychopathological symptoms in a sample of 91 bulimics, in whom axis II diagnoses were established with the aid of structured interviews (76). As in the study of Wonderlich and Swift, borderlines evinced more pronounced anomalies on diverse measures of general psychopathology without showing more severe eating symptoms. Thus, while it is undeniably associated with greater generalized psychopathology in BN sufferers, PD may not have a marked connotation for severity of ED symptoms. In apparent contrast, personality pathology has been associated with more severe binge eating in BED (33,77).

Outcome

Comorbid personality pathology has been associated with poorer global outcome from AN, BN, and BED.

Anorexia Nervosa

Following an extensive review (encompassing 119 studies and 5590 patients), Steinhausen (78) concluded that obsessive-compulsive PD is associated with an unfavorable prognosis in AN. Intriguingly, he noted hysterical personality features (somewhat the antithesis of obsessive-compulsive features) to coincide with favorable prognosis. Several results suggest the prognostic utility in AN of other personality measures. A recent study reported response in 42 restricter anorexics after 180 days of multimodal therapy (79). Categorical PD diagnoses did not predict improvement, but dimensional measure (low novelty seeking, and high asceticism and maturity fears) were systematically linked to poorer response. Suggesting similar effects at long-term follow-up, Bulik and her colleagues (36) found anorexics who remained ill after 12 years to be characterized partly by more severe eating disturbances and partly by greater harm avoidance (i.e., anxious avoidance and overcontrol) and lower self-directedness. In a similar 4-year prospective study for AN, lower self-esteem and stronger maturity fears were associated with poorer outcome (80).

Bulimia Nervosa

Results for BN also seem to associate personality pathology with poorer global treatment response: Herzog et al. (81) linked comorbid PD (diagnosed using structured interview in 179 bulimics) with lower probability of abstinence from BN after 9 or more months. Similarly, Rossiter et al. (82) reported that Dramatic–Erratic personality traits predicted greater chance of persistent vomiting in BN after one year. Other studies corroborate the same trend: One shows BN patients with high initial Borderline Syndrome Index scores to be more likely to remain bulimic after one year than patients with initially lower scores (83). Another reports that bulimic patients who showed persistent "borderline features" over the first 3 months of therapy showed poorest response of bulimic symptoms after 6 and 12 months (84).

When finer grained outcome dimensions (rather than "global ED outcome") are assayed, however, subtler effects sometimes emerge. Wonderlich et al. (85) reported that PD comorbidity predicted poorer global response, but only weak differences on indices of bulimic symptoms, in 30 bulimics followed for 4–5 years. Our group studied progress in treatment, in function of interview-based PD diagnoses, of bulimics after 3, 6, and then 12 and more months. Borderline bulimics showed greater psychiatric symptoms than did nonborderline bulimics at all points in time but limited differences on measures reflecting the course of eating symptoms (76,86). Norring (87) reported similar findings in heterogeneous ED cases. Patients showing a "borderline organization" showed poorest response after 2 and 3 years—but differences were more pronounced on comorbid symptoms than on eating-specific ones. Such tendencies led Grilo (27), after an excellent and comprehensive review, to conclude that PD may be more closely associated with the longtudinal course of general psychiatric symptoms or psychosocial functioning in ED patients than with fluctuations in the course of eating symptoms.

It is possible that "impulsivity" measures may yield more reliable prognostic effects. After an extensive literature review, Keel and Mitchell (88) concluded that impulsivity was foremost among prognostic indices for BN, with PD having inconsistent effects. In addition, isolated personality dimensions have emerged as having prognostic value for BN: Joiner et al. (89) found "maturity fears" and "perfectionism" to be weak long-term (10-year) predictors of bulimic symptoms. Bulik and her colleagues (90) examined predictors of outcome one year after completion of a randomized psychotherapy trial. PD symptoms were not predictive, but a measure reflecting self-directedness was associated with lower postreatment frequency of bingeing and purging.

Binge Eating Disorder

Available studies have suggested that PD may also predict poorer outcome for BED. For example, Wilfley and colleagues (33) found that presence of a Dramatic–Erratic PD predicted significantly more binge eating in BED patients at one year after treatment. Likewise, Stice and colleagues documented poorer treatment response in BED patients with a concurrent PD (77).

Treatment Usage

Personality pathology apparently has an additional clinical relevance as a predictor of treatment usage: Several studies document more frequent hospitalizations and medication usage in bulimics with Dramatic–Erratic or borderline PDs than in those with lesser PD comorbidity (74,75,86). Suggesting that this trend cuts across ED subtypes, Keel and colleagues (91) reported a link, in 294 women treated for AN or BN, between presence of a PD and use of psychotherapy and medication after 5 years.

WITHIN-SUBTYPE HETEROGENEITY AS TO PERSONALITY FEATURES

The patterning of association between personality and eating symptom variations has inspired various speculations on the "shaping" role, in ED expression, of personality factors. Relatively circumscribed comorbidity of a compulsive type in restrictive AN makes an obvious appeal to the idea that obstinacy, constriction, and hypersensitivity to social approval may "power" rigid dieting and driven pursuit of thinness. Likewise, affinities between bulimic behaviors and tendencies toward behavioral dyscontrol encourages the view that bingeing and purging may only be isolated instances, in affected individuals, of a more generalized dysregulation. Although intuitively appealing, the latter view is challenged by the reality that individuals who binge-eat display heterogeneous personality characteristics—sometimes impulsive, sometimes compulsive.

Diversity of personality characteristics seen in bulimic syndromes has (as discussed earlier) been thought to correspond to different etiological paths to binge eating—sometimes reflecting a primary and rather pervasive disruption of controls over mood, impulses, and appetite, and sometimes a more circumscribed erosion of appetitive controls, following prolonged dieting (5, 31,92,93). The idea that binge eating results from prolonged dietary restraint is established clinically and empirically, and fundamental to Polivy and Herman's (94) well-known restraint theory. However, recent studies reveal a subgroup of BN and BED sufferers in whom binge eating seems not to follow from antecedent dieting (95)—and to whom restraint theory seems to be less applicable. This "binge-first" subgroup is furthermore reported to show more marked personality pathology than do more traditional "diet-first" bulimics— which supports the conjecture that personality pathology might (sometimes) directly enhance susceptibility to binge eating (via emotion- or impulse-linked pathways). Recent data from our group resonate with this idea. We had 51 bulimic women record ongoing emotions and behaviors over a roughly 3-week span (96). Findings suggested that restraint may have been a weaker hour-to-hour binge antecedent in impulsive than in nonimpulsive bulimics—or that impulsivity may have been intrinsically conducive to binge eating in the relative absence of antecedent dietary restraint.

Other findings are similarly relevant to the notion that personality trait variations might help define meaningful ED subtype distinctions: Studies applying cluster-analytical techniques to personality indices obtained in eating-disordered samples indicate that there may be something quite repeatable about a tripartite classification of ED patients into the following subgroups: (a) "psychologically relatively intact", (b) "overregulated (compulsive)" and (c) "dysregulated (impulsive)" (93). Furthermore, these findings link AN-restrictive subtype consistently with the overcontrolled personality profile, but associate bulimic ED variants about equiprobably with any of the three personality profiles. Assuming that this is so, we find it intriguing to contemplate the ways in which such distinctions may correspond to data on neurobiological variations and developmental typologies. For example, the spectrum from over- to underregulated personality characteristics could, in theory, span a continuum from hyperactivity to hypoactivity of serotonin mechanisms. Similarly, the overregulated subtype could correspond to familial overinvolvement (with low risk of childhood trauma), whereas the dysregulated subtype might be linked to familial incohesion (and greater risk of childhood abuse).

INTEGRATION AND CLINICAL APPLICATIONS

Findings in the EDs converge on the idea that personality variables correspond to meaningful variations as to developmental, familial, and neurobiological typologies. Furthermore, findings suggest that personality factors may be relevant to global functioning, treatment outcome, and prognosis in ED sufferers. These trends suggest that personality-linked considerations may have an important contribution to make in clinical formulation and clinical decision making in this area. To illustrate how this may be so, we offer a few general conceptual and clinical guidelines:

(1) *Eating and personality disturbances are separate but interdependent entities.* There are reasons to assume that eating and personality pathologies are independently determined. For example, one can be severe, whereas the other is mild; one can resolve, whereas the other persists. This implies, as suggested by available outcome literature, that eating problems can to some extent be treated independently of associated personality characteristics. However, that eating and personality disturbances co-occur so frequently also suggests nonnegligible measures of causal overlap. Consider the following: Neurobiological vulnerabilities (e.g., altered serotonin neurotransmission) may, along with predictable effects on personality manifestations (e.g.,

heightened impulsivity), confer vulnerability to impaired satiety. If so, having a particular personality trait (like impulsivity) might increase vulnerability to a particular disturbance in eating behavior (like binge eating) because of neuro-biological propensities that are linked to both the trait and the appetitive behavior. Given this notion, it becomes fascinating to contemplate all of the possible sources of influence that may act upon the neurobiological status in a given individual at a given moment in time (e.g., heredity, nutritional state, effects of developmental and current stressors, etc.)—and, in turn, to con-template the complexity of processes that determine whether or not a given personality trait (e.g., impulsivity) or eating symptom (e.g., binge eating) is likely to come to expression. We address such convergences elsewhere (31,60,68,70). In a related vein, common developmental factors (e.g., child-hood sexual abuse) can be thought to impact, not only upon interpersonal expectations and functioning, but also upon the sense of bodily integrity, control, and esteem. Such effects might, in turn, heighten susceptibility to concurrent interpersonal difficulties and maladaptive weight control practices or food avoidances.

(2) *Eating disturbances worsen personality disturbances.* The view that ED sequelae exacerbate obsessionality, impulsivity, or other apparent per-sonality problems in ED sufferers has a simple wisdom. Evidence indicates that EDs can exaggerate personality problems, and this certainly explains recent practice preferences leaning toward symptom-focused models of ther-apy for the EDs. A rationale (aside from the obvious aim of reducing pres-enting symptoms) is that improving nutritional status in an ED sufferer often improves her personality and general functioning. Consequently, we urge that it is never appropriate to ignore eating disturbances and focus on underlying personality issues alone. At the same time, primacy of personality disturban-ces, and persistence following recovery, suggests that it is untenable to regard personality factors solely as ED sequelae and hence (swinging to the other extreme) to ignore them in treatment. In a closely related vein:

(3) *Eating and personality problems have mutual "pathoplastic effects" (30)—pathology of one sort "shaping" variations in the other.* For example, impulse control problems may exacerbate intensive vomiting, self-image dis-turbances may amplify body dissatisfaction, and general compulsivity may support compulsive dieting. This means that work aimed at generalized behavioral or self-image problems can often have "spinoff" benefits, as far as resolution of eating symptoms is concerned. As patients learn to manage anxiety and impulsive responses, they become less reliant on binge episodes to sooth eating-induced anxiety. As they learn to be less angry, they become less reliant on binge episodes as a means of diffusing angry affects. As they learn to process social experiences more adaptively, they become less prone to injury in interpersonal experiences and to recourse to eating symptoms as a means of regulating negative "self" experiences (97).

We introduce a fourth point, not yet treated in our review but one that (we believe) is essential to any adequate discussion of the clinical implications of personality pathology in the EDs.

(4) *Personality pathology has powerful interpersonal repercussions.* PDs impact on all relationship experiences, including therapeutic ones. For this reason, we advocate close attention to relational aspects in therapy of ED patients. We propose that you cannot manage eating disturbances without caring for the relationship experience—not only because it is the vehicle of alliance, but also, because (we believe) it is a direct ingredient of change. To illustrate, we bring in a concept proposed by clinician-theorists who concern themselves with the impact of therapeutic alliance upon therapy outcome (98). The concept holds that when patients have dysfunctional beliefs and expectancies about interpersonal experiences (a given with comorbid personality pathology), they can invite dysfunctional behaviors from others—including their therapists. For example, the hostile patient (depending on the therapist's own proclivities) can evoke complementary hostility (or defensive withdrawal); the regressive patient can evoke excessive nurturance (or unrealistic demands for autonomous functioning); the grandiose patient can evoke competitiveness (or adoration); and the compulsive patient can stimulate struggles around power and control (or excessive acquiescence and gentleness). It is an obvious point that, to be therapeutic, therapists need not "complement" patients' dysfunctional interpersonal responses (in the ways described), but should evoke healthy interpersonal experiences that disconfirm dysfunctional relationship expectancies.

CONCLUSIONS

Our thinking in this chapter has been structured around the concept that eating and personality pathologies have multiple and (often) shared biological, psychological, and social determinants. This means that personality cannot be conceptualized as a unidimensional psychological aspect of what occurs in people with EDs—but rather, needs to be understood as an integral part of the ED syndrome, tightly woven into its complex of causes and symptoms, and relevant as both an expression of, and influence on, the ED's biopsychosocial "mix."

This perspective asks that we revise our thinking about psychopathological syndromes and traits, especially as far as the idea of separating "syndromic" and "personality" components is concerned. It may be that we can never fully segregate "having an eating disorder" (in either phenomenological or etiological respects) from "concurrent personality tendencies." Rather, "personality" phenomena (like impulsivity, compulsivity, or perfectionism) may be at least as relevant to defining ED syndrome "variants" as any one of a number of superficially more relevant aspects of ED phenomenology (e.g., presence of binge eating or laxative abuse). Indeed, available data argue that the personality variations may be the stronger predictors of clinical phenomenology, neurobiological substrates, sexual abuse history, treatment outcome, prognosis, and other aspects. This argues for a more central attention to personality trait variations in the development of ED diagnostic classifications—a view that has been advocated by several others (30,31,93).

The same concept is relevant to treatment considerations. To date, ED specialists have succeeded in standardizing and formalizing interventions aimed at eating disturbances. A next step, we would urge, is to be equally rigorous in our efforts to develop, integrate, and perfect interventions aimed at personality components in the EDs (and their inextricable consequences for the therapeutic alliance). We are thinking here not of an "adjunctive" use of personality concepts—treating personality features as some sort of "grease on the wheels" of eating-focused interventions—but of a central attention to the ways in which personality may shape expression of eating symptoms, the relational aspects of the therapeutic experience and, in turn, the process of change.

Various theorists have argued that eating symptoms need to be contextualized in light of comorbid personality characteristics (5,30,31,93). For example, a symptom like vomiting may have quite a different meaning when it arises in (a) the emotionally constricted and weight gain–phobic patient, or (b) the highly dysregulated or posttraumatic patient. In the former, vomiting may serve as a phobic avoidance, driven by relatively circumscribed weight gain fears–in the latter, as a desparate response to felt emptiness, posttraumatic memories, or overwhelming rage. Until equipped to process such experiences adaptively, encouraging the very highly dysregulated patients to defer vomiting seems barely adequate and risks "missing the mark." In other words, therapeutic prescriptions need to be tailored to the personality context. In summary, if we hope to understand the EDs' phenomenological complexity, we believe that it is heuristic to minimize the conceptual distance between eating-specific aspects of phenomenology and more generalized aspects usually thought to define "personality." This, we believe, is because eating-specific and personality-linked components of the ED may become quite inextricably intermingled once the eating syndrome becomes instated.

REFERENCES

1. Gordon RA. Anatomy of a social epidemic. Oxford: Basil Blackwell, 1990:12.
2. Ziolko H-U. Bulimia: a historical outline. Int J Eat Disord 1996; 20:345–358.
3. American Psychiatric Association. Diagnostic and Statistical Manual of Mental Disorders 4th ed. Washington, DC: DSM-IV, 1994.

4. Sohlberg S, Strober M. Personality in anorexia nervosa: an update and a theoretical integration. Acta Psychiatr Scand 1994; 89(Suppl 378):1–15.
5. Vitousek K, Manke F. Personality variables and disorders in anorexia nervosa and bulimia nervosa. J Abnorm Psychol 1994; 103:137–147.
6. Casper RC, Hedeker D, McClough JF. Personality dimensions in eating disorders and their relevance for subtyping. J Am Acad Child Adol Psychiatry 1992; 31:830–840.
7. Norman DK, Blais D, Herzog D. Personality characteristics of eating-disordered patients as identified by the Millon Clinical Multiaxial inventory. J Pers Disord 1993; 7:1–9.
8. Bulik CM, Sullivan PF, Weltzin TF, Kaye WH. Temperament in eating disorders. Int J Eat Disord 1995; 17:251–261.
9. Brewerton TD, Hand JD, Bishop EM. The Tridimensional Personality Questionnaire in patients with eating disorders. Int J Eat Disord 1993; 14:213–218.
10. Diaz-Marsa M, Carrasco JL, Saiz J. A study of temperament and personality in anorexia and bulimia nervosa. J Pers Disord 2000; 14:352–359.
11. Cumella EJ, Wall AD, Kerr-Almeida N. MMPI-2 in the inpatient assessment of women with eating disorders. J Pers Assess 2000; 75:387–403.
12. Halmi KA, Sunday SR, Strober M, Kaplan A, Woodside DB, Fichter M, Treaure J, Berrettini W, Kaye WH. Perfectionsim in anorexia nervosa: variation by clinical subtype, obsessionality, and pathological eating behavior. Am J Psychiatry 2000; 157:1799–1805.
13. Srinivasagam NM, Kaye WH, Plotnicov KH, Greeno C, Weltzin TE, Rao R. Persistent perfectionism, symmetry, and exactness after long-term recovery from anorexia nervosa. Am J Psychiatry 1995; 152:1630–1634.
14. Lilenfeld LR, Stein D, Bulik CM, Strober M, Plotnicov K, Pollice C, Rao R, Merikangas KR, Nagy L, Kaye WH. Personality traits among currently eating disordered, recovered and never ill first-degree female relatives of bulimic and control women. Psychol Med 2000; 30:1399–1410.
15. Pratt EM, Telch CF, Labouvie EW, Wilson GT, Agras WS. Perfectionism in women with binge eating disorder. Int J Eat Disord 2001; 29:177–186.
16. Fairburn CG, Doll HA, Welch SL, Hay PJ, Davies BA, O'Connor ME. Risk factors for binge eating disorders: a community-based study. Arch Gen Psychiatry 1998; 55:425–432.
17. Fairburn CG, Cooper Z, Doll HA, Welch SL. Risk factors for anorexia nervosa: three integrated case-controlled comparisons. Arch Gen Psychiatry 1999; 56: 468–476.
18. Woodside DB, Bulik CM, Halmi KA, Fichter MM, Kaplan A, Berrettini WH, Strober M, Treasure J, Lilenfeld L, Klump K, Kaye WH. Personality, perfectionism, and attitudes toward eating in parents of individuals with eating disorders. Int J Eat Disord 2002; 31:290–299.
19. Wolfe BE, Jimerson DC, Levine JM. Impulsivity ratings in bulimia nervosa: relationship to binge eating behaviours. Int J Eat Disord 1994; 15:289–292.
20. Mitchell JE, Hatsukami D, Pyle RL, Eckert ED. The bulimia syndrome: course of the illness and associated problems. Comp Psychiatry 1986; 27:165–170.
21. Newton JR, Freeman CP, Munro J. Impulsivity and dyscontrol in bulimia

nervosa: is impulsivity an independent phenomenon or a marker of severity? Acta Psychiatr Scand 1993; 87:389–394.

22. Crosby RD, Wonderlich SA, Redlin J, Engel SG, Simonich H, Jones-Paxton M, Myers T, Norton M, Thompson KM, Mitchell JE. Impulsive behavior patterns in a sample of females with bulimia nervosa. Poster presented at the annual meeting of the Eating Disorders Research Society, Bernalillo, New Mexico, 2001.

23. Lacey JH, Evans CD. The impulsivist: a multi-impulsive personality disorder. Br J Addict 1986; 81:641–649.

24. Herzog DB, Dorer DJ, Keel PK, Selwyn SE, Ekeblad ER, Flores AT, Greenwood DN, Burwell RA, Keller MB. Recovery and relapse in anorexia and bulimia nervosa: a 7.5-year follow-up study. J Am Acad Child Adol Psychiatry 1999; 38:829–837.

25. Favaro A, Santonastaso P. Suicidality in eating disorders: clinical and psychological correlates. Acta Psychiatr Scand 1997; 95:508–514.

26. Paul T, Schroeter K, Dahme B, Nutzinger DO. Self-injurious behavior in women with eating disorders. Am J Psychiatry 2002; 159:408–411.

27. Grilo CM. Recent research of relationships among eating disorders and personality disorders. Curr Psychiatry Rep 2002; 4:18–24.

28. Johnson C, Wonderlich S. Personality characteristics as a risk factor in the development of eating disorders. In: Crowther JH, Tennenbaum DL, Hobfell SE, Stephens MAP, eds. The Etiology of Bulimia Nervosa: The Individual and Family Context. New York: Hemisphere Publishing, 1992.

29. Rosenvinge JH, Martinussen M, Ostensen E. The comorbidity of eating disorders and personality disorders: a meta-analytic review of studies published between 1983 and 1998. Eat Weight Disord 2000; 5:52–61.

30. Wonderlich SA, Mitchell JE. Eating disorders and comorbidity: empirical, conceptual and clinical implications. Psychopharmacol Bull 1997; 33:381–390.

31. Steiger H, Bruce K, Israël M. Eating Disorders. In: Stricker G, Widiger TA, Wiener IB, eds. Comprehensive Handbook of Psychology. New York: John Wiley and Sons, 2003:173–194.

32. Yanovski SZ, Nelson JE, Dubbert BK, Spitzer RL. Association of binge eating disorder and psychiatric comorbidity in obese subjects. Am J Psychiatry 1993; 150:1472–1479.

33. Wilfley DE, Friedman MA, Dounchis JZ, Stein RI, Welch RR, Ball SA. Comorbid psychopathology in binge eating disorder: relation to eating disorder severity at baseline and following treatment. J Consult Clin Psychol 2000; 68:641–649.

34. Grilo CM, Masheb RM. DSM-IV psychiatric comorbidity in binge eating disorder: relation to gender and eating disorder symptomatology. Paper presented at the annual meeting of the Association for the Advancement of Behaviour Therapy. Philadelphia, November 2001.

35. Keys A, Brozek J, Henschel A, Mickelson O, Taylor H. The Biology of Human Starvation. Minneapolis: University of Minnesota Press, 1950.

36. Bulik CM, Sullivan PF, Fear JL, Pickering A. Outcome of anorexia nervosa: eating attitudes, personality, and parental bonding. Int J Eat Disord 2000; 28: 139–147.

37. Garner DM, Olmsted R, Davis R, Rockect W, Goldbloom D, Eagle M. The association between bulimic symptoms and reported psychopathology. Int J Eat Disord 1990; 9:1–16.
38. Råstam M. Anorexia nervosa in 51 swedish adolescents: Premorbid problems and comorbidity. J Am Acad Child Adol Psychiatry 1992; 31:819–829.
39. Nagata T, Kawarada Y, Kiriike N, Iketani T. Multi-impulsivity of Japanese patients with eating disorders: primary and secondary impulsivity. Psychiatry Res 2000; 94:239–250.
40. Matsunaga H, Kaye WH, McConaha C, Plotnicov K, Pollice C, Rao R, Stein D. Psychopathological characteristics of recovered bulimics who have a history of physical or sexual abuse. J Nerv Ment Dis 1999; 187:472–477.
41. Nilsson EW, Gillberg C, Gillberg IC, Rastam M. Ten-year follow-up of adolescent onset anorexia nervosa: Personality disorders. J Am Acad Child Adol Psychiatry 1999; 38:1389–1395.
42. Pla C, Toro J. Anorexia nervosa in a Spanish adolescent sample: an 8-year longitudinal study. Acta Psychiatr Scand 1999; 100:441–446.
43. Nordahl HM, Stiles TC. Perceptions of parental bonding in patients with various personality disorders, lifetime depressive disorders, and healthy controls. J Pers Disord 1997; 11:391–402.
44. Nickell AD, Waudby CJ, Trull TJ. Attachment, parental bonding and borderline personality disorder features in young adults. J Pers Disord 2002; 16:148–159.
45. Wonderlich SA. Relationship of family and personality factors in bulimia. In: Crowther JH, Tennenbaum DL, Hobfell SE, Stephens MAP, eds. The Etiology of Bulimia Nervosa: The Individual and Family Context. New York: Hemisphere Publishing, 1992.
46. Hodges EL, Cochrane CE, Brewerton TD. Family characteristics of binge-eating disorder patients. Int J Eat Disord 1998; 23:145–151.
47. Tachi T. Family environment in eating disorders: a study of the familiar factors influencing the onset and course of eating disorders. Seishin Shinkeigaku Zasshi 1999; 101:427–445.
48. Dominy NL, Johnson W-B, Koch C. Perception of parental acceptance in women with binge-eating disorder. J Psychol 2000; 134:23–36.
49. Schmidt U, Humfress H, Treasure J. The role of general family environment and sexual and physical abuse in the origins of eating disorders. Eur Eat Disord Rev 1997; 5:184–207.
50. Steiger H, Liquornik K, Chapman J, Hussain N. Personality and family disturbances in eating-disorder patients: comparison of "restricters" and "bingers" to normal controls. Int J Eat Disord 1991; 10:501–512.
51. Herman JL, Perry C, van der Kolk BA. Childhood trauma in borderline personality disorder. Am J Psychiatry 1989; 146:490–495.
52. Paris J, Zweig-Frank H, Guzder J. Psychological risk factors for borderline personality disorder in female patients. Compr Psyhiatry 1994; 35:301–305.
53. Everill J, Waller G. Reported sexual abuse and eating psychopathology: a review of evidence for a causal link. Int J Eat Disord 1995; 18:1–11.
54. Wonderlich SA, Brewerton TD, Jocic Z, Dansky B, Abbott DW. Relationship of

childhood sexual abuse and eating disorders. J Am Acad Child Adolesc Psychiatry 1997; 36:1107–1115.

55. Steiger H, Zanko M. Sexual traumata in eating-disordered, psychiatric and normal female groups: comparison of prevalences and defense styles. J Interpers Violence 1990; 5:74–86.

56. Bushnell JA, Wells JE, Oakley-Brown MA. Long term effects of intrafamilial sexual abuse in childhood. Acta Psychiatr Scand 1992; 85:36–142.

57. Dansky BS, Brewerton TD, Kilpatrick DG, O'Neil PM. The National Women's Study: relationship of victimization and posttraumatic stress disorder to bulimia nervosa. Int J Eat Disord 1997; 21:213–228.

58. Moreno JK, Selby MJ, Neal S. Psychopathology in sexually abused and nonsexually abused eating-disordered women. Psychother Private Pract 1998; 17:1–9.

59. Steiger H, Jabalpurwala S, Champagne J. Axis-II comorbidity and developmental adversity in bulimia nervosa. J Nerv Ment Dis 1996; 184:555–560.

60. Steiger H, Gauvin L, Israël M, Koerner N, Ng Ying Kin NMK, Paris J, Young SN. Association of serotonin and cortisol indices with childhood abuse in bulimia nervosa. Arch Gen Psychiatry 2001; 58:837–843.

61. Léonard S, Steiger H, Kao A, Childhood and adulthood abuse in bulimic and nonbulimic women: prevalence and psychological correlates. Int J Eat Disord 2003; 33:397–405.

62. Wonderlich SA, Crosby R, Mitchell J, Thompson K, Redlin J, Demuth G, Smyth J, Haseltine B. Eating disturbance and sexual trauma in childhood and adulthood. Int J Eat Disord 2001; 30:401–412.

63. Brewerton TD. Toward a unified theory of serotonin dysregulation in eating and related disorders. Psychoneuroendocrinology 1995; 20:561–590.

64. Kaye WH, Ebert MH, Gwirtsman HE, Weiss SR. Differences in brain serotonergic metabolism between bulimic and nonbulimic patients with anorexia nervosa. Am J Psychiatry 1984; 141:1598–1601.

65. Åsberg M, Schalling D, Träskman-Bendz L, Wägner A. Psychobiology of suicide, impulsivity and related phenomena. In: Meltzer HY, ed. Psychopharmacology: Third Generation of Progress. New York: Raven Press, 1987:655–688.

66. Cloninger CR, Svrakic DM, Przybeck TR. A psychobiological model of temperament and character. Arch Gen Psychiatry 1993; 50:975–990.

67. Waller DA, Sheinberg AL, Gullion C, Moeller FG, Cannon DS, Petty F, Hardy BW, Orsulak P, Rush A. Impulsivity and neuroendocrine response to buspirone in bulimia nervosa. Biol Psychiatry 1996; 39:371–374.

68. Steiger H, Koerner NM, Enghleberg M, Israël M, Ng Ying Kin NMK, Young SN. Self-destructiveness and serotonin function in bulimia nervosa. Psychiatry Res 2001; 103:15–26.

69. Carrasco JL, Diaz-Marsa M, Hollander E, Cesar J, Saiz-Ruiz J. Decreased platelet monoamine oxidase activity in female bulimia nervosa. Eur Neuropsychopharmacol 2000; 10:113–117.

70. Steiger H, Young SN, Kin NM, Koerner N, Israel M, Lageix P, Paris J. Implications of impulsive and affective symptoms for serotonin function in bulimia nervosa. Psychol Med 2001; 31:85–95.

71. Steiger H, Gauvin L, Israel M, Ng Ying Kin NMK, Young S, Walsh S, Hudon N. Serotonin indices predict personality traits and likelihood of sexual abuse in bulimia nervosa. Paper presented at the 2002 Annual Meeting of the Eating Disorders Research Society, Charleston, South Carolina, Nov. 21–23, 2002.

72. Nishiguchi N, Matsushita S, Suzuki K, Murayama M, Shirakawa O, Higuchi S. Association between 5HT2A receptor gene promoter region polymorphism and eating disorders in Japanese patients. Biol Psychiatry 2001 Jul 15; 50:123–128.

73. Devlin B, Bacanu SA, Klump KL, Bulik CM, Fichter MM, Halmi KA, Kaplan AS, Strober M, Treasure J, Woodside DB, Berrettini WH, Kaye WH. Linkage analysis of anorexia nervosa incorporating behavioral covariates. Hum Mol Genet 2002; 11:689–696.

74. Johnson C, Tobin D, Enright A. Prevalence and clinical characteristics of borderline patients in an eating-disordered population. J Clin Psychiatry 1989; 50:9–15.

75. Wonderlich SA, Swift WJ. Borderline versus other personality disorders in the eating disorders clinical description. Int J Eat Disord 1990; 9:629–638.

76. Steiger H, Thibaudeau J, Leung F, Houle L, Ghadirian AM. Eating and psychiatric symptoms as a function of axis II comorbidity in bulimic patients: three-month and six-month responses after therapy. Psychosomatics 1994; 35: 41–49.

77. Stice E, Agras WS, Telch CF, Halmi KA, Mitchell JE, Wilson T. Subtyping binge eating-disordered women along dieting and negative affect dimensions. Int J Eat Disord 2001; 30:11–27.

78. Steinhausen HC. The outcome of anorexia nervosa in the 20th century. Am J Psychiatry 2002; 159:1284–1293.

79. Fassino S, Abbate Dagga G, Amianto F, Leombruni P, Fornas B, Garzaro L, D'Ambrosio G, Rovera GG. Outcome predictors in anorexic patients after 6 months of multimodal treatment. Psychother Psychosom 2001; 70:201–208.

80. Van der Ham T, van Strien DC, van England H. Personality characteristics predict outcome of eating disorders in adolescents: a 4-year prospective study. Eur Child Adol Psychiatry 1998; 7:79–84.

81. Herzog DB, Keller MB, Sacks NR, Yeh CJ, Lavori PW. Psychiatric comorbidity in treatment-seeking anorexics and bulimics. J Am Acad Child Adol Psychiatry 1992; 31:810–818.

82. Rossiter EM, Agras WS, Telch CF, Schneider JA. Cluster B personality disorder characteristics predict outcome in the treatment of bulimia nervosa. Int J Eat Disord 1993; 13:349–357.

83. Johnson C, Tobin DL, Dennis A. Differences in treatment outcome between borderline and nonborderline bulimics at one-year follow-up. Int J Eat Disord 1990; 9:617–627.

84. Steiger H, Stotland S, Houle L. Prognostic implications of stable versus transient "borderline features" in bulimic patients. J Clin Psychiatry 1994; 55:206–214.

85. Wonderlich SA, Fullerton D, Swift WJ, Klein MH. Five-year outcome from eating disorders: Relevance of personality disorders. Int J Eat Disord 1994; 15:233–244.

86. Steiger H, Stotland S. Prospective study of outcome in bulimics as a function of

axis-II comorbidity: long-term responses on eating and psychiatric symptoms. Int J Eat Disord 1996; 20:149–161.

87. Norring C. Borderline personality organization and prognosis in eating disorders. Psychoanal Psychol 1993; 10:551–572.

88. Keel PK, Mitchell JE. Outcome in bulimia nervosa. Am J Psychiatry 1997; 154:313–321.

89. Joiner TE Jr, Heatherton TF, Keel PK. Ten-year stability and predictive validity of five bulimia-related indicators. Am J Psychiatry 1997; 154:1133–1138.

90. Bulik CM, Sullivan PF, Joyce PR, Carter FA, McIntosh VV. Predictors of 1-year treatment outcome in bulimia nervosa. Compr Psychiatry 1998; 39:206–214.

91. Keel PK, Dorer DJ, Eddy KT, Delinsky SS, Franko DL, Blais MA, Keller MB, Herzog DB. Predictors of treatment utilization among women with anorexia and bulimia nervosa. Am J Psychiatry 2002; 159:140–142.

92. Meyers C, Waller G, Waters A. Emotional states and bulimic psychopathology. In: Hoek H, Treasure J, Katzman M, eds. Neurobiology in the Treatment of Eating Disorders. New York: John Wiley and Sons, 1998:263–279.

93. Westen D, Harnden-Fischer J. Personality profiles in eating disorders: rethinking the distinction between axis I and axis II. Am J Psychiatry 2001; 158:547–562.

94. Polivy J, Herman CP. Dieting and binging: a causal analysis. Am Psychol 1985; 40:193–201.

95. Borman Spurrell E, Wilfley DE, Tanofsky MB, Brownell KD. Age of onset for binge eating: Are there different pathways to binge eating. Int J Eat Disord 1997; 21:55–65.

96. Steiger H, Lehoux P, Gauvin L. Impulsivity, dietary restraint, and the urge to binge in bulimic eating syndromes. Int J Eat Disord 1999; 26:261–274.

97. Steiger H, Gauvin L, Jabalpurwala S, Séguin JR, Stotland S. Hypersensitivity to social interactions in bulimic eating syndromes: relationship to binge-eating. J Consult Clin Psychol 1999; 67:765–775.

98. Safran J, Segal ZV. Interpersonal Process in Cognitive Therapy. Northvale, NJ: Aronson, 1996.

10

Medical Comorbidity of Anorexia Nervosa, Bulimia Nervosa, and Binge Eating Disorder

Pauline S. Powers and Yvonne Bannon
University of South Florida
Tampa, Florida, U.S.A.

Anorexia nervosa (AN), bulimia nervosa (BN), and binge eating disorder (BED) are the three major eating disorders, affecting between 5 million and 10 million people in the United States (1–3). More people have eating disorders than have Alzheimer's disease (4), and patients typically fall ill early in their life rather than at the end of their life. Eating disorders are more common than schizophrenia, which affects 2.2 million people in the United States (5). The eating disorders are expensive to treat, in part because of the multiple medical complications associated with them. The average yearly cost of treating eating disorders in the United States is about $6 billion (6) compared to the global cost of antipsychotic medication, which is about $7 billion (7). AN is the least common eating disorder but the most expensive to treat: the average annual cost of treating a patient with AN is $6045 compared to $4824 for a patient with schizophrenia (6). BN and BED are somewhat less expensive to treat than AN, similar to or more expensive than the treatment of obsessive-compulsive disorder (8).

The eating disorders have high rates of medical comorbidity. AN has the highest premature mortality rate of any psychiatric disorder. Untreated, after 20 years, the mortality rate is 18–20% (9). Since the typical patient falls ill in midadolescence, by age 35 one-fifth of untreated patients have died.

Approximately two-thirds of the deaths are due to cardiac or renal complications and about one-third due to suicide. Less is known about the mortality
for BN, but after 15–20 years 5% may have died (10). The premature mortality rate for BED is poorly understood, but since most patients are obese,
the medical risks are probably those associated with obesity. These risks include type 2 diabetes mellitus, hypertension, dyslipidemia, cardiovascular disease, stroke, sleep apnea, gallbladder disease, hyperuricemia and gout, and
osteoarthritis. Although BED was described in 1959 (11), studies specific to
the complication of BED are only now being undertaken; the most work has
been done on the relationship between BED and diabetes mellitus. Although
the night eating syndrome was described by Stunkard nearly 50 years ago
(12), it is only recently that the physiological concomitants of this condition
have been investigated.

DIAGNOSTIC ISSUES

The current diagnostic nomenclature for eating disorders includes AN, BN,
and eating disorders–not otherwise specified (ED-NOS). Under the current
system (13), BED is technically classified as an ED-NOS, along with sub-
syndromal and atypical cases of AN and BN. It is likely that the next revision
of the *Diagnostic and Statistical Manual* (DSM) will include BED. The night
eating syndrome, often associated with obesity, is currently under study and
may eventually be classified as an eating disorder. The night eating syndrome
is usually defined as having three main features: morning anorexia, hyperphagia at night, and insomnia (12,14). Nocturnal sleep-related eating disorder
is a condition in which night eating occurs during total or partial uncon-
sciousness, often during stage 3 or 4 sleep (14). One report (15) found that
60% of patients with nocturnal sleep-related eating disorder had sleepwalking
(somnambulism).
    One important issue that has not been resolved is whether or not obesity
should be considered an eating disorder. Although obesity is often associated
with abnormalities in both food consumption and energy expenditure, early
studies found that there were no typical psychological symptoms associated
with obesity and therefore obesity was not considered a psychiatric disorder.
However, recent evidence documenting some of biological underpinnings of
the typical eating disorders and evidence documenting multiple psychological
problems in many individuals with obesity may result in obesity eventually
being considered an eating disorder.
    Figure 1 illustrates some of the relationships between AN, BN, BED,
and other forms of obesity. As weight increases, the condition becomes more
common (e.g., AN is less common than BN, which is less common than BED,

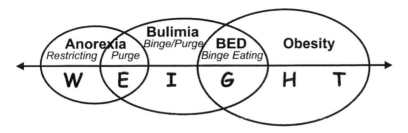

FIGURE 1 Eating Disorders Continuum.

which is less common than obesity unassociated with binge eating). With increasing weight, more males are affected. For example, less than 10% of patients with AN are male, about 20% of patients with BN are male, and about 30% of patients with BED are male.

ASSESSMENT

Ideally, the initial evaluation of patients with eating disorders includes an assessment of the common medical complications. Many of the physiological complications are associated with signs and symptoms. For example, patients with BN may have enlarged parotid glands on physical examination, and laboratory testing may reveal elevated salivary amylase levels; patients with BED may have headaches and elevated blood pressure. However, many of the serious complications of eating disorders are not associated with symptoms or signs. For example, osteopenia, which occurs in more than 60% of AN patients, may be silent for years. Dyslipidemias that occur in BED may be unassociated with signs or symptoms. Table 1 lists the laboratory tests that should be done for all patients with eating disorders and specific tests for patients with AN, BN, or BED.

During the assessment procedure, it is often helpful to engage the patient and family in a discussion of the common medical complications that have been identified. It is helpful to assist the patient in recognizing the relationship between his or her behavior and the medical complication. For example, a patient who is abusing laxatives may develop chest pain, have an arrhythmia on physical examination, have an abnormal electrocardiogram with a prolonged QT interval, and have hypokalemia. Helping the patient to see the relationship between laxative abuse and the chest pain along with the risk of a fatal arrhythmia may allow the patient to enter treatment and participate meaningfully in the recovery process. This therapeutic use of signs

TABLE 1 Laboratory Testing. SGPT (ALT) = Serum Glutamic Pyruvic Transaminase, SGOT (AST) = Serum Glutamic Oxaloacetic Transaminase, DEXA = Dual Energy X-ray Absorptiometry

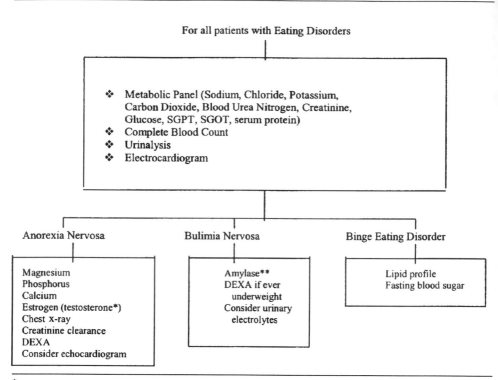

For all patients with Eating Disorders

- ❖ Metabolic Panel (Sodium, Chloride, Potassium, Carbon Dioxide, Blood Urea Nitrogen, Creatinine, Glucose, SGPT, SGOT, serum protein)
- ❖ Complete Blood Count
- ❖ Urinalysis
- ❖ Electrocardiogram

Anorexia Nervosa | Bulimia Nervosa | Binge Eating Disorder

Magnesium
Phosphorus
Calcium
Estrogen (testosterone*)
Chest x-ray
Creatinine clearance
DEXA
Consider echocardiogram

Amylase**
DEXA if ever
   underweight
Consider urinary
   electrolytes

Lipid profile
Fasting blood sugar

* For males.
** If purging with laxatives, obtain amylase isoenzymes.

and symptoms is often best accomplished by the physician who initially assesses the patient and makes the diagnosis.

The exact nature of the medical comorbidity depends on the patient's age and underlying physiological vulnerability, the intensity and type of purge behavior, rapidity and extent of weight change, and duration of the eating disorder. For example, a patient who loses 30% of her body weight in a 6-month period is likely to be at greater risk than a patient who loses 30% of her body weight over a 3-year period. If other factors are equal, use of prescription diuretics and certain types of laxatives appears to pose greater risk than similar intensity of purging by vomiting.

MEDICAL COMPLICATIONS

Cardiac Complications

Cardiac complications are common in patients with eating disorders and are associated with significant mortality and morbidity. About one-third of the deaths in patients with AN are due to cardiac complications (16), and many of the unexpected deaths in patients with BN are probably due to cardiac arrhythmias. BED patients have higher psychophysiological arousal levels than controls (17), and this may increase cardiac risk. Also, since most BED patients are overweight or obese, they have an increased risk for cardiac comorbidity, including hypertension and atherosclerosis.

Patients with AN or BN frequently have symptoms or signs of cardiac malfunction, although patients with BED often do not. Common symptoms suggesting cardiac abnormalities in AN or BN include light-headedness or dizziness, coldness, palpitations, and chest pain. Associated symptoms include orthostatic hypotension, hypothermia, acrocyanosis, arrhythmias, and midsystolic click. An example of the relationship between symptoms, signs, and laboratory data is as follows: A patient with chest pain may have a midsystolic click and on echocardiogram have evidence of mitral valve prolapse.

Cardiac arrhythmias are a particularly important issue for patients with AN and some patients with BN. QTc (corrected QT) interval prolongation and dispersion are indicators of increased risk for cardiac arrhythmia and sudden death, and is present in many patients with AN and some patients with BN (18). QTc is a measure of repolarization of the heart, and prolongation or dispersion (differences in various leads on the electrocardiagram) predisposes to a number of arrhythmias, including torsade de pointes (TDP), which is a ventricular tachycardia that can result in sudden death. Females are at greater risk for QT prolongation and for TDP (19), and patients with AN or BN have an even greater risk. Hypokalemia appears to increase the risk even more, although some eating disorder patients without electrolyte disturbances may have prolonged QTc intervals and TDP. This may be because serum potassium levels may be normal even when total body potassium stores are decreased (20). Certain medications are associated with prolonged QTc, including ziprasadone (Geodon) and thioridazine (Mellaril). These and other medications that prolong QTc should be avoided in eating disorder patients.

Mitral valve prolapse (MVP) occurs in a large percentage of patients (21). Although there may be no symptoms, the presence of chest pain or a midsystolic click is an indication for an echocardiogram, that may reveal MVP with or without regurgitation. Tricuspid valve prolapse also occurs but is less common. The etiology of the prolapse appears to be related to a decrease in size of the heart with semistarvation and development of a so-called valvular-ventricular disproportion (22). When chest pain occurs with

MVP it may be particularly difficult to treat. For patients with MVP, antibiotics should be taken prior to procedures that result in a bacterial shower (e.g., dental procedures).

Ipecac is used to induce vomiting after accidental poisonings and is available over the counter. About 1.3% of patients with eating disorders utilize ipecac to induce vomiting (23). Ipecac is toxic to muscle (including the muscle of the heart) and may result in a cardiomyopathy that can be fatal. Emetine, one of the alkaloid constituents of ipecac, is particular dangerous. Patients who present with proximal muscle weakness and a waddling gait should be assessed for use of ipecac.

The refeeding syndrome (24) may occur during the early treatment of patients with AN. The refeeding syndrome is the cardiovascular collapse that can occur with refeeding and is very serious. Several factors contribute to this syndrome including reduced myocardial mass, which makes it hard for the heart to handle the increased circulatory load during refeeding and changes in serum levels of phosphate, potassium, and magnesium. The immediate etiologic factor appears to be that glucose in the food causes phosphate to enter the intracellular space leading to low phosphate, which can affect contractility of the heart and lead to heart failure. The symptoms include swollen ankles, shortness of breath, tiredness, and anxiety. Signs include pedal edema, rales in the lungs, elevated jugular venous pressure, and a midsystolic click. The chest radiograph reveals an enlarged heart and evidence of congestive heart failure. Treatment includes correcting electrolytes, decreasing fluid and caloric intake, diuretics, and sometimes digitalis. Patients with the refeeding syndrome usually should be in the coronary care unit with telemetry.

The key to preventing the refeeding syndrome is conservative management for seriously underweight patients. Caloric intake should be low initially coupled with correction of dehydration and electrolytes. Phosphorus and electrolytes should be obtained every other day for the first 7–10 days and then weekly. Calories should be increased slowly by 100–200 calories once or twice a week during the first 2 weeks.

Renal Complications

Among AN patients, kidney failure accounts for about one-third of deaths. Herzog and colleagues (25) have shown that high serum creatinine levels and elevated uric acid levels predict a chronic course in AN patients. Although less well understood, a number of BN patients also develop chronic renal abnormalities. Several factors have been implicated in the kidney abnormalities that develop, particularly electrolyte abnormalities. Hypokalemia and metabolic acidosis that can result from persistent vomiting or laxative abuse are implicated in the catabolism that occurs in uremia (26). End-stage renal disease has been reported in patients with longstanding eating disorders; hypokalemic nephropathy has been implicated in these cases (27). Volume depletion with repeated dehydration from either semistarvation or purging or both contributes to elevated blood urea nitrogen and elevated creatinine levels. Many patients with eating disorders, especially AN, have decreased creatinine clearance as well. Elevated levels of uric acid may account for the occasional patient who develops gout. AN associated with rhabdomyolysis has been associated with hypophosphatemia and renal failure (28). Nephrolithiasis may be more common in patients with AN because chronic dehydration is known to contribute to the development of renal stones (29). One study has found a lower filtration factor in AN as well as a decreased urinary concentration capacity following fluid deprivation both before and after administration of vasopressin (30).

Electrolyte Abnormalities

Electrolyte abnormalities occur with semistarvation and various types of purging behavior, including vomiting, diuretic and laxative abuse, and ipecac abuse. About half of AN and BN patients have electrolyte abnormalities (31); the most common abnormality is elevated serum bicarbonate (metabolic alkalosis). Potassium and chloride abnormalities also occur. Potassium depletion can occur during semistarvation if there is inadequate potassium intake. During vomiting, hydrochloric acid is vomited and there is compensatory excretion of potassium through the kidneys, resulting in a decrease in potassium. Total body potassium is often decreased even when serum potassium is normal (20); thus, a random test of serum potassium may not detect abnormally low total body potassium and the patient may still be at risk for various cardiac complications related to hypokalemia. Abnormalities of chloride and bicarbonate may be present prior to the detection of hypokalemia. Among patients who are dehydrated, potassium may be in the normal range, but when hydration occurs the hypokalemia may become apparent.

Clinical findings suggestive of electrolyte abnormalities include weakness, constipation, dizziness, and depression. Patients with hypokalemia may develop leg cramps. Patients with either hypomagnesemia or hypocalcemia may develop tetany (sharp flexion of the ankle or wrist joints).

Many patients with bulimia nervosa are very secretive about use of self-induced vomiting, laxatives, or diuretics. Sometimes it is helpful to assess both serum and urinary electrolytes to determine the type of purge behavior that has occurred. Self-induced vomiting or diuretic abuse typically results in metabolic alkalosis with decreased serum potassium and chloride and elevated bicarbonate, whereas laxative abuse more typically results in metabolic acidosis.

Endocrine Abnormalities

Multiple endocrine abnormalities occur in the eating disorders (32). AN is the best studied (see Table 2), but there are similar if less pronounced abnormalities in BN. The endocrine abnormalities seen in BED are usually those seen in patients with obesity, including type 2 diabetes mellitus, but other endocrine abnormalities also occur.

The key symptom reflecting abnormalities in the hypothalamic–pituitary–gonadotropin (HPG) axis among AN patients is amenorrhea or irregular menses. Nearly one-third of patients with AN develop amenorrhea prior to the onset of weight loss and this finding is unexplained. It may relate to stress, but may also indicate a vulnerability of the endocrine system in patients with anorexia nervosa. Patients with AN have decreased gonadotropin-releasing hormone, decreased follicle stimulating hormone, and decreased estrogen levels which contribute to the development of osteopenia.

Abnormalities in the hypothalamic–pituitary–adrenal (HPA) axis are also very common. A key endocrine finding in patients with AN is hypercortisolism (which probably promotes the development of osteoporosis); elevated corticotropin-releasing hormone (CRH) is also characteristic, but typically there are normal adrenocorticotrophic hormone (ACTH) levels. Some patients with BN have normal cortisol levels, but some have findings similar to those seen in AN. Abnormal dexamethasone suppression tests are common in patients with BN. The HPA axis has also been shown to be disturbed among patients with the night eating syndrome. In these patients, there is an increased diurnal secretion of cortisol and an attenuated response of ACTH and cortisol in plasma after injection of CRH (33).

Among patients with BED, the emergence of non-insulin-dependent diabetes mellitus (type 2 diabetes mellitus) is probably common. One study (34) found that among obese type 2 diabetic adult patients, one-fourth had BED, although it is unclear if BED preceded or followed onset of the diabetes. One method of assessing diabetic control is measurement of glycosylated hemoglobin (HbA1c), which gives an estimate of blood sugar over the previous 3 months. The principle behind this is that the amount of hemoglobin that has become conjugated with glucose is proportional to the average level of blood glucose during the life of the red blood cell (an average of 3 months). Surprisingly, one study found that patients with type 2 diabetes mellitus who also had BED did not have evidence of higher glycosylated hemoglobin levels than type 2 diabetes mellitus patients without BED (33). However, several studies have shown that body mass index is positively correlated with increased levels

TABLE 2 Neuroendocrine Abnormalities in Anorexia Nervosa

Hormone	Level	Clinical effect
ACTH	Normal	None
Cortisol	Increased	Osteopenia
CRH	Increased	Suppression of appetite-stimulating effect of NPY
β-Endorphin	Decreased[a]	Abnormal feeding behavior and inhibition of antral contractility
Estradiol	Decreased	Amenorrhea, osteopenia, dyspareunia, decreased libido
FSH	Decreased	Amenorrhea
GH	Increased	GH resistance
GHRH	Increased	GH resistance
GIH	Increased	Delayed gastric emptying and altered satiety
GnRH	Decreased	Amenorrhea and osteopenia
HVA	Decreased[a]	Unknown
5-HIAA	Decreased[a]	Influences feeding behavior and satiety; increased levels after weight gain
IGF-1	Decreased	GH resistance
Leptin	Decreased	Amenorrhea and appetite
LH	Decreased	Amenorrhea
NPY	Increased[a]	Amenorrhea and abnormal feeding behavior
Norepinephrine	Decreased	Bradycardia, hypothermia, hypotension, and depression
Oxytocin	Decreased[a]	Unknown
T_3	Decreased	Low T_3 syndrome and decreased resting energy expenditure
T_4	Normal or decreased	Decreased resting energy expenditure
Testosterone	Decreased	Osteopenia, delayed puberty, and decreased libido and sexual functioning
TSH	Normal	None
Vasopressin	Decreased	Hypotension

ACTH, adrenocorticotrophic hormone; CRH, corticotropin-releasing hormone; GH, growth hormone; FSH, follicle-stimulating hormone; GHRH, GH-releasing hormone; GIH, somatostatin; GnRH, gonadotropin-releasing hormone; 5-HIAA, 5-hydroxyindoleacetic acid, a serotonin metabolite; HVA, homovanillic acid; IGF, insulin-like growth factor; LH, lutenizing hormone; TSH, thyroid-stimulating hormone; GH, growth hormone; NPY, neuropeptide Y.
[a] CSF level rather than serum level.
Source: Chial HJ and McAlpine DE. Anorexia nervosa: Manifestations and Management for the Gastroenterologist. Reprinted with permission from the American College of Gastroenterology, (Am J Gastroenterol 2002; 97:225–269).

of HbA1c, and since some studies have shown that obese BED patients consume more calories than obese non-BED patients, indirectly BED may result in elevated levels of HbA1c (35).

Among patients with type 1 diabetes mellitus, the presence of BN or AN is associated with higher levels of HbA1c than type 1 diabetic patients without these conditions (36). Furthermore, patients with type 1 diabetes who have either AN or BN have an increased risk of diabetic complications (37).

Leptin levels have been shown to be low in AN and normal-weight BN patients but elevated in BED patients (38). Brewerton and colleagues (39) have shown that plasma leptin levels are low in BN when compared to normal controls; the differences do not appear related to body weight but may be related to HPA axis activation and serotonin dysregulation. Among patients with night eating syndrome, there is an attenuation of the nocturnal rise in leptin and melatonin (40).

Gastrointestinal Complications

Gastrointestinal complaints occur in more than 50% of patients with eating disorders and include bloating, flatulence, constipation, decreased appetite, abdominal pain, borborygmi, and nausea (41,42). Multiple complications can occur involving the entire gastrointestinal track. The most common complications include dental caries, enlarged parotid glands, gastroesophageal reflux disorder, delayed gastric emptying, and delayed colonic transit. Semistarvation and various types of purge behavior affect metabolic and hormonal processes that influence gastrointestinal functioning. The complications depend in part on the type and intensity of the behavior. For example, an underweight patient who utilizes large quantities of stimulant-type laxatives (e.g., senna) on a daily basis is likely to be at greater risk than a normal-weight patient who utilizes bulk agents (e.g., docusate) infrequently.

Oral and dental complications are common among patients who binge eat and purge by vomiting. A common dental problem is enamel erosion (perimolysis) due to chronic exposure of tooth structures to hydrochloric acid from vomiting; this is particularly pronounced on the lingual side of the teeth. Dental caries (cavities) occur because of consumption of high-calorie binge foods and weakened tooth structure. Hypersensitivity of the teeth to hot, cold, and sweet foods occurs because of exposed dentin and root surfaces. Fillings and other restorations may fail because of exposure to hydrochloric acid. Periodontitis (gum disease) with gingival recession occurs due to nutritional deficiencies and trauma to the mucosa. Salivary abnormalities include reduced salivary flow (zerostomia) experienced symptomatically as a dry mouth and enlarged parotid and submandibular glands.

Management of dental and oral problems begins with a full assessment. The dentist may be the first health care professional to recognize the problem (43,44). Dental care includes emergency treatment and management of pain, basic fillings, and other routine care. If possible, restorative cosmetic dental care should be postponed until the eating disorder is under control; however, if this is not possible, porcelain and ceramics may be less likely to fail than resins in patients with active BN. Educating patients who are still binge-eating and purging can often help prevent some dental problems (45). For example, it may help decrease dental complications if the patient uses antiacids after vomiting and delays brushing. Application of fluoride and use of zylitol chewing gum may also prevent some problems.

Parotid gland enlargement (sialadenosis) is common among patients with BN and also occasionally occurs in those with restricting AN. Sialadenosis is a noninflammatory recurrent enlargement of the salivary glands, most commonly the parotids, which is almost always associated with an underlying systemic disorder, including diabetes, alcoholism, malnutrition, and eating disorders. The cause is thought to be a peripheral autonomic neuropathy resulting in disordered metabolism and secretion (46). Serum amylase concentration is elevated in patients with parotid gland enlargement and is correlated with frequency of bulimic symptoms (47).

Delayed gastric emptying is common among patients with AN and also occurs in BN patients (48). Most AN patients have delayed emptying of both solid and liquids associated with decreased frequency, intensity, and coordination of gastric contractions. Symptoms of nausea, vomiting, and gastric fullness correlate with slowed gastric emptying. With weight gain most patients have an improvement in gastric emptying as well as a decrease in gastrointestinal symptoms. During weight restoration, liquids may be better tolerated than solids, and weight gain alone usually results in improved gastric emptying. Metoclopramide has been shown to improve gastric emptying and reduce gastrointestinal symptoms in anorexic patients (49). One problem with metoclopramide is that it crosses the blood–brain barrier and can result in extrapyramidal symptoms; underweight patients seem to be particularly vulnerable to this side effect. Patients with BN also may have delayed gastric emptying as well as larger mean stomach capacity and blunted postprandial cholecystokinin (CCK) release (50). The delayed CCK release may contribute to the impaired satiety seen in BN patients.

Few studies of gastrointestinal functioning have been undertaken among either BED or night eating syndrome patients. However, one study has found that obese BED patients have an increase in gastric capacity compared to non-BED obese patients (51).

Multiple *esophageal problems* can occur ranging from mild esophagitis to esophageal rupture (52). Exposure to stomach acid secondary to self-induced vomiting can lead to esophagitis, erosion, ulcerations, esophageal strictures, gastroesophageal reflux disease (GERD), or Barrett's esophagus (characterized by columnar-lined cells at the distal end of the esophagus). Four case reports have suggested that BN may lead to Barrett's esophagus and the eventual development of carcinoma (53).

GERD symptoms are common among eating disorder patients, especially those who purge by vomiting, although the incidence has not been fully established (54). Symptoms include heartburn, regurgitation, dysphagia, and angina-like chest pain. Treatment includes elevation of the head of the bed and use of antacids. The next step of treatment is H_2 antagonists that inhibit the action of histamine at the H_2 receptors of the parietal cells of the stomach. The H_2 antagonists include cimetidine (Tagamet) given 400–800 mg twice daily and rantidine (Zantac) given 150 mg twice daily. Proton pump inhibitors can be utilized to suppress the H^+K^+-ATPase enzyme. These medications include omeprazole (Prilosec) 20 mg/day and lansoprazole (Prevacid) 30 mg/day; these medications should be continued for 2 weeks after symptoms subside. It may be that chronic GERD can result in Barrett's esophagus.

Constipation is a very common problem that can result from semi-starvation or the long-term use of stimulant laxatives. Whole-gut transit times as well as colonic transit time is delayed in both AN and BN patients (55,56). Weight and eating normalization improves constipation. For patients who abuse laxatives, several strategies can be helpful. Preparing the patient for the consequences of stopping laxatives can be helpful. Most patients develop constipation, fluid retention, bloating, and temporary weight gain. The patient should be advised to discontinue use of all laxatives (including herbal remedies), drink 8–10 cups of water per day (and no caffeinated fluids since they may act as a diuretic), to exercise regularly and moderately, and to eat normally. Dietary changes that promote normal bowel function include (a) consumption of whole-grain breads, cereals, and crackers and wheat bran or foods with wheat bran added; (b) addition of fruits and vegetables; and (c) avoidance of prunes, which contain an ingredient that is actually an irritant laxative. When laxatives are required for patients with chronic constipation or who are withdrawing from laxatives, psyllium or docusate, both of which are bulk agents, can be used.

Hunger and satiety functions are frequently disturbed in eating disorder patients. Multiple factors contribute to these problems. For example, increased growth hormone, increased cortisol-releasing hormone, decreased β-endorphin, and autonomic insufficiency all contribute to delayed gastric emptying, which leads to an increase in satiety. Similarly, a decrease in 5-HT, an increase in neuropeptide Y, and a decrease in leptin also increase satiety. Ghrelin, a hormone produced by the endocrine cells of the stomach, that is a potent appetite stimulant, and is present at higher levels in BN patients than in normal controls (57), may partly account for the impaired satiety seen in these patients.

Central Nervous System Complications

There is much interest in the effects of starvation and malnutrition on the brain and the nervous system. Several abnormalities have been noted. *Structural abnormalities* in the brain have been identified in AN patients. Specifically, ventricular and sulcal enlargement have been identified, which may not be fully reversible with weight gain (58). Enlarged cerebrospinal fluid spaces have been associated with sleep disruption and sleep-onset insomnia; sleep studies of patients with enlarged cerebrospinal fluid spaces have shown an increased amount of time spent in slow-wave sleep, and the duration of rapid eye movement sleep is reduced (59). It is unclear if this is a result of nutritional deficiencies or a particular cerebral dysfunction. Underweight patients with AN have decreases in both the gray and white matter of the brain; white matter volume appears to return to normal with weight gain, but the gray matter has not been shown return to normal with weight gain (60). Cortisol has been postulated to have a role in these abnormalities; urinary free cortisol is positively correlated with total cerebral spinal fluid volume and inversely correlated with total gray matter volume (61). Various studies have found an incidence of cerebral atrophy in AN patients ranging from 25% to 75% (62). When these abnormalities are suspected or confirmation is needed, magnetic resonance imaging, rather than computed tomography, provides the most information at the least risk to the patient.

It has been recognized for decades that patients with eating disorders have abnormalities in cognition that have typically been classified as cognitive distortions such as dichotomization or personalization (63); these abnormalities have been generally thought to be due to psychological developmental delay or regression. However, several studies have found *neurocognitive abnormalities* in AN patients, including attention deficits, difficulty with abstraction and flexibility of thought, abnormalities in executive function, visual spatial abnormalities, and impaired memory (64–67). The relationships between these neurocognitive abnormalities and the structural abnormalities and cortisol abnormalities are unclear but may be important. There may also be a relationship between neurocognitive abnormalities and body image (68), but the exact nature of this relationship is unknown. Although many of the neurocognitive abnormalities resolve with weight gain (69), subtle abnormalities remain and may predispose to relapse (70).

A few studies have looked at various types of *abnormalities in functional imaging*. Positron emission tomography (PET) has revealed that BN patients do not have the right cortical activation seen in normal women (71). Brain imaging has found a hypometabolism of glucose in several cerebral regions in both AN and BN patients (72,73). In a study by Troop and colleagues (74), 74 patients with a variety of eating disorders were compared to normal patients using PET to assess activation during presentation of items expected to elicit the reaction of disgust; disgust was found to be positively related to eating disorder symptoms in the patients but not in the controls.

Many AN patients drink large quantities of water to assuage hunger, and some patients with AN surreptitiously drink large quantities of water to gain weight prior to being weighed by their physician. Occasionally this results in severe water intoxication and electrolyte imbalance (particularly hyponatremia) that can lead to neurological deficits including ataxia, cerebral edema, seizures, central pontine myelinolysis, coma, and even death (75). Even when patients do not have water intoxication, seizures can occur in about 5% of patients with AN (76), probably due to electrolyte disturbances or hypoglycemia.

Peripheral Nervous System Complications

Peripheral neuropathies occur in 8–13% of anorexia nervosa patients (76,77). The likely cause is chronic malnutrition including repeated episodes of hypoglycemia. Patients with AN are also at increased risk for developing localized compression neuropathies due to loss of subcutaneous tissue.

In AN and BN there is a reduction in noradrenergic activity in the central and peripheral nervous systems. The clinical complications of this reduction are hypotension, bradycardia, hypothermia, and depression (78).

In BN and BED elevated pain thresholds have been found. This may be another partial explanation of the abnormal satiety response seen in both groups of patients since the feeling of fullness and subsequent termination of a meal are activated by the vagus nerve (79). In addition, Brewerton and colleagues (80) have shown that BN patients have lower cerebral spinal fluid concentrations of β-endorphin than normal controls; furthermore, β-endorphin concentrations were inversely correlated with measures of depression.

Musculoskeletal Complications

Tendons and muscles are also affected by AN. Diminished or absent tendon reflexes may be found on physical examination. An early report (76) found that generalized muscle weakness was present in 43% of 47 patients with AN. Proximal muscle weakness that is associated with a selective disturbance of the skeletal muscle metabolism is often seen. This is due to a diminished lactate response to ischemic exercise (81) and is associated with reduced serum carnosinase activity. This myopathy is associated with selective type 2 fiber atrophy with abnormal accumulation of glycogen within the muscle fibers (82).

Short stature is a common finding among AN patients. One explanation has been that if AN develops in adolescence prior to the closure of the epiphyses there may be a potential irreversible growth retardation resulting in short stature. However, it has also been suggested (83) that the observed short stature seen in many AN patients may have a different etiology. Among 85 patients, 80% developed AN after menarche, but, compared to a control group, 76% of the patients were below the 50th height percentile and nearly 15% were below the 5th percentile.

Scoliosis may also be more common in patients with AN. Forty-four young women with idiopathic scoliosis were found to be similar in height to controls, but they had significantly lower body mass indices than controls and 25% were in the range considered to represent anorexia (84). The reasons for this finding are unknown.

Osteoporosis or *osteopenia* affects up to 90% of patients with AN and many patients with BN who have a past history of AN (85). Among obese BED patients, osteoporosis may be less common because obesity seems to be a relative protective factor against loss of bone mineral density. Furthermore, osteopenia develops early in the course of AN, often within the first year. Men are affected as well, and there is some evidence that the loss may be greater in men than in women (86). Furthermore, the loss of bone mineral density has long-term consequences. Among a group of 208 patients followed an average of 40 years after diagnosis, the cumulative incidence of any fracture was 57% (87). Among a group of 19 women who had been fully recovered for a mean of 21 years, femur BMD was still significantly less than among controls (88). Although the cause of this significant bone loss is poorly understood, it is clear that it is different from postmenopausal osteoporosis, which affects primarily bone resorption; the osteoporosis of AN is related to both bone formation and bone resorption.

The World Health Organization criteria for osteoporosis (89) is based on a system of T scores that indicate the standard deviation (SD) from the mean derived from a young normal sex-matched reference population. Normal bone mineral density is defined as less than 1 SD below the normal mean; osteopenia (low bone mass) is defined as 1 SD below to 2.5 SD below normal; osteoporosis is defined as more than 2.5 SD below the normal mean, and severe osteoporosis is more than 2.5 SD below the mean with one or more fractures. *Z* scores compare the bone density of a subject with that of an age- and sex-matched control.

The majority of peak bone mass is achieved by age 20, although there is some continuing accumulation until age 30. AN typically develops during adolescence at a time when peak bone mass has not been achieved. The osteoporosis that occurs in AN affects both trabecular bone (found mainly in the spine) and cortical bone (found mainly in the long bones). The spine and hip seem to be particularly vulnerable.

Bone is constantly in a state of remodeling, which involves balanced coupling of bone formation and bone resorption. Osteoblasts are cells involved in bone formation and osteoclasts are cells involved in bone-resorption. Serum and urinary markers of bone formation include osteocalcin, bone-specific alkaline phosphatase, and procollagen-I carboxy terminal propeptide; bone resorption markers include urine deoxypyridinoline and serum carboxy terminal type I propeptide and N-telopeptide. In AN, there is an increase in resorption accompanied by a decrease or no change in the rate of bone formation.

The cause of this uncoupling of bone formation and resorption is unknown but a number of factors have been implicated. In AN, there are decreased levels of insulin-like growth factor-1 (IGF-1), which is a bone tropic factor, and levels of IGF-1 increase with weight gain (90). Although not proven, elevated cortisol levels (a very common finding in AN) may facilitate trabecular bone loss by suppressing osteoblast proliferation. The exact role of amenorrhea and hypoestrogenemia in the pathogenesis of osteoporosis is unclear. Although bone density has been shown to be related to the length of amenorrhea (91), and mean serum estrogen and progesterone levels are consistently low in underweight anorexics, estrogen administration has not been consistently shown to improve bone density (92,93).

At present, a dual-energy X-ray absorptiometry (DEXA) is the gold standard for detection of osteoporosis (94). Patients who have osteopenia should have repeat tests every 18–20 months. Although ultrasound is less expensive and avoids radiation exposure, it has not yet been shown to be effective in detecting osteoporosis at the sites most vulnerable in AN patients.

Unfortunately, treatments have not been shown to be completely effective in restoring normal bone mineral density (91,95). Weight gain prevents further loss of BMD and after time may improve bone mineral density. Short-term nutrition rehabilitation has been shown to improve bone formation markers as well as IGF-1 and leptin, but whether this translates into improved bone mineral density is not yet known (96). Although it seems reasonable that estrogen supplementation would improve bone mineral density, its efficacy has not been established despite many attempts to do so. One study has shown that recombinant human IGF-1 has some benefit in restoring BMD and that administration with oral contraceptive may be of additional benefit (97). However, this treatment is still experimental. At present, the most reasonable approach is to restore normal weight and normal menses while ensuring adequate calcium intake (1000–1500 mg/day) and vitamin D (600 IU daily).

Some patients may benefit from estrogen supplementation, and some patients with osteoporosis may benefit from biphosphates which reduce bone resorption. Alendronate or risendronate sodium might be considered, although they both cause gastrointestinal side effects, including esophagitis, and must be used carefully. Alendronate (Fosamax) is currently available in a once-a-week preparation, which may make it easier for selected patients to use.

Gynecological and Obstetrical Complications

Eating disorder patients have multiple gynecological and obstetrical complications. Amenorrhea is a key finding in most AN patients, and many patients with BN also have amenorrhea or irregular menses. Multiple factors contribute to the amenorrhea, including weight loss, decrease in body fat, stress, excessive exercise, and decreased estrogen and follicle stimulating hormone levels.

Among AN patients and some BN patients, the ovarian and uterine volume is decreased, depth of endometrial thickness is decreased, and atrophic changes occur in the vaginal mucosa (98). Multifollicular ovaries also occur in AN (99). The change from microfollicular to multifollicular to dominant follicle and finally to ovulatory follicle occurs during puberty. Many underweight AN patients have multifollicular ovaries; with weight gain there is progression to the ovulatory stage. Some of these findings can be helpful in establishing a goal weight during treatment of AN patients (100). For example, increase to normal thickness of the endometrium and progression to a single ovulatory follicle have been used to signal achievement of normal body weight. Polycystic ovaries have also been reported in patients with BN (101) and with BED (102).

Many women with AN are infertile, but most women with BN are fertile. Complications for both the mother and the baby are common when the eating disorder is active. Many patients with AN do not gain adequate weight during pregnancy. Some patients are able to gain adequate weight or interrupt purge behavior for the safety of the baby, but the eating disorder frequently recurs after delivery (103); women with chronic AN or those with BN with a past history of AN were more likely to relapse after delivery (104). Women with active eating disorders are at greater risk for cesarean section and for postpartum depression (105). Complications for the infant include preterm delivery, low birthweight, intrauterine growth restriction, and low Apgar scores (106). If possible, it is wise for the patient to delay pregnancy until her eating disorder is in remission. For patients who become pregnant while their eating disorder is still active, a multidisciplinary team is usually needed and should include an obstetrician who specializes in high-risk pregnancies, a neonatologist, and a psychiatrist (107).

There may be effects on the infants of women with eating disorders. One study compared infants of mothers who had an eating disorder during the first year postpartum to infants of mothers without such a history (108). Mothers with a history of an eating disorder postpartum were more intrusive with their infants during mealtimes and during play, and their infants had more negative emotional tones, and the mealtimes were more conflicted than those of infants of normal mothers. Furthermore, infants of these mothers tended to be lighter in weight during their second year of life than infants of control mothers.

CONCLUSIONS

Multiple medical complications are associated with the three major eating disorders. These complications frequently require treatment by several specialists at various points in the recovery process. It is important for the many physicians and other care providers involved to work collaboratively to address the problems in an organized way utilizing an agreed-upon timeline. For example, during the initial management of AN, the cardiologist and psychiatrist may need to work together to design a program that prevents emergence of the refeeding syndrome. Later in the course of treatment when the patient is near ideal body weight, the activity therapist may have to be actively involved in designing an appropriate exercise program to reduce the impact of osteoporosis. Once the patient has achieved ideal body weight, the gynecologist may be needed to assess possible need for hormonal intervention if menses have not resumed. During the entire course of treatment from initial assessment to eventual discharge from treatment (often several years later), there needs to be a team leader organizing the delivery of care. When this occurs, outcome is often improved.

REFERENCES

1. Yager J, Andersen A, Devlin M, Egger H, Herzog D, Mitchell J, Powers P, Yates A, Zerbe K. American Psychiatric Association Work Group on Eating Disorders: practice guideline for the treatment of patients with eating disorders (revision). Am J Psychiatry 2000; 157(suppl):1–39.
2. Garfinkel PE, Lin E, Goering P, Spegg C, Goldbloom D, Kennedy S, Kaplan AS, Woodside DB. Should amenorrhea be necessary for the diagnosis of anorexia nervosa? Br J Psychiatry 1996; 168:500–506.
3. National Institute of Mental Health. The Numbers Count. 2002. Web Address Http//www.nimh.nih.gov/publicat/numbers.cfm.
4. McDowell I. Alzheimer's disease: insights from epidemiology. Aging (Milano) 2001; 13:143–162.

5. Narrow WE. One-year prevalence of mental disorders, excluding substance use disorders, in the US: NIMH ECA prospective data. Population estimates based on US Census estimated residential population age 18 and over on July 1, 1998. Unpublished.

6. Striegel-Moore RH, Leslie D, Petrill SA, Garvin V, Rosenheck RA. One year use and cost of inpatient and outpatient services among female and male patients with an eating disorder: evidence from a national database of health insurance claims. Int J Eat Disord 2000; 27:381–389.

7. Tamminga CA, Lieberman JA. Schizophrenia research series: from molecule to public policy. Biol Psychiatry 1999; 46:3.

8. Agras WS. The consequences and costs of the eating disorders. Psychiatr Clin North Am 2001; 24:371–379.

9. Theander S. Anorexia nervosa. A psychiatric investigatio of 94 female patients. Arch Psychiatr Scand Suppl 1970; 214:1–194.

10. Nielsen S, Moller-Madsen S, Isager T, Jorgensen J, Pagsberg K, Theander S. Standardized morality in eating disorders—a quantitative summary of previously published and new evidence. J Psychosom Res 1998; 44:413–434.

11. Stunkard AJ. Eating patterns and obesity. Psychiatr Q 1959; 33:284–294.

12. Stunkard AJ, Grace WJ, Wolff HG. The night-eating syndrome: a pattern of food intake among certain obese patients. Am J Med 1955; 19:78–86.

13. American Psychiatric Association. Diagnostic and Statistical Manual of Mental Disorders. 4th ed. Washington, DC: Text Revision (DSM-IVTR), 2000: 583–586, 785–787.

14. Stunkard AJ, Allison KC. Two forms of disordered eating in obesity: binge eating and night eating. Obesity 2003; 27:1–12.

15. Schenck C, Mahowald MW. Review of nocturnal sleep-related eating disorders. Int J Eat Disord 1994; 15:343–356.

16. Schocken DD, Holoway JD, Powers PS. Weight loss and the heart: effects of anorexia nervosa and starvation. Arch Intern Med 1989; 149:877–881.

17. Vogele C, Florin I. Psychophysiological responses to food exposure: an experimental study in binge eaters. Int J Eat Disord 1997; 21:147–157.

18. Swenne I, Larsson PT. Heart risk associated with weight loss in anorexia nervosa and eating disorders: risk factors for QTc interval prolongation and dispersion. Acta Paediatr 1999; 88:304–309.

19. Wolbrette D. Gender differences in the proarrhythmic potential of QT-prolonging drugs. Curr Womens Health Rep 2002; 2:105–109.

20. Powers PS, Tyson IB, Stevens BA, Heal AV. Total body potassium and serum potassium among eating disorder patients. Int J Eat Disord 1995; 18:269–276.

21. de Simone G, Scalfi L, Galderisi M, Celentano A, Di Biase G, Tammaro P, Garofalo M, Mureddu GF, de Divitiis O, Contaldo F. Cardiac abnormalities in young women with anorexia nervosa. Br Heart J 1994; 71:287–292.

22. Oka Y, Ito T, Matsumoto S, et al. Mitral valve prolapse in patients with anorexia nervosa. Two-dimensional echocardiographic study. Jpn Heart J 1987; 28:873–882.

23. Powers PS, Mitchell JE, Garner DM, Monson N. International eating disorders

database: preliminary findings. Presented at Academy for Eating Disorders, 2001 International Conference on Eating Disorders, April 27, 2001, Boston.

24. Mehler PS. Eating disorders: 1. Anorexia nervosa. Hosp Pract 1996; 31:109–113.

25. Herzog W, Deter HC, Fiehn W, Petzold E. Medical findings and predictors of long-term physical outcome in anorexia nervosa: a prospective, 12-year follow-up study. Psychol Med 1997; 27:269–279.

26. Franch HA, Mitch WE. Catabolism in uremia: the impact of metabolic acidosis. J Am Soc Nephrol 1998; 9:S78–81.

27. Abdel-Rahman EM, Moorthy AV. End-stage renal disease (ESD + RD in patients with eating disorders. Clin Nephrol 1997; 47:106–111.

28. Wada S, Nagase T, Koike Y, Kugai N, Nagata N. A case of anorexia nervosa with acute renal failure induced by rhabdomyolysis: possible involvement of hypophosphatemia or phosphate depletion. Intern Med 1992; 31:478–482.

29. Silber TJ, Kass EJ. Anorexia nervosa and nephrolithiasis. J Adol Health Care 1984; 5:50–52.

30. Aperia A, Broberger O, Fohlin L. Renal function in anorexia nervosa. Acta Paediatr Scand 1978; 67:219–224.

31. Mitchell JE, Pyle RL, Eckert ED, Hatsukami D, Lentz R. Electrolyte and other physiological abnormalities in patients with bulimia. Psychol Med 1983; 14:273–278.

32. Chial HJ, McAlpine DE, Camilleri M. Anorexia nervosa: manifestations and management for the gastroenterologist. Am J Gastroenterol 2002; 97:255–269.

33. Birketvedt GS, Sundsfjord J, Florholmen JR. Hypothalamic-pituitary-adrenal axis in night eating syndrome. Am J Physiol Endocrinol Metab 2002; 282(2):366–369.

34. Crow S, Kendall D, Praus B, Thuras P. Binge eating and other psychopathology in patients with type II diabetes mellitus. Int J Eat Disord 2001; 30:222–226.

35. Goebel-fabbri AE, Fikkan JL, Connell A, Vangsness L, Anerson B. J Binge eating, BMI, emotional distress, and health status in women with type 2 diabetes. Presented at the Academy for Eating Disorders 2002 International Conference on Eating Disorders and Clinical Teaching Day, Boston.

36. Birk R, Spencer ML. The prevalence of anorexia nervosa, bulimia, and induced glycosuria in IDDM females. Diabetes Educator, 1989, 336–341.

37. Rydall A, Rodin G, Olmsted M, Devenyi R, Daneman D. A four year follow-up study of eating disorders and medical complications in young women with insulin-dependent diabetes mellitus [Abstr]. Psychosom Med 1994; 56:179.

38. Monteleone P, DiLieto A, Tortorella A, Longobardi N, Maj M. Circulating leptin in patients with anorexia nervosa, bulimia nervosa or binge-eating disorder: relationship to body weight, eating patterns, psychopathology and endocrine changes. Psychiatry Res 2000; 94(2):121–129.

39. Brewerton TD, Lesem MD, Kennedy A, Garvey WT. Reduced plasma leptin concentrations in bulimia nervosa. Psychoneuroendocrinology 2000; 25:548–649.

40. Birketvedt GS, Florholmen J, Sundsfjord J, Osterud B, Dinges D, Bilker W,

Stunkard A. Behavioral and neuroendocrine characteristics of the night-eating syndrome. JAMA 1999; 282:657–663.

41. Chami TN, Anderson AE, Crowell MD, Schuster MM, Whitehead WE. Gastrointestional symptoms in bulimia nervosa: effects of treatment. Am J Gastroenterology 1995; 90:88–92.

42. McClain CJ, Humphries LL, Hill KK, Nicki NJ. Gastrointestinal and nutritional aspects of eating disorders. J Am Coll Nutr 1993; 12:466–474.

43. Steel AW, Mehler PS. Oral and dental complications. In Eating Disorders: A Guide to Medical Care and Complications. Baltimore: Johns Hopkins University Press, 1999:144–152.

44. Schwartz MI. Dentistry and eating disorders. In AABA Newsletter, Fall 1997.

45. Sundaram G, Bartlett D. Preventative measures for bulimic patients with dental erosion. Eur J Prosthodont Restor Dent 2001; 9:25–29.

46. Coleman H, Altini M, Nayler S, Richards A. Sialadenosis: a presenting sign in bulimia. Head Neck 1998; 20:758–760.

47. Metzger ED, Levine JM, McArdle CR, Wolfe BE, Jimerson DC. Salivary gland enlargement and elevated serum amylase in bulimia nervosa. Biol Psychiatry 1999; 45:1520–1522.

48. Rigaud D, Bedig G, Merrouche M, Vulpillat M, Bonfils S, Apfelbaum M. Delayed gastric emptying in anorexia nervosa is improved by completion of a renutrition program. Dig Dis Sci 1988; 33:919–925.

49. Saleh JW, Lebwohl P. Metoclopramide-induced gastric emptying in patients with anorexia nervosa. Am J Gastroenterol 1980; 74:27–32.

50. Devlin MJ, Walsh BT, Guss JL, Kissileff HR, Liddle RA, Petkova E. Postprandial cholecystokinin release and gastric emptying in patients with bulimia nervosa. Am J Clin Nutr 1997; 65:114–120.

51. Geliebter A, Hashim SA. Gastric capacity in normal, obese and bulimic women. Physiol Behav 2001; 74:743–746.

52. Kiss A, Wiesnagrotski S, Abatzi TA, Meryn S, Haubenstock A, Base W. Upper gastrointestinal endoscopy findings in patients with long-standing bulimia nervosa. Gastrointest Endos 1989; 35:516–518.

53. Dessureault S, Coppola D, Weitzner M, Powers P, Karl RC. Barrett's oesophagus and squamous cell carcinoma with psychogenic vomiting. Int J Gastrointest Cancer 2002; 32:57–61.

54. Bartlett DW, Evans DF, Smith BG. The relationship between gastroesophageal reflux disease and dental erosion. J Oral Rehabil 1996; 23:289–297.

55. Kamal N, Chami T, Andersen A, Rosell FA, Schuster MM, Whitehead WE. Delayed gastrointestinal transit times in anorexia nervosa and bulimia nervosa. Gastroenterology 1991; 101:1320–1324, 1991.

56. Chun AB, Sokol MS, Kaye WH, Hutson WR, Wald A. Colonic and anorectal function in constipated patients with anorexia nervosa. Am J Gastroenterol 1997; 92:879–883.

57. Tanaka M, Naruo T, Muranaga T, Yasuhara D, Shiiya T, Nakazato M, Matsukura S, Nozoe S. Increased fasting plasma ghrelin levels in patients with bulimia nervosa. Eur J Endocrin 2002; 146:R1–R3.

58. Katzman DK, Zipursky RB, Lambe EK, Mikulis DJ. A longitudinal magnetic

resonance imaging study of brain changes in adolescents with anorexia nervosa. Arch Pediatr Adolesc Med 1997; 151:793–797.

59. Eiber R, Friedman S. Correlation between eating disorders and sleep disturbances. Encephale 2001; 27:429–434.
60. Lambe EK, Katzman DK, Mikulis DJ, Kennedy SH, Zipursky RB. Cerebral gray matter volume deficits after weight recovery from anorexia nervosa. Arch Gen Psychiatry 1997; 54:537–542.
61. Katzman DK, Lambe EK, Mikulis DJ, Ridgley JN, Goldbloom DS, Zipursky RB. Cerebral gray matter and white matter volume deficits in adolescent girls with anorexia nervosa. J Pediatr 1996; 129:794–803.
62. di Pietralata GM. Imaging techniques in the management of anorexia and bulimia nervosa. Eat Weight Disord 2002; 7:146–151.
63. Garner DM, Fairburn CG, Davis R. Cognitive-behavioral treatment of bulimia nervosa. A critical appraisal. Behav Modif 1987; 11:398–431.
64. Fassino S, Piero A, Daga GA, Leombruni P, Mortara P, Rovera GG. Attentional biases and frontal functioning in anorexia nervosa. Int J Eat Disord 2002; 31:274–283.
65. Neumarker KJ, Bzufka WM, Dudeck U, Hein J, Neumarker U. Are there specific disabilities of mnumber processing in adolescent patients with anorexia nervosa? Evidence from clinical and neuropsychological data when compared to morphometric measures from magnetic resonance imaging. Eur Child Adol Psychiatry 2000; 9:111–121.
66. Seed JA, Dixon RA, McCluskey SE, Young AH. Basal activity of the hypothalamic-pituitary-adrenal axis and cognitive function in anorexia nervosa. Eur Arch Psychiatry Clin Neurosci 2000; 250:11–15.
67. Mathias JL, Kent PS. Neuropsychological consequences of extreme weight loss and dietary restriction in patients with anorexia nervosa. J Clin Exp Neuropsychol 1998; 20:548–564.
68. Epstein J, Wiseman CV, Sunday SR, Klapper F, Alkalay L, Halmi KA. Neurocognitive evidence favors "topdown" over "bottom up" mechanisms in the pathogenesis of body size distortions in anorexia nervosa. Eat Weight Disord 2001; 6:140–147.
69. Lauer CJ, Gorzewski B, Gerlinghoff M, Backmund H, Zihl J. Neuropsychological assessments before and after treatment in patients with anorexia nervosa and bulimia nervosa. J Psychiatr Res 1999; 33:129–138.
70. Green MW, Elliman NA, Wakeling A, Rogers PJ. Cognitive functioning, weight change and therapy in anorexia nervosa. J Psychiatr Res 1996; 30:401–410.
71. Wu JC, Hagman J, Buchsbaum MS, Blinder B, Derrfler M, Tai WY, Hazlett E, Sicotte N. Greater left cerbral hemispheric metabolism in bulimia assessed by positron emission tomography. Am J Psychiatry 1990; 147:309–312.
72. Delvenne V, Lostra F, Goldman S, Biver F, DeMaertelaer V, Appelboom-Fondu J, Schoutens A, Bidaut LM, Luxen A, Mendelwicz J. Brain hypometabolism of glucose in anorexia nervosa: A PET-scan study. Biol Psychiatry 1995; 37:161–169.

73. Delvenne V, Goldman S, Simon Y, De Maertelaer V, Lotstra F. Brain hypometabolism of glucose in bulimia nervosa. Int J Eat Disord 1997; 21:313–326.
74. Troop NA, Murphy F, Bramon E, Treasure JL. Disgust sensitivity in eating disorders: a preliminary investigation. Int J Eat Disord 2000; 27:446–451.
75. Amann B, Schafer M, Sterr A, Arnold S, Grunze H. Central pontine myelinolysis in a patient with anorexia nervosa. Int J Eat Disord 2001; 30:462–466.
76. Patchell RA, Fellows HA, Humphries LL. Neurologic complications of anorexia nervosa. Acta Neurol Scand 1994; 89:111–116.
77. MacKenzie JR, LaBan MM, Sackeyfio AH. The prevalence of peripheral neuropathy in patients with anorexia nervosa. Arch Phys Med Rehab 1989; 70:827–830.
78. Pirke KM. Central and peripheral noradrenalin regulation in eating disorders. Psychiatry Res 1996; 16:43–49.
79. Raymond NC, deZwaan M, Faris PL, Nugent SM, Achard DM, Crosby RD, Mitchell JE. Pain thresholds in obese binge-eating disorder subjects. Biol Psychiatry 1995; 37:202–204.
80. Brewerton TD, Lydiara RB, Laraia MT, Shook JE, Ballenger JC. CSF beta-endorphin and dynorphin in bulimia nervosa. Am J Psychiatry 1992; 149:1086–1090.
81. McLoughlin DM, Wassif WS, Morton J, Spargo E, Peters TJ, Russell GF. Metabolic abnormalities associated with skeletal myopathy in severe anorexia nervosa. Nutirtion 2000; 16:192–196.
82. McLoughlin DM, Spargo E, Wassif WS, et al. Structural and functional changes in skeletal muscle in anorexia nervosa. Act Neuropathol 1998; 95:632.
83. Nussbaum M, Baird D, Sonnenblick M, Cowan K, Shenker IR. Short stature in anorexia nervosa patients. J Adol Health Care 1985; 6:453–455.
84. Smith FM, Latchford G, Hall RM, Millner PA, Dickson RA. Indications of disordered eating behaviour in adolescent patients with idiopathic scoliosis. J Bone Joint Surg Br 2002; 84:392–394.
85. Grinspoon S, Thomas E, Pitts S, Gross E, Mickley D, Miller K, Herzog D, Klibanski A. Prevalence and predictive factors for regional osteopenia in women with anorexia nervosa. Ann Intern Med 2000; 133:790–794.
86. Andersen AE, Watson T, Schlechte J. Osteoporosis and osteopenia in men with eating disorders. Lancet 2000; 355:1967–1968.
87. Lucas AR, Melton LJ III, Crowson CS, O'Fallon WM. Long-term fracture risk among women with anorexia nervosa: a population-based cohort study. Mayo Clin Proc 1999; 74:972–977.
88. Hartman D, Crisp A, Rooney B, Rackow C, Atkinson R, Patel S. Bone density of women who have recovered from anorexia nervosa. Int J Eat Disord 2000; 28:1007–1112.
89. Kanis JAWHO Study Group. Assessment of fracture risk and its application for screening post-menopausal osteoporosis. Osteoporos Int 1994; 4:368–381.
90. Soyka LA, Grinspoon S, Levitsky LL, Herzog DB, Klibanksi A. The effects of

AN on bone meabolism in female adolescents. J Clin Endocrinol Metab 1999; 84:4489–4496.

91. Andersen AE, Woodward PJ, LaFrance N. Bone mineral density of eating disorder subgroups. Int J Eat Disord 1995; 18:335–342.

92. Klibanski A, Biller BM, Schoenfeld DA, Herzog DB, Saxe VC. The effects of estrogen administration on trabecular bone loss in young women with AN. J Clin Endocrinol Metab 1995; 80:898–904.

93. Karlsson MK, Weigall SJ, Duan Y, Seeman E. Bone size and volumetric density in women with AN receiving estrogen replacement therapy and in women recovered from AN. J Encocrinol Metab 2000; 85:3177–3182.

94. Wolfert A, Mehler PS. Osteoporosis: prevention and treatment in anorexia nervosa. Eat Weight Disord 2002; 7:72–81.

95. Bachrach LK, Katzman DK, Litt IF, Guido D, Marcus R. Recovery from osteopenia in adolescent girls with AN. J Clin Endocrinol Metab 1991; 72:602–606.

96. Heer M, Mika C, Grzella I, Drummer C, Herpertz-Dahlmann B. Changes in bone turnover in patients with anorexia nervosa during eleven weeks of inpatient dietary treatment. Clin Chem 2002; 48:754–760.

97. Grinspoon S, Thomas L, Miller K, Herzog D. Klibanski A Effects of recombinant human IGF-I and oral contraceptive administration on bone density in anorexia nervosa. J Clin Endocrinol Meab 2002; 87:2883–2891.

98. Lai KY, de Bruyn R, Lask B, Bryant-Waugh R, Hankins M. Use of pelvic ultrasound to monitor ovarian and uterine maturity in childhood onset anorexia nervosa. Arch Dis Child 1994; 71:228–231.

99. Treasure JL, Gordon PA, King EA, Wheeler M, Russell GF. Cystic ovaries: a phase of anorexia nervosa. Lancet 1985; 2:1379–1382.

100. Treasure JL. The ultrasonographic features in anorexia nervosa and bulimia nervosa: a simplified method of monitoring hormonal states during weight gain. J Psychosom Res 1988; 32:623–634.

101. Jahanafar S, Eden JA, Nguyent TV. Bulimia nervosa and polycystic ovary syndrome. Gynecol Endocrinol 1995; 9:113–117.

102. Johnson JG, Spitzer RL, Williams JB. Health problems, impairment and illnesses associated with bulimia nervosa and binge eating disorder among primary care and obstetric gynaecology patients. Psychol Med 2001; 31:1455–1466.

103. Blais MA, Becker AE, Burwell RA, Flores AT, Nussbaum KM, Greenwood DN, Ekeblad ER, Herzog DB. Pregnancy: outcome and impact on symptomatology in a cohort of eating-disordered women. Int J Eat Disord 2000; 27: 140–149.

104. Morgan JF, Lacey JH, Sedgwick PM. Impact of pregnancy on bulimia nervosa. Br J Psychiatry 1999; 174:278.

105. Franko DL, Blais MA, Becker AE, Delinsky SS, Greenwood DN, Flores AT, Ekeblad ER, Eddy KT, Herzog DB. Pregnancy complications and neonatal outcomes in women with eating disorders. Am J Psychiatry 2000; 158:1461–1466.

106. James DC. Eating disorders, fertility, and pregnancy: relationships and complications. J Perinat Neonat Nurs 2001; 15:36–48.
107. Franko DL, Spurrell EB. Detection and management of eating disorders during pregnancy. Obstet Gynecol 2000; 95:942–946.
108. Stein A, Woolley H, Cooper SD, Fairburn CG. An observational study of mothers with eating disorders and their infants. J Child Psychol Psychiatry 1994; 35:733–748.

11

Neurotransmitter Dysregulation in Anorexia Nervosa, Bulimia Nervosa, and Binge Eating Disorder

Timothy D. Brewerton
Medical University of South Carolina
Charleston, South Carolina, U.S.A.

Howard Steiger
Douglas Hospital
Montreal, Quebec, Canada

The current system of psychiatric diagnosis, DSM-IV (1), addresses two official eating disorder (ED) syndromes—anorexia nervosa (AN) and bulimia nervosa (BN)—and a third (still provisional) diagnostic entity—binge eating disorder (BED). However, BED has all but officially been recognized as a distinct eating syndrome. AN, BN, and BED are all polysymptomatic syndromes, defined by maladaptive attitudes and behaviors around eating, weight, and body image, but typically including "nonspecific" disturbances of self-image, mood, impulse regulation, and interpersonal functioning. All three syndromes are known to be associated with significant mortality and morbidity, both medical and psychiatric (2,3). Despite popular beliefs, there is no convincing evidence that cultural factors alone cause eating disorders. Indeed, during the past few years (and especially the last decade) investigations into the role of neurotransmitters and other neuromodulators in the eating disorders have been highly productive, and have implicated primary neurotransmitter disturbances in the etiology of both AN and BN. Furthermore, recent data clearly identify strong genetic factors in AN and BN, which appear to share common genetic vulnerabilities (4,5) linked to obsessionality, perfectionism, anxiety, and/or behavioral inhibition (6,7). One powerful piece of evidence to support monoamine involvement in the eating disorders is the observation that antidepressant medications can be beneficial in controlled studies, not only in BN patients but in recovered AN patients as well (8).

However, it is also clear that some disturbances are consequences of the abnormal eating practices and nutritional disturbances that characterize these disorders (9), which in turn exacerbate or perpetuate signs and symptoms (10). This perspective, taken together with the disorders' consequences, challenges, and costs, compels us toward a better understanding of the biological mechanisms underlying all stages and types of eating disorders. The identification of the psychobiological underpinnings of these conditions may be useful in many ways, including the development of improved medical and psychopharmacological interventions, improved education and psychotherapy for patients and their families, and improved prevention efforts at a primary level.

It must be emphasized that most measurements of neurotransmitter function provide only a glimpse into the state of the organism at that moment. Sorting out what is trait and what is state related has been a challenging focus of neurotransmitter research in the eating disorders.

MONOAMINES

The classical monoaminergic neurotransmitter systems, including serotonin (5-hydroxytryptamine, 5-HT), norepinephrine (NE), and dopamine (DA), have been fairly extensively studied in the eating disorders using available techniques in biological psychiatry. Most of these studies have been conducted during the active state of illness, during which severe nutritional compromise may represent an important confound. Dieting and/or semi-starvation clearly depletes central monoamines and leads to altered neurotransmitter levels and receptor sensitivity in animals and humans (11–15). To avoid this problem, a more recent strategy has been to study "recovered" patients, i.e., AN and BN patients who have attained normalization of eating and weight, resumption of menses and/or normalization of gonadal hormone levels, and abatement of typical cognitive features to subclinical levels. This strategy attempts to minimize starvation state–related effects and to reveal potential trait-related disturbances or vulnerabilities. However, the long-term effects of chronic malnutrition and disordered eating behaviors on the brain (similar to substance use disorders) should not be minimized. Studies of transmitter function in at-risk premorbid individuals as well as nonaffected identical and fraternal twins, siblings, and other first-degree relatives of ED patients could begin to confirm trait-related disturbances.

Neurotransmitter function in patients with EDs have been investigated using a variety of existing techniques and methodologies, each of which has its own advantages and disadvantages. Studies of cerebrospinal fluid (CSF) concentrations of the major metabolites have been a popular strategy and include measures of 5-hydroxyindoleacetic acid (5-HIAA) for 5-HT, 3-methoxy-4-hydroxyphenylglycol (MHPG) for NE, and homovanillic acid (HVA) for DA. Some studies have also examined actual concentrations of 5-HT and NE, but not DA. Such studies measure transmitter metabolism of the whole brain and spinal cord and lack any anatomical specificity.

Neuroendocrine and other psychobiological response measures have been studied following acute challenges with various agents, including amino acid precursors, e.g., L-tryptophan (L-TRP) and 5-hydroxytryptophan (5-HTP) for 5-HT, presynaptic receptor agonists, e.g., dl-fenfluramine (dl-FEN) or d-fenfluramine (d-FEN) for 5-HT, postsynaptic receptor agonists, e.g., m-chlorophenylpiperazine (m-CPP) for 5-HT, and isoproterenol (ISOP) for NE. Longer term challenges with receptor antagonists, e.g., antipsychotics for DA and 5-HT, and antidepressants, especially the serotonin-specific reuptake inhibitors (SSRIs), also illuminate the role of neurotransmitters in the eating disorders. Acute amino acid precursor depletion, most notably of L-TRP (16–19), has been another important source of information about the role of central 5-HT function in eating and related disorders.

Platelet (PLT) and leukocyte studies are possibly reflective of central neurotransmitter function but are always at least one step removed from the nervous system, e.g., platelet 5-HT reuptake, ^{3}H-imipramine binding, ^{3}H-paroxetine binding, platelet monoamine oxidase (MAO), platelet 5-HT content, as well as platelet receptor–mediated aggregation (5-HT$_2$ and α-adrenergic).

Plasma concentrations of neurotransmitter precursors, e.g., L-TRP, L-tyrosine (L-TYR), and their competing large neutral amino acids (LNAAs), neurotransmitters themselves, e.g., NE, DA, and whole-blood serotonin (WBS), as well as the usual metabolites, MHPG, HVA, and 5-HIAA.

Brain imaging receptor-binding studies are a promising avenue but remain relatively unexplored in the eating disorders.

For each neurotransmitter, the results from controlled studies in humans will be reviewed and summarized for both AN and BN. Where applicable, comparisons between restricting AN patients, bingeing–purging AN patients, and normal-weight BN patients will be made. Very little work of this nature has been done in BED patients but when available will be mentioned.

NOREPINEPHRINE

There are a number of reasons to suspect NE involvement in the eating disorders. Most notably, NE pathways at the level of the hypothalamus are known to be involved in the initiation of feeding (20). Disturbances in these pathways may therefore be involved in the pathophysiology of the profoundly altered feeding behaviors classically associated with the eating disorders. In addition, NE's role in the modulation of mood, anxiety, neuroendocrine control, metabolic rate, sympathetic tone, and temperature make it a likely candidate for study (21–26). It has been recognized for some time that low-weight anorexic patients, and to some degree bulimic patients, have reduced body temperature, blood pressure, pulse, and metabolic rate (25,27,28). Investigations in this area have shown that low-weight AN patients have reduced measures of plasma, urinary, and CSF MHPG (27,29–31). In contrast, reports of plasma NE levels in the eating disorders has been more variable (32,33), and this appears to be linked not only to weight but to the stresses associated with the illness (25). AN patients tend to have higher plasma NE levels at admission, which then decrease as treatment and weight gain progresses (25,34).

When ill, BN patients demonstrate lower values of plasma NE at baseline (21,28) and in response to abstinence (35), standing (36), test meal challenge (37), and mental challenge (37). They also have other evidence of blunted sympathetic activation in response to mental stress (38). However, despite low baseline plasma NE levels, BN patients show normal responses to exercise (39) but reduced responses to orthostasis (40).

In AN patients, depression has been found to be significantly worse in those patients with the lowest Δ change in plasma NE concentrations to orthostasis (41). Reduced urinary MHPG levels have also been related to the presence of comorbid major depression (29,42). It is therefore important in such studies to control for psychiatric comorbidity.

Like the plasma NE studies, CSF NE levels have been reported to be no different in AN patients than controls at low weight and after short-term weight gain, but then significantly lower after weight recovery of at least 6 months (26,31,32). In BN patients, reduced CSF NE levels have been reported during the active state of the illness (23,43). However, upon long-term recovery, concentrations of CSF MHPG have been reported to normalize in both AN and BN (7) despite earlier reports of lower levels (32). Given that CSF NE concentrations have not yet been reported in long-term (> 1 year) recovered AN or BN patients, the extent to which adrenergic alterations seen in the eating disorders are trait related remains unclear. Nevertheless, available evidence suggests exquisite sensitivity of this system to malnutrition or stress.

Challenge studies using the β-adrenergic agonist isoproterenol in underweight anorexic patients revealed erratic secretion of plasma NE in response to increasing doses (24). Bulimic patients demonstrated significantly increased chronotropic responses to isoproterenol (44). Challenge studies with adrenergic agents in recovered patients have not been reported.

The number of platelet α_2 receptors has been reported to be reduced in both AN and BN compared to controls (33,45), suggesting increased postsynaptic receptor sensitivity that is probably secondary to dieting or semi-starvation. In summary, peripheral and central sympathetic nervous activity is reduced in both AN and BN, although it tends to normalize with recovery. Taken together, the preponderance of the evidence so far leads to the conclusion that these changes are a result of chronic starvation or intermittent dieting (26). However, a trait-related disturbance of the adrenergic system cannot be ruled out at this time (35).

Studies of adrenergic receptors on human leukocytes have been another strategy to investigate adrenergic function in the eating disorders. Buckholtz et al. (46) reported altered β-adrenergic receptor affinity on circulating lymphocytes of BN patients compared to those of controls. However, in a similar study of a mixed group of eating disorder patients, Lonati-Galligani and Pirke (40) reported lower receptor number (B_{max}) but normal affinity (K_d) in low-weight AN patients, whereas both measures were no different from controls in the BN patients and the weight-recovered AN patients. Gill and colleagues (47) reported differential changes in α- and β-adrenoceptor linked ($^{45}Ca^{2+}$) uptake in platelets from patients with AN, further documenting an adrenergic disturbance in eating disorder patients. However, the issue of cause versus effect remains unanswered in platelet and leukocyte studies.

DOPAMINE

DA is also suspect in the neuropathophysiology of the eating disorders given its reported involvement in the regulation of feeding, mood, activity, perception, sexual/social behavior, hormone and peptide release, and to some extent aggression (48–51). Notably, DA is involved in the hedonic reward responses to eating and its maintenance as well as to other pleasurable activities (52–54).

The majority of studies of DA metabolism in the eating disorders have consistently shown that low-weight AN patients have reduced measures of peripheral and central DA activity, including decreased plasma (27) and CSF HVA (31). In BN patients, reduced CSF HVA levels also have been reported in BN patients with frequent binge–purge episodes (23,50) but not in those less severely ill. Furthermore, binge frequency was inversely correlated with CSF HVA levels in one study (50). Upon long-term recovery, concentrations of CSF HVA have been reported to normalize in BN (8), whereas a trend for decreased CSF HVA levels persisted in six restricting AN patients compared to controls and to bingeing and/or purging AN patients (7). This suggests a possible trait-related disturbance specific to restricting AN, although this finding needs replication given the small sample size. These results could also still be due to nutritional factors given that patients in this study weighed significantly less than those in the BN group and may still have been at the low end of the normal weight range.

Anecdotal reports of the successful use of dopaminergic antagonists (typical antipsychotic agents) in the treatment of AN patients (55) have been generally followed by equivocal results in controlled studies (56,57). Atypical antipsychotic agents may show more promise in the adjunctive treatment of AN given their combined antidopaminergic and antiserotonergic effects (58–60), but the results of placebo-controlled studies remain to be seen.

Genetic investigations into the role of DA have been limited to the Bal I DRD3 receptor polymorphisms in which no differences were found between AN patients and controls (61). However, the polymorphisms of other genes coding for DA receptors could be tested. Interestingly, Corcos and colleagues (62) reported significantly lower IgG and IgM autoantibodies to DA in BN patients compared to controls. There was also a trend for lower levels of IgM autoantibodies to DA in the eating-disordered group. The relevance of these findings to the pathophysiology of the eating disorders remains uncertain but invokes possible autoimmune mechanisms.

SEROTONIN

Several lines of reasoning point to disturbances of 5-HT function in the pathophysiology and neuropsychopharmacology of the EDs (8,9,63), including serotonin's role in feeding (64,65), satiety (66,67), dieting/fasting (11,12), mood regulation (16), anxiety (68), obsessive-compulsiveness/perfectionism/behavioral inhibition (69), harm avoidance (70,71), impulsivity/aggression (72,73), motor activity (74,75), gender (76,77), seasonality (66,78,79), body image/perception (80), and social behavior (81–83) (see Table 1).

Reductions in a variety of 5-HT parameters have been consistently reported in low-weight AN patients. Although no significant differences have been found in absolute plasma L-TRP levels (84–86), the plasma L-TRP/LNAA ratio is reduced in the low weight state (30,87,88) but normalizes upon short-term weight recovery (22,30). In BN, Gendal and Joyce (89) reported that the L-TRP/LNAA ratio inversely correlated with the desire to binge-eat. In addition, symptomatic bulimic relapse or worsening of symptoms has been reported following acute L-TRP depletion in BN (17–19).

TABLE 1 Monoamines and the Phenomenology of the Eating Disorders

Factor	Norepinephrine	Dopamine	Serotonin
Activity/exercise	X	X	X
Fasting effects	X	X	X
Mood regulation	X	X	X
Hormone regulation	X	X	X
Neuropeptide regulation	X	X	X
Trauma effects	X	X	X
Temperature	X		X
Anxiety	X		X
Blood pressure/pulse	X		X
Metabolic rate	X		
Feeding initiation/hunger	X		
Body image/perception		X	X
Impulsivity/aggression		X	X
Sexual behavior		X	X
Feeding maintenance/hedonic reward		X	
Novelty/sensation seeking		X	
Harm avoidance			X
Behavioral inhibition			X
Feeding termination/satiety			X
Obsessive-compulsiveness/perfectionism			X
Social hierarchy/rank			X
Gender differences			X
Seasonality/light effects			X
Circadian rhythmicity			X
Age/developmental effects			X

Other significant findings include decreased CSF L-TRP levels (90) and decreased CSF 5-HIAA levels (22,88,91) during low weight status with normalization of these levels with short-term weight recovery (STWR, goal weight maintenance ≥3 weeks). Strikingly, Kaye and colleagues (69,92) have reported abnormally elevated CSF 5-HIAA levels following long-term weight recovery (LTWR, goal weight maintenance >6–12 months), and interpret these findings as indicating that AN may correspond to a primary state of excessive 5-HT tone, which is then masked by malnutrition-induced *reductions* in 5-HT activity during active illness. In other words, they propose that the pathophysiology of AN actually involves a hyperserotonergic trait and, furthermore, postulate that this trait may correspond to behavioral traits of obsessionality and inhibition. Corroborating the notion of hyperserotonergic status in AN, Kaye and colleagues have noted long-term weight-restored anorexics to display *elevated* 5-HT_{1a} receptor binding, measured by positron emission tomography (PET) (93).

In BN, reduced levels of CSF 5-HIAA are consistently reported only in the subgroup of patients displaying more frequent binge–purge episodes (23,50). Suggesting a possible link to severity of bulimic symptomatology, binge frequency has been found to correlate inversely with CSF 5-HIAA concentrations (50). In a small pilot study, Brewerton and colleagues (94) have reported no difference in CSF 5-HT levels between BN patients and controls. However, upon recovery for at least a year, BN patients have been reported to have elevated CSF 5-HIAA levels compared to healthy controls (95), much like those described earlier as being characteristic of long-term recovered anorexics. As in AN, this finding has been linked to obsessive-compulsive personality traits, perfectionism, and behavioral inhibition, associated with a hypothetical tendency toward hyperserotonergic status. However, we note, that the Kaye et al. study of recovered BN may be confounded by small weight discrepancies between their (heavier) recovered bulimics and lighter comparison controls. Such weight differentials could underlie discrepant levels of 5-HT metabolism.

Decreased prolactin (PRL) responses following *m*-CPP (96–98), L-TRP (96,97), and fenfluramine (FEN) (99–101) have been reported in AN and indicate an anatomically specific alteration in 5-HT receptor sensitivity at the level of the hypothalamus, which could conceivably also occur in other brain pathways (9). Blunting of PRL following *m*-CPP persists into short-term weight recovery, although trends toward normalization of PRL responses, after refeeding and weight gain, have been reported (97). With at least a year of recovery, neurohormonal responses to *m*-CPP normalize in restricting AN patients (92). Apparently, full normalization of PRL responsivity to serotonergic agents occurs after full weight restoration, normalization of hypothalamic-pituitary-gonadal function, and abatement of overt eating disorder symptoms (7). However, the appetite-suppressing effect of FEN is significantly diminished in recovered AN patients despite normalization of hormonal release (102).

Platelet (PLT) studies contribute to the demonstration of serotonergic dysfunction in AN. Significant increases/reductions in PLT imipramine (IMI) binding (103), but not PLT 5-HT uptake (103,104) or PLT MAO content (42), have been reported in low-weight AN patients. However, a more recent study reported decreased PLT MAO in AN (105), which was inversely correlated with impulsivity and positively correlated with persistence (which is similar to rigidity). In a related vein, Finocchiaro and colleagues (106) conducted a novel study of indole metabolism and reported altered phytohemagglutinin stimulated, light-induced [^{3}H]thymidine incorporation into the DNA of peripheral blood mononuclear leukocytes in AN patients compared to controls. The authors concluded that the white cells of AN patients show a failure in the regulation of 5-HT and melatonin metabolism in response to light.

As in AN, neurobiological indices in active BN are often consistent with reduced 5-HT tone. For example, findings in BN show a consistent pattern of PRL blunting following m-CPP (107–110), fenfluramine (99,101,111–113), and 5-hydroxytryptophan (5-HPT) (114), but not L-TRP (9,107). PRL responses following L-TRP are low only in the BN patients with concurrent major depression, again emphasizing the need to control for comorbidity. PRL responses following m-CPP are inversely correlated to baseline cortisol (CORT) (9). Self-reported binge frequency also has been shown to be inversely correlated to PRL responses following m-CPP (9) and fenfluramine (101,111,113) in BN patients. Given that this presumed alteration in hypothalamic postsynaptic 5-HT functioning normalizes with recovery from BN (8,95,115), these serotonergic abnormalities could be understood to be a *result* of bingeing, purging, and/or dieting rather than a *cause* of these behaviors, although other vulnerabilities of the 5-HT system may also exist and interact with these psychosomatic behaviors. There is only one serotonergic challenge study reported in BED (101), which found that PRL responses following d-FEN were no different in patients with BED than in controls. This lends support to the idea that purging, dieting, and weight loss (rather than bingeing per se) have greater roles in creating the serotonergic abnormalities noted above. Dieting, bingeing, and vomiting all may affect central 5-HT synthesis (13,14,22,116,117) and could conceivably result in down-regulation of post-synaptic 5-HT receptors and blunted PRL responses. In addition, these behaviors may involve activation of the HPA axis, which in turn appears to dampen 5-HT receptor sensitivity (9,107). Despite findings linking recovery from BN to normalization of blunted endocrine responses after 5-HT agonists (95,115), other findings (based on PET techniques) suggest persistent reductions in postsynaptic 5-HT$_{2a}$ receptor activity even in fully recovered bulimics (118). Such findings associate BN with a stable reduction in 5-HT neurotransmission at some central sites and present the possibility that such tendencies exist independently of disorder sequelae in BN patients.

In BN, platelet studies indicate reduced PLT IMI binding (119) and PLT MAO (120). PLT 5-HT uptake has been reported to be increased in one study (121) but not another (120). Steiger et al. (110,122) reported reduced PLT paroxetine binding in groups of BN patients compared to healthy controls.

Possible Trait-Linked Effects

Independently of dietary factors, personality trait variations might explain some of the variations in 5-HT status seen in eating disorder sufferers. In non-eating-disordered populations, correspondence between 5-HT function and personality trait variations has been well established. For example, impulsivity has been consistently linked to decreased 5-HT activity; suicide, fire setting, violence, and borderline personality disorder (BPD, for which impulsivity is pathognomonic) have all been linked to decreased 5-HT metabolism (as indicated by reduced CSF 5-HIAA) (123,124). Likewise, impulsive suicidality and aggression have been linked to low platelet 5-HT content and reduced PRL response to 5-HT agonists (123,124). On the opposite side of the same coin, findings in non eating-disordered samples have (at least inconsistently) associated anxiety or compulsivity with *increased* 5-HT tone. For example, patients with obsessive-compulsive disorder have been reported to display elevated CSF 5-HIAA (125) and increased PRL response after the 5-HT agonist fenfluramine (126). Furthermore, the partial 5-HT agonist *m*-CPP has been observed to increase obsessionality in obsessive-compulsive patients, and anxiety in patients with generalized anxiety disorder (127–129). Likewise, heightened anxiety has been associated with elevated 5-HT activity in both generalized anxiety disorder (130) and AN (131). Such findings have encouraged some theorists to propose that "impulsive" and "compulsive" traits occupy opposite poles of a continuum of 5-HT under- to overactivation (132,133). While this notion remains controversial, it is tempting to contemplate the possibility that 5-HT findings in restrictive versus bulimic ED variants may reflect variations associated with differential loadings of compulsive or impulsive traits in these ED subgroups.

In keeping with the notion outlined above, various studies report that personality trait variations account for variations of 5-HT indices in ED patients, at least when actively eating disordered. Waller and colleagues (134) observed that hostile bulimics, compared to less hostile ones (by self report), showed smaller neuroendocrine responses following buspirone (which they presumed to be a $5-HT_{1a}$ agonist). Likewise, Carrasco and colleagues (135) observed systematically lower platelet MAO concentrations (taken as a proxy for reduced 5-HT activity) in bulimics with impulsive or "borderline" traits. Results of several studies by Steiger and his colleagues are comparable. In one study, PRL responses after *m*-CPP were measured in bulimic women who reported, or who denied, a history of self-mutilative or suicidal impulsivity (136). (Incidentally, these two groups of women, were quite comparable on indices of binge and purge frequency and body mass). Compared to normal eaters, the self-harming bulimics were clearly blunted, as far as 5-HT function was concerned; the non-self-harming bulimics were not. In other words, an association was observed between blunting of the *m*-CPP-stimulated PRL response and self-destructiveness, comparable to that obtained in non-eating-disordered populations (137). This observation suggests that hypoactivity of the 5-HT system in BN may be more strongly linked to self-aggressive impulsivity than it is to binge–purge symptoms per se. However, in the study by Brewerton et al. (107), no such differences were found between bulimic patients with and without a history of suicidality. Another study by Steiger's group examined platelet ^{3}H-paroxetine binding in normal women and in bulimic women, and assessed effects of "nonplanning impulsivity" (i.e., the tendency to act without considering consequences) (110). Both bulimic groups displayed reductions in density (B_{max}) of paroxetine binding sites. However, in bulimics, the extent of reduction in binding site density was inversely correlated with "nonplanning." In other words, reduced peripheral 5-HT reuptake corresponded to increased impulsivity. This effect parallels inverse relationships noted between platelet 5-HT binding and aggressive impulsivity (138) or self-mutilation (138) in personality-disordered subjects, raising the notion that in BN we could be observing a constitutional (trait-linked) susceptibility to underactivity of the 5-HT system. Furthermore, if exacerbated by effects of dieting, such susceptibilities could cause certain people to become especially impulsive and/or prone to binge eating.

Taken together, research findings from plasma, CSF, and pharmacological challenge studies suggest reduced 5-HT synthesis, uptake, and turnover, as well as altered postsynaptic 5-HT receptor sensitivity during the active phases of both AN and BN. Consequently, many reported alterations in 5-HT function appear to be state dependent, although they may have important biological roles in the perpetuation of symptoms, particularly mood dysregulation, increased anxiety, obsessionality, impulsivity, self-aggression, and perhaps the resistance to and difficulty in learning healthier coping strategies (139).

However, to avoid presenting an oversimplified, unidirectional hypothesis of 5-HT alterations in the eating disorders, it is necessary to note some findings suggesting heightened 5-HT receptor sensitivity at certain central sites in eating disorder patients with active symptoms. For example, Brewerton (9) reported enhanced temperature and migraine headache responses to m-CPP but not L-TRP in BN patients (regardless of the comorbid presence of AN or MD) (9,140,141). As discussed in detail elsewhere (141), the enhanced migraine-like HA responses in the BN patients may indicate enhanced 5-HT$_2$ receptor sensitivity in CNS vascular tissues. Enhanced 5-HT-mediated platelet aggregation, a 5-HT$_2$ receptor–mediated phenomenon, has also been reported in BN (142) and AN (99,112,142) and lends further support to this hypothesis. The normal cortisol responses following m-CPP and L-TRP in AN and BN are compatible with this view given the involvement of both 5-HT$_1$ (facilitative) and 5-HT$_2$ receptors (inhibitive) in cortisol secretion. These presumed alterations in 5-HT receptor sensitivity, whether primary or secondary, demonstrate that 5-HT receptor sensitivity can be both decreased and increased in the same subjects depending on the anatomical location of the receptor as well as the receptor subtype. We (9,143) have argued in favor of a dysregulation hypothesis of serotonin dysfunction in the eating and related disorders, proposing that there is a failure in transmitter regulation in the face of a variety of psychobiological perturbations potentially affecting monoamine function, including dieting, fasting, purging, substance abuse, excessive exercising, medical illnesses, family stresses or losses, sociocultural pressures, traumatic events, puberty, other developmental tasks/challenges, and changes in the seasons. Certainly, evidence suggests that a model of neurotransmitter alterations in the eating disorders stated in terms of a unidirectional (high versus low activity) concept will not be adequate.

Interest in 5-HT activity in the EDs has led to quite a catalogue of studies on 5-HT system genes—controlling activity of 5-HT receptors, tryptophan hydroxylase (TPH, the rate-limiting enzyme for 5-HT synthesis), and 5-HT transporter (reuptake) mechanisms (144). Collier et al. (145) reported a statistically significant 5-HT2A-1438G/A receptor gene polymorphism in a group of restricting AN patients compared to healthy controls. This finding has been replicated in at least two other studies in AN (146,147) as well as in OCD (147), but not in BN (147). Nacmias et al. (146) reported that other serotonergic polymorphisms of the 5-HT_{2a} as well as those of the 5-HT_{2c} receptors showed no differences in AN patients compared to controls. Likewise, no differences between AN patients and controls have been reported for serotonin transporter gene–linked polymorphisms (5-HTTLPR) (148,149), tryptophan hydroxylase polymorphisms (150), and 5-HT1Dbeta and 5-HT7 gene polymorphisms (151).

For BN, there have been various association studies: Studies on 5-HT_{2c} polymorphisms in BN detect no syndrome-linked associations (144). Similarly, three of four available studies on the 5-HT_{2a} receptor gene indicate absence of association with BN (146,147,152). However, a fourth (in a heterogeneous anorexic–bulimic sample) associates the 5-HT_{2a} "G" allele with proneness to bulimic symptoms, borderline personality, and generalized impulsivity (153). Such findings imply that common genetic factors might mediate concurrence of bulimic eating patterns and traits of a borderline/impulsive type. Yet another recent study, first to examine the 5-HT transporter gene (promoter region, 5HTTLPR) in BN, indicates a short-allele variation to confer sevenfold risk of BN (154). The short (s) allele of 5HTTLPR has been linked to reduced transcription of 5-HT transporter protein, decreased 5-HT reuptake in lymphoblasts (155), and traits like suicidality (156), neuroticism, and impulsivity (157). Preliminary findings from our lab provide a second indication of relevance of the 5-HT transporter (5-HTT) gene to binge eating and impulsivity (158). Results in 48 women with binge eating syndromes showed individuals carrying the short (s) allele of 5HTTLPR (either s/s or s/l genotypes) to show more impulsivity and lower density of paroxetine-binding sites than did long (l) allele homozygotes. These results, if they hold up, would cross-validate (at a genetic level) a link between impulse control problems and hyposerotonergic status, indicating convergence among impulsive traits, low 5-HT transporter activity, and the s allele.

Evidence from Pharmacological Effects

It is well known that serotonin-specific antidepressant medications can be beneficial in controlled studies of BN patients (159) but not in low-weight AN patients (160,161). More recent data indicate a prophylactic effect of fluoxetine following weight gain in recovered AN patients (8). SSRIs don't work during the low-weight state, presumably because of central depletion of 5-HT and other monoamines with starvation. There is significantly less 5-HT centrally to be inhibited by SSRIs.

Finally, recent evidence indicates significant antibulimic responses to 5-HT_3 antagonists, such as ondansetron (162,163). Although the authors attribute this therapeutic response to the drug's ability to reduce vagal tone, the role of the 5-HT_3 receptor remains intriguing given its antianxiety effects (164). These findings open important new arenas for future research involving possible serotonergic-cholinergic mechanisms, which has been a relatively unexplored area in the eating disorders.

MAO/ISATIN

Isatin, or tribulin, is an endogenous indole associated with stress, which inhibits MAO (165). Brewerton et al. (94) reported significantly higher CSF concentrations of isatin in BN patients compared to healthy controls. There was also a trend for CSF isatin concentrations to be inversely correlated with CSF concentrations of the serotonin metabolite 5-HIAA ($n = 14$, $\rho = -0.51$, $p = 0.06$), although CSF isatin levels were not significantly correlated with CSF MHPG or HVA. The increase in isatin levels has been hypothesized to be in response to the resultant monoamine depletion secondary to the effects of the illness on monoaminergic function. As noted previously, platelet MAO has been reported to be decreased in BN (120) and in AN (105). This decrease may represent a compensatory change in response to monoamine depletion during the active state of the disorders.

RELATIONSHIP TO OTHER SYSTEMS

Neurotransmitter systems do not exist in a vacuum but are exquisitely interdependent with other brain and body systems and the environment as well. It is important to think about systems (e.g., 5-HT) and their subsystems (presynaptic, postsynaptic, receptor subtypes) in the context of larger systems (brain, environment) and interacting systems/subsystems (e.g., NE, DA, neurohormones, neuropeptides) with complex feedback and counterfeedback mechanisms at multiple anatomical levels. An extensive discussion of this rather far-reaching topic is beyond the scope of this chapter but is discussed in more detail elsewhere (9).

CONCLUSIONS

Taken together, available findings implicate abnormalities of all monoamine neurotransmitter systems during the active phases of both AN and BN. Upon normalization of weight and neurohormonal function, most transmitter anomalies resolve or atleast improve. Some data show persistent particularities of the 5-HT system, and suggest that observed tendencies may reflect psychological traits found in both AN and BN, including obsessionality, perfectionism, high harm avoidance, and behavioral inhibition, on the one hand, and recklessness, failure to consider consequences of actions, self-destructiveness, and behavioral disinhibition, on the other. Furthermore, some evidence may be consistent with association between greater behavioral inhibition and excessive 5-HT activity (at some loci in the system), and behavioral disinhibition and reduced 5-HT neurotransmission (also at some loci in the system). The findings in question create a case for the idea that any given individuals' 5-HT functioning probably varies in function of constitutionally determined (latent or manifest) personality trait tendencies. In this light, it is intriguing to contemplate the ways in which constitutional traits associated with hypoactivity of the 5-HT system (e.g., impulsivity) may predispose to binge eating—and traits associated with elevated 5-HT tone (like compulsivity or harm avoidance) may predispose to dietary restriction.

Some evidence suggests prolonged alterations in NE metabolism, but this is most likely due to persistent low-grade dietary restraint following recovery. Preliminary data indicate a DA deficit in restricting AN patients, but this result remains to be replicated in larger samples. Recent findings also emphasize the importance of neurotransmitter precursor substrate availability to normal brain function and especially to the process of recovery from an eating disorder. Future research directions will include further exploration of neurotransmitter-related gene candidates, in vivo receptor imaging studies, and improved psychopharmacological interventions based on biological alterations characteristic of the different stages and features of these dangerous disorders.

REFERENCES

1. American Psychiatric Association. Diagnostic and Statistical Manual of Mental Disorders, 4th ed. Washington, DC: American Psychiatric Press, 1994.
2. Becker AE, Grinspoon SK, Klibanski A, Herzog DB. Eating disorders. N Engl J Med 1999; 340:1092–1098.

3. Walsh BT, Devlin MJ. Eating disorders: progress and problems. Science 1998; 280:1387–1390.

4. Lilenfeld LR, Kaye WH, Greeno CG, Merikangas KR, Plotnicov K, Pollice C, Radhika R, Strober M, Bulik C, Nagy L. A controlled family study of anorexia nervosa and bulimia nervosa. Arch Gen Psychiatry 1998; 55:603–610.

5. Strober M, Freeman R, Lampert C, Diamond J, Kaye WH. Controlled family study of anorexia nervosa and bulimia nervosa: evidence of shared liability and transmission of partial syndromes. Am J Psychiatry 2000; 157:393–401.

6. Halmi KA, Sunday SR, Strober M, Kaplan A, Woodside DB, Fichter M, Treasure J, Berrettini WH, Kaye WH. Perfectionism in anorexia nervosa: variation by clinical subtype, obsessionality, and pathological eating behavior. Am J Psychiatry 2000; 157:1799–1805.

7. Kaye W, Strober M, Stein D, Gendall K. New directions in treatment research of anorexia and bulimia nervosa. Biol Psychiatry 1999b; 45:1285–1292.

8. Kaye WH, Gendall KA, Strober M. Serotonin neuronal function and selective reuptake inhibitor treatment in anorexia nervosa and bulimia nervosa. Biol Psychiatry 1998a; 44:825–838.

9. Brewerton TD. Toward a unified theory of serotonin dysregulation in eating and related disorders. Psychoneuroendocrinology 1995; 20:561–590.

10. Pollice C, Kaye WH, Greeno CG, Weltzin TE. Relationship of depression, anxiety, and obsessionality to state of illness in anorexia nervosa. Int J Eat Disord 1997; 21:367–376.

11. Cowen PJ, Clifford EM, Walsh AE, Williams C, Fairburn CG. Moderate dieting causes 5-HT$_{2C}$ receptor supersensitivity. Psychol Med 1996; 26:1155–1159.

12. Cowen PJ, Smith KA. Serotonin, dieting, and bulimia nervosa. Adv Exp Med Biol 1999; 467:101–104.

13. Goodwin GM, Fairburn CG, Cowen PJ. Dieting changes serotonergic function in women, not men: implications for the etiology of anorexia nervosa. Psychol Med 1987a; 17:839–842.

14. Goodwin GM, Fairburn CG, Cowen PJ. The effects of dieting and weight loss upon neuroendocrine responses to tryptophan, clonidine and apomorphine in volunteers: important implications for neuroendocrine investigations in depression. Arch Gen Psychiatry 1987b; 44:952–957.

15. Goodwin GM, Cowen PJ, Fairburn CG, Parry-Billings M, Calder PC, Newsholme EA. Plasma concentrations of tryptophan and dieting. Br Med J 1990; 300:1499–1500.

16. Deldago PL, Charney DS, Price LH, Aghajanian GK, Landis H, Henninger GR. Serotonin function and the mechanism of antidepressant action: reversal of antidepressant-induced remission by rapid depletion of plasma tryptophan. Arch Gen Psychiatry 1990; 47:411–418.

17. Kaye WH, Gendall KA, Fernstrom MH, Fernstrom JD, McConaha CW, Weltzin TE. Effects of acute tryptophan depletion on mood in bulimia nervosa. Biol Psychiatry 2000; 47:151–157.

18. Smith KA, Fairburn CG, Cowen PJ. Symptomatic relapse in bulimia nervosa following acute tryptophan depletion. Arch Gen Psychiatry 1999; 56:171–176.
19. Weltzin TE, Fernstrom MH, Fernstrom JD, Neuberger SK, Kaye WH. Acute tryptophan depletion and increased food intake and irritability in bulimia nervosa. Am J Psychiatry 1995; 152:1668–1671.
20. Rowland NE, Morien A, Li BH. The physiology and brain mechanisms of feeding. Nutrition 1996; 12:626–639.
21. Jimerson DC, George DT, Kaye W, Brewerton TD, Goldstein DS. Norepinephrine regulation in bulimia. In: Hudson JI, Pope HG, eds. Psychobiology of Bulimia. Washington, DC: American Psychiatric Press, 1987: 145–156.
22. Kaye WH, Gwirtsman HE, George DT, Jimerson DC, Ebert MH. CSF 5-HIAA concentrations in anorexia nervosa: reduced values in underweight subjects normalize after weight gain. Biol Psychiatry 1988b; 23:102–105.
23. Kaye WH, Ballenger JC, Lydiard RB, Stuart GW, Laraia MT, O'Neil P, Fossey MD, Stevens V, Lesser S, Hsu G. CSF monoamine levels in normal-weight bulimia: evidence for abnormal noradrenergic activity. Am J Psychiatry 1990; 147:225–229.
24. Kaye WH, George DT, Gwirtsman HE, Jimerson DC, Goldstein DS, Ebert MH, Lake CR. Isoproterenol infusion test in anorexia nervosa: assessment of pre- and post-beta-noradrenergic receptor activity. Psychopharmacol Bull 1990; 26:355–359.
25. Lesem MD, George DT, Kaye WH, Goldstein DS, Jimerson DC. State-related changes in norepinephrine regulation in anorexia nervosa. Biol Psychiatry 1989; 25:509–512.
26. Pirke KM. Central and peripheral noradrenalin regulation in eating disorders. Psychiatry Res 1996; 62:43–49.
27. Gross HA, Lake CR, Ebert MH, Ziegler MG, Kopin IJ. Catecholamine metabolism in primary anorexia nervosa. J Clin Endocrinol Metab 1979; 49:805–809.
28. Obarzanek E, Lesem MD, Goldstein DS, Jimerson DC. Reduced resting metabolic rate in patients with bulimia nervosa. Arch Gen Psychiatry 1991; 48:456–462.
29. Halmi KA, Dekirmenjian H, Dav JM, Casper R, Goldberg S. Catecholamine metabolism in anorexia nervosa. Arch Gen Psychiatry 1978; 35:458–460.
30. Johnston JL, Leiter LA, Burrow GN, Garfinkel PE, Anderson GH. Excretion of urinary catecholamine metabolites in anorexia nervosa: effect of body composition and energy intake. Am J Clin Nutr 1984; 40:1001–1006.
31. Kaye WH, Ebert MH, Raleigh M, Lake CR. Abnormalities in CNS monoamine metabolism in anorexia nervosa. Arch Gen Psychiatry 1984; 41:350–355.
32. Kaye WH, Jimerson DC, Lake CR, Ebert MH. Altered norepinephrine metabolism following long-term weight recovery in patients with anorexia nervosa. Psychiatry Res 1985; 14:333–342.
33. Luck P, Mikhailid DP, Dashwood MR, Barradas MA, Sever PS, Dandona P, Wakeling A. Platelet hyperaggregability and increased alpha-adrenoceptor density in anorexia nervosa. J Clin Endocrinol Metab 1983; 57:911–914.

34. Pahl J, Pirke KM, Schweiger U, Warnhoff M, Gerlinghoff M, Brinkmann W, Berger M, Krieg C. Anorectic behavior, mood, and metabolic and endocrine adaptation to starvation in anorexia nervosa during inpatient treatment. Biol Psychiatry 1985; 20:874–887.

35. Kaye WH, Gwirtsman HE, George DT, Jimerson DC, Ebert MH, Lake CR. Disturbances of noradrenergic systems in normal weight bulimia: relationship to diet and menses. Biol Psychiatry 1990; 27:4–21.

36. Pirke KM, Jorg P, Schweiger U, Warnhoff M. Metabolic and endocrine indices of starvation in bulimia: a comparison with anorexia nervosa. Psychiatry Res 1985; 15:33–39.

37. Pirke KM, Kellner M, Philipp E, Laessle R, Krieg JC, Fichter MM. Plasma norepinephrine after a standardized test meal in acute and remitted patients with anorexia nervosa and in healthy controls. Biol Psychiatry 1992; 31:1074–1077.

38. Koo-Loeb JH, Pedersen C, Girdler SS. Blunted cardiovascular and catecholamine stress reactivity in women with bulimia nervosa. Psychiatry Res 1998; 80:13–27.

39. Pirke KM, Eckert M, Ofers B, Goebl G, Spyra B, Schweiger U, Tuschl RJ, Fichter MM. Plasma norepinephrine response to exercise in bulimia, anorexia nervosa, and controls. Biol Psychiatry 1989; 25:799–802.

40. Lonati-Galligani M, Pirke KM. Beta 2-adrenergic receptor regulation in circulating mononuclear leukocytes in anorexia nervosa and bulimia. Psychiatry Res 1986; 19:189–198.

41. Laessle RG, Schweiger U, Pirke KM. Mood and orthostatic norepinephrine response in anorexia nervosa. Psychiatry Res 1988; 24:87–94.

42. Biederman J, Herzog DB, Rivinus TM, Ferber RA, Harper GP, Onsulak PJ, Schildkraut JJ. Urinary MHPG in anorexia nervosa patients with and without a concomitant major depressive disorder. J Psychiatr Res 1984; 18:149–160.

43. Kaye WH, George DT, Gwirtsman HE, Jimerson DC, Goldstein DS, Ebert MH, Lake CR. Isoproterenol infusion test in anorexia nervosa: assessment of pre- and post-beta-noradrenergic receptor activity. Psychopharmacol Bull 1990; 26:355–359.

44. George DT, Kaye WH, Goldstein DS, Brewerton TD, Jimerson DC. Altered norepinephrine regulation in bulimia: effects of pharmacological challenge with isoproterenol. Psychiatry Res 1990; 33:1–10.

45. Heufelder A, Warnhoff M, Pirke KM. Platelet alpha 2-adrenoceptor and adenylate cyclase in patients with anorexia nervosa and bulimia. J Clin Endocrinol Metab 1985; 61:1053–1060.

46. Buckholtz NS, George DT, Davies AO, Jimerson DC, Potter WZ. Lymphocyte beta-adrenergic receptor modification in bulimia. Arch Gen Psychiatry 1988; 45:479–482.

47. Gill J, DeSouza V, Wakeling A, Dandona P, Jeremy JY. Differential changes in alpha- and beta-adrenoceptor linked [45Ca^{2+}] uptake in platelets from patients with anorexia nervosa. J Clin Endocrinol Metab 1992; 74:441–446.

48. Engstrom G, Alling C, Blennow K, Regnell G, Traskman-Bendz L. Reduced

cerebrospinal HVA concentrations and HVA/5-HIAA ratios in suicide attempters: monoamine metabolites in 120 suicide attempters and 47 controls. Eur Neuropsychopharmacol 1999; 9:399–405.

49. Hoebel BG. Brain neurotransmitters in food and drug reward. Am J Clin Nutr 1985; 42:1133–1150.

50. Jimerson DC, Lesem MD, Kaye WH, Brewerton TD. Low serotonin and dopamine metabolite concentrations in CSF from bulimic patients with frequent binge episodes. Arch Gen Psychiatry 1992; 49:132–138.

51. Kaye WH, Guido KWF, Frank GK, McConaha C. Altered dopamine activity after recovery from restricting anorexia nervosa. Neuropsychopharmacology 1999; 21:503–506.

52. Schultz W. Reward signaling by dopamine neurons. Neuroscientist 2001; 7: 293–302.

53. Hoebel BG, Hernandez L, Schwartz DH, Mark P, Hunter GA. Microdialysis studies of brain norepinephrine, serotonin, and dopamine release during ingestive behavior. The Psychobiology of Human Eating Disorders. Ann N Y Acad Sci 1989; 575:71–193.

54. Dayan P, Balleine BW. Reward, motivation, and reinforcement learning. Neuron 2002; 36:285–298.

55. Dally P, Sargant W. Treatment and outcome of anorexia nervosa. Br Med J 1966; 2:793–795.

56. Vandereycken W, Pierloot R. Pimozide combined with behavior therapy in the short-term treatment of anorexia nervosa. A double-blind placebo-controlled cross-over study. Acta Psychiatr Scand 1982; 66:445–450.

57. Vandereycken W. Neuroleptics in the short-term treatment of anorexia nervosa: a double-blind placebo-controlled, cross-over trial with sulpride. Br J Psychiatry 1984; 144:288–292.

58. Hansen L. Olanzapine in the treatment of anorexia nervosa. Br J Psychiatry 1999; 175:592.

59. Jensen VS, Mejlhede A. Anorexia nervosa: treatment with olanzapine. Br J Psychiatry 2000; 177:87.

60. LaVia M, Gray N, Kaye WH. Case reports of olanzapine treatment of anorexia nervosa. Int J Eat Disord 2000; 27:363–366.

61. Bruins-Slot L, Gorwood P, Bouvard M, Blot P, Ades J, Feingold J, Schwartz JC, Mouren-Simeoni MC. Lack of association between anorexia nervosa and D_3 dopamine receptor gene. Biol Psychiatry 1998; 43:76–78.

62. Corcos M, Atger F, Levy-Soussan P, Avrameas S, Guilbert B, Cayol V, Jeammet P. Bulimia nervosa and autoimmunity. Psychiatry Res 1999; 87:77–82.

63. Kaye WH, Weltzin TE. Serotonin activity in anorexia and bulimia nervosa: relationship to the modulation of feeding and mood. J Clin Psychiatry 1991; 52(suppl):41–48.

64. Dourish CT, Cooper SJ, Gilbert F, Coughlan J, Iversen SD. The 5-HT$_{1A}$ agonist 8-OH-DPAT increases consumption of palatable wet mash and liquid diets in the rat. Psychopharmacology 1988; 94:58–63.

65. De Vry J, Schreiber R. Effects of selected serotonin 5-HT(1) and 5-HT(2)

receptor agonists on feeding behavior: possible mechanisms of action. Neurosci Biobehav Rev 2000; 24:341–353.

66. Brewerton TD, Murphy DL, Jimerson DC. Testmeal responses following *m*-chlorophenylpiperazine and L-tryptophan in bulimics and controls. Neuropsychopharmacology 1994; 11:63–71.

67. Leibowitz SF, Alexander JT. Hypothalamic serotonin in control of eating behavior, meal size, and body weight. Biol Psychiatry 1998; 44:851–864.

68. Anderson IM, Mortimore C. 5-HT and human anxiety: evidence from studies using acute tryptophan depletion. Adv Exp Med Biol 1999; 467:43–55.

69. Kaye WH, Gwirtsman HE, George DT, Ebert MH. Altered serotonin activity in anorexia nervosa after long-term weight restoration. Arch Gen Psychiatry 1991a; 48:556–562.

70. Brewerton TD, Hand LD, Bishop ER. The Tridimensional Personality Questionnaire in eating disorder patients. Int J Eat Disord 1993; 14:213–218.

71. Waller DA, Gullion CM, Petty F, Hardy BW, Murdock MV, Rush AJ. Tridimensional Personality Questionnaire and serotonin in bulimia nervosa. Psychiatry Res 1993; 48:9–15.

72. Linnoila M, Virkhunen M, Scheinin M, Nuutila A, Rimon R, Goodwin FK. Low cerebrospinal fluid 5-hydroxyindoleacetic acid concentration differentiates impulsive from nonimpulsive violent behavior. Life Sci 1983; 33:2609–2614.

73. Coccaro EF, Siever LJ, Klar H, Maurer G, Cochrane K, Cooper TB, Mohr RC, Davis KL. Serotonergic studies in affective and personality disorder patients: correlates with suicidal and impulsive aggressive behavior. Arch Gen Psychiatry 1989; 46:587–599.

74. Brewerton TD, Stellefson EJ, Hibbs N, Hodges EJ, Cochrane CE. A comparison of eating disorder patients with and without compulsive exercising. Int J Eat Disord 1995; 17:413–416.

75. Epling F, Pierci D. Activity-based anorexia: a biological perspective. Int J Eat Disord 1988; 7:475–485.

76. Carlsson M, Svensson K, Eriksson E, Carlsson A. Rat brain serotonin: biochemical and functional evidence for a sex difference. J Neural Transm 1985; 63:297–313.

77. Goodwin GM, Fraser S, Stump K, Fairburn CG, Elliott JM, Cowen PJ. Dieting and weight loss in volunteers increases the number of alpha$_2$-adrenoceptors and 5-HT receptors on blood platelets without effect on [^{3}H]imipramine binding. J Affect Disord 1987; 12:267–274.

78. Brewerton TD. Seasonal variation of serotonin function in humans: research and clinical implications. Ann Clin Psychiatry 1989; 1:153–164.

79. Brewerton TD, Berrettini W, Nurnburger J, Linnoila M. An analysis of seasonal fluctuations of CSF monoamines and neuropeptides in normal controls: findings with 5-HIAA and HVA. Psychiatry Res 1988; 23:257–265.

80. Goldbloom DS, Olmsted MP. Pharmacotherapy of bulimia nervosa with fluoxetine: assessment of clinically significant attitudinal change. Am J Psychiatry 1993; 50:770–774.

81. Raleigh MJ, McGuire MT, Brammer GL, Yuwiler A. Social and environmental

influences on blood serotonin concentrations in monkeys. Arch Gen Psychiatry 1984; 41:405–410.

82. Raleigh MJ, Brammer GL, McGuire MT, Yuwiler A. Dominant social status facilitates the behavioral effects of serotonergic agonists. Brain Res 1985; 348:274–282.

83. McQuire MT, Raleigh MJ. Serotonin–behavior interactions in vervet monkeys. Psychopharmacol Bull 1985; 21:458–463.

84. Russell GF. The nutritional disorder in anorexia nervosa. J Psychosom Res 1967; 11:141–149.

85. Coppen AJ, Gupta RK, Eccleston EG, Wood KM, Wakeling A, de Sousa VF. Plasma tryptophan in anorexia nervosa. Lancet 1976; 1:961.

86. Hassanyeh F, Marshall EF. Measures of serotonin metabolism in anorexia nervosa. Acta Psychiatr Scand 1991; 84:561–563.

87. Askenazy F, Candito M, Caci H, Myquel M, Chambon P, Darcourt G, Puech AJ. Whole blood serotonin content, tryptophan concentrations, and impulsivity in anorexia nervosa. Biol Psychiatry 1998; 43:188–195.

88. Kaye WH, Ebert MH, Gwirtsman HE, Weiss SR. Differences in brain serotonergic metabolism between nonbulimic and bulimic patients with anorexia nervosa. Am J Psychiatry 1984; 141:1598–1601.

89. Gendall KA, Joyce PR. Meal-induced changes in tryptophan:LNAA ratio: effects on craving and binge eating. Eat Behav 2000; 1:53–62.

90. Gerner RH, Cohen DJ, Fairbanks L, Anderson GM, Young JG, Scheinin M, Linnoila M, Shaywitz BA, Hare TA. CSF neurochemistry of women with anorexia nervosa and normal women. Am J Psychiatry 1984; 141:948–949.

91. Gillberg C. Low dopamine and serotonin levels in anorexia nervosa. Am J Psychiatry 1983; 140:948–949.

92. Kaye WH. Persistent alterations in behavior and serotonin activity after recovery from anorexia and bulimia nervosa. Ann N Y Acad Sci 1997; 817:162–178.

93. Kaye W, Frank G. Gene-environment interactions: Brain and behavior in anorexia nervosa. Paper presented at the annual meeting of the Eating Disorder Research Society, November 20–23, 2002, Charleston, South Carolina.

94. Brewerton TD, Zealberg JL, Lydiard RB, Glover V, Sandler M, Ballenger JC. CSF isatin is elevated in bulimia nervosa. Biol Psychiatry 1995; 37:481–483.

95. Kaye WH, Greeno CG, Moss H, Fernstrom J, Fernstrom M, Lilenfeld LR, Weltzin TE, Mann JJ. Alterations in serotonin activity and psychiatric symptoms after recovery from bulimia nervosa. Arch Gen Psychiatry 1998; 55:927–935.

96. Brewerton TD, Brandt HA, Lesem DT, Murphy DL, Jimerson DC. Serotonin in eating disorders. In: Coccaro E, Murphy D, eds. Serotonin in Major Psychiatric Disorders. Washington, DC: American Psychiatric Press, 1990:153–184.

97. Brewerton TD, Jimerson DC. Studies of serotonin function in anorexia nervosa. Psychiatry Res 1996; 62:31–42.

98. Hadigan CM, Walsh BT, Buttinger C, Hollander E. Behavioral and neuro-

endocrine responses to metaCPP in anorexia nervosa. Biol Psychiatry 1995; 37:504–511.

99. Halmi KA, McBride PA, Sunday SR. Serotonin responsivity and hunger and satiety in eating disorders. Primary and Secondary Eating Disorders: A Psychoneuroendocrine and Metabolic Approach. Proceedings of the 2nd International Symposium on Disorders of Eating Behaviour, Pavia, Italy, September 15–19, 1992:123–131.

100. Monteleone P, Brambilla F, Bortolot F, La Rocca A, Maj M. Prolactin response to d-fenfluramine blunted in people with anorexia nervosa. Br J Psychiatry 1998; 172:439–442.

101. Monteleone P, Brambilla F, Bortolotti G, Maj M. Serotonergic dysfunction across the eating disorders: relationship to eating behaviour, purging behaviour, nutritional status and general psychopathology. Psychol Med 2000; 30:1099–1110.

102. Ward A, Brown N, Lightman S, Campbell IC, Treasure J. Neuroendocrine, appetitive and behavioural responses to d-fenfluramine in women recovered from anorexia nervosa. Br J Psychiatry 1998; 172:351–358.

103. Weizman R, Carmi M, Tyano S, Apter A, Rehavi M. High affinity [³H]imipramine binding and serotonin uptake to platelets of adolescent females suffering from anorexia nervosa. Life Sci 1986b; 38:1235–1242.

104. Zemishlany Z, Modai I, Apter A, Jerushalmy Z, Samuel E, Tyano S. Serotonin (5-HT) uptake by blood platelets in anorexia nervosa. Acta Psychiatr Scand 1987; 75:127–130.

105. Diaz-Marsa M, Carrasco JL, Hollander E, Cesar J, Saiz-Ruiz J. Decreased platelet monoamine oxidase activity in female anorexia nervosa. Acta Psychiatr Scand 2000; 101:226–230.

106. Finocchiaro LM, Polack E, Nahmod VE, Glikin GC. Cultured peripheral blood mononuclear leukocytes from anorexia nervosa patients are refractory to visible light. Life Sci 1995; 57:559–569.

107. Brewerton TD, Mueller EA, Lesem MD, Brandt HA, Quearry B, George DT, Murphy DL, Jimerson DC. Neuroendocrine responses to m-chlorophenylpiperazine and L tryptophan in bulimia. Arch Gen Psychiatry 1992b; 49:852–861.

108. Levitan RD, Kaplan AS, Joffe RT, Levitt AJ. Hormonal and subjective responses to intravenous meta-chlorophenylpiperazine in bulimia nervosa. Arch Gen Psychiatry 1997; 54:521–527.

109. Steiger H, Gauvin L, Israël M, Koerner N, Ng Ying Kin NMK, Paris K, Young SN. Association of serotonin and cortisol indices with childhood abuse in bulimia nervosa. Arch Gen Psychiatry 2001; 58:837–843.

110. Steiger H, Young SN, Kin NM, Koener N, Israël M, Lageix P, Paris J. Implications of impulsive and affective symptoms for serotonin function in bulimia nervosa. Psychol Med 2001; 31:85–95.

111. Jimerson DC, Wolfe BE, Metzger ED, Finkelstein DM, Cooper TB, Levine JM. Decreased serotonin function in bulimia nervosa. Arch Gen Psychiatry 1997; 54:529–534.

112. McBride PA, Anderson GM, Khait VD, Sunday SR, Halmi KA. Serotonergic responsivity in eating disorders. Psychopharmacol Bull 1991; 27:365–372.
113. Monteleone P, Brambilla F, Bortolot F, Ferraro C, Maj M. Plasma prolactin response to D-fenfluramine blunted in bulimic patients with frequent binge episodes. Psychol Med 1998; 28:975–983.
114. Goldbloom DS, Garfinkel PE, Katz R, Brown GM. The hormonal response to intravenous 5-hydroxytryptophan in bulimia nervosa. J Psychosom Res 1996; 40:289–297.
115. Wolfe BE, Metzger ED, Levine JM, Finkelstein DM, Cooper TB, Jimerson DC. Serotonin function following remission from bulimia nervosa. Neuropsychopharmacology 2000; 22:257–263.
116. Fernstrom JD. Dietary effects on brain serotonin synthesis: relationship to appetite regulation. Am J Clin Nutr 1985; 42:1072–1082.
117. Kaye WH, Gwirtsman HE, Brewerton TD, George DT, Jimerson DC, Wurtman RJ. Bingeing behavior and plasma amino acids: a possible involvement of brain serotonin in bulimia. Psychiatry Res 1988; 23:31–43.
118. Kay WH, Frank GK, Meltzer CM, Price JC, McConaha CW, Crossan PJ, Klump K, Rhodes L. Altered serotonin 2A receptor activity in women who have recovered from bulimia nervosa. Am J Psychiatry 2001; 158:1152–1155.
119. Marazziti D, Macchi E, Rotondo A, Placidi GF, Cassano GB. Involvement of serotonin system in bulimia. Life Sci 1988; 43:2123–2126.
120. Hallman J, Sakurai E, Oreland L. Blood platelet monoamine oxidase activity, serotonin uptake and release rates in anorexia and bulimia patients and in healthy controls. Acta Psychiatr Scand 1989; 81:73–77.
121. Goldbloom DS, Hicks LK, Garfinkel PE. Platelet serotonin uptake in bulimia nervosa. Biol Psychiatry 1988; 28:644–647.
122. Steiger H, Leonard S, Kin NY, Ladouceur C, Ramdoyal D, Young SN. Childhood abuse and platelet tritiated-paroxetine binding in bulimia nervosa: implications of borderline personality disorder. J Clin Psychiatry 2000;61:428–435.
123. Asberg M, Schalling D, Träskman-Bendz L, Wägner A. Psychobiology of suicide, impulsivity and related phenomena. In: Meltzer HY, ed. Psychopharmacology: Third Generation of Progress. New York: Raven Press, 1987:655–688.
124. Coccaro EF, Siever LJ, Klar HM, Cochrane K, Cooper TB, Mohs RC, Davis KL. Serotonergic studies in patients with affective and personality disorders: correlates with suicidal and impulsive aggressive behaviour. Arch Gen Psychiatry 1989; 46:587–599.
125. Swedo SE, Leonard HL, Krusei MJP, Rettew DC, Listwak SJ, Berrettini W, Stipetic M, Hamburger S, Gold PW, Potter WZ, Rapoport JL. Cerebrospinal fluid neurochemistry in children and adolescents with obsessive-compulsive disorder. Arch Gen Psychiatry 1992; 49:29–36.
126. Fineberg NA, Roberts A, Montgomery SA, Cowen PJ. Brain 5-HT function in obsessive-compulsive disorder. Prolactin responses to d-fenfluramine. Br J Psychiatry 1998; 171:280–282.
127. Altemus M, Swedo SE, Leonard HL, Richter D, Rubinow DR, Potter WZ, Rapaport JL. Changes in cerebrospinal fluid neurochemistry during treatment

of obsessive-compulsive disorder with clomipramine. Arch Gen Psychiatry 1994; 51:846–849.

128. Germine RH, Goddard AW, Woods SW, Charnet DS, Henninger GR. Anger and anxiety response to *m*-chlorophenylpiperazine in generalized anxiety disorder. Biol Psychiatry 1992; 32:457–461.

129. Mundo E, Bellodi L, Smeraldy E. Effects of acute intravenous clominpramine in obsessive-compulsive symptoms and response to chronic treatment. Biol Psychiatry 1995; 28:525–531.

130. Garvey MJ, Nowyes R Jr, Woodman C, Laukes C. Relationship of generalized anxiety symptoms to urinary 5-hydroxyindoleacetic acid and vanyllylmandelic acid. Psychol Res 1995; 57:1–5.

131. Askenazy F, Candito M, Caci H, Myquel M, Chambon P, Darcourt G, Puech AJ. Whole blood serotonin content, tryptophan concentrations, and impulsivity in anorexia nervosa. Biol Psychiatry 1998; 43:188–195.

132. Cloninger CR, Svrakic DM, Przybeck TR. A psychobiological model of temperament and character. Arch Gen Psychiatry 1993; 50:975–990.

133. Hollander E. Treatment of obsessive-compulsive spectrum disorder with SSRIs. Br J Psychiatry 1998; 35(suppl):7–12.

134. Waller DA, Sheinberg AL, Gullion C, Moeller FG, Cannon DS, Petty F, Hardy BW, Orsulak P, Ruch AJ. Impulsivity and neuroendocrine response to buspirone in bulimia nervosa. Biol Psychiatry 1996; 39:371–374.

135. Carrasco JL, Diaz-Marsa M, Hollander E, Cesar J, Saiz-Ruiz J. Decreased platelet monoamine oxidase activity in female bulimia nervosa. Eur Neuropsychopharmacol 2000; 10:113–117.

136. Steiger H, Koerner NM, Engleberg M, Israël M, Ng Ying Kin NMK, Young SN. Self-destructiveness and serotonin function in bulimia nervosa. Psychiatry Res 2001; 103:15–26.

137. Coccaro EF, Kavoussi RJ, Sheline YI, Lish JD, Cszwenansky JG. Impulsive aggression in personality disorder correlates with tritiated paroxetine binding in the platelet. Arch Gen Psychiatry 1996; 53:531–536.

138. Simeon D, Stanley B, Frances A, Mann JJ, Winchel R, Stanley M. Self-mutilation in personality disorders: psychological and biological correlates. Am J Psychiatry 1992; 149:221–226.

139. Riedel WJ, Klaassen T, Deutz NE, van Someren A, van Praag HM. Tryptophan depletion in normal volunteers produces selective impairment in memory consolidation. Psychopharmacology 1999; 141:362–369.

140. Brewerton TD, Murphy DL, Mueller EA, Jimerson DC. The induction of migraine-like headaches by the serotonin agonist, *m*-chlorophenylpiperazine. Clin Pharmacol Ther 1988; 43:605–609.

141. Brewerton TD, Murphy DL, Lesem MD, Brandt HA, Jimerson DC. Headache responses to *m*-chlorophenylpiperazine and L-tryptophan in bulimia nervosa. Headache 1992; 32:217–222.

142. Spigset O, Andersen T, Hagg S, Mjondal T. Enhanced platelet serotonin 5-HT_2A receptor binding in anorexia nervosa and bulimia nervosa. Eur Neuropsychopharmacol 1999; 9:469–473.

143. Steiger H. Eating disorders and the serotonin connection: states, traits and developmental effects. J Psychiatry Neurosci. In press.

144. Hinney A, Remschimidt H, Hebebrand J. Candidate gene polymorphisms in eating disorders. Eur J Pharmacol 2000; 410:147–159.

145. Collier DA, Arranz MJ, Mupita D, Brown N, Treasure J. Association between the 5-HT$_{2A}$ receptor gene polymorphism and anorexia nervosa. Lancet 1997; 350:412.

146. Nacmias B, Ricca V, Tedde A, Mezzani B, Rotella CM, Sorbi S. 5-HT$_{2A}$ receptor gene polymorphisms in anorexia nervosa and bulimia nervosa. Neurosci Lett 1999; 277:134–136.

147. Enoch MA, Kaye WH, Rotondo A, Greenberg BD, Murphy DL, Goldman D. 5-HT$_{2A}$ promoter polymorphism −1438G/A, anorexia nervosa, and obsessive-compulsive disorder. Lancet 1998; 351:1785.

148. Hinney A, Barth N, Ziegler A, vonPrittwitz S, Hamann A, Hennighausen K, Pirke KM, Heils A, Rosenkranz K, Roth H, Coners H, Mayer H, Herzog W, Siegfried A, Lehmkuhl G, Poustka F, Schmidt MH, Schafer H, Grzeschik KH, Lesch KP, Lentes KU, Remschmidt H, Hebebrand J. Serotonin transporter gene–linked polymorphic region, allele distributions in relationship to body weight and in anorexia nervosa. Life Sci 1997; 61:295–303.

149. Sundaramurthy D, Pieri LF, Gape H, Markham AF, Campbell DA. Analysis of serotonin transporter gene linked polymorphism (5-HTTLPR) in anorexia nervosa. Am J Med Genet 2000; 96:53–55.

150. Han L, Nielsen DA, Rosenthal NE, Jefferson K, Kaye W, Murphy D, Altemus M, Humphries J, Cassano G, Rotondo A, Virkkunen M, Linnoila M, Goldman D. No coding variant of the tryptophan hydroxylase gene detected in seasonal affective disorder, obsessive-compulsive disorder, anorexia nervosa, and alcoholism. Biol Psychiatry 1999; 45:615–619.

151. Hinney A, Herrmann H, Lohr T, Rosenkranz K, Ziegler A, Lehmkuhl G, Poustka F, Schmidt MH, Mayer H, Siegfried W, Remschmidt H, Hebebrand J. No evidence for an involvement of alleles of polymorphisms in the serotonin1Dbeta and 7 receptor genes in obesity, underweight or anorexia nervosa. Int J Obes Relat Metab Disord 1999; 23:760–763.

152. Ziegler A, Hebebrand J, Gorg R, Rosenkranz K, Fichter MM, Herpertz-Dahlmann B, Remschmidt H, Hinney A. Further lack of association between the 5-HT$_{2A}$ gene promoter polymorphism and susceptibility to eating disorders and a meta-analysis pertaining to anorexia nervosa. Mol Psychiatry 1999; 4:410–412.

153. Nishiguchi N, Matsuchita S, Suzuki K, Murayama M, Shirakawa O, Higuchi S. Association between 5HT$_{2A}$ receptor gene promoter region polymorphism and eating disorders in Japanese patients. Biol Psychiatry 2001; 50:123–128.

154. Di Bella DD, Catalano M, Cavallini MC, Riboldi C, Bellodi I. Serotonin transporter linked polymorphic region in anorexia nervosa and bulimia nervosa. Mol Psychiatry 2000; 5:233–241.

155. Heils A, Teufel A, Petri S, Stober G, Riederer P, Bengel D. Lesch KP: Allelic variations of human serotonin transporter gene expression. J Neurochem 1996; 66:2621–2624.

156. Bondy B, Erfurth A, de Jonge S, Krüger M, Meyer H. Possible association of the short allele of the serotonin transporter promoter gene polymorphism (5-HTTLPR) with violent suicide. Mol Psychiatry 2000; 5:193–195.

157. Lesch KP, Wolozin BL, Murphy DL, Reiderer P. Primary structure of the human platelet serotonin uptake site: identity with the brain serotonin transporter. J Neurochem 1993; 60:2319–2322.

158. Steiger H, Joober R, Israël M, Bruce K, NG Ying Kin NMK, Gauvin L, Young SN, Joncas J, Torkaman-Xehi A. A polymorphism in the promoter region of the serotonin transporter gene (5-HTTLPR) corresponds to impulsivity and reduced paroxetine binding in eating-disordered and normal-eater woman. Presented at the Annual Meeting of the Eating Disorders Research Society, Charleston, South Carolina, November 23, 2002.

159. Fluoxetine Bulimia Nervosa Collaborative Group. Fluoxetine in the treatment of bulimia nervosa: a multicenter, placebo-controlled, double-blind trial. Arch Gen Psychiatry 1992; 49:139–147.

160. Attia E, Haiman C, Walsh BT, Flater SR. Does fluoxetine augment the inpatient treatment of anorexia nervosa? Am J Psychiatry 1998; 155:548–551.

161. Strober M, Pataki C, Freeman R, DeAntonio M. No effect of adjunctive fluoxetine on eating behavior or weight phobia during the inpatient treatment of anorexia nervosa: an historical case-control study. J Child Adol Psychopharmacol 1999; 9:195–201.

162. Faris PL, Kim SW, Meller WH, Goodale RL, Hofbauer RD, Oakman SA, Howard LA, Stevens ER, Eckert ED, Hartman BK. Effect of ondansetron, a 5-HT$_3$ receptor antagonist, on the dynamic association between bulimic behaviors and pain thresholds. Pain 1998; 77:297–303.

163. Faris PL, Kim SW, Meller WH, Goodale RL, Oakman SA, Hofbauer RD, Marshall AM, Daughters RS, Banerjee-Stevens D, Eckert ED, Hartman BK. Effect of decreasing afferent vagal activity with ondansetron on symptoms of bulimia nervosa: a randomised, double-blind trial. Lancet 2000; 355:792–797.

164. Roychoudhury M, Kulkarni SK. Anti-anxiety profile of ondansetron, a selective 5-HT$_3$ antagonist, in a novel animal model. Methods Find Exp Clin Pharmacol 1997; 19:107–111.

165. Glover V, Halket JM, Watkins PJ, Clow A, Goodwin BL, Sandler M. Isatin: identity with the purified endogenous monoamine oxidase inhibitor tribulin. J Neurochem 1988; 51:656–659.

12

Neuroendocrine and Neuropeptide Dysregulation in Anorexia Nervosa, Bulimia Nervosa, and Binge Eating Disorder

Ursula F. Bailer and Walter H. Kaye
Western Psychiatric Institute and Clinic,
   University of Pittsburgh School of Medicine
Pittsburgh, Pennsylvania, U.S.A.

NEUROENDOCRINOLOGY

Abnormal hormone profiles and responses to challenge are closely related to the "starvation" status of anorexia nervosa (AN) and bulimia nervosa (BN) patients. Hormone abnormalities may also be present, but to a lesser extent, in normal-weight women with BN. The presence of starvation in AN is evident from the weight loss, but it may not be recognized in normal-weight bulimics. Although bulimic women often maintain a normal weight, they do so by restricting food intake when not bingeing and purging, and they may have monotonous and poorly balanced meals. Starvation-induced depletion of hepatic glycogen stores results in free fatty acids and ketone bodies replacing glucose as the primary energy source. This shift from glycogenolysis to lipolysis and ketogenesis is associated with an increase in free fatty acids and their metabolites. β-Hydroxybutyric acid levels are elevated in both AN and BN (1), indicating that bulimic patients are nutritionally depleted in spite of their normal body weight.

The relationship of starvation and eating disorders to neuroendocrine function is most clearly seen for the pituitary gonadal axis. Secondary

283

amenorrhea is one of the criteria for AN in postmenarcheal women, and oligomenorrhea occurs in about 50% of bulimics. The secondary amenorrhea is a direct result of altered gonadotropin secretion. Serum sex hormone–binding globulin may be increased, and both estrogen and testosterone are decreased (2). The luteinizing hormone response to luteinizing hormone–releasing hormone stimulation is blunted, but the follicle-stimulating hormone response is usually normal.

With reference to the hypothalamic–pituitary–adreno-cortical (HPA) axis, it is well known that plasma cortisol is increased at all times of the day and night, but its circadian rhythm is preserved in terms of amplitude and timing. Stimulation and suppression tests of the HPA axis have been conducted mainly in AN, and they are in accord with the baseline hormone findings. Adrenocorticotropic hormone (ACTH) response to corticotropin-releasing hormone (CRH) administration is reduced, undoubtedly secondary to enhanced negative feedback on the pituitary corticotrophs exerted by elevated circulating cortisol. The cortisol response to ACTH administration is increased, suggesting increased secretory capacity of the adrenal cortex. The low-dose dexamethasone suppression test is abnormal in 50–90% of anorexics and in 20% to 60% of bulimics, depending on the weight loss. Because dexamethasone acts primarily at the pituitary, ACTH and cortisol escape from dexamethasone suppression, suggesting increased suprapituitary stimulation of corticotrophs by CRH and vasopressin. Taken together, the pituitary–adrenocortical findings indicate a mild to moderate activation of this hormone axis in AN and BN. Interestingly, the abnormalities in AN and in reduced-weight BN (3,4) are strikingly similar to those occurring in 30–50% of patients with major depression, although malnutrition, and not mood disturbances, are likely to be most contributory.

Obese women with binge eating disorder do not show abnormalities of dexamethasone suppression, either before or after weight loss (5). Data are not available on prolactin, growth hormone (GH) secretion, or 24-h cortisol secretion in subjects with binge eating disorder (6). Among obese binge eaters who do not purge, no abnormalities of glucose or insulin have been reported relative to weight-matched controls (7). However, sophisticated methodologies to evaluate cephalic-phase insulin release (CPIR) and glucose metabolism have not been applied to this population.

With reference to the pituitary–thyroid axis, starvation leads to considerably decreased plasma free triiodothyronine (T_3) concentrations, along with somewhat decreased plasma free thyroxine (T_4) and increased plasma reverse T_3 concentrations. This represents the "euthyroid sick syndrome" hormone profile (8,9). The decreased circulating T_3 helps reduce energy expenditure and minimizes muscle protein catabolism into amino acids for gluconeogenesis. Cerebrospinal fluid (CSF) thyrotropin-releasing hormone also appears to be reduced in AN (10). When bingeing, bulimic patients generally have normal thyroid indices with perhaps reduced T_3 and thyroid-stimulating hormone concentrations; however, when they become abstinent, their pituitary–thyroid axis function resembles that of anorexic patients (11–13). Thyroid hormone levels are similar in obese binge eaters and weight-matched controls (7,14).

Insulinlike growth factor, type I (IGF-1) concentrations are low in both AN and BN, and circulating GH is increased, perhaps owing to diminished feedback of IGF-1 on GH secretion. Circulating prolactin is usually unchanged in AN and may be reduced in BN. Prolactin responses to serotonergic challenges such as *meta*-chlorophenylpiperazine, fenfluramine, L-tryptophan, and 5-OH-tryptophan are diminished in both AN and BN.

NEUROPEPTIDES

The past decade has witnessed accelerating basic research on the role of neuropeptides in the regulation of feeding behavior and obesity. The mechanisms for controlling food intake involve a complicated interplay between peripheral systems (including gustatory stimulation, gastrointestinal peptide secretion, and vagal afferent nerve responses) and central nervous system (CNS) neuropeptides and/or monoamines. Thus, studies in animals show that neuropeptides, such as cholecystokinin, the endogenous opioids (such as β-endorphin), and neuropeptide Y regulate the rate, duration, and size of meals, as well as macronutrient selection (15,16). In addition to regulating eating behavior, a number of CNS neuropeptides participate in the regulation of neuroendocrine pathways. Thus, clinical studies have evaluated the possibility that CNS neuropeptide alterations may contribute to dysregulated secretion of the gonadal hormones, cortisol, thyroid hormones, and growth hormone in the eating disorders (17,18).

While there are relatively few studies to date, most of the neuroendocrine and neuropeptide alterations apparent during symptomatic episodes of AN and BN tend to normalize after recovery. This observation suggests that most of the disturbances are consequences rather than causes of malnutrition, weight loss, and/or altered meal patterns. Still, an understanding of these neuropeptide disturbances may shed light on why many people with AN or BN cannot easily "reverse" their illness. In AN, malnutrition may contribute to a downward spiral sustaining and perpetuating the desire for more weight loss and dieting. Symptoms such as increased satiety, obsessions, and dysphoric mood may be exaggerated by these neuropeptide alterations and thus contribute to the downward spiral. In addition, mutual interactions between neuropeptide, neuroendocrine, and neurotransmitter pathways may contribute to the constellation of psychiatric comorbidity often observed in these disorders. Even after weight gain and normalization of eating patterns, many individuals who have recovered from AN or BN have physiological, behavioral, and psychological symptoms that persist for extended periods. Menstrual cycle dysregulation, for example, may persist for several months after weight restoration. The following sections provide a brief overview of studies of neuropeptides in AN and BN.

Corticotropin-Releasing Hormone

When underweight, patients with AN have increased plasma cortisol secretion, which is thought to be at least in part a consequence of hypersecretion of endogenous CRH (3,19–21). In that the plasma and CSF measures return to normal, it appears likely that activation of the HPA axis is precipitated by weight loss. The observation of increased CRH activity is of great theoretical interest in AN since intracerebroventricular CRH administration in experimental animals produces many of the physiological and behavioral changes associated with AN, including markedly decreased eating behavior (22), hypothalamic hypogonadism (23), decreased sexual activity (24), and hyperactivity (25).

Opioid Peptides

Studies in laboratory animals raise the possibility that altered endogenous opioid activity might contribute to pathological feeding behavior in eating disorders since opioid agonists generally increase, and opioid antagonists decrease, food intake (26). State-related reductions in concentrations of CSF β-endorphin and related opiate concentrations have been found in both underweight AN and ill BN subjects (27–29). In contrast, using the T lymphocyte as a model system, Brambilla et al. (30) found elevated β-endorphin levels in AN, although the levels were normal in BN (31). If β-endorphin activity is a facilitator of feeding behavior, then reduced CSF concentrations could reflect decreased central activity of this system, which then maintains or facilitates inhibition of feeding behavior in the eating disorders.

A disturbance in CNS opioid function may also contribute to the neuroendocrine abnormalities in AN and BN (e.g., disturbances in HPA and pituitary–gonadal axis function) (32,33). Brain opioid pathways inhibit ACTH and cortisol release in humans, and they suppress pulsatile gonadotropin secretion in rats and in sexually mature humans. Underweight anorexics frequently have a blunted response of LH secretion to opiate antagonists (34), and weight restoration tends to normalize this response. The failure of opioid antagonists to increase luteinizing hormone secretion in underweight anorexics suggests that another neurotransmitter system (or systems) may be responsible for this neuroendocrine disturbance.

Vasopressin and Oxytocin

In addition to the effects of vasopressin on HPA axis regulation and free-water clearance by the kidney and the effects of oxytocin during the puerperium, these structurally related neuropeptides are distributed throughout the CNS and function as long-acting neuromodulators of complex behaviors. The effects of vasopressin appear to be reciprocal to those of oxytocin; central administration of vasopressin to rats enhances memory consolidation and retrieval, whereas administration of oxytocin disrupts memory (35).

In addition to abnormally high CSF vasopressin concentrations and impaired osmoregulation of plasma vasopressin (36), AN patients have reduced CSF oxytocin concentrations and impaired plasma oxytocin responses to stimulation (37). Underweight anorexics also have an impaired plasma oxytocin response to challenging stimuli (38). These abnormalities tend to normalize after weight restoration, suggesting that they are secondary to malnutrition or abnormal fluid balance, or both. In underweight anorexics, low CNS oxytocin might interact with high CNS vasopressin to enhance the retention of cognitive distortions of the aversive consequences of eating, thereby reinforcing these patients' perseverative preoccupation with the adverse consequences of food intake.

Normal-weight bulimics were found to have elevated CSF vasopressin concentrations but normal CSF oxytocin both on admission and after 1 month of nutritional stabilization and abstinence from bingeing and purging. In these patients as well, CNS vasopressin might contribute to their obsessional preoccupation with the aversive consequences of weight gain (39).

Neuropeptide Y and Peptide YY

Neuropeptide Y (NPY) and Peptide YY (PYY) are of considerable theoretical interest since they are among the most potent endogenous stimulants of feeding behavior in the CNS (16,26,40). PYY is more potent than NPY in stimulating food intake; both are selective for carbohydrate-rich foods. Underweight individuals with AN have been shown to have elevations of CSF NPY but normal PYY (41). Clearly, elevated NPY does not result in increased feeding in underweight individuals with AN; however, the possibility that increased NPY activity underlies the obsessive and paradoxical interest in dietary intake and food preparation is a hypothesis worth exploring. On the other hand, CSF levels of NPY and PYY have been reported to be normal in women with BN when measured while subjects were acutely ill. Although levels of PYY increased above normal when subjects were reassessed after one month of abstinence from bingeing and vomiting, levels of the peptides were similar to control values in long-term recovered individuals

(42). More recently, it has been reported that the plasma concentration of NPY was lower in AN patients than in controls, whereas BN patients had elevated NPY levels (43). Additional studies to assess the potential behavioral correlates of these findings are needed.

Cholecystokinin

Cholecystokinin (CCK) is a peptide secreted by the gastrointestinal system in response to food intake. Release of CCK is thought to be one means of transmitting satiety signals to the brain by way of vagal afferents (44). In parallel to its role in satiety in rodents, exogenously administered CCK reduces food intake in humans. The preponderance of data suggests that patients with BN, in comparison to controls, have diminished release of CCK following ingestion of a standardized test meal (45–48). Measurements of basal CCK values in blood lymphocytes and in CSF also appear to be decreased in patients with BN (31,49). It has been suggested that the diminished CCK response to a meal may have a role in diminished post-ingestive satiety observed in BN. The CCK response in BN patients was found to return to normal following treatment (45).

Studies of CCK in AN have yielded less consistent findings. Some studies have found elevations in basal levels of plasma CCK (46,50), as well as increased peptide release following a test meal (46,51). One study found that blunting of CCK response to an oral glucose load normalized in AN patients after partial restoration of body weight (50). Other studies have found that measures of CCK function in AN were similar to or lower than control values (30,47,52,53). Further studies are needed to evaluate the relationship between altered CCK regulation and other indices of abnormal gastric function in symptomatic BN and AN patients (54).

Leptin

Leptin, the protein product of the *ob* gene, is secreted predominantly by adipose tissue cells and acts in the CNS to decrease food intake, thus regulating body fat stores. In rodent models, defects in the leptin coding sequence resulting in leptin deficiency or defects in leptin receptor function are associated with obesity. In humans, serum and CSF concentrations of leptin are positively correlated with fat mass in individuals across a broad range of body weight, including obesity (55,56). Thus, obesity in humans is not thought to be a result of leptin deficiency per se, although rare genetic deficiencies in leptin production have been associated with familial obesity (57).

Underweight patients with AN have consistently been found to have significantly reduced serum leptin concentrations in comparison to normal weight controls (53,58–61). Based on studies in laboratory animals, it has been suggested that low leptin levels may contribute to amenorrhea and other hormonal changes in the disorder (60). Although the reduction in fasting serum leptin levels in AN is correlated with reduction in body mass index (BMI), there has been some discussion of the possibility that leptin levels in AN patients may be higher than expected based on the extent of weight loss (62,63). Mantzoros et al. (60) reported an elevated CSF to serum leptin ratio in AN compared to controls, suggesting that the proportional decrease in leptin levels with weight loss is greater in serum than in CSF. A longitudinal investigation during refeeding in AN patients has shown that CSF leptin concentrations reach normal values before full weight restoration, possibly as a consequence of the relatively rapid and disproportionate accumulation of fat during refeeding (60). This finding led the authors to suggest that premature normalization of leptin concentration might contribute to difficulty in achieving and sustaining a normal weight in AN. Plasma and CSF leptin levels appear to be similar to control values in long-term recovered AN subjects (42).

Recent studies indicate that patients with BN, in comparison to carefully matched controls, have significantly decreased leptin concentrations in serum samples obtained after overnight fast (43,62,64–66). Initial findings in individuals who have achieved sustained recovery from BN, when compared to controls with closely matched percent body fat, suggest that serum leptin levels remain decreased. This finding may be related to evidence for a persistent decrease in activity in the hypothalamic–pituitary–thyroid axis in long-term recovered BN individuals. These alterations could be associated with decreased metabolic rate and a tendency to weight gain, contributing to the preoccupation with body weight characteristic of BN.

Ghrelin

Ghrelin was originally discovered in the rat and the human stomach, and stimulates GH secretion in rodents. This petide that antagonizes leptin action has a role in the regulation of feeding behavior and energy metabolism in the CNS (67). Ghrelin-producing neurons are located in the hypothalamus, whrereas ghrelin receptors are expressed in various regions of the brain. Intracerebroventricular injections of ghrelin strongly stimulated feeding in rats and increased body weight gain. In addition, it has been reported that fasting plasma ghrelin concentrations in humans are negatively correlated with BMI (68,69), percentage body fat and fasting leptin and insulin concentrations (70), which have an important role in the pathophysiology of AN (71). In the latter study it could be shown that ghrelin was elevated in AN patients and returned to normal levels after weight recovery. The possibility of ghrelin resistance in cachectic states as caused by eating disorders could be suggested. Fasting plasma ghrelin concentrations in patients with BN were significantly higher than those in controls (69), although the BMIs between bulimics and controls were not significantly different, suggesting that not only BMI, but also abnormal eating behavior with bingeing and purging, had an influence on circulating ghrelin level in BN patients.

Gastrin-Releasing Peptide

Human gastrin-releasing peptide (GRP) is a 27-amino-acid peptide that shares similar decapeptide with bombesin (BBS) (72). Peripheral and central administration of GRP attenuates food intake in mammals and humans (73,74). In the CNS, distinct BBS-like receptor subtypes have been identified in brain tissue such as the bed nucleus of the stria terminalis, the olfactory tubercle, the putamen, and the neocortex, with a neuromedin B- and a GRP-preferring subtype (75,76). Both subtypes have been implicated in the modulation of BBS-like peptide-induced food suppression (77). CSF GRP was significantly lower in recovered bulimic patients (>1 year, normal weight, and regular menstrual cycles, no bingeing or purging) compared to normal controls and recovered anorectic patients (78). Lower CSF GRP in this group could be a trait-related disturbance that might add to hyperphagic behavior, and thus to the pathophysiology of this illness.

CONCLUSIONS AND PERSPECTIVES

The increase in understanding of neuropeptide modulation of appetite and weight control also resulted in new insights into endocrine and neuropepetide disturbances in AN and BN. Obviously, there are still many methodological problems to be taken into consideration when interpreting the endocrinological observations. Animal models that focus on one facet of behavior, such as motor activity or sexual receptivity, are not necessarily suitable models for AN. The serum concentrations of monoamines and peptides reflect pituitary secretion but may provide a limited perspective on higher brain function. CSF measures reflect some general pool of chemicals but offers limited understanding of specific pathways. Minor weight changes in patients with AN are associated with significant responses in serum catecholamines, leptin, cortisol, gonadotropin, and GH, indicating that the timing of the respective investigations is of critical importance and may be a cause of discrepant findings in several studies (18).

Among individuals who engage in binge eating without purging, few biological correlates of binge eating have been identified. Neuroendocrine function does not differ from weight-matched controls in nonpurging binge eaters (6).

Determining whether abnormalities are a consequence or a potential antecedent of pathological feeding behavior is a major question in eating disorders. When studying patients who had recovered from their eating disorder, any persistent psychobiological abnormalities might be trait related and potentially have contributed to the pathogenesis of the disorder.

Last but not least, most models describe only one or two specific systems out of many, while our knowledge about the interactions between these systems is limited and, at the present time, it is not possible to map the sum of numerous interactive pathways.

REFERENCES

1. Pirke KM, Pahl J, Schweiger U. Metabolic and endocrine indices of starvation in bulimia: a comparison with anorexia nervosa. Psychiatry Res 1985; 15:33–39.
2. Tomova A, Kumanov P, Kirilov G. Factors related to sex hormone binding globulin concentrations in women with anorexia nervosa. Psychosom Med 1995; 40:499–506.
3. Gold PW, Gwirtsman H, Avgerinos PC, Nieman LK, Gallucci WT, Kaye W, Jimerson D, Ebert M, Rittmaster R, Loriaux DL. Abnormal hypothalamic-pituitary-adrenal function in anorexia nervosa. Pathophysiologic mechanisms in underweight and weight-corrected patients. N Engl J Med 1986; 314:1335–1342.
4. Fichter MM, Pirke KM, Pollinger J, et al. Disturbances in the hypothalamo-pituitary-adrenal and other neuroendocrine axes in bulimia. Biol Psychiatry 1990; 27:1021–1037.
5. Yanovski SZ, Yanovski JA, Gwirtsman HE, Bernat A, Gold PG, Chrousos GP. Normal dexamethasone suppression in obese binge and nonbinge eaters with rapid weight loss. J Clin Endocrinol Metab 1993; 76:675–679.
6. Yanovski SZ. Biological correlates of binge eating. Addict Behav 1995; 20:705–712.
7. Adami GF, Gandolfo P, Campostano A, Cocchi F, Bauer B, Scopinaro N. Obese binge eaters: metabolic characteristics, energy expenditure, and dieting. Psychol Med 1995; 25:195–198.
8. Wartofsky L, Burman KD. Alterations in throid function in patients with systemic illness: the "euthyroid sick syndrome." Endocr Rev 1982; 3:164–217.
9. Altemus M, Hetherington M, Kennedy B, et al. Thyroid function in bulimia nervosa. Psychoneuroendocrinology 1996; 21:249–261.
10. Lesem MD, Kaye WII, Bissette G, et al. Cerebrospinal fluid TRH immunoreactivity in anorexia nervosa. Biol Psychiatry 1994; 35:48–53.
11. Devlin MJ, Walsh BT, Kral JG, et al. Metabolic abnormalities in bulimia nervosa. Arch Gen Psychiatry 1990; 47:144–148.
12. Altemus M, Hetherington M, Flood M. Decrease in resting metabolic rate during abstinence from bulimic behavior. Am J Psychiatry 1991; 148:1071–1072.
13. Spalter AR, Gwirtsman HE, Demitrack MA, et al. Throid function in bulimia nervosa. Biol Psychiatry 1993; 33:408–414.

14. Wadden TA, Foster GD, Letizia KA, Wilk JE. Metabolic, anthropometric, and psychological characteristics of obese binge eaters. Int J Eat Disord 1993; 14: 127–135.

15. Morley JE, Blundell JE. The neurobiological basis of eating disorders: some formulations. Biol Psychiatry 1988; 23:53–78.

16. Schwartz MW, Woods SC, Porte D Jr, Seeley RJ, Baskin DG. Central nervous system control of food intake. Nature 2000; 404:661–671.

17. Jimerson DC, Wolfe BE, Naab S. In: Anorexia nervosa and bulimia nervosa. CE, Brumback RA, eds. Textbook of Pediatric Neuropsychiatry Coffee Washington, DC: American Psychiatric Press, 1998:563–578.

18. Stoving RK, Hangaard J, Hansen-Nord M, Hagen C. A review of endocrine changes in anorexia nervosa. J Psychiatr Res 1999; 33:139–152.

19. Kaye WH, Gwirtsman HE, George DT, Ebert MH, Jimerson DC, Tomai TP, Chrousos GP, Gold PW. Elevated cerebrospinal fluid levels of immunoreactive corticotropin-releasing hormone in anorexia nervosa: relation to state of nutrition, adrenal function, and intensity of depression. J Clin Endocrinol Metab 1987; 64:203–208.

20. Walsh BT, Roose SP, Katz JL, Dyrenfurth I, Wright L, Vande Wiele R, Glassman AH. Hypothalamic-pituitary-adrenal-cortical activity in anorexia nervosa and bulimia. Psychoneuroendocrinology 1987; 12:131–140.

21. Licinio J, Wong ML, Gold PW. The hypothalamic-pituitary-adrenal axis in anorexia nervosa. Psychiatry Res 1996; 62:75–83.

22. Glowa JR, Gold PW. Corticotropin releasing hormone produces profound anorexigenic effects in the rhesus monkey. Neuropeptides 1991; 18:55–61.

23. Rivier C, Vale W. Influence of corticotropin releasing factor on reproductive functions in the rat. Endocrinology 1984; 114:914–921.

24. Sirinathsinghji DJ, Rees LH, Rivier J. Corticotropin-releasing factor is a potent inhibitor of sexual receptivity in the female rat. Nature 1983; 305:232–235.

25. Sutton RE, Koob GF, LeMoal M. Corticotropin-releasing factor produces behavioral activation in rats. Nature 1982; 297:331–333.

26. Morley JE, Levine AS, Gosnell BA, Mitchell JE, Krahn DD, Nizielski SE. Peptides and feeding. Peptides 1985; 6:181–192.

27. Kaye WH, Berrettini WH, Gwirtsman HE, Chretien M, Gold PW, George DT, Jimerson DC, Ebert MH. Reduced cerebrospinal fluid levels of immunoreactive pro-opiomelanocortin related peptides (including beta-endorphin) in anorexia nervosa. Biol Psychiatry 1987; 41:2147–2155.

28. Lesem MD, Berrettini W, Kaye WH, Jimerson DC. Measurement of CSF dynorphin A 1–8 immunoreactivity in anorexia nervosa and normal-weight bulimia. Biol Psychiatry 1991; 29:244–252.

29. Brewerton TD, Lydiard RB, Laraia MT, Shook JE, Ballenger JC. CSF beta-endorphin and dynorphin in bulimia nervosa. Am J Psychiatry 1992; 149:1086–1090.

30. Brambilla F, Brunetta M, Peirone A, Perna G, Sacerdote P, Manfredi B, Panerai AE. T-lymphocyte cholecystokinin-8 and beta-endorphin concentrations in eating disorders: I. Anorexia nervosa. Psychiatry Res 1995; 59:43–50.

31. Brambilla F, Brunetta M, Draisci A, Manfredi B, Panerai AE, Peirone A, Perna G, Sacerdote P. T-lymphocyte cholecystokinin-8 and beta-endorphin in eating disorders: II. Bulimia nervosa. Psychiatry Res 1995; 59:51–56.

32. Grossman A. Brain opiates and neuroendocrine function. Clin Endocrinol Metab 1983; 12:725–746.

33. Pfeiffer A, Herz A. Endocrine actions of opioids. Horm Metab Res 1984; 16: 386–397.

34. Armeanu M, Berkhout GMJ, Schoemaker J. Pulsatile luteinizing hormone secretion in hypothalamic amenorrhea, anorexia nervosa, and polycystic ovarian disease during naltrexone treatment. Fertil Steril 1992; 57:762–770.

35. Bohus B, Kovacs GL, De Weid D. Oxytocin, vasopressin and memory: opposite effects on consolidation and retrial process. Brain Res 1978; 157:414–417.

36. Nishita JK, Ellinwood EH Jr, Rockwell WJ. Abnormalities in the response of plasma arginine vasopressin durinh hypertonic saline infusion in patients with eating disorders. Biol Psychiatry 1989; 26:73–86.

37. Demitrack MA, Lesem MD, Listwak SJ. CSF oxytocin in anorexia nervosa and bilimia nervosa: clinical and pathophysiological considerations. Am J Psychiatry 1990; 147:882–886.

38. Chiodera P, Volpi R, Capretti L. Effect of estrogen or insulin-induced hypoglyccmia on plasma oxytocin levels in bulimia and anorexia nervosa. Metabolism 1991; 40:1226–1230.

39. Gold PW, Kaye WH, Robertson GL, et al. Abnormalities in plasma and cerebrospinal-fluid arginine vasopressin in patients with anorexia nervosa. N Engl J Med 1983; 308:1117–1123.

40. Kalra SP, Dube MG, Sahu A, Phelps CP, Kalra PS. Neuropeptide Y secretion increases in the paraventricular nucleus in association with increased appetite for food. Proc Natl Acad Sci USA 1991; 88:10931–10935.

41. Kaye WH, Berrettini W, Gwirtsman H, George DT. Altered cerebrospinal fluid neuropeptide Y and peptide YY immunoreactivity in anorexia and bulimia nervosa. Arch Gen Psychiatry 1990; 47:548–556.

42. Gendall K. Leptin, neuropeptide Y, and peptide YY in long-term recovered eating disorder patients. Biol Psychiatry 1999; 46:292–299.

43. Baranowska B, Wolinska-Witort E, Wasilewska-Dziubinska E, Roguski K, Chmielowska M. Plasma leptin, neuropeptide Y (NPY) and galanin concentrations in bulimia nervosa and in anorexia nervosa. Neuroendocrinol Lett 2001; 22:356–358.

44. Gibbs J, Young RC, Smith GP. Cholecystokinin decreases food intake in rats. J Comp Physiol Psychology 1973, 84:488–495.

45. Geracioti TD Jr, Liddle RA. Impaired cholecystokinin secretion in bulimia nervosa. N Engl J Med 1988; 319:683–688.

46. Phillipp E, Pirke KM, Kellner MB, Krieg JC. Disturbed cholecystokinin secretion in patients with eating disorders. Life Sci 1991; 48:2443–2450.

47. Pirke KM, Kellner MB, Friess E, Krieg JC, Fichter MM. Satiety and cholecystokinin. Int J Eat Disord 1994; 15:63–69.

48. Devlin MJ, Walsh BT, Guss JL, Kissileff HR, Liddle RA, Petkova E. Post-

prandial cholecystokinin release and gastric emptying in patients with bulimia nervosa. Am J Clin Nutr 1997; 65:114–120.

49. Lydiard RB, Brewerton TD, Fossey MD, Laraia MT, Stuart G, Beinfeld MC, Ballenger JC. CSF cholecystokinin octapeptide in patients with bulimia nervosa and in normal comparison subjects. Am J Psychiatry 1993; 150:1099–1101.

50. Tamai H, Takemura J, Kobayashi N, Matsubayashi S, Matsukura S, Nakagawa T. Changes in plasma cholecystokinin concentrations after oral glucose tolerance test in anorexia nervosa before and after therapy. Metab Clin Exp 1993; 42:581–584.

51. Harty RF, Pearson PH, Solomon TE, McGuigan JE. Cholecystokinin, vasoactive intestinal peptide and peptide histidine methionine responses to feeding in anorexia nervosa. Regul Peptides 1991; 36:141–150.

52. Geracioti TD Jr, Liddle RA, Altemus M, Demitrack MA, Gold PW. Regulation of appetite and cholecystokinin secretion in anorexia nervosa. Am J Psychiatry 1992; 149:958–961.

53. Baranowska B, Radzikowska M, Wasilewska-Dziubinska E, Roguski K, Borowiec M. Disturbed release of gastrointestinal peptides in anorexia nervosa and in obesity. Diabetes Obes Metab 2000; 2:99–103.

54. Geliebter A, Melton PM, McCray RS, Gallagher DR, Gage D, Hashim SA. Gastric capacity, gastric emptying, and test-meal intake in normal and bulimic women. Am J Clin Nutr 1992; 56:656–661.

55. Considine RV, Considine EL, Williams CJ, Hyde TM, Caro JF. The hypothalamic leptin receptor in humans: identification of incidental sequence polymorphisms and absence of the db/db mouse and fa/fa rat mutations. Diabetes 1996; 45:992–994.

56. Schwartz MW, Peskind E, Raskind M, Boyko EJ, Porte D Jr. Cerebrospinal fluid leptin levels: relationship to plasma levels and to adiposity in humans. Nature Med 1996; 2:589–593.

57. Farooqi IS, Keogh JM, Kamath S, Jones S, Gibson WT, Trussell R, Jebb SA, Lip GY, O'Rahilly S. Partial leptin deficiency and human adiposity. Nature 2001; 414:34–35.

58. Hebebrand J, van der Heyden J, Devos R, Kopp W, Herpertz S, Remschmidt H, Herzog W. Plasma concentrations of obese protein in anorexia nervosa. Lancet 1995; 346:1624–1625.

59. Grinspoon S, Gulick T, Askari H, Landt M, Lee K, Anderson E, Ma Z, Vignati L, Bowsher R, Herzog D, Klibanski A. Serum leptin levels in women with anorexia nervosa. J Clin Endocrinol Metab 1996; 81:3861–3863.

60. Mantzoros C, Flier JS, Lesem MD, Brewerton TD, Jimerson DC. Cerebrospinal fluid leptin in anorexia nervosa: correlation with nutritional status and potential role in resistance to weight gain. J Clin Endocrinol Metab 1997; 82: 1845–1851.

61. Eckert ED, Pomeroy C, Raymond N, Kohler PF, Thuras P, Bowers CY. Leptin in anorexia nervosa. J Clin Endocrinol Metab 1998; 83:791–795.

62. Frederich R, Hu S, Raymond N, Pomeroy C. Leptin in anorexia nervosa and

bulimia nervosa: importance of assay technique and method of interpretation. J Lab Clin Med 2002; 139:72–79.

63. Jimerson DC. Leptin and the neurobiology of eating disorders. J Lab Clin Med 2002; 139:70–71.
64. Brewerton TD, Lesem MD, Kennedy A, Garvey WT. Reduced plasma leptin concentration in bulimia nervosa. Psychoneuroendocrinology 2000; 25:649–658.
65. Jimerson DC, Mantzoros C, Wolfe BE, Metzger ED. Decreased serum leptin in bulimia nervosa. J Clin Endocrinol Metab 2000; 85:4511–4514.
66. Monteleone P, Bortolotti F, Fabrazzo M, La Rocca A, Fuschino A, Maj M. Plasma leptin response to acute fasting and refeeding in untreated women with bulimia nervosa. J Clin Endocrinol Metab 2000; 85:2499–2503.
67. Nakazato M, Murakami N, Date Y, Kojima M, Matsuo H, Kangawa K, Matsukura S. A role for ghrelin in the central regultion of feeding. Nature 2001; 409: 194–198.
68. Shiiya T, Nakazato M, Mizuta M, Date Y, Mondal MS, Tanaka M, Nozoe S, Hosoda H, Kangawa K, Matsukura S. Plasma ghrelin levels in lean and obese humans and the effect of glucose on ghrelin secretion. J Endocrinol Metab 2002; 87:240–244.
69. Tanaka M, Naruo T, Muranaga T, Yasuhara D, Shiiya T, Nakazato M, Matsukura S, Nozoe S. Increased fasting plasma ghrelin levels in patients with bulimia nervosa. Eur J Endocrinol 2002; 146:R1–R3.
70. Tschöp M, Weyer C, Tataranni AP, Devanarayan V, Ravussin B, Heiman ML. Circulating ghrelin levels are decreased in human obesity. Diabetes 2001; 50: 707–709.
71. Otto B, Cuntz U, Fruehauf E, Wawarta R, Folwaczny C, Riepl RL, Heiman ML, Lehnert P, Fichter M, Tschöp M. Weight gain decrease elevated plasma ghrelin concentrations of patients with anorexia nervosa. Eur J Endocrinol 2001; 145:669–673.
72. Brown M, Marki W, Rivier J. Is gastrin releasing peptide mammalian bombesin? Life Sci 1980; 27:125–128.
73. Bray GA. Nutrient intake is modulated by peripheral petide aministration. Obesity Res 1995; 3(Suppl. 4):569S–572S.
74. Flynn FW. Bombesin-like peptides in the reglation of ingestive behavior. Ann NY Acad Sci 1994; 739:120–134.
75. Ladenheim EE, Jensen RT, Mantey SA, Moran TH. Distinct distributions of two bombesin receptor subtypes in the rat central nervous system. Brain Res 1992; 593:168–178.
76. Wolf SS, Moody TW. Receptors for GRP/bombesin-like peptides in the rat forebrain. Peptides 1985; 6(Suppl. 1):111–114.
77. Ladenheim EE, Wirth KE, Moran TH. Receptor subtype mediation of feeding suppression by bombesin-like peptides. Pharmacol Biochem Behav 1996; 54: 705–711.
78. Frank GK, Kaye WH, Ladenheim EE, McConaha C. Reduced gastrin releasing peptide in cerebrospinal fluid after recovery from bulimia nervosa. Appetite 2001; 37:9–14.

13

Neuroimaging of the Eating Disorders

Janet Treasure

Thomas Guy House
London, England

Rudolf Uher

Institute of Psychiatry
London, England

It has been an unfortunate fact that eating disorders are all too often dismissed as trivial complaints of spoilt princesses who are merely being stubborn and willful. However, it will be difficult to continue to hold such a position in the face of the evidence that is coming from research into brain imaging. Pictures can be worth a thousand words, and the brain images, which show both structural and functional brain changes, cannot be easily dismissed. Food provokes a unique pattern of brain activation in people with eating disorders. Moreover, food-induced activation of the orbitofrontal cortex continues after recovery. Also structural abnormalities persist after recovery. Are these effects scars from the illness or markers of a neuro-developmental diathesis? The answers may have implications for clinical evaluation, diagnostics, treatment, and outcome. We therefore argue that brain imaging is not just an interesting application of modern technology but an essential and exciting tool that can be used to clarify the confusing tapestry of eating disorders.

Interest in imaging applied to eating disorders began with the increased resolution offered by computed tomography (CT). This revealed that the brain, in parallel with all other organs of the body, was shrunken especially in AN. However, this was somewhat dismissed as a nonspecific side effect of starvation and added to the list of numerous clinical consequences. However, the second phase of this research, which relates to brain function, can be and has been hypothesis driven. We predict that this may have a more profound effect on thinking in the field.

GENERAL ASPECTS OF METHODOLOGY

There are several aspects of the technology and methodology of brain imaging that are of importance in understanding and interpreting research in this field. For example, the level of resolution and the balance between cost, utility, and acceptability varies among the different technologies. Functional magnetic resonance scanning has the best resolution and does not involve injections of radioactive substances; however, the design at the moment is limited to rapid changes in blood flow. The other two technologies allow for investigation into the chemistry of the brain but the time course and resolution are slower. Each of the technologies is best suited to answering different questions, and there can be useful synergy between the approaches.

Scanning experiments have to be carefully designed. They are expensive and can be difficult to interpret. The experimental conditions (both internal and external) need to be clearly defined. For example, if food is used as the paradigm under investigation it is important to control for metabolic factors such as time since the last meal. In earlier studies, all patients with an eating disorder (anorexia nervosa or bulimia) were analyzed as a group with no attempt to subcategorize according to eating behaviors. However, bingeing/disinhibited eating appears to be associated with a distinct pattern of brain activation to food whereas weight causes less of a differential response. Thus, the subcategorization as defined in DSM-IV has some utility.

As in all aspects of science it helps to have a clear, specific hypothesis. Here we have an advantage over those working in different fields of psychopathology as the brain physiology and biochemistry of appetite control has been clearly defined in animal models. Furthermore, it has been possible to develop this research further in man. Thus, it is possible to develop testable hypotheses in relationship to food, drawing from this body of research.

The statistical techniques used to analyze clusters of activation are complex, but in the end all methods need to follow the basic principles of eliminating type 1 and 2 errors and adjusting for multiple testing. Unfortunately, in many scanning studies, especially those in the first wave, these principles were neglected. However, in later studies the statistical methods are more robust.

In this chapter we have focused on those studies that are of higher quality in terms of all the features outlined above. However, as this is a new line of investigation we have also included some studies, that would fail these quality criteria but are important first steps into this area.

BACKGROUND: BRAIN DEVELOPMENT

Eating disorders have their onset at a crucial time for development: biologically, cognitively, and socially. Adolescence is a critical phase of brain development. Although the total brain size does not increase significantly from the age of 5 a large number of changes occur before mature, adult function emerges. White matter volume increases significantly during childhood and adulthood, as axons are gradually myelinated. A reciprocal decrease in gray matter volume occurs [for review, see (1)]. A wave of synaptic proliferation takes place in the frontal lobes at around the time of puberty. This is followed by dramatic reductions in cortical–cortical connectivity in especially in frontal regions during adolescence (2). This synaptic pruning is thought to be the central neurodevelopment event, which leads to full adult functioning. The gender dimorphism in brain development is of particular relevance for eating disorders. Interestingly there is differential growth in the areas of the brain implicated in appetite control. For example, the amygdala is smaller in females whereas the hippocampus and caudate nucleus are larger.

These developmental changes in brain structure are associated with changes in brain function. For instance, the reaction time for emotional recognition increases during adolescence. This is thought to be due to a relative inefficiency in frontal circuitry prior to the pruning of excess synaptic contacts (3). Furthermore, links between structure and function have been demonstrated. For example, the speed with normal children switch attentional set is linked to the size of the anterior cingulate gyrus (4). In conclusion, the timing of the onset of eating disorders during this rapid flux in brain structure and function may have profound implications for both the etiology and course of the illness. In particular, the frontal lobes with their key role in appetite as well as cognitive and emotional control are of great relevance.

BRAIN STRUCTURE AND EATING DISORDERS

Anorexia Nervosa

Reduced total cerebral volume is a consistent finding in AN (5–9). The majority of these studies were undertaken before AN was subdivided into the restricting and the binge–purge subtypes, and often the generic term "eating disorders" was used so it is not easy to relate anatomical changes to symptoms. The greater the absolute weight loss and the faster the rate of weight loss, the smaller the brain volume. Two small longitudinal studies examined the structural changes in the brain of adolescents after full weight gain (10,11). Both found persistent deficits in gray matter (cell bodies of neurons and glial cells), although there was recovery of white matter (mainly myelinated axons). This supports the finding of gray matter deficits in people who have made a full recovery from their eating disorder (12). One post-mortem study reported that there was a reduction in basal dendritic fields and dendritic spine density (13). Similar findings have been reported in schizo-phrenia and mood disorders where these changes are most apparent in those with a positive family history (14).

Brain shrinkage may be localized to specific regions. For instance, the pituitary gland (15) and the amygdala–hippocampal complex are decreased in size (16).

Bulimia Nervosa

The cerebral sulci are also widened in BN although the cerebral ventricles are normal in size as are the thalamus and midbrain areas (17–19). One magnetic resonance imaging (MRI) study found that the inferior frontal lobe cortex was reduced in size (18). To our knowledge there are no data on brain structure in binge eating disorder.

Brain Biochemistry

Brain biochemistry assessed using proton magnetic resonance spectroscopy is perturbed in people with eating disorders. For example, lipid signals in the frontal lobe were reduced to half of those seen in the normal population (20). Lipid levels correlated with body mass index.

Brain Damage and Eating Symptoms

Reports that relate eating disorder symptoms and syndromes with structural changes in the brain have been recently reviewed (21). Lesions in the prefrontal and temporal cortices and mesiotemporal structures and hypo-thalamus predominantly on the right-hand side are particularly linked with eating disorder symptoms. These case studies are of interest in testing and generating hypotheses about the central control of appetite, nutrition, and metabolism; however, in the majority of cases of AN there is no macroscopic brain lesion.

BRAIN FUNCTION IN EATING DISORDERS

In the absence of specific, structural abnormalities in eating disorders there has been interest in examining how the brain works. Several studies have examined the activity of the brain at rest. However, the resting state in the context of these experimental procedures probably varies between individual and site depending on the subjective reaction to the experimental maneuver and the precise metabolic state. Therefore, studies in the resting state can be difficult to interpret. Other investigators have studied brain activity in response to emotional and eating disorder–specific stimuli such as food and body shape.

Studies on Eating Disorders in the Resting State

Several studies have examined people with eating disorders in the resting state using positron emission tomography (PET). As might be expected given the poor nutritional state in AN with low glucose and high levels of ketones, there is a global reduction in cerebral glucose metabolism most marked in the frontal and parietal areas. However, glucose metabolism is relatively increased in the basal ganglia (22–24). There have also been reports of regional, relative hypoperfusion using single photon emission computed tomography (SPECT). A study in children and adolescents with AN found poor flow in the temporal lobe (25). Adults with the restricting form of AN had decreased flow in the frontal and anterior cingulate region (26,27). Flow in the thalamus, amygdala, and hippocampus was increased (27). This differential pattern of resting activity was not found in those with the binge–purge subtype of AN. In BN no clear findings have been found in resting blood flow in either the acute state (22,28) or after recovery (28,29).

In conclusion, there may be basal differences in brain activity in people with eating disorders, but this appears to vary according to clinical features such as age, symptom pattern, and metabolic state.

The Brain in Relation to Food and Appetite

One of the obvious paradigms to be investigated in functional studies in people with eating disorders is the response to food. This system has been studied both in animals and in humans. We are therefore digressing from the focus on people with eating disorders to discuss what is known about the central control of appetite.

Animal Models

The control of food intake is of central importance to all living beings and requires a complex integration between the individual and the environment. The central information processing pathways for food stimuli in the visual, olfactory, and gustatory modalities in the primate brain have been studied in depth. Rolls (30,31) has summarized the findings from his meticulous series of experiments involving electrophysiological recording from individual neurons. The initial processing of food stimuli occurs in the inferior temporal visual cortex (visual), olfactory bulb and piriform cortex (smell), and nucleus of the solitary tract, thalamus, and insula (taste). These areas project to the amygdala, orbitofrontal cortex, lateral hypothalamus, and striatum where the reward value of the stimuli is calibrated (Fig. 1).

The reward value assigned to food-related stimuli is modulated by integrated information from peripheral metabolism and the gastrointestinal tract. Dopaminergic projections to the ventral striatum and other limbic structures play a major role in food reward- and food-driven behavior (32). The lateral hypothalamus, in particular the perifornical area, is also implicated in the modulation of the rewarding aspect of food. For example, weight loss (25% body weight) enhances the rewarding effect of stimulation in this area whereas leptin administration produces the opposite effect and attenuates the effectiveness of the rewarding stimulus for up to 4 days (33). Thus, this

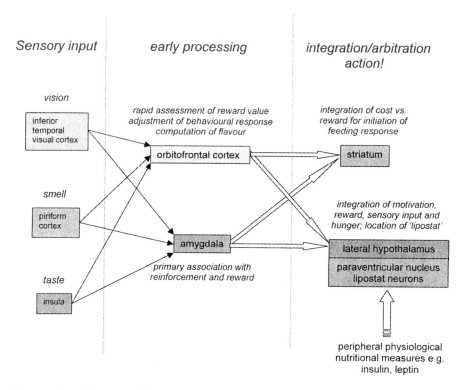

FIGURE 1 Schematic illustration of the processing of food-related stimuli. It is based on data from Rolls (30,31).

particular reward system is only responsive to long-term shifts in energy balance. Acute food deprivation for up to 48 h does not have an effect on these neurons. This suggests that in states of chronic starvation with low leptin, such as AN, areas of the brain associated with food reward should become more sensitive to food stimuli.

In conclusion, research into the central reaction to food needs to consider both the background metabolic state and the hedonic properties.

Brain Imaging of the Appetite Control System in Humans

Food

Extrinsic food cues in a variety of sensory modalities lead to brain activation. Visual images of food contrasted with nonfood produced changes in activation in the left temperoinsular cortical region. The level of activation correlated with the subjective rating of hunger (34,35). Taste and olfactory stimuli activated the orbitofrontal cortex (36).

Hunger and Satiety

Several studies have investigated brain activation in response to various tates of hunger and satiation and the sites of activation are shown in Table 1. Tataranni and colleagues have done a series of studies in which they have used PET scanning after a 36 h fast in men (37) and women (42) at normal weight and in people with obesity (44). The design of this study was limited in that there was no direct evidence that the activation in the fasting state was related to hunger. Others have used different designs to ensure that focus of brain activity is on food or appetite in the fasting state. Thus, Morris and Dolan had an interesting design in that they used a cognitive task (memory for food/nonfood items) as a marker for hunger (induced by fasting for 16 h) (39). They thus were able to correlate activation in PET scanning in various brain areas both with hunger and performance on this task. LaBar used visual food-related cues (38). In summary, many of these studies find that the orbitofrontal cortex, anterior cingulate, amygdala, insula, and hypothalamus are more activated in states of hunger (Fig. 2).

Studies examining the process of satiation are easier to design in that they follow differences in activation after food consumption (for summary, see Table 1). Several studies show increased activation in the dorsolateral and anteror medial prefrontal cortex, posterior insula, and hypothalamus after satiation (Fig. 3). This change in activation during satiation parallels changes in metabolic factors. The increase in insulin is linked to changes in cerebral blood flow in the hypothalamus, insula, and orbitofrontal cortex (40). Quantitative rather then qualitative differences were found between genders in that the women appeared to have less hunger and were more satiated. In the

TABLE 1   Changes in Brain Activation Relating to States of Hunger and Satiation

Stimulus	Site	Change	Author
Hunger (36-h fast)	Hypothalamus	↑ activation	37
Hunger (36-h fast)	Posterior orbitofrontal cortex	↑ activation	37
Hunger (36-h fast)	Anterior cingulate	↑ activation	37
Hunger (36-h fast)	Insula	↑ activation	37
Hunger (visual food cues)	Amygdala	↑ activation	38
Hunger (visual food cues)	Anterior fusiform gryrus	↑ activation	38
Hunger (visual food cues)	Parahippocampus	↑ activation	38
Hunger (memory food)	R lateral orbitofrontal cortex	↑ activation	39
Hunger (memory food)	L amygdala	↑ activation	39
Hunger (memory food)	L dorsal insula R ant insula	↑ activation	39
Hunger (memory food)	R nucleus accumbens	↑ activation	39
Satiation	Hypothalamus	↓ activation <20 min	40
Satiation (post food and memory food)	R posterior insula x	↑ activation	39
Satiation	Hypothalamus	↑ activation 8–13 min	40
Satiation	Dorsolateral and anterior ventromedial prefrontal	↑ activation	37
Satiation	L Inferior parietal lobule	↑ activation	37
Satiation	Dorsolateral prefrontal cortex	↑ activation F > M	41
Satiation	Precuneus	↑ activation F > M	41
Satiation	Parietal:angula gyrus	↑ activation F > M	41,42
Satiation	Occipitotemporal	↑ activation F > M	41
Satiation	Ventromedial prefrontal	↑ activation M > F	41
Satiation	Medial orbitofrontal cortex	↓ activation	43
Satiation	Insula	↓ activation	43
Satiation	lateral orbitofrontal	↑ activation	43
Satiation	Prefrontal	↑ activation	43
Satiation	Parahippocampal	↑ activation	43

Orexogenic Circuit

Hunger

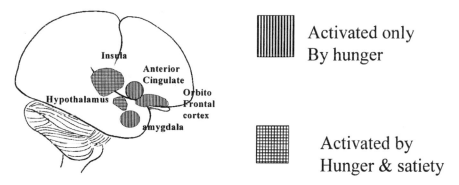

FIGURE 2   Areas of the brain activated in states of hunger (the orexogenic network). The vertical lines are areas activated by hunger only and the cross-hatched areas are those activated by both hunger and satiety.

Anorexogenic Circuit

Satiation

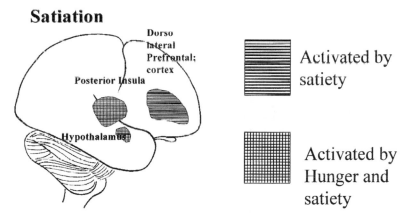

FIGURE 3   Areas of the brain activated by satiation (the anorexogenic network). The horizontal lines are areas activated by hunger only and the cross-hatched areas are those activated by both hunger and satiety.

hungry state men had greater activation in the frontotemporal and paralimbic areas. After satiation women had greater activation in the dorsolateral prefrontal cortex and the occipital and parietal sensory association areas (42).

There are hedonic as well as metabolic components to the process of satiation. Sensory-specific satiety is the process by which a food substance becomes less rewarding after a substantial amount of it has been eaten independent of the calorie content eaten and the metabolic state (45). Several loci in the orbitofrontal and medial prefrontal cortex are activated by olfactory food stimuli in a sensory-specific manner, i.e., they are activated only to food that has not been eaten to satiety (46). This emphasizes the role of the orbitofrontal and medial prefrontal cortex in modulating the reward associated with food.

In summary, the human central appetite control system is composed of an orexigenic (i.e., appetite promoting) network and an anorexigenic (i.e. inhibitory conrol) circuit; the balance between these two subsystems determines eating behavior. Both external (visual, taste, or olfactory) and internal appetite cues are associated with changes in blood flow in the orexogenic system. The orexigenic network (consisting of orbitofrontal and insular cortices, amygdala, and hypothalamus) activates with fasting and promotes feeding behavior. The inhibitory, anorexigenic circuit consists of anterior ventromedial and dorsolateral prefrontal cortices and acts to terminate eating, probably by direct inhibition of the orexigenic system (8,12,15,16, 47,48).

Food Challenges in Eating Disorders

External and internal stimuli (food cues or eating) have been used as specific challenges in people with an eating disorder. The first specific-challenge, neuroimaging study, using SPECT, reported a significant increase in perfusion of the frontal lobes in reaction to eating a cake in people with AN (49). In a later study people with AN were shown to have the opposite patterns of regional cerebral blood flow (rCBF) to those with BN: in BN there was increased frontotemporal perfusion in the resting state which decreased when the patient ate a cake; in the AN group decreased perfusion at rest was followed by increased perfusion after eating (again most markedly in frontal and temporal lobe) (50). More recently, the diagnostic subgroups of binge-ing–purging, anorexia nervosa (BPAN), and restricting anorexia nervosa (RAN) were also found to have contrasting patterns of brain activity in response to food. BPAN but not RAN showed increases in glucose metabolism in the right prefrontal and parietal regions in response to the sight of a custard cake (51). The importance of specifying between the different subtypes of eating disorders may explain the negative results of an earlier study (52).

Karhunen and colleagues (53), also using SPECT, found that exposure to food was associated with different changes in the cerebral blood flow in obese women who binge-ate compared to either normal-weight or obese controls with no binge eating. The binge eating group had increased flow in the left hemisphere, especially in the frontal and prefrontal regions. There were strong correlations between frontal flow and hunger during exposure to the food. In a different study following a person with binge eating disorder over time in the binge eating state there was a bilateral increase in global blood flow whereas in the restrictive phase flow on the right-hand side of the brain was diminished relative to that on the left (54). This suggests that food stimuli elicit frontal/temporal activation in the bulimic disorders across the weight spectrum. This pattern is different from that found in people with restricting AN who have reduced activation. Unfortunately, the resolution of SPECT studies is not sufficient to distinguish specifically between the orexogenic and anorexogenic pathways.

Recently, functional MRI (fMRI) has been introduced into eating disorder research, bringing the potential of better spatial-temporal resolution. High-calorie drinks versus low calorie drinks elicited activity in the orexogenic circuit including amygdala, prefrontal cortex, and insula (55). On the other hand, there was no differential activation in this circuit when high- and low-calorie foods were used both in MRI (Ellison, personal communication) and in PET (34). One possible explanation for this finding is that there is no dose–response relationship between activation of the orexogenic circuit to visual cues of foods that differ in terms of calorie content. The hedonic properties between foods, which may vary among individuals, may have a greater impact on activation than calorie content. Thus food/nonfood or liked/not-liked food may be a better experimental design for such studies.

In an fMRI study using food/nonfood stimuli (color photographs), the medial orbitofrontal cortex was activated by food in AN patients but not in healthy controls (56). The same paradigm was used to investigate the response to food cues in various subtypes of eating disorder and in people who have recovered from AN (57). The results from this study are summarized in Table 2 and Figure 3. In response to food stimuli, patients with eating disorder (either AN or BN) recruit the orbitofrontal cortex and the anterior cingulate instead of the lateral prefrontal cortex, inferior parietal lobule, precuneus, and posterior cerebellum, which are activated in the comparison group; most of these differences are left sided. The anterior cingulate is not activated by food in those currently ill with restricting AN. Activation of the dorsolateral prefrontal area differs across eating disorder subtypes and is reduced in BN. People who had recovered from AN activated the same lateral prefrontal area as did the healthy comparison group. Failure to activate this area with food may be considered as a state marker of an eating disorder (Figure 4).

TABLE 2 Brain Regions Significantly Differentially Activated in ED and Its Subgroups as Compared to Controls

	No.	MO-PFC	ACC	PCC	L-PFC	IPL	Precuneus	Cerebell.
ED	26	↑	↑		↓	↓	↓	↓
BN	10	↑	↑	↑	↓		↓	
AN	16	↑	↑			↓	↓	↓
BPAN	7	↑	↑		↓			↓
RAN	9	↑						
Rec RAN	9	↑	↑			↓		↑

Brain regions: MO-PFC, medial and orbital prefrontal cortex; ACC, anterior cingulate cortex; PCC, posterior cingulate cortex; L-PFC, lateral prefrontal cortex; IPL, inferior parietal lobule; cerebell, cerebellum. ↑ significantly more active than in controls; ↓ significantly less active than in controls.

BODY IMAGE CHALLENGE

The concept of body image is less easy to study than food as there are no animal models on which to base experimental work in order to test a hypothesis. Damasio conceptualizes body image as a complex function of a widely distributed network spanning structures from the brainstem to the associative cortices (58).

In a preliminary study people with AN were challenged with an image of their own body distorted to maximal unacceptability. There was activation of the right amygdala, right fusiform, and brainstem. The authors interpreted this to be activation of the fear network (59). Thus, it may be possible to examine this controversial aspect of the psychopathology of eating disorders in more detail using scanning techniques.

NEUROTRANSMISSION

Neuroimaging techniques have recently been used to examine the neuropharmacology of eating disorders. The monoamines dopamine and serotonin have an important role in feeding behavior in animals and humans. Dopamine is linked to reward and it may modulate the hedonic response to food. Serotonin inhibits feeding. The serotonin hypothesis of eating disorders has as its essence the idea that abnormal 5-HT function may be a trait vulnerability for eating disorders.

People with bulimia nervosa were found to have a 17% reduction in the levels of serotonin transporter in the hypothalamus and thalamus and a 15% reduction in levels of dopamine transporter in the striatum (60). A reduction in serotonin transporter was also found in obese binge eaters (61).

Food Activation in Eating Disorders

Anterior Cingulate
↑ BN, AN & recovered AN

Dorsolateral Prefrontal cortex
↓ in BN & BPAN

Medial Orbitofrontal cortex
↑ BN, AN & recovered AN

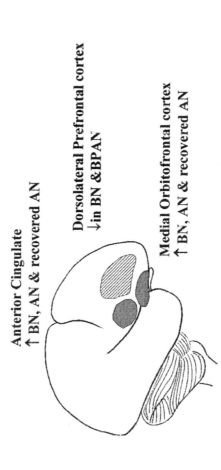

FIGURE 4 Areas of the brain activated by visual food stimuli in people with eating disorders. It is based on functional fMRI studies (56,57).

In people with obesity an inverse relationship was found between BMI and striatal dopamine receptor availability. Thus, this preliminary evidence suggests that abnormal monamine systems may be associated with disinhibited eating.

The serotonin theory has also been tested by examining 5-HT receptor levels in people who have recovered from an eating disorder. Reduced levels of 5-HT_{2A} binding were found in the mesial temporal cortex (including the amygdala and hippocampus) and to a lesser degree in the cingulate of women with a history of restricting AN (62). The mechanism underlying this phenomenon is unknown. The reduced receptor binding may be a process compensating for increased extracellular 5-HT. (Earlier research had indeed found increased 5-HT in the CSF of people who had recovered from AN; 63).

A similar study was undertaken with a smaller group of patients who had recovered from BN. These people had reduced 5-HT_{2A} in the lateral and medial orbitofrontal cortex (64). Furthermore, this group of patients did not have the expected age-related decline in 5-HT_{2A} receptors. In conclusion, abnormal levels of 5-HT_{2A} receptor are found in various sites of the orexogenic network after recovery from an eating disorder.

WHAT CAN WE UNDERSTAND FROM THE FUNCTIONAL STUDIES?

Across the spectrum of eating disorders, in response to either extrinsic or intrinsic food-related cues, there are changes in activity in the frontal and limbic areas that form the orexogenic and anorexogenic systems. The functional imaging studies implicate, in particular, the orbitofrontal cortex and the lateral prefrontal cortex as key areas of differential activity in people with eating disorders. The functional response to food differs between the subtypes of eating disorders in both SPECT and fMRI studies. People with bulimic symptoms had reduced activation of the dorsolateral prefrontal cortex.

Interestingly, people who had recovered from restricting AN had some activation (in the orbitofrontal cortex and anterior cingulate) similar to that found in people with a current eating disorders but also activated parts of the brain responsive to food cues in non–eating disorder controls (such as the apical and lateral prefrontal cortex). This suggests that there are both state and trait functional differences in response to food in people with eating disorders.

LINKING STRUCTURE AND FUNCTION

The orbitofrontal cortex and lateral frontal areas are of key importance in many other aspects of brain function beside the control of appetite (65), e.g., psychopathology (65) and personality (66). It is interesting to examine whether this can enrich theories that explain the mechanisms that underlie eating disorders.

The Orbitofrontal Cortex

The orbitofrontal cortex is involved in the appraisal and processing of subjectively salient and self-related stimuli and is critically involved in the motivational control of goal-directed behavior (67,68). Thus, apart from the primary reinforcers, such as food and touch, in humans, secondary reinforcers, such as money and drugs of abuse (e.g., cocaine) activate this area (69).

Activation in the orbitofrontal cortex occurs to both positive and negative rewards (70). There is some preliminary evidence of anatomical specificity between positive and negative reinforcement for touch (36). However, the resolution of fMRI may be insufficient to distinguish between positive and negative rewards for other stimuli such as food because in animals positive and negative rewards are computed on individual neurons.

There are interesting parallels between people with damage to the orbitofrontal cortex and people with AN. For example, people with ventral frontal lobe damage have impaired identification of facial and vocal expression. This disability correlates with the degree of alteration of their emotional experience (68). Impaired identification of facial and vocal expression is present also in AN (71). Animals with lesions of the prefrontal cortex experience an interceptive agnosia, i.e., an inability to determine how the body is reacting when faced with contrasting behavioral options. This resonates with the clinical descriptions of alexithymia (72,73) and poor interoceptive awareness in AN (74).

The Lateral Prefrontal Cortex

The dorsolateral prefrontal circuit is involved in executive functions (75). For example, lesions in the right lateral prefrontal cortex produce defects in working memory (76). These areas are activated in set shifting tasks (77). This is of interest as we have found people with eating disorders to be impaired in these types of tasks. Abnormal activation in these circuits has also been found in depression, obsessive-compulsive disorder, schizophrenia, and substance abuse (75).

POSSIBLE MECHANISMS UNDERPINNING THE STRUCTURAL AND FUNCTIONAL BRAIN ABNORMALITIES IN EATING DISORDERS

The state and trait abnormalities found in both brain structure and function have implications for etiological models. The trait abnormalities may result from neurodevelopmental mechanisms or from damage or "scaring" from the illness.

The neurodevelopmental theory posits that programming either from genetic mechanisms or from early environmental experiences causes the structural and functional abnormalities in the brain. These may be linked to variations in neurotransmitter function, e.g., 5-HT.

Eating Behaviors as Part of a Neurodevelopmental Process

Research into the development of the central control of appetite is burgeoning. Many of the genetic causes of obesity that are now being described result from abnormalities in the central control of appetite with overeating as a consequence. For example, one of the commonest monogenic causes of obesity relates to mutations in the melanocortin receptor (78). It means that phenotypes of obesity that focus on abnormal eating behaviors may be more pertinent than those with a focus on metabolic abnormalities.

Eating behaviors run in families. In a study on the Amish the heritability for disinhibition of eating was found to be 40% and for restraint 30% (79). The mechanisms underpinning these effects are uncertain. Extreme eating behaviors may be caused by increased hypothalamic drive, but also they may be moderated by variations in olfactory and gustatory sensory perception (80) or in the reward system (81).

Also, early environmental effects may set the level of activity of the appetite system, a type of metabolic imprinting or programming (82,83). One such theory is that poor fetal growth with malnutrition early in development may predispose to a thrifty phenotype (84), whereas poor nutrition later in pregnancy or in early development may protect people from developing obesity (85,86). Continuities in the patterns of eating persist over childhood. For example, poor sucking in infancy is associated with picky eating at ages of 3.5 and 5.5 (87).

Anorexia Nervosa as a Neurodevelopmental Disorder

Gillberg has suggested that eating disorders, in particular AN, should be considered to be a neurodevelopmental disorder (88). He bases this argument on the presence of neurological soft signs. He found dysdiadochokinesis in some 16-year-olds with AN, which was still present when they were 21. We have also found that dysdiadokinesis is present in a proportion of adults with AN. This is present in the context of other abnormalities in neuropsychological testing such as a difficulty in set shifting tasks that also remain after recovery (89,90).

Early environmental adversities, such as maternal stress and anxiety during pregnancy, perinatal hypoxic injury, or postinfective autoimmune reactions, are associated with aberrant brain development (91,92). People with AN have a higher exposure to these risk factors. Maternal anxiety, complications during pregnancy, birth injury, being small for date, and a seasonal birth pattern have all been implicated as risk factors in case control studies (93–96). Links with later infective etiology have also been made such as the association between AN and pediatric autoimmune neuropsychiatric disorder (PANDAS) (97,98). Further research that links functional neuroimaging with research into genetic and childhood risk factors is needed to develop these ideas further.

Brain Abnormalities in Anorexia Nervosa Consequent on the Illness (Scars)

Severe malnutrition during the critical period of adolescence may arrest brain maturation or cause the dysfunctional development of brain structure and function. An obvious possibility is that it is caused by vitamin or essential fatty acid deficiencies. Alternatively, it may result from an epiphenomenona of AN, such as high levels of cortisol, which has been implicated in the neuropathological changes in mood disorders (99) and schizophrenia. No clear relationships between structural and functional brain changes and any putative etiological factor have been reported. However, these studies often use data from cross-sectional measures, and it is likely that it is the integrated effect of deficiencies over time, that is the relevant factor.

CONCLUSION

The information produced by brain scanning has implications for models used in attempts to explain the etiology and maintenance of eating disorders. The findings are consistent with a neurodevelopmental etiologic process. However, there is also substantial evidence to suggest that many of the changes represent acquired damage. Eating disorders occur at a critical time of brain development, and toxic effects from malnutrition or stress may cause atrophic or dystrophic changes. There is no doubt that these studies have generated many new ideas about symptoms, causes, and consequences of eating disorders, and further research linking genetics, precise definitions of the phenotypes of eating disorders, and scanning has great potential to increase our knowledge about these confusing conditions.

SUMMARY

- The technologies used to image the brain have a different balance of strengths and weaknesses. Each of them is suited to answer different types of questions.

- The onset of eating disorders coincides with a transitional flux in brain structure and function that may have implications for both etiology and prognosis.
- Cerebral volume is reduced and the gray matter loss may persist in AN. Smaller structural changes are seen in BN.
- Lesions in the prefrontal and temporal cortices and mesiotemporal structures and hypothalamus predominantly on the right-hand side are particularly linked with eating disorder symptoms. However, in the majority of cases of AN there is no macroscopic brain lesion.
- The central control of appetite, nutrition, and metabolism involves pathways that recognize food in the environment and modulate the response to these cues depending-on the current metabolic state and expected hedonic effect.
- The orbito frontal cortex, anterior cingulate, amygdala, insula and hypothalamus form the orexogenic system, which is activated by hunger.
- The dorsolateral and anterior medial prefrontal cortex, posterior insula and the hypothalamus form the anorexogenic system activated by satiation.
- The orbitofrontal cortex and the lateral prefrontal cortex are key areas of differential activity between people with eating disorders and those without in one fMRI study.
- In studies using SPECT the pattern of activation in response to food cues differed between people who binge ate in comparison to pure restrictors. People with bulimic symptoms had reduced activation of the dorso lateral prefrontal cortex in one fMRI study.
- People who had recovered from restricting anorexia nervosa had some activation (in the orbitofrontal cortex and anterior cingulate) similar to that found in people with a current eating disorders but also activated parts of the brain responsive to food cues in non eating disorder controls (such as the apical and lateral prefrontal cortex).
- There are two theories that may account for abnormal brain structure or function in people with eating disorders. (a) Neuro-developmental disorders and brain abnormalities precede the onset of the illness. (b) The brain abnormalities are consequent to the illness and result from starvation or other aspects of the illness.

ACKNOWLEDGMENTS

This study was supported by grant QLK1-1999-916 from the European Commission Framework V program http://www.cordis.lu/life/home.html), the Nina Jackson Eating Disorders Research Charity, and a Wellcome Trust Travelling Fellowship for Dr. R. Uher.

REFERENCES

1. Durston S, Hulshoff Pol HE, Casey BJ, Giedd JN, Buitelaar JK, van Engeland H. Anatomical MRI of the developing human brain: what have we learned? J Am Acad Child Adol Psychiatry 2001; 40(9):1012–1020.
2. Huttenlocher PR. Synaptic density in human frontal cortex: developmental changes and the effects of aging. Brain Res 1979; 163(2):195–205.
3. McGivern R, Andersen J, Byrd D, Mutter K, Reilly J. Cognitive efficiency on a match to sample task decreases at the onset of puberty in children. Brain Cogn 2002; 50(1):73.
4. Casey BJ, Trainor R, Giedd J, Vauss Y, Vaituzis CK, Hamburger S, et al. The role of the anterior cingulate in automatic and controlled processes: a developmental neuroanatomical study. Dev Psychobiol 1997; 30(1):61–69.
5. Dolan RJ, Mitchell J, Wakeling A. Structural brain changes in patients with anorexia nervosa. Psychol Med 1988; 18(2):349–353.
6. Kohn MR, Ashtari M, Golden NH, Schebendach J, Patel M, Jacobson MS, et al. Structural brain changes and malnutrition in anorexia nervosa. Ann N Y Acad Sci 1997; 817:398–399.
7. Kingston K, Szmukler G, Andrewes D, Tress B, Desmond P. Neuropsychological and structural brain changes in anorexia nervosa before and after refeeding. Psychol Med 1996; 26(1):15–28.
8. Krieg JC, Pirke KM, Lauer C, Backmund H. Endocrine, metabolic, and cranial computed tomographic findings in anorexia nervosa. Biol Psychiatry 1988; 23(4):377–387.
9. Swayze VW, Andersen A, Arndt S, Rajarethinam R, Fleming F, Sato Y, et al. Reversibility of brain tissue loss in anorexia nervosa assessed with a computerized Talairach 3-D proportional grid. Psychol Med 1996; 26(2):381–390.
10. Katzman DK, Lambe EK, Mikulis DJ, Ridgley JN, Goldbloom DS, Zipursky RB. Cerebral gray matter and white matter volume deficits in adolescent girls with anorexia nervosa. J Pediatr 1996; 129(6):794–803.
11. Golden NH, Ashtari M, Kohn MR, Patel M, Jacobson MS, Fletcher A, et al. Reversibility of cerebral ventricular enlargement in anorexia nervosa, demonstrated by quantitative magnetic resonance imaging. J Pediatr 1996; 128(2):296–301.
12. Lambe EK, Katzman DK, Mikulis DJ, Kennedy SH, Zipursky RB. Cerebral gray matter volume deficits after weight recovery from anorexia nervosa. Arch Gen Psychiatry 1997; 54(6):537–542.
13. Neumarker KJ, Dudeck U, Meyer U, Neumarker U, Schulz E, Schonheit B. Anorexia nervosa and sudden death in childhood: clinical data and results obtained from quantitative neurohistological investigations of cortical neurons. Eur Arch Psychiatry Clin Neurosci 1997; 247(1):16–22.
14. Rosoklija G, Toomayan G, Ellis SP, Keilp J, Mann JJ, Latov N, et al. Structural

abnormalities of subicular dendrites in subjects with schizophrenia and mood disorders: preliminary findings. Arch Gen Psychiatry 2000; 57(4):349–356.

15. Doraiswamy PM, Krishnan KR, Figiel GS, Husain MM, Boyko OB, Rockwell WJ, et al. A brain magnetic resonance imaging study of pituitary gland morphology in anorexia nervosa and bulimia. Biol Psychiatry 1990; 28(2):110–116.

16. Giordano GD, Renzetti P, Parodi RC, Foppiani L, Zandrino F, Giordano Gm, et al. Volume measurement with magnetic resonance imaging of hippocampus–amygdala formation in patients with anorexia nervosa. J Endocrinol Invest 2001; 24(7):510–514.

17. Krieg JC, Backmund H, Pirke KM. Cranial computed tomography findings in bulimia. Acta Psychiatr Scand 1987; 75(2):144–149.

18. Hoffman GW, Ellinwood EH Jr, Rockwell WJ, Herfkens RJ, Nishita JK, Guthrie LF. Cerebral atrophy in bulimia. Biol Psychiatry 1989; 25(7):894–902.

19. Hoffman GW, Ellinwood EH Jr, Rockwell WJ, Herfkens RJ, Nishita JK, Guthrie LF. Brain T1 measured by magnetic resonance imaging in bulimia. Biol Psychiatry 1990; 27(1):116–119.

20. Roser W, Bubl R, Buergin D, Seelig J, Radue EW, Rost B. Metabolic changes in the brain of patients with anorexia and bulimia nervosa as detected by proton magnetic resonance spectroscopy. Int J Eat Disord 1999; 26(2):119–136.

21. Uher R, Treasure J, Campbell IC. Neuranatomical bases of eating disorders. In: H'haenen HA, den Boer JA, Willner P, eds. Biological Psychiatry. John Wiley & Sons: Chichester, 2002:1173–1180.

22. Delvenne V, Goldman S, De MV, Lotstra F. Brain glucose metabolism in eating disorders assessed by positron emission tomography. Int J Eat Disord 1999; 25(1):29–37.

23. Delvenne V, Goldman S, Simon Y, De MV, Lotstra F. Brain hypometabolism of glucose in bulimia nervosa. Int J Eat Disord 1997; 21(4):313–320.

24. Herholz K, Krieg JC, Emrich HM, Pawlik G, Beil C, Pirke KM, et al. Regional cerebral glucose metabolism in anorexia nervosa measured by positron emission tomography. Biol Psychiatry 1987; 22(1):43–51.

25. Gordon I, Lask B, Bryant-Waugh R, Christie D, Timimi S. Childhood-onset anorexia nervosa: towards identifying a biological substrate. Int J Eat Disord 1997; 22(2):159–165.

26. Naruo T, Nakabeppu Y, Deguchi D, Nagai N, Tsutsui J, Nakajo M, et al. Decreases in blood perfusion of the anterior cingulate gyri in anorexia nervosa restricters assessed by SPECT image analysis. BMC Psychiatry 2001; 1(1):22.

27. Takano A, Shiga T, Kitagawa N, Koyama T, Katoh C, Tsukamoto E, et al. Abnormal neuronal network in anorexia nervosa studied with I-123-IMP SPECT. Psychiatry Res 2001; 107(1):45–50.

28. Andreason PJ, Altemus M, Zametkin AJ, King AC, Lucinio J, Cohen RM. Regional cerebral glucose metabolism in bulimia nervosa. Am J Psychiatry 1992; 149(11):1506–1513.

29. Frank GK, Kaye WH, Greer P, Meltzer CC, Price JC. Regional cerebral blood flow after recovery from bulimia nervosa. Psychiatry Res 2000; 100(1):31–39.

30. Rolls ET, Baylis LL. Gustatory, olfactory, and visual convergence within the primate orbitofrontal cortex. J Neurosci 1994; 14(9):5437–5452.

31. Rolls ET, Critchley HD, Browning A, Hernadi I. The neurophysiology of taste and olfaction in primates, and umami flavor. Ann N Y Acad Sci 1998; 855:426–437.
32. Wise RA, Rompre PP. Brain dopamine and reward. Annu Rev Psychol 1989; 40:191–225.
33. Fulton S, Woodside B, Shizgal P. Modulation of brain reward circuitry by leptin. Science 2000; 287(5450):125–128.
34. Gordon CM, Dougherty DD, Fischman AJ, Emans SJ, Grace E, Lamm R, et al. Neural substrates of anorexia nervosa: a behavioral challenge study with positron emission tomography. J Pediatr 2001; 139(1):51–57.
35. Gordon CM, Dougherty DD, Rauch SL, Emans SJ, Grace E, Lamm R, et al. Neuroanatomy of human appetitive function: a positron emission tomography investigation. Int J Eat Disord 2000; 27(2):163–171.
36. Francis S, Rolls ET, Bowtell R, McGlone F, O'Doherty J, Browning A, et al. The representation of pleasant touch in the brain and its relationship with taste and olfactory areas. Neuroreport 1999; 10(3):453–459.
37. Tataranni PA, Gautier JF, Chen K, Uecker A, Bandy D, Salbe AD, et al. Neuroanatomical correlates of hunger and satiation in humans using positron emission tomography. Proc Natl Acad Sci USA 1999; 96 AB(8):4569–4574.
38. LaBar KS, Gitelman DR, Parrish TB, Kim YH, Nobre AC, Mesulam MM. Hunger selectively modulates corticolimbic activation to food stimuli in humans. Behav Neurosci 2001; 115(2):493–500.
39. Morris JS, Dolan RJ. Involvement of human amygdala and orbitofrontal cortex in hunger-enhanced memory for food stimuli. J Neurosci 2001; 21(14):5304–5310.
40. Liu Y, Gao JH, Liu HL, Fox PT. The temporal response of the brain after eating revealed by functional MRI. Nature 2000; 405(6790):1058–1062.
41. Del Parigi A, Gautier JF, Chen K, Salbe AD, Ravussin E, Reiman E, et al. Neuroimaging and obesity: mapping the brain responses to hunger and satiation in humans using positron emission tomography. Ann N Y Acad Sci 2002; 967: 389–397.
42. Del Parigi A, Chen K, Gautier JF, Salbe AD, Pratley RE, Ravussin E, et al. Sex differences in the human brain's response to hunger and satiation. Am J Clin Nutr 2002; 75(6):1017–1022.
43. Small DM, Zatorre RJ, Dagher A, Evans AC, Jones-Gotman M. Changes in brain activity related to eating chocolate: from pleasure to aversion. Brain 2001; 124; (Pt 9):1720–1733.
44. Gautier JF, Chen K, Uecker A, Bandy D, Frost J, Salbe AD, et al. Regions of the human brain affected during a liquid-meal taste perception in the fasting state: a positron emission tomography study. Am J Clin Nutr 1999; 70(5):806–810.
45. Raynor HA, Epstein LH. Dietary variety, energy regulation, and obesity. Psychol Bull 2001; 127(3):325–341.
46. O'Doherty J, Rolls ET, Francis S, Bowtell R, McGlone F, Kobal G, et al. Sensory-specific satiety-related olfactory activation of the human orbitofrontal cortex. Neuroreport 2000; 11(4):893–897.
47. Katzman DK, Lambe EK, Mikulis DJ, Ridgley JN, Goldbloom DS, Zipursky

RB. Cerebral gray matter and white matter volume deficits in adolescent girls with anorexia nervosa [see comments]. J Pediatr 1996; 129(6):794–803.
48. Kingston K, Szmukler G, Andrewes D, Tress B, Desmond P. Neuropsychological and structural brain changes in anorexia nervosa before and after refeeding. Psychol Med 1996; 26(1):15–28.
49. Nozoe S, Naruo T, Nakabeppu Y, Soejima Y, Nakajo M, Tanaka H. Changes in regional cerebral blood flow in patients with anorexia nervosa detected through single photon emission tomography imaging. Biol Psychiatry 1993; 34(8):578–580.
50. Nozoe S, Naruo T, Yonekura R, Nakabeppu Y, Soejima Y, Nagai N, et al. Comparison of regional cerebral blood flow in patients with eating disorders. Brain Res Bull 1995; 36(3):251–255.
51. Naruo T, Nakabeppu Y, Sagiyama K, Munemoto T, Homan N, Deguchi D, et al. Characteristic regional cerebral blood flow patterns in anorexia nervosa patients with binge/purge behavior. Am J Psychiatry 2000; 157(9):1520–1522.
52. Krieg JC, Lauer C, Leinsinger G, Pahl J, Schreiber W, Pirke KM, et al. Brain morphology and regional cerebral blood flow in anorexia nervosa. Biol Psychiatry 1989; 25(8):1041–1048.
53. Karhunen LJ, Vanninen EJ, Kuikka JT, Lappalainen RI, Tiihonen J, Uusitupa MI. Regional cerebral blood flow during exposure to food in obese binge eating women. Psychiatry Res 2000; 99(1):29–42.
54. Hirano H, Tomura N, Okane K, Watarai J, Tashiro T. Changes in cerebral blood flow in bulimia nervosa. J Comput Assist Tomogr 1999; 23(2):280–282.
55. Ellison Z, Foong J, Howard R, Bullmore E, Williams S, Treasure J. Functional anatomy of calorie fear in anorexia nervosa. Lancet 1998; 352(9135):1192.
56. Uher R, Murphy T, Brammer M, Dalgleish T, Phillips M, Ng V, et al. Functional neural correlates of eating disorders, personal communication, 2002
57. Uher R. Recovery and chronicity in anorexia nervosa: brain activity associated with differential outcomes. Biol Psychiatry. (In press).
58. Damasio AR. How the brain creates the mind. Sci Am 1999; 281(6):112–117.
59. Seeger G, Braus DF, Ruf M, Goldberger U, Schmidt MH. Body image distortion reveals amygdala activation in patients with anorexia nervosa—a functional magnetic resonance imaging study. Neurosci Lett 2002; 326(1):25–28.
60. Tauscher J, Pirker W, Willeit M, de Zwaan M, Bailer U, Neumeister A, et al. [123I] Beta-CIT and single photon emission computed tomography reveal reduced brain serotonin transporter availability in bulimia nervosa. Biol Psychiatry 2001; 49(4):326–332.
61. Kuikka JT, Tammela L, Karhunen L, Rissanen A, Bergstrom KA, Naukkarinen H, et al. Reduced serotonin transporter binding in binge eating women. Psychopharmacology (Berl) 2001; 155(3):310–314.
62. Frank GK, Kaye WH, Meltzer CC, Price JC, Greer P, McConaha C, et al. Reduced 5-HT2A receptor binding after recovery from anorexia nervosa. Biol Psychiatry 2002; 52(9):896–906.
63. Kaye WH, Gwirtsman HE, George DT, Ebert MH. Altered serotonin activity in anorexia nervosa after long-term weight restoration. Does elevated cerebrospinal

fluid 5-hydroxyindoleacetic acid level correlate with rigid and obsessive behavior? Arch Gen Psychiatry 1991; 48(6):556–562.

64. Kaye WH, Frank GK, Meltzer CC, Price JC, McConaha CW, Crossan PJ, et al. Altered serotonin 2A receptor activity in women who have recovered from bulimia nervosa. Am J Psychiatry 2001; 158(7):1152–1155.

65. Joseph R. Frontal lobe psychopathology: mania, depression, confabulation, catatonia, perseveration, obsessive compulsions, and schizophrenia. Psychiatry 1999; 62(2):138–172.

66. Cloninger RC. Functional neuroanatomy and brain imaging of personality and its disorders. In: D'haenen H, den Boer JA, Willner P, eds. Biological Psychiatry. Chichester: John Wiley & Sons Ltd, 2002:1377–1385.

67. Damasio AR. The somatic marker hypothesis and the possible functions of the prefrontal cortex. Philos Trans R Soc Lond B Biol Sci 1996; 351(1346):1413–1420.

68. Hornak J, Rolls ET, Wade D. Face and voice expression identification in patients with emotional and behavioural changes following ventral frontal lobe damage. Neuropsychologia 1996; 34(4):247–261.

69. Volkow ND, Fowler JS. Addiction, a disease of compulsion and drive: involvement of the orbitofrontal cortex. Cereb Cortex 2000; 10(3):318–325.

70. Rolls ET. The orbitofrontal cortex and reward. Cereb Cortex 2000; 10(3):284–294.

71. Kucharska-Pietura K, Nikolaou V, Masiak M, Treasure J. The recognition of emotion in faces and voice in anorexia nervosa. Int J Eat Disord. In press.

72. Troop NA, Schmidt UH, Treasure JL. Feelings and fantasy in eating disorders: a factor analysis of the Toronto Alexithymia Scale. Int J Eat Disord 1995; 18(2):151–157.

73. Cochrane CE, Brewerton TD, Wilson DB, Hodges EL. Alexithymia in the eating disorders. Int J Eat Disord 1993; 14(2):219–222.

74. Bruch H. Eating Disorders: Obesity, Anorexia Nervosa, and the Person Within. New York: Basic Books, 1973.

75. Tekin S, Cummings JL. Frontal-subcortical neuronal circuits and clinical neuropsychiatry: an update. J Psychosom Res 2002; 53(2):647–654

76. Bechara A, Damasio H, Damasio AR. Emotion, decision making and the orbitofrontal cortex. Cereb Cortex 2000; 10(3):295–307.

77. Konishi S, Hayashi T, Uchida I, Kikyo H, Takahashi E, Miyashita Y. Hemispheric asymmetry in human lateral prefrontal cortex during cognitive set shifting. Proc Natl Acad Sci USA 2002; 99(11):7803–7808.

78. Farooqi IS, Yeo GS, Keogh JM, Aminian S, Jebb SA, Butler G, et al. Dominant and recessive inheritance of morbid obesity associated with melanocortin 4 receptor deficiency. J Clin Invest 2000; 106(2):271–279.

79. Steinle NI, Hsueh WC, Snitker S, Pollin TI, Sakul H, St Jean PL, et al. Eating behavior in the Old Order Amish: heritability analysis and a genome-wide linkage analysis. Am J Clin Nutr 2002; 75(6):1098–1106.

80. Lindemann B. Receptors and transduction in taste. Nature 2001; 413 (6852):219–225.

81. Pelchat ML. Of human bondage: food craving, obsession, compulsion, and addiction. Physiol Behav 2002; 76(3):347–352.

82. Barker DJ. In utero programming of chronic disease. Clin Sci (Lond) 1998; 95(2):115–128.

83. Waterland RA, Garza C. Potential mechanisms of metabolic imprinting that lead to chronic disease. Am J Clin Nutr 1999; 69(2):179–197.

84. Hales CN, Barker DJ. The thrifty phenotype hypothesis. Br Med Bull 2001; 60:5–20.

85. Ravelli AC, Der Meulen JH, Osmond C, Barker DJ, Bleker OP. Obesity at the age of 50 y in men and women exposed to famine prenatally. Am J Clin Nutr 1999; 70(5):811–816.

86. Ravelli GP, Stein ZA, Susser MW. Obesity in young men after famine exposure in utero and early infancy. N Engl J Med 1976; 295(7):349–353.

87. Jacobi C, Agras WS, Bryson S, Hammer LD. Behavioral validation, precursors, and concomitants of picky eating in childhood. J Am Acad Child Adol Psychiatry 2003; 42(1):76–84.

88. Gillberg C, Rastam M, Gillberg IC. Anorexia nervosa: physical health and neurodevelopment at 16 and 21 years. Dev Med Child Neurol 1994; 36(7):567–575.

89. Tchanturia, Morris RG, Brecelj Anderluh, B, Nikolaou V, Treasure J. An examination of set shifting in anorexia nervosa before and after weight gain and in full recovery and links to childhood and adult OCPD Traits. Br J Psychiatry. In press.

90. Tchanturia K, Serpell L, Troop N, Treasure J. Perceptual illusions in eating disorders: rigid and fluctuating styles. J Behav Ther Exp Psychiatry 2001; 32(3):107–115.

91. Lou HC, Hansen D, Nordentoft M, Pryds O, Jensen F, Nim J, et al. Prenatal stressors of human life affect fetal brain development. Dev Med Child Neurol 1994; 36(9):826–832.

92. O'Connor TG, Heron J, Golding J, Beveridge M, Glover V. Maternal antenatal anxiety and children's behavioural/emotional problems at 4 years. Report from the Avon Longitudinal Study of Parents and Children. Br J Psychiatry 2002; 180:502–508.

93. Cnattingius S, Hultman CM, Dahl M, Sparen P. Very preterm birth, birth trauma, and the risk of anorexia nervosa among girls. Arch Gen Psychiatry 1999; 56(7):634–638.

94. Eagles JM, Andrew JE, Johnston MI, Easton EA, Millar HR. Season of birth in females with anorexia nervosa in Northeast Scotland. Int J Eat Disord 2001; 30(2):167–175.

95. Foley DL, Thacker LR, Aggen SH, Neale MC, Kendler KS. Pregnancy and perinatal complications associated with risks for common psychiatric disorders in a population-based sample of female twins. Am J Med Genet 2001; 105(5):426–431.

96. Shoebridge P, Gowers SG. Parental high concern and adolescent-onset anorexia nervosa. A case-control study to investigate direction of causality. Br J Psychiatry 2000; 176:132–137.

97. Sokol MS, Ward PE, Tamiya H, Kondo DG, Houston D, Zabriskie JB. D8/17 expression on B lymphocytes in anorexia nervosa. Am J Psychiatry 2002; 159(8): 1430–1432.
98. Sokol MS. Infection-triggered anorexia nervosa in children: clinical description of four cases. J Child Adol Psychopharmacol 2000; 10(2):133–145.
99. Cotter DR, Pariante CM, Everall IP. Glial cell abnormalities in major psychiatric disorders: the evidence and implications. Brain Res Bull 2001; 55(5):585–595.

14

Molecular Biology of Anorexia Nervosa, Bulimia Nervosa, Binge Eating Disorder, and Obesity

Dorothy Grice*

University of Pennsylvania
Philadelphia, Pennsylvania, U.S.A.

Eating disorders reflect a wide range of abnormal eating behaviors and unhealthy attitudes toward food, food consumption, body shape, and body size. Eating disorders such as anorexia nervosa (AN) and bulimia nervosa (BN) have been well defined clinically and generally fall under the purview of psychiatric disorders [see *Diagnostic and Statistical Manual of Mental Disorders*, 4th ed. DSM-IV(1)], although less well-studied disorders such as binge eating disorder (BED) and eating disorder–not otherwise specified (ED–NOS), are also found in this domain. With the rising appreciation of the biological and genetic basis of psychiatric disorders and, specific to this chapter, eating disorders, many researchers have sought to identify the genetic contributions to complex disorders such as these. This chapter will briefly review molecular genetic approaches to the study of complex disorders and focus on recent molecular genetic studies of eating disorders. The preponderance of this literature is based on studies of AN and BN: however, when possible, studies that examine other phenotypes, such as BED, will be included. Lastly, we will

---

* *Current affiliation*: University of Medicine and Dentistry of New Jersey, New Jersey Medical School, Newark, New Jersey, U.S.A.

consider how genetic research on obesity may inform studies in the psychiatrically defined eating disorders.

A critical aspect of genetic studies is determining an accurate phenotype, e.g., the clinical, behavioral, or biological indicators that comprise core feature(s) of the disorder under study. Phenotypes for eating disorders have emerged from decades, if not centuries, of in-depth and thoughtful clinical examinations and interviews. Of the DSM-IV eating disorders, AN and BN are the most studied. AN is a serious psychiatric disorder characterized by severely restricted eating, obsessive fears of weight gain, and distorted attitudes toward eating, food, and body image. As symptoms progress, individuals with AN fail to maintain a minimally normal body weight (or fail to progress through developmentally appropriate growth phases). Often presenting as a waxing-and-waning disorder, AN typically has its onset during adolescence. BN, a related eating disorder, is characterized by recurrent episodes of binge eating followed by various inappropriate compensatory behaviors of weight control (such as self-induced vomiting), and a persistent and pathological preoccupation with body weight and shape. Similar to AN, BN usually has its onset during adolescence, not uncommonly after an episode of dieting and/or food restriction. The vast majority of individuals diagnosed with AN or BN are female, with the lifetime prevalence of AN estimated to be 0.5–1.6% (2,3) and of BN 1.0–3.0 % (4,5). In women, AN has the highest mortality of the psychiatric disorders (6). AN and BN have high rates of co-occurrence. During their lifetime, almost 40% of individuals with AN will also meet criteria for BN (7–9). From this perspective, AN and BN can be considered heritable eating disorders that likely have both disease-specific and overlapping genetic components.

GENETICS

Genetic study of disease yields evidence about the transmission and underlying biology of the illness, two important factors related to treatment and prevention. Psychiatric genetics is a very young field and thus far genes for psychiatric disorders have been difficult to isolate. Eating disorders are complex disorders, as are most psychiatric diagnoses. Genetic, biological, developmental, and sociocultural forces contribute to vulnerabilities to and etiologies of these disorders. These various influences are thought to have direct and indirect effects, including synergistic influences, on the onset and continuation of pathological eating disorders. Although clinical descriptions of anorexic syndromes can be found in the literature dating back to the early 1870s (10,11), it is only in the past few decades that the genetic basis of eating disorders has come to be appreciated and examined.

Understanding the genetic contributors to eating disorders presents particular challenges. For example, there are strong social and cultural presentations of ideal body weight and shape that influence an individual's self-perception of body size, in addition to any existing inherent genetic vulnerabilities in this regard. Inheritance patterns of eating disorders in families, useful in performing some genetic analyses, are often unclear and do not follow traditional mendelian patterns. The often secretive and isolated nature of pathological behaviors associated with eating disorders, particularly when affected individuals display a normal or near-normal body mass index (BMI), may compound the difficulty in identifying clinical cases and family patterns of affectedness. These features, compounded by variability in clinical expression, can obscure phenotype classification. Lastly, from the clinical perspective there is a spectrum of eating disorder diagnoses and pathology. AN and BN are considered the most severe eating disorder diagnoses, each with diagnostic subtypes; however, there is a residual category in DSM-IV that identifies eating disorders not otherwise specified (ED-NOS), including subthreshold AN, BN, and BED. Beyond DSM-IV diagnostic categories, many other pathological eating behaviors and attitudes are associated with disruptions in psychological and/or physical health, although the specific genetic factors that may contribute to these states are largely unexamined (12).

GENETIC METHODS

Traditional methods of determining the role of genetic factors in the etiology of a given disorder are twin, family, and adoption studies. Heritability (the proportion of the population variance of a trait that can be explained by genetic transmission) can be estimated from these types of studies. Once heritability is established for a given disorder, genetic linkage analysis, association studies, and candidate gene surveys are used to search for genes that underlie a particular disorder. The bases for sound genetic studies include homogeneous phenotype classification, unbiased ascertainment of index patients (probands), and accurate clinical assessments. As discussed above, accurate assessment and definition of AN and BN phenotypes requires particular attention. Study design should also include appropriate ascertainment strategies to identify probands and families and mimimize ascertainment bias (e.g., epidemiological studies or, lacking that, multiple recruitment strategies to minimize ascertainment influence from a single referral source) and to gather sufficient numbers of subjects for sound statistical analysis. In addition to defined homogeneous phenotypes, it is also important that the specific clinical assessment of study subjects be free from inadvertent bias, such as can occur when subjects are assessed by multiple researchers or phenotyped without structured criteria.

IDENTIFYING GENES

Several genetic analysis methods have been used to search for susceptibility genes for eating disorders. Genetic association analyses, including case-control studies, of candidate genes can identify gene variants that are statistically associated with illness by comparing allele frequencies of presumably biologically relevant genes in affected individuals (cases) and control individuals. In a case-control study, when the allele frequencies of affected individuals are compared to those of nonfamily controls, the control population should be carefully selected since there are natural variations in gene frequencies that occur between ethnic groups. This phenomenon, known as population stratification, can introduce errors into gene frequency analyses. Differences in allele frequencies between an affected group and a mismatched control group can be misinterpreted as an indication of genetic association, or lack thereof, when in fact the results are due to population stratification. An alternative to case-control association studies are family-based (rather than population-based) association methods.

One example of a family-based method is the transmission disequilibrium test (TDT) (13). The TDT measures linkage in the presence of association. In the TDT method, candidate gene allele determinations (genotypes) are done on affected individuals and their biological parents (about whom no clinical or diagnostic data is needed). From this group of families, in order to have unambiguous determination of allele transmissions from parent to child, only those families with parents having heterozygous genotypes are selected for further analysis, (Because the child's genotype is derived from one allele transmitted from the mother and one allele transmitted from the father, in the case of a homozygous parent it is not possible to resolve the exact allele transmission pattern.) The transmission frequency of the targeted allele is then calculated in the affected subjects and compared to the frequency of its nontransmission. In this way, the parental allele group of nontransmitted alleles becomes a perfectly matched genetic control for the transmitted alleles, bypassing the issue of population stratification.

Candidate gene studies focus on specific, known genes that are hypothesized to underlie the biology of the disorder being studied; thus, by design, candidate gene studies do not function at the genomic level. In contrast, genetic linkage analysis is atheoretical about specific gene involvement in a disorder. Instead, this method relies on anonymous genetic markers dispersed at fairly close intervals through the entire genome, making no assumptions about regions of interest. Typically in a genetic linkage study, multigenerational families are identified in which there are multiple affected individuals. Family members are phenotyped and then genotyped with a set of genetic markers. These markers are usually short tandem repeats (STRs) that are located at about 10-cM intervals through the genome. STRs are chosen because they have significant variability but no functionality. In a commonly used linkage method, STR marker alleles that display a higher frequency of sharing (than expected by chance) in affected family members are presumed to be linked to a nearby susceptibility gene for the disorder under study. The linkage signal is measured as an LOD score [log_{10} of the likelihood ratio that two loci are linked versus nonlinked (i.e. independent assortment)]. Once linkage is found [LOD score >3.6, the presently accepted threshold for linkage in a complex trait (14)], additional markers are used to narrow the region of interest and positional cloning is used to identify genes for further study.

In each of these molecular genetic approaches, proband and family assessments for phenotypical classification must be rigorous and controlled, using instruments with good reliability and validity. Confidentiality must be scrupulously guarded, both between family members and in general, with adequate precautions taken to blind data and ensure protection of subjects' privacy. The importance of control group selection is discussed above. Also central to study integrity is sample size. Current hypotheses suggest that as complex traits many psychiatric disorders are caused by several to many susceptibility genes, each of small to modest effect, that likely interact to render susceptibility to the disorder. Since this genetic susceptibility is parsed over several to many genetic loci, large study populations are needed to generate sufficient power to detect these genes (15,16). In uncommon disorders such as eating disorders, large sample sizes are very difficult to achieve such that multiple collaborative sites are necessary to generate a sufficient patient population for genetic studies.

CANDIDATE GENE STUDIES IN EATING DISORDERS

In order to identify candidate genes for a genetic study, a significant amount must be known about the underlying biology of the disorder of interest. The serotonergic, dopaminergic, leptinergic, noradrenergic, and opioid systems are implicated in eating behaviors, appetite, weight control, mood, obsessionality, impulse regulation, and energy regulation—all features of the clinical presentation of eating disorders. Alterations in these biological systems are found during an acute phase of illness or in the midst of treatment or recovery. While causal links can be inferred from these findings (and, in many cases, supported by studies of animal models), it should be done with the caveat that these are not prospective clinical studies. The following section will summa-

TABLE 1 Association Studies (Population-Based and Family-Based) of Eating Disorders and the 5-HT$_{2A}$ Promoter Polymorphism −1438A/G

Clinical groups	N	5-HT$_{2A}$ polymorphism		P value	Comments	Authors
		−1438A frequency	−1438G frequency			
AN	81	0.51*	0.49	= 0.02*	Population association	Collier et al., 1997 (18)
Controls	226	0.41*	0.59			
AN	100	0.40	0.60	NS	Population association[a]	Hinney et al., 1997 (23)
Obese	254	0.42	0.58			
Underweight	101	0.43	0.57			
AN	152	0.48	0.52	NS	Population association	Campbell et al., 1998 (24)
Controls	150	0.42	0.58			
AN	77	0.56*	0.43	<0.0001*	Population association[b,c]	Sorbi et al., 1998 (19)
Controls	107	0.36*	0.64			
AN (US)	68	0.51*	0.49	<0.005*	Population association	Enoch et al., 1998 (20)
BN	22	0.34	0.66			
Controls	69	0.36*	0.64			
AN (Italy)	20	0.65**	0.35	*0.005		
BN	37	0.38**	0.62			
AN	78	0.29	0.71		Population association[b]	Ziegler et al., 1999 (25)
BN	99	0.31	0.59			

Controls	170	0.30	0.70	<0.0001*	Population association[b,c]	Nacmias et al., 1999 (21)
AN	109	0.55*	0.45			
BN	59	0.47	0.53			
Controls	107	0.36*	0.64	NS	Population association[b]	Ando et al., 2001 (26)
AN	75	0.55	0.45			
Controls	127	0.50	0.50	NS	Population association[b,d]	Nishiguchi et al., 2001 (28)
AN	62	0.46	0.54			
BN	110	0.44	0.54			
Controls	374	0.54	0.46	NS	Family-based association	Gorwood et al., 2002 (27)
AN	316	0.40	0.60			
Controls	316	0.43	0.57		Population association[b,c]	Ricca et al., 2002 (22)
AN	148	0.52*	0.48	= 0.007*		
BN	86	0.54**	0.47	= 0.02*		
BED	54	0.51	0.49			
Obese	132	0.51	0.49			
Controls	115	0.36*,**	0.64			

[a] TDT method applied to a sample subset.

[b] In the AN group, restricting and binge–purge subtypes were studied.

[c] RAN subtype significantly associated with −1438A allele, or the −1438 AA genotype.

[d] Significant association ($p < 0.01$) was found between −1438G allele and BN.

*,** Denotes comparison groups that yielded a p value ≤ 0.05.

NS, Nonsignificant; $p > 0.05$.

rize candidate gene studies (organized by gene class when appropriate) in eating disorders and offer some perspectives on the often-mixed findings that have emerged.

SEROTONINERGIC GENES IN EATING DISORDERS

Serotonin (5-HT) produces its effects by acting at a number of membrane-bound serotonin receptors, which, for the most part, belong to the G-protein-coupled receptor superfamily (for a review, see 17). The major regulators of the serotonergic system in the brain are tryptophan hydroxylase, the 5-HT transporter, and 5-HT receptors. The 5-HT receptor family is composed of at least 14 distinct types and is one of the most complex families of neurotransmitter receptors. In addition to being found in the central nervous system, 5-HT receptors are also located in the peripheral nervous system as well as other tissues, including the cardiovascular system, blood, and gut. Serotonin dysregulation has been implicated in many psychiatric disorders, including eating disorders, major depression, schizophrenia, obsessive-compulsive disorder, as well as other anxiety disorders such as panic disorder and social phobia. Beyond psychiatric disorders, serotonin is also thought to play a role in migraine headaches, hypertension, irritable bowel syndrome, and vomiting. Given the fundamental role of 5-HT in a multitude of biological and behavioral functions related to eating behaviors, considerable interest is focused on the role serotonergic system candidate genes may play in eating disorders. (Table 1 summarizes findings related to the 5-HT_{2A} receptor nucleotide -1438 variations; Table 2 summarizes all other association studies of serotonergic genes in eating disorders.)

THE 5-HT_2 RECEPTORS

5-HT_{2A} Subclass

The 5-HT_2 receptor class is composed of the 5-HT_{2A}, 5-HT_{2B}, and 5-HT_{2C} receptors. These receptors demonstrate 46–50% sequence homology and have been mapped to chromosome 13q14-q21, 2q36.3-37.1, and Xq24, respectively. The 5-HT_{2A} receptor is expressed in many peripheral and central tissues. In the central nervous system, the cortex, basal ganglia, and claustrum are primary sights for 5-HT_{2A} expression. In genetic studies of eating disorders, the 5-HT_{2A} receptor is the most extensively studied serotonin-related gene. Several polymorphisms have been reported in the 5-HT_{2A} receptor gene. The variant that has received the most attention is a polymorphism in the promoter (regulatory) region of the gene in which there is an A or G at nucleotide -1438.

TABLE 2 Association Studies of Eating Disorders and Serotonin-Related Genes[a]

Candidate gene	Variant	Comparison groups	p value	Comment	Author
5-HT$_{2A}$ receptor	Thr25Asn	Obese, underweight, nonpsychiatric controls	NS	Population based; TDT on subset	Hinney et al., 1997 (23); Nacmias et al., 1999 (21)
	His452Tyr	Obese, underweight, nonpsychiatric controls	NS	Population based; TDT on subset	Hinney et al., 1997 (23); Nacmias et al., 1999 (21)
	102 T/C	Nonpsychiatric controls	NS	Population based	Nacmias et al., 1999 (21)
	516 C/T	Nonpsychiatric controls	NS	Population based	Nacmias et al., 1999 (21)
5-HT$_{2C}$ receptor	Cys23Ser	Nonpsychiatric controls; weight loss spectrum*	<0.0002*	Population based	Nacmias et al., 1999 (21); Westberg et al., 2002 (36)
5-HT transporter	Long/short (44bp INS/DEL)	Obese, underweight, bulimics, nonpsychiatric controls, normal weight**, score on Eating Attitudes Test**	NS <0.05 <0.003#	Population based; TDT on subset	Hinney et al., 1997 (44); Sundaramurthy et al., 2000 (45); Di Bella et al., 2000 (46); Fumeron et al., 2002 (43);*,** Matsushita et al., 2002 (47)#
5-HT$_{1D\beta}$ receptor	Phe124Cys G861C	Obese; underweight; BMI spectrum##	NS <0.0001	Population based	Hinney et al., 1999 (38); Levitan et al., 2001 (39)##
5-HT$_7$ receptor	Pro279Leu	Obese; underweight	NS	Population based	Hinney et al., 1999 (38)
Tryptophan hydroxylase	1095 T/C	OCD; SAD; panic disorder; bipolar; alcoholism; nonpsychiatric controls	NS	Population based	Han et al., 1999 (48)

[a] Studies of the 5-HT$_{2A}$ −1438 A/G promoter polymorphism are summarized in Table 1.
*,**,#,## Denotes comparison group that yielded a p value ≤ 0.05 and associated authorship.
NS, Nonsignificant; p > 0.05.

A series of association studies (both population based using obese, underweight, normal-weight, and non–psychiatrically ill controls, and family based using the TDT) have examined the serotonin receptor 5-HT_{2A} promoter polymorphism -1438A/G. Five studies have found a positive association between the 5-HT_{2A} -1438A allele and eating disorders (18–22). The two studies that focused solely on AN phenotypes found evidence for a positive association between the -1438A allele and AN (all subtypes) (18,19) and/or the AN restricting subtype (19). Three studies examined a broader range of eating disorder phenotypes (20–22). One study demonstrated a significant association of the -1438A allele with AN but not BN (20). One study found an association between the -1438A allele and the AN restricting subtype but not AN binge–purge subtype or BN (21). And the third study found a positive association between the -1438A allele in AN, the AN restricting subtype, and the BN purging subtype but not in binge eating disorder (22). In contrast to the above positive findings, five additional studies have examined the 5-HT_{2A} -1438A/G polymorphism and found no significant associations with AN and/or BN using a variety of population-based controls (23–26), the family-based TDT (27), as well as subphenotypes (the AN restricting subtype, age of illness onset, minimal lifetime BMI; 25,27). Interestingly, in a study of Japanese patients, the alternative G allele at nucleotide -1438 was associated with BN (but not AN) (28); this study further suggests an association between binge eating and/or purging behavior and comorbid borderline personality disorder with increased frequency of the G allele, although this type of analysis has not been replicated.

Finally, four other polymorphisms in the 5-HT_{2A} receptor gene have been examined in eating disorders. Two variants are in the coding region of the gene (Thr25Asn and His452Tyr) and two are located in the noncoding region of the gene (102 T/C and 516 C/T). A range of comparison groups were used in these analyses (including the TDT on a subset of individuals); however, none of these studies produced a significant finding in AN or BN (21,23).

At this stage, it is difficult to draw clear interpretations from the studies of 5-HT_{2A} polymorphisms and eating disorders. All in all, evidence is accumulating that the AN restricting subtype may be genetically distinct from other AN subtypes or BN (19–22). This theory is supported by clinical studies (29,30) as well as recent genetic linkage study of AN (31). Other issues that may cloud our understanding of the role of the 5-HT_{2A} gene in eating disorders have been discussed above. For example, in molecular genetic studies, it is important to use large enough sample sizes (and control groups) to garner sufficient power to detect genes of small to modest effect, and the effect of a particular candidate gene is also an estimated value. We do not definitively know if all of these studies were sufficiently powerful to detect association (or lack thereof) with confidence, although several studies did have robust sample sizes.

In part to address some of these methodological issues, a meta-analysis to examine association between the 5-HT_{2A} -1438 polymorphism and AN was done and found no significant relationship between -1438A/G polymorphism and AN (25). Genetic heterogeneity and ethnic admixture leading to population stratification could have obscured positive findings from this meta-analysis. However, using the family-based TDT to control population stratification bias, a multicenter collaborative study identified a large number of AN subjects ($n > 300$) but found neither an association between AN and 5-HT_{2A} -1438A allele nor evidence of an interaction of this allele with age of onset of AN or minimum lifetime BMI (27). Although the sample size in this study is the largest to date, we still do not know for sure if it generates sufficient power when the odds ratio associated with the A allele is small. Of note, however, is a follow-up study based in part on this sample that used a quantitative TDT approach to suggest that the A allele may act as a modifying factor, delaying age of AN onset (32). Thus, the definitive role of the 5-HT_{2A} polymorphisms in eating disorders remains unclear but of great interest. There are some very interesting findings and leads to follow, particularly related to the AN restricting subtype and the 5-HT_{2A} -1438A allele. We must await verification of these results, likely through large-scale controlled studies, before firm conclusions can be drawn about the ultimate relevance of the 5-HT_{2A} gene to the genetics of eating disorders.

5-HT_{2C} Subclass

Similar to the 5-HT_{2A} receptor, the 5-HT_{2C} receptor has been implicated in the regulation of feeding-related behaviors such as satiety and eating continuity (33). Supportive evidence also comes from mouse models in which transgenic mice lacking the 5-HT_{2C} receptor demonstrate abnormal feeding behavior (34). A small number of studies have examined allele frequencies of the 5-HT_{2C} Cys23Ser polymorphism in subjects with a range of eating disorder phenotypes. Although no association was found between Cys23Ser variants and DSM-IV diagnoses of AN (neither restricting nor purging subtypes) (21), BN (21,35), or BED (35), there was a significant association between the Ser23 allele and a clinically defined group of underweight teenage girls (some of whom met criteria for AN) (36). If confirmed these data suggest that 5-HT_{2C} may be involved in the regulation of food intake or proneness to weight loss rather than an eating disorder diagnosis per se.

5-HT_1 Subclass

The 5-HT_1 receptor class comprises five receptor subtypes (5-HT_{1A}, 5-HT_{1B}, 5-HT_{1D}, 5-HT_{1E}, and 5-HT_{1F}), which share 40–63% sequence homology in humans (17). The $5\text{-HT}_{1D\beta}$ receptor, also known as 5-HT_{1B}, has been mapped to chromosome 6q13. $5\text{-HT}_{1D\beta}$ is expressed in the central nervous system, particularly in the basal ganglia, striatum, and frontal cortex, and is thought to function as an autoreceptor as well as a heteroreceptor that effects release of acetylcholine, glutamate, dopamine, noradrenaline, and γ-aminobutyric acid (for review, see 37). Population-based studies of the 5-HT$_{1D\beta}$ receptor gene have examined its possible role in both AN and BN. In a study of AN individuals, the Phe124Cys variant was studied using obese and underweight individuals as comparison but found no significant association (38). A study of the 5-HT$_{1B}$ G681C polymorphism examined the distribution of genotypes in women with BN (39). When the minimum and maximum lifetime BMIs were compared across the three genotypic groups (G/G, G/C, and CC) both the G/C and C/C genotypes were associated with lower minimum lifetime BMIs (and unrelated to lifetime AN rates), perhaps suggesting a role for 5-HT$_{1B}$ in a subphenotype not defined by DSM-IV schemas.

5-HT$_7$ Subclass

The 5-HT$_7$ receptor is located on chromosome 10q23.3-24.4 and shows less than 50% homology to other receptors in the 5-HT family. 5-HT$_7$ receptors are found in the limbic and thalamocortical brain regions, regions implicated in central regulation of feeding behavior (40). These localizations, together with evidence that atypical antipsychotics have a high affinity for 5-HT$_7$ (41), make it an attractive candidate gene for psychiatric disorders. However, the sole study of the 5-HT$_7$ receptor in eating disorders examined the Pro279Leu polymorphism in AN subjects and found no significant association between allele frequencies in AN compared to obese and underweight controls (38).

OTHER SEROTONERGIC-RELATED GENES

Serotonin Transporter

The serotonin transporter is an integral component in regulating serotonin function in the central nervous system and is the site of action for the serotonin reuptake inhibitors. A 44-base-pair insertion/deletion (5-HTTLPR) polymorphism in the promoter region of the 5-HT transporter gene (5-HTT) confers differential transcription rates on gene expression. The so-called short variant of 5-HTTLPR (the deletion variant) is associated with significant decreases in 5-HTT expression and 5-HT uptake (42), making 5-HTT a candidate gene of great interest for many psychiatric disorders, including eating disorders. Several groups have examined this variant, using population-based methods and a variety of control groups, and found conflicting results regarding the role of 5-HTT in a range of eating disorders phenotypes. One positive association was found between the 5-HTTLPR deletion (short) variant in AN compared to obese and normal-weight controls (43). Three studies did not support this finding (44–46), although one group found a positive association between this same variant and BN (46). Also of note is a positive association between the 5-HTTLPR insertion (long) variant and abnormal eating behaviors (defined by high scores on the Eating Attitudes Test) in nonclinical subjects (47). Since these studies have not been replicated, as with other candidate genes, we will have to await further research on 5-HTTLPR to show us how, if at all, this gene influences susceptibility to abnormal eating behaviors or clinically defined eating disorder diagnoses.

Tryptophan Hydroxylase

Since tryptophan hydroxylase (TPH) is the rate-limiting enzyme in the serotonin synthesis pathway it has been seen as a potential candidate gene in eating disorders. TPH is mapped to chromosome 11p15.3-p14. In the one published study on TPH and AN, there was no evidence for association (48).

CANDIDATE GENES BEYOND SEROTONIN

Beyond the serotonergic hypotheses underlying the biology and heritability of AN, other genes from a variety of biological classes have been examined (49–63) primarily through the case-control association method. Due to methodological issues (e.g., sample sizes, risk of population stratification) these studies may have limited power to detect differences between affected individuals and controls. In addition, it is important to recall that although the genes chosen do have theoretical or functional roles in eating behavior, weight regulation, or related phenomenon, these studies are exploratory and the actual role of these genes in eating disorder phenotypes is, for the most part, not completely understood. With these caveats, however, there are several positive findings associating eating disorder phenotypes with specific genes, e.g., estrogen receptor β (52,61), uncoupling protein 2,3 (UCP 2/UCP-3) (56), catechol O-methyltransferase (58), agouti-related protein (59), small-conductance calcium-activated potassium channel 3 (hSKCa3) (60), norepinephrine transporter gene (62), and melanocortin-4 receptor gene (MC-4r) (63), which is reviewed briefly below and summarized in Table 3.

Estrogen Receptors

There are two types of estrogen receptors: ER-α and ER-β mapped to chromosomes 6q25.1 and 14q23.2, respectively. ERs belong to the nuclear hormone receptor family and are found in brain areas involved in regulation of food intake (for review, see 64). Since high estrogen levels are known to inhibit food intake (65) and in the brain, ERs colocalize with corticotropin-releasing factor (CRF), it is theorized that interactions between estrogen and

TABLE 3 Association Studies of Eating Disorders and Candidate Genes Displayed in Chronological Order[a]

Candidate gene	Variant	Comparison group	p value	Comment	Authors
β-3 adrenergic receptor	Trp64Arg	Obese; underweight; normal weight; and family based	NS	Population based and TDT	Hinney et al., 1997 (49)
Pro-opiomelanocortin	9bp insertion (codon 73–74)	Obese; underweight	NS	Population based	Hinney et al., 1998 (50)
D_3 dopamine receptor	Bal I RFLP[b]	Nonpsychiatric controls	NS	Population based	Bruins-Slot et al., 1998 (51)
Estrogen receptor β	1082 G/A	Obese; underweight; BN	0.04	Population based	Rosenkranz et al., 1998 (52)
	1730 A/G	Obese; underweight; BN	NS		
Neuropeptide Y Y1 receptor	Pst I RFLP[b]	Obese; underweight; and family based	NS	Population based and TDT	Rosenkranz et al., 1998 (53)
Neuropeptide Y Y5 receptor	Gly426Gly	Obese; underweight; and family based	NS	Population based and TDT	Rosenkranz et al., 1998 (53)
Leptin gene	LEGLUR[c] 1387 G/A	Obese; underweight; normal weight; BN; and family based	NS	Population based and TDT	Hinney et al., 1998 (54)
D_4 dopamine receptor	48 bp VNTR[d] 13 bp deletion	Obese; underweight; and family based	NS	Population based and TDT	Hinney et al., 1999 (55)
Uncoupling protein 2,3	D11S911[e] D11S916[e]	Nonpsychiatric controls	0.0013 NS	Population based	Campbell et al., 1999 (56)

Gene	Polymorphism	Controls	p	Study	Reference
Tumor necrosis factor-α	−1031 T/C	Nonpsychiatric controls	NS	Population based	Ando et al., 2001 (57)
	−836 C/A		NS		
	−857 C/T		NS		
Catechol-O-methyltransferase	Val158Met	Family based	0.015	TDT	Frisch et al., 2001 (58)
Agouti-related protein gene	Ala67Thr	Volunteer controls	0.015	Population based	Vink et al., 2001 (59)
	650 C/T		NS		
hSKCa3[f]	CAG repeat	Volunteer controls	<0.001	Population based and TDT	Koronyo-Hamaoui et al., 2002 (60)
Estrogen receptor α	Pvu II RFLP	Family based	0.0013	Population based	Eastwood et al., 2002 (61)
		Non-eating-disordered controls	NS		
	Xbal RFLP	Non-eating-disordered controls	NS		
Estrogen receptor β	1082 G/A	Non-eating-disordered controls	0.003	Population based	Eastwood et al., 2002 (61)
	1730 A/G		NS		
Norepinephrine transporter gene	AAGG repeat	Family based	0.0052	TDT	Urwin et al., 2002 (62)

a Studies of the 5-HT$_{2A}$ −1438 A/G promoter polymorphism and other serotonin-related genes are summarized in Table 1 and Table 2, respectively.
b RFLP, restriction fragment length polymorphism.
c LEGLUR, leptin gene–linked upstream region.
d VNTR, variable number of tandem repeats.
e Microsatellite markers that flank the gene.
f hSKCa3, small-conductance calcium-activated potassium channel 3.
NS, Nonsignificant; $p > 0.05$.

CRF may modulate the hypothalamic–pituitary–adrenal axis and be involved in the molecular basis of feeding, satiety, and, perhaps, eating disorders, especially AN (66). Two studies have looked specifically at the association between ERs and eating disorders (52,61). ER-β was screened for variations in subjects with a range of weight extremes (extremely obese, AN, BN, healthy underweight) (52). Although five different sequence variants were identified, the association results were negative except for a suggestive association between a G/A polymorphism at nucleotide 1082 and the AN phenotype. A second study examined ER-α and ER-β in AN subjects (61). There were no significant findings related to ER-α, but in ER-β the heterozygous genotype GA at nucleotide 1082 was associated with AN.

Uncoupling Protein-2/Uncoupling Protein-3

Uncoupling protein-2 and uncoupling protein-3 (UCP-2/UCP-3) are involved in resting metabolic rate and energy expenditure (67,68). The UCP-2/UCP-3 locus is on chromosome 11q13; UCP-2 has been linked to obesity and hyperinsulinemia, making it an interesting candidate gene for other abnormal weight disorders (69). In a study of AN subjects and markers located in the UCP-2/UCP-3 locus a significant association between a marker (D11S911) and AN was found (56). Further work in this area will elucidate if UCPs are involved in the genetic basis of eating disorders beyond obesity.

Catechol-O-Methyltransferase

Catechol-O-methyltransferase (COMT) catalyzes the transfer of a methyl group to catecholamines (dopamine, epinephrine, and norepinephrine) and is the major degradative pathway of these neurotransmitters. COMT has been mapped to chromosome 22q11.21. In humans there is a functional polymorphism (Val/Met158) that determines high and low enzymatic activity. COMT has been considered a candidate gene for several psychiatric disorders and associated with positive findings in a subset of these studies (e.g., substance use disorders, schizophrenia, attention deficit disorder). Relevant to this summary, the Val/Met polymorphism was studied in a family-based association study and the high-activity allele was significantly associated with AN, indicating a possible role in eating disorders (58).

Melanocortinergic System Genes

The central melanocortinergic system is involved in regulation of food intake, body weight, and eating behavior and is a major pathway in leptin signaling (for review, see 70). There are at least two melanocortin receptors; melanocortin-3 receptor (MC3-r) and melanocortin-4 receptor (MC4-r). Hormones in this system are the melanocortins, products of the proopiomelanocortin gene (POMC), that act as MC receptor agonists, such as ACTH, β endorphin, and MSH, and the orexigenic neuropeptide agouti-related protein (AGRP) that acts as an MC receptor antagonist. In this system, leptin stimulates POMC expression and suppresses AGRP expression in brain regions involved in feeding and satiety. Leptin also regulates other important hormones involved in food intake, neuroendocrine balance, and energy expenditure, e.g., neuropeptide Y (NPY, another orexigenic neuropeptide), thyrotropin-releasing hormone, and corticotropin-realeasing hormone. Many components of the central melanocortinergic system are candidate genes for disordered weight and eating phenotypes. MC-4r (mapped to chromosome 18q22), POMC (mapped to chromosome 2p23.3), AGRP (mapped to chromosome 16q22), NPY Y1 (mapped to chromosome 4q31.3-q32), NPY Y5 (mapped to chromosome 4q31-q32), and the leptin gene (mapped to chromosome 7q32.1) have been studied in eating disorder phenotypes in population-based and family-based association studies. From these studies, one positive association was found between AGRP and AN (59), and one subject with BN (out of 81 screened) had a haplo insufficiency mutation in MC4-r (63).

OTHER CANDIDATE GENES

hSKCa3

hSKCa3 is a small-conductance calcium-activated potassium channel involved in regulating neural excitability. hSKCa3 has been mapped to chromosome 1q21. In one model, small-conductance calcium-activated potassium channels may contribute to the genetic susceptibility to bipolar disorder and schizophrenia (71,72). To date, one study has examined hSKCa3 polymorphisms in AN (60). Using a family-based association method, a positive association was found, with longer alleles from the hSKCa3 gene found at higher rates in the AN sample compared to controls.

Norepinephrine Transporter

Norepinephrine transporter (NET) expression is regulated by norepinephrine; thus, it has an important role in noradrenergic transmission. This system regulates many neuroendocrine systems implicated in the pathophysiology of eating disorders as well as anxiety disorders. In clinical research, reduced noradrenergic activity is found in AN patients following normal-weight restoration (73,74) although the mechanism underlying these findings are unknown. Using a family-based association method, a polymorphic region in the promoter of the NET gene was studied in the restricting subtype of AN

(62). A significant association was found between an insertion in this region and the restricting AN subtype, suggesting that this NET gene variant, or a variant in linkage disequilibrium with it, increases risk for restricting AN.

LINKAGE ANALYSIS IN EATING DISORDERS

Three genetic linkage studies of eating disorders are in the literature (31,75,76). The two linkage studies of AN are based on the same sample of about 200 affected families. These families contained at least two family members affected with an eating disorder, all ascertained through a proband with AN. Both studies used an allele-sharing linkage strategy to identify genetic loci that contribute to AN. In the first linkage study of AN, the linkage analysis of the entire sample did not yield any statistically significant results (31). However, when the phenotype was narrowed to include only those families ascertained through a proband with the restricting subtype of AN, a significant linkage signal of 3.45 was found on chromosome 1p. Several interesting candidate genes related to eating phenotypes are found in this region, including an orexin receptor gene (Hcrtr1), the delta opioid receptor, and the 5-HT_{1D} receptor. Further studies will determine if there are specific associations between these candidate genes, or other genes in this region that have not yet been identified, and restricting AN. The second linkage study of AN used two clinically based covariates, drive for thinness and obsessionality, which were shown to discriminate subsets in the clinical sample (75). When these covariates were incorporated into the linkage analysis, the genome region with greatest statistical significance showed linkage on chromosome 1q (LOD = 3.46), a different region from that seen in the first AN linkage study, and two weaker signals on chromosome 2 and 13.

The BN linkage study examined about 300 families affected with eating disorders, all ascertained through a proband with the purging subtype of BN (76). Purging methods must have at least included regular vomiting, and a lifetime or current history of AN was acceptable. Using this phenotype, the highest linkage signal of 2.92 was found on chromosome 10p. A second peak in this same region of 10p approached significance and a smaller suggestive linkage signal was found on chromosome 14. The sample was then narrowed by selecting only those families in which at last one other affected relative had regular vomiting behavior (by design, the proband had already met this criteria). When this subset of 133 families was studied, the initial linkage signal at chromosome 10p increased to 3.39. This chromosomal region has been implicated in other disorders, such as obesity, alcoholism, schizophrenia, and bipolar disorder, perhaps reflecting that this region harbors a gene(s) that generically increases susceptibility to a range of psychiatric and related disorders (as summarized in (76)). It is also possible that a gene(s) in this region may specifically alter susceptibility to BN and obesity, two disorders that may have overlapping vulnerabilities and/or manifestations.

OBESITY

Compared to the genetic studies of DSM-IV-defined eating disorders, there are a plethora of studies of human obesity. This intensity of research has identified putative regions affecting obesity phenotypes on all chromosomes except chromosome Y and with over 250 significant regions of interest in the genome under study, a summary of which is beyond the scope of this chapter (for review, see 77). Well over 150 studies covering approximately 60 candidate genes have reported significant associations with obesity. Genome-wide linkage analyses of obesity-related phenotypes have uncovered similar numbers of loci linked to obesity indicators. As in eating disorders, a variety of phenotypes related to obesity have been defined, including BMI, body fat mass, percentage of body fat, fat-free mass, skinfolds, resting metabolic rates, and plasma leptin levels—again indicating the importance of phenotypical definition beyond absolute clinical categories. Relevant to this review of the genetics of eating disorders, many of the genes discussed in this chapter also have been examined in obesity. Significant findings in obesity genetics have been associated with serotonergic genes ($5-HT_{1B}$, $5-HT_{2C}$, $5-HT_{2A}$), melanocortinergic genes (MC4-r, POMC, NPY, AGRP), ER-α, UCP-2/UCP-3, and tumor necrosis factor-α. As research continues to delve into the genetic basis of eating disorders we should expect to see greater understanding of which pathways (e.g., those related to feeding behavior, satiety, and/or energy metabolism) are affected in both obesity disorders and eating disorders. Delineation of the specific genetic variations associated with relevant phenotypes will allow us to discover if abnormal eating behaviors can be seen as a spectrum of disorders ranging from obesity to anorexia or if the genetic bases for these disorders are in fact distinct.

SUMMARY

Although research in the genetics of obesity syndromes far outdistances research in the genetics of eating disorders at this time, our knowledge and research in AN and BN far exceeds that for other eating disorder syndromes or diagnoses. It is apparent that AN and BN are heritable eating disorders that result from complex interactions of genetic liabilities and environmental factors. The positive case-control studies associated with several genes of interest (e.g., the $5-HT_{2A}$ receptor, melanocortinergic system genes) have piqued interest in the molecular genetic basis of eating disorders. Recent findings of significant linkage peaks on chromosome 1p and 1q (related to an

AN subtype) and on chromosome 10p (related to a BN subtype) have spurred the field forward with new enthusiasm. Thus, many promising leads are emerging from genetic linkage studies and candidate gene analyses; however, we must await further molecular studies to confirm the specific genes that confer heritability to eating disorders. Impediments to progress are due in part to the low population prevalence of eating disorders and perhaps also the low rates of clinical identification of eating disorder phenotypes, both of which make it very difficult to ascertain samples sufficiently powerful to detect genes of less than major effect. In addition, it is only in the past few years that molecular geneticists have had the means to examine the human genome with the level of specificity and detail required for human genetic studies. As a result of these technological and methodological advances, the field of molecular genetics in eating disorders is growing rapidly. The large-scale linkage studies of AN and BN and the larger TDT and association studies are evidence of the more methodologically robust and controlled analyses that have recently been undertaken. Collaborations such as these, combined with ongoing developments in molecular genetic and genomic analytical tools, will further strengthen genetically based studies and bring us closer still to the identification of specific genes that confer susceptibility to eating disorders.

REFERENCES

1. American Psychiatric Association. Diagnostic and Statistical Manual of Mental Disorders. 4th ed. Washington, DC, 1994:544–545.
2. Walters EE, Kendler KS. Anorexia nervosa and anorexic-like syndromes in a population-based female twin sample. Am J Psychiatry 1995; 152:64–71.
3. Hoek HW, van Harten PN, van Hoeken D, Susser E. Lack of relation between culture and anorexia nervosa-results of an incidence study on Curacao. N Engl J Med 1998; 338(17):1231–1232.
4. Timmerman MG, Wells LA, Chen SP. Bulimia nervosa and associated alcohol abuse among secondary school students. J Am Acad Child Adol Psychiatry 1990; 29(1):118–122.
5. Kendler KS, MacLean C, Neale M, Kessler R, Heath A, Eaves L. The genetic epidemiology of bulimia nervosa. Am J Psychiatry 1992; 48:1627–1637.
6. Sullivan PF. Mortality in anorexia nervosa. Am J Psychiatry 1995; 152:1073–1074.
7. Hsu LKG, Crisp AH, Harding B. Outcome of anorexia nervosa. Lancet 1979; 1(8107):61–65.
8. Caspar RC, Eckert ED, Halmi KA, et al. Bulimia: its incidence in patients with anorexia nervosa. Arch Gen Psychiatry 1980; 37:1030–1035.
9. Strober M, Salkin B, Burroughs J, Morrell W. Validity of the bulimia-restricter distinction in anorexia nervosa. J Nerv Ment Dis 1982; 170:345–351.

10. Gull WW. Anorexia nervosa (apepsia hysterica, anorexia hysterica). Trans Clin Soc London 1874; 7:22–28.
11. Lasègue E-C. On hysterical anorexia. Med Times Gazette, 1873:265–266:367–369.
12. Gerson ES, Cloninger CR. Genetic approaches to mental disorders. Washington, DC: American Psychiatric Press, 1994.
13. Spielman RS, McGinnis RE, Ewens WJ. Transmission test for linkage disequilibrium: the insulin gene region and insulin-dependent diabetes mellitus (IDDM). Am J Hum Genet 1993; 52:506–516.
14. Lander E, Kruglyak L. Genetic dissection of complex traits: guidelines for interpreting and reporting linkage results. Nat Genet 1995; 11(3):241–247.
15. Risch N, Merikangas K. The future of genetic studies of complex human diseases. Science 1996; 273:1516–1517.
16. Risch N. Searching for genetic determinants in the new millennium. Nature 2000; 405:847–856.
17. Hoyer D, Hannon JP, Martin GR. Molecular, pharmacological and functional diversity of 5-HT receptors. Pharmacol Biochem Behav 2002; 71(4):533–554.
18. Collier DA, Arranz MJ, Li T Mupita D, Brown N, Treasure J. Association between 5-HT$_{2A}$ gene promoter polymorphism and anorexia nervosa. Lancet 1997; 350:412.
19. Sorbi S, Nacmias B, Tedde A, Ricca V, Mezzani B, Rotella CM. 5-HT$_{2A}$ promoter polymorphism in anorexia nervosa. Lancet 1998; 351:1785.
20. Enoch MA, Kaye WH, Rotondo A, Greenberg BD, Murphy DL, Goldman D. 5 HT$_{2A}$ promoter polymorphism -1438G/A, anorexia nervosa, and obsessive compulsive disorder. Lancet 1998; 351:1785–1786.
21. Nacmias B, Ricca V, Tedde A, Mezzani B, Rotella CM, Sorbi S. 5-HT$_{2A}$ receptor gene polymorphisms in anorexia nervosa and bulimia nervosa. Neurosci Lett. 1999; 277(2):134–136.
22. Ricca V, Nacmias B, Cellini E, Di Bernardo M, Rotella CM, Sorbi S. 5-HT$_{2A}$ receptor gene polymorphism and eating disorders. Neurosci Lett 2002; 323(2):105–108.
23. Hinney A, Ziegler A, Nother MM, Remschmidt H, Hebebrand J. 5-HT$_{2A}$ receptor gene polymorphisms, anorexia, and obesity. Lancet 1997; 350:1324–1325.
24. Campbell DA, Sundaramurthy D, Markham AF, Pieri LF. Lack of association between 5-HT$_{2A}$ gene promoter polymorphism and susceptibility to anorexia nervosa. Lancet 1998; 351:499.
25. Ziegler A, Hebebrand J, Gorg T, Rosenkranz K, Fichter M, Herpertz Dahlmann B, Remschmidt H, Hinney A. Further lack of association between the 5-HT$_{2A}$ gene promoter polymorphism and susceptibility to eating disorders and a meta-analysis pertaining to anorexia nervosa. Mol Psychiatry 1999; 4(5):410–412.
26. Ando T, Komaki G, Karibe M, Kawamura N, Hara S, Takii M, Naruo T, Kurokawa N, Takei M, Tatsuta N, Ohba M, Nozoe S, Kubo C, Ishikawa T. 5-HT$_{2A}$ promoter polymorphism is not associated with anorexia nervosa in Japanese patients. Psychiatr Genet 2001; 11(3):157–160.
27. Gorwood P, Ades J, Bellodi L, Cellini E, Collier DA, Di Bella D, Di Bernardo M, Estivill X, Fernandez-Aranda F, Gratacos M, Hebebrand J, Hinney A, Hu X,

Karwautz A, Kipman A, Mouren-Simeoni MC, Nacmias B, Ribases M, Remschmidt H, Ricca V, Rotella CM, Sorbi S, Treasure J. The 5-HT(2A) −1438G/A polymorphism in anorexia nervosa: a combined analysis of 316 trios from six European centres. Mol Psychiatry 2002; 7(1):90–94.

28. Nishiguchi N, Matsushita S, Suzuki K, Murayama M, Shirakawa O, Higuchi S. Association between $5HT_{2A}$ receptor gene promoter region polymorphism and eating disorders in Japanese patients. Biol Psychiatry 2001; 50(2):123–128.

29. Kaye WH, Ebert MH, Gwirtsman HE, Weiss SR. Differences in brain serotonergic metabolism between nonbulimic and bulimic patients with anorexia nervosa. Am J Psychiatry 1984; 141(12):1598–1601.

30. Herzog DB, Field AE, Keller MB, West JC, Robbins WM, Staley J, Colditz GA. Subtyping eating disorders: is it justified? J Am Acad Child Adol Psychiatry 1996; 35(7):928–936.

31. Grice DE, Halmi KA, Fichter MM, Strober M, Woodside DB, Treasure JT, Kaplan AS, Magistretti PJ, Goldman D, Bulik CM, Kaye WH, Berrettini WH. Evidence for a susceptibility gene for anorexia nervosa on chromosome 1. Am J Hum Genet 2002; 70(3):787–792.

32. Kipman A, Bruins-Slot L, Boni C, Hanoun N, Ades J, Blot P, Hamon M, Mouren-Simeoni M, Gorwood P. 5-HT(2A) gene promoter polymorphism as a modifying rather than a vulnerability factor in anorexia nervosa. Eur Psychiatry 2002; 17(4):227–279.

33. Simansky KJ. Serotonergic control of the organization of feeding and satiety. Behav Brain Res 1996; 73(1–2):37–42.

34. Tecott LH, Sun LM, Akana SF, Strack AM, Lowenstein DH, Dallman MF, Julius D. Eating disorder and epilepsy in mice lacking 5-HT_{2c} serotonin receptors. Nature 1995; 374(6522):542–546.

35. Burnet PW, Smith KA, Cowen PJ, Fairburn CG, Harrison PJ. Allelic variation of the 5-HT_{2C} receptor (HTR2C) in bulimia nervosa and binge eating disorder. Psychiatr Genet 1999; 9(2):101–104.

36. Westberg L, Bah J, Rastam M, Gillberg C, Wentz E, Melke J, Hellstrand M, Eriksson E. Association between a polymorphism of the 5-HT_{2C} receptor and weight loss in teenage girls. Neuropsychopharmacology 2002; 26(6):789–793.

37. Pauwels PJ. 5-HT 1B/D receptor antagonists. Gen Pharmacol 1997; 29(3):293–303.

38. Hinney A, Herrmann H, Lohr T, Rosenkranz K, Ziegler A, Lehmkuhl G, Poustka F, Schmidt MH, Mayer H, Siegfried W, Remschmidt H, Hebebrand J. No evidence for an involvement of alleles of polymorphisms in the serotonin[1Dbeta] and 7 receptor genes in obesity, underweight or anorexia nervosa. Int J Obes Relat Metab Disord 1999; 23(7):760–763.

39. Levitan RD, Kaplan AS, Masellis M, Basile VS, Walker ML, Lipson N, Siegel GI, Woodside DB, Macciardi FM, Kennedy SH, Kennedy JL. Polymorphism of the serotonin 5-HT_{1B} receptor gene (HTR1B) associated with minimum lifetime body mass index in women with bulimia nervosa. Biol Psychiatry 2001; 50(8): 640–643.

40. Bernardis LL, Bellinger LL. The lateral hypothalamic area revisited: neuro-

anatomy, body weight regulation, neuroendocrinology and metabolism. Neurosci Biobehav Rev 1993; 17(2):141–193.

41. Roth BL, Craigo SC, Choudhary MS, Uluer A, Monsma FJ Jr, Shen Y, Meltzer HY, Sibley DR. Binding of typical and atypical antipsychotic agents to 5-hydroxytryptamine-6 and 5-hydroxytryptamine-7 receptors. J Pharmacol Exp Ther 1994; 268(3):1403–1410.

42. Lesch KP, Bengel D, Heils A, Sabol SZ, Greenberg BD, Petri S, Benjamin J, Muller CR, Hamer DH, Murphy DL. Association of anxiety-related traits with a polymorphism in the serotonin transporter gene regulatory region. Science 1996; 274(5292):1527–1531.

43. Fumeron F, Betoulle D, Aubert R, Herbeth B, Siest G, Rigaud D. Association of a functional 5-HT transporter gene polymorphism with anorexia nervosa and food intake. Mol Psychiatry 2001; 6(1):9–10.

44. Hinney A, Barth N, Ziegler A, von Prittwitz S, Hamann A, Hennighausen K, Pirke KM, Heils A, Rosenkranz K, Roth H, Coners H, Mayer H, Herzog W, Siegfried A, Lehmkuhl G, Poustka F, Schmidt MH, Schafer H, Grzeschik KH, Lesch KP, Lentes KU, Remschmidt H, Hebebrand J. Serotonin transporter gene-linked polymorphic region: allele distributions in relationship to body weight and in anorexia nervosa. Life Sci 1997; 61:PL 295–303.

45. Sundaramurthy D, Pieri LF, Gape H, Markham AF, Campbell DA. Analysis of the serotonin transporter gene linked polymorphism (5-HTTLPR) in anorexia nervosa. Am J Med Genet 2000; 96(1):53–55.

46. Di Bella DD, Catalano M, Cavallini MC, Riboldi C, Bellodi L. Serotonin transporter linked polymorphic region in anorexia nervosa and bulimia nervosa. Mol Psychiatry 2000; 5(3):233–234.

47. Matsushita S, Nakamura T, Nishiguchi N, Higuchi S. Association of serotonin transporter regulatory region polymorphism and abnormal eating behaviors. Mol Psychiatry 2002; 7:538–540.

48. Han L, Nielsen DA, Rosenthal NE, Jefferson K, Kaye W, Murphy D, Altemus M, Humphries J, Cassano G, Rotondo A, Virkkunen M, Linnoila M, Goldman D. No coding variant of the tryptophan hydroxylase gene detected in seasonal affective disorder, obsessive-compulsive disorder, anorexia nervosa, and alcoholism. Biol Psychiatry 1999; 45(5):615–619.

49. Hinney A, Lentes K-U, Rosenkranz K, Barth N, Roth H, Ziegler A, Hennighausen K, Coners H, Wurmser H, Jacob K, Romer G, Winnikes U, Mayer H, Herzog W, Lehmkuhl G, Poustka F, Schmidt MH, Blum WF, Pirke KM, Schafer H, Grzeschik KH, Remschmidt H, Hebebrand J. Beta$_3$ adrenergic receptor allele distributions in children, adolescents, and young adults with obesity, underweight, and anorexia nervosa. Int J Obesity 1997; 21:224–230.

50. Hinney A, Becker I, Heibult O, Nottebom K, Schmidt A, Ziegler A, Mayer H, Siegfried W, Blum WF, Remschmidt H, Hebebrand J. Systematic mutation screening of the pro-opiomelanocortin gene: identification of several genetic variants including three different insertions, one nonsense and two missense point mutations in probands of different weight extremes. J Clin Endocrinol Metab 1998; 83(10):3737–3741.

51. Bruins-Slot L, Gorwood P, Bouvard M, Blot P, Ades J, Feingold J, Schwartz JC, Mouren-Simeoni MC. Lack of association between anorexia nervosa and D3 dopamine receptor gene. Biol Psychiatry 1998; 43:76–78.

52. Rosenkranz K, Hinney A, Ziegler A, Hermann H, Fichter M, Mayer H, Siegfried W, Young JK, Remschmidt H, Hebebrand J. Systematic mutation screening of the estrogen receptor beta gene in probands of different weight extremes: identification of several genetic variants. J Clin Endocrinol Metab 1998; 83(12):4524–4527.

53. Rosenkranz K, Hinney A, Ziegler A, von Prittwitz S, Barth N, Roth H, Mayer H, Siegfried W, Lehmkuhl G, Poustka F, Schmidt M, Schafer H, Remschmidt H, Hebebrand J. Screening for mutations in the neuropeptide Y Y5 receptor gene in cohorts belonging to different weight extremes. Int J Obesity Relat Metab Disord 1998; 22(2):157–163.

54. Hinney A, Bornscheuer A, Depenbusch M, Mierke B, Tolle A, Middeke K, Ziegler A, Roth H, Gerber G, Zamzow K, Ballauff A, Hamann A, Mayer H, Siegfried W, Lehmkuhl G, Poustka F, Schmidt MH, Hermann H, Herpertz-Dahlmann BM, Fichter M, Remschmidt H, Hebebrand J. No evidence for involvement of the leptin gene in anorexia nervosa, bulimia nervosa, underweight or early onset extreme obesity: identification of two novel mutations in the coding sequence and a novel polymorphism in the leptin gene linked upstream region. Mol Psychiatry 1998; 3(6):539–543.

55. Hinney A, Schneider J, Ziegler A, Lehmkuhl G, Poustka F, Schmidt MH, Mayer H, Siegfried W, Remschmidt H, Hebebrand J. No evidence for involvement of polymorphisms of the dopamine D4 receptor gene in anorexia nervosa, underweight, and obesity. Am J Med Genet 1999; 88(6):594–597.

56. Campbell DA, Sundaramurthy D, Gordon D, Markham AF, Pieri LF. Association between a marker in the UCP-2/UCP-3 gene cluster and genetic susceptibility to anorexia nervosa. Mol Psychiatry 1999; 4(1):68–70.

57. Ando T, Ishikawa T, Kawamura N, Karibe M, Oba M, Tatsuta N, Hara S, Takii M, Naruo T, Takei M, Kurokawa N, Nozoe S, Kubo C, Komaki G. Analysis of tumor necrosis factor-alpha gene promoter polymorphisms in anorexia nervosa. Psychiatr Genet 200; 11(3):161–164.

58. Frisch A, Laufer N, Danziger Y, Michaelovsky E, Leor S, Carel C, Stein D, Fenig S, Mimouni M, Apter A, Weizman A. Association of anorexia nervosa with the high activity allele of the COMT gene: a family-based study in Israeli patients. Mol Psychiatry 2001; 6(2):243–245.

59. Vink T, Hinney A, van Elburg AA, van Goozen SH, Sandkuijl LA, Sinke RJ, Herpertz-Dahlmann BM, Hebebrand J, Remschmidt H, van Engeland H, Adan RA. Association between an agouti-related protein gene polymorphism and anorexia nervosa. Mol Psychiatry 2001; 6(3):325–328.

60. Koronyo-Hamaoui M, Danziger Y, Frisch A, Stein D, Leor S, Laufer N, Carel C, Fennig S, Minoumi M, Apter A, Goldman B, Barkai G, Weizman A, Gak E. Association between anorexia nervosa and the hsKCa3 gene: a family-based and case control study. Mol Psychiatry 2002; 7(1):82–85.

61. Eastwood H, Brown KM, Markovic D, Pieri LF. Variation in the ESR1 and

ESR2 genes and genetic susceptibility to anorexia nervosa. Mol Psychiatry 2002; 7(1):86–89.

62. Urwin RE, Bennetts B, Wilcken B, Lampropoulos B, Beumont P, Clarke S, Russell J, Tanner S, Nunn KP. Anorexia nervosa (restrictive subtype) is associated with a polymorphism in the novel norepinephrine transporter gene promoter polymorphic region. Mol Psychiatry 2002; 7(6):652–657.

63. Hebebrand J, Fichter M, Gerber G, Gorg G, Hermann H, Geller F, Schafer H, Remschmidt H, Hinney A. Genetic predisposition to obesity in bulimia nervosa: a mutation screen of the melanocortin-4 receptor gene. Mol Psychiatry 2002; 7:647–651.

64. Pettersson K, Gustafsson JA. Role of estrogen receptor beta in estrogen action. Annu Rev Physiol 2001; 63:165–192.

65. Wade GN, Gray JM. Gonadal effects on food intake and adiposity. A metabolic hypothesis. Physiol Behav 1979; 22:593.

66. Dagnault A, Richard D. Involvement of the medial preoptic area in the anorectic action of estrogens. Am J Physiol 1997; 272:R311–R317.

67. Boss O, Samec S, Paoloni-Giacobino A, Rossier C, Dulloo A, Seydoux J, Muzzin P, Giacobino JP. Uncoupling protein −3: a new member of the mitochondrial carrier family with tissue-specific expression. FEBS Lett 1997; 408:39–42.

68. Del Mar Gonzalez-Barroso M, Ricquier D, Cassard-Doulcier AM. The human uncoupling protein-1 gene (UCP1): present status and perspectives in obesity research. Obes Rev 2000; 1(2):61–72.

69. Fleury C, Neverova M, Collins S, Raimbault S, Champigny O, Levi-Meyrueis C, Bouillaud F, Seldin MF, Surwit RS, Ricquier D, Warden CH. Uncoupling protein-2: a novel gene linked to obesity and hyperinsulinemia. Nat Genet 1997; 15:269–272.

70. Lu XY. Role of central melanocortin signaling in eating disorders. Psychopharmacol Bull 2001; 35(4):45–65.

71. Chandy KG, Fantino E, Wittekindt O, Kalman K, Tong L-L, Ho T-H, et al. Isolation of a novel potassium channel gene kSKCa3 containing a polymorphic CAG repeat: a candidate for schizophrenia and bipolar disorder? Mol Psychiatry 1998; 3:32–37.

72. Dror V, Shamir E, Ghanshani S, Kimhi R, Swartz M, Barak Y, et al. hSKca3/KCNN3 potassium channel gene: association of longer CAG repeats with schizophrenia in Israeli Ashkenazai Jews, expression in human tissues and localization to chromosome 1q21. Mol Psychiatry 1999; 4:254–260.

73. Kaye WH, Jimeson DC, Lake CR, Ebert MH. Altered norepinephrine metabolism following long-term weight recovery in patients with anorexia nervosa. Psychiatry Res 1985; 14:333–342.

74. Pirke KM, Kellner M, Phillip E, Laessle R, Krieg JC, Fichter MM. Plasma norepinephrine after a standardized test meal in acute and remitted patients with anorexia nervosa and healthy controls. Biol Psychiatry 1992; 31:1074–1077.

75. Devlin B, Bacanu SA, Klump KL, Bulik CM, Fichter MM, Halmi KA, Kaplan AS, Strober M, Treasure J, Woodside DB, Berrettini WH, Kaye WH. Linkage

analysis of anorexia nervosa incorporating behavioral covariates. Hum Mol Genet 2002; 11(6):689–696.

76. Bulik CM, Devlin B, Bacanu SA, Thornton L, Klump KL, Fichter MM, Halmi KA, Kaplan AS, Strober M, Woodside DB, Bergen AW, Ganjei JK, Crow S, Mitchell J, Rotondo A, Mauri M, Cassano G, Kellp P, Berrettini WH, Kaye WH. Significant linkage on chromosome 10p in families with bulimia nervosa. Am J Hum Genet 2003; 72:200–207.

77. Rankinen T, Perusse L, Weisnagel SJ, Snyder EE, Chagnon YC, Bouchard C. The human obesity gene map: the 2001 update. Obesity Res 2002; 10(3):196–243.

15

Management of Eating Disorders: Inpatient and Partial Hospital Programs

Wayne A. Bowers, Arnold E. Andersen, and Kay Evans
University of Iowa Hospital & Clinics
Iowa City, Iowa, U.S.A.

It was the best of times; it was the worst of times. One might use that phrase when examining the current state in the management of eating disorders, especially when management occurs in an inpatient or partial hospitalization setting. Inpatient treatments for eating disorders have evolved considerably, with increasing acceptance of a multidisciplinary approach, but still remain overly variable even with the current amount of evidence-based information. Earlier hospital-based treatments included one or several of the following: high doses of antipsychotic medications, tube feeding, nursing management, bed rest with a high-calorie diet, strict behavioral contingency management, hyperalimentation, and a variety of medical regimes (1–5). The literature also describes a variety of variably successful psychological interventions to restore weight among persons with an eating disorder. Several controlled trials of behavior therapy have been reported (6–8). Strict behavioral interventions have recently been criticized as being narrow minded, leading to short-term compliance but frequent relapse. Long-term outcome studies suggested that weight restoration alone by strictly medical or behavioral methods was a temporary phenomenon, which at times produced negative effects (9).

A multidimensional perspective to the management of eating disorders was developed (10–13) that advocated that weight gain achieved by comprehensive management of eating disorders in the context of identifying, challenging, and changing distorted cognitions was more enduring. Behavior therapy was best seen as one aspect of a total treatment program that included additionally required cognitive, family, and medical interventions (14,15). The complex nature of eating disorders suggested the need for a coordinated, multidisciplinary approach to treatment, focusing on the combined biological, social, behavioral, and psychological needs of the patient. Successful treatment was described as a skillful blend of weight restoration, psychotherapy (individual, group, family), psychoeducational interventions, medical management, and, at times, pharmacotherapy (10,14). Pharmacotherapy was seen as an adjunct to the other therapies. Low-dose antipsychotics and anti-anxiety agents are at times useful to reduce anxiety associated with fear of loss of control surrounding meals and weight gain, but are not used to increase hunger. While antidepressant medication was suggested to treat concomitant depressive symptoms or to reduce obsessive-compulsive symptoms sometimes seen in these patients, such agents are relatively ineffective in starved patients (16,17). Some classes of antidepressants have been found to be useful in maintenance of weight after restoration (18).

Over the past 15 years the most progress has been made in creating effective outpatient treatments for bulimia nervosa (19,20). The use of cognitive–behavioral therapy and interpersonal therapy has been shown to be effective in both short- and long-term treatment (21,22) and have reduced the need for hospitalization for many individuals with bulimia nervosa. In a similar manner, the use of psychopharmacological agents, often layered on top of manual-based proven psychotherapies, have been shown to be effective in the management of bulimia nervosa (18,23,24). With a greater understanding of treatment options for bulimia nervosa the need for hospital-based intervention has decreased except where outpatient treatments have failed or patients have severe comorbidity.

In the same time period, less progress has been made in the effective management of anorexia nervosa. Although the use of family therapy has been shown to work effectively with adolescents and this approach has been manualized (25), it is still not widely used in practice. However, it may be very effective in a limited number of younger patients. Although many patients are successfully treated in an outpatient setting, hospital-based care by a skilled team remains the intervention of choice for those individuals who fail outpatient treatment settings or are too ill. The literature has shown that inpatient care is an effective method to manage both the physical and psychological aspects of anorexia nervosa (14). However, the change in health care influenced by health maintenance organizations (HMOs) has altered the face of inpatient treatment. The pressure to reduce length of stay (LOS) for hospitalized patients and reduced insurance coverage for the management of eating disorders has limited treatment. Bezold et al. (26) reported that the average length of stay in a psychiatric hospital decreased 25% between 1988 and 1992. The pressure to reduce cost is translated into reductions in LOS for individuals with an eating disorder. The same type of decrease in LOS has been reported regarding hospitalization for eating disorders. Over a 15-year period from 1984 to 1998, the length of stay for a hospitalized eating disorder patient went from 149.5 days in 1984 to 22.7 days in 1998 (27). The reduction in LOS affects the health of the patient, adversely influencing long-term care, and contributing to high readmission rates (28).

One positive result of managed care creating pressure to reduce LOS has been the development of day treatment or partial hospitalization programs (PHPs) (29). Although these programs are influenced by their own health care climates, there are similarities among PHPs (30). Among the common elements are use of a multidisciplinary staff, group treatment as a primary method of treatment, and the use of the PHP as part of a continuum of care for some programs. The design of the program often reflects the area in which the program works, such as a freestanding program or as part of a hospital-based treatment model. Most programs run from 3 to 5 days a week and integrate some form of cognitive–behavioral therapy, readiness, or motivational therapy into the treatment (31). Empirical data about the effectiveness of PHPs is sparse. However, there is an indication that these programs can be effective in continuing gains from an inpatient treatment program as well as assist reduction in symptoms when patients "step up" from outpatient status (28,32). One study (28) documented empirical decision rules for optimizing successful transition from inpatient to PHP.

The American Psychiatric Association guidelines for the management of eating disorders (33) give both specific and broad recommendations for evidence-based, current best-practice treatment of eating disorders resulting from research studies and clinical consensus (34). The revised guidelines have detailed the necessity of integrating nutritional rehabilitation, psychosocial treatments, medical procedures, and psychopharmacological interventions, and summarize levels of care for a treatment continuum. This continuum includes outpatient, intensive outpatient, partial hospitalization and full-day programming, and residential and inpatient care. The remainder of the chapter presents a prototype for inpatient and partial hospitalization based on APA guidelines in the management of eating disorders.

INPATIENT TREATMENT

The comprehensive treatment of anorexia nervosa often requires inpatient care as part of a continuum of care to restore healthy mental, physical, and social functioning. This type of program must achieve safe, prompt, and effective short-term hospital-based improvement. It must also prepare patients for transition to a less intense, step-down, partial hospitalization treatment, followed by long-term continued outpatient care emphasizing relapse prevention and health promotion. The conceptual model most appropriate for guiding the management of anorexia nervosa is that of a multifactorial etiologic process. Eating disorders have never been adequately explained by single etiologic factors but require a more complex, multifactorial understanding of both origin and treatment. Since treatments logically grow out of assumptions of the nature of the disorder, the clearest possible description of known contributing factors is important for guiding effective management of eating disorders.

Admission to hospital for management of anorexia nervosa or bulimia nervosa remains a clinical decision based on multiple factors, summarized in Table 1. Many of these factors interact with or potentiate each other. For example, a very rapid weight loss of 25 pounds may be medically more dangerous than a slower weight loss of 40 pounds. Hypokalemia with an irregular but nonbradycardic heartbeat may be more medically serious than a very slow regular heartbeat of 40, gradually attained.

The broad goals of inpatient care are weight restoration and beginning treatment for the psychological and environmental factors that contribute to maintenance of the disorder, especially overvalued beliefs and cognitive distortions, and dysfunctional family systems. Table 2 summarizes significant but achievable goals for the inpatient care of persons with anorexia nervosa. Weight restoration (a vital but not exclusive goal) means restoration of a fully

TABLE 1   Criteria for Admission to Inpatient Care for Eating Disorders

1. Severe or rapid self-induced weight loss (or lack of normal gain), usually to less than 85% of normal weight or with significant medical, psychological, and social abnormality.
2. Lack of response to a reasonable trial of outpatient treatment with lack of improvement in weight or binge–purge symptoms.
3. Significant psychiatric comorbidity, including major depressive illness, severe OCD, borderline personality with impulsive behaviors, substance abuse, self-harm plans or behaviors.
4. Significant medical complications, including hypokalemia, cardiac abnormalities, comorbid diabetes mellitus, etc.
5. Lack of outpatient facilities, or a toxic/barren family or psychosocial environment.
6. Diagnosis and treatment of weight loss/low weight or binge–purge behavior in atypical cases from medical or psychiatric referrals where diagnosis is uncertain but significant problems exist in eating behavior or weight control.

TABLE 2   Goals of Treatment

1. Healthy body weight:
   (a) adequate weight
   (b) stable weight
   (c) healthy body composition
2. Normal eating behavior in time, manner, content
3. Development of social comfort, personal confidence, knowledge of balanced nutrition with practice in eating meals in a wide variety of situations
4. Management of comorbid psychiatric disorders
5. Moderate, appropriate exercise behavior
6. Resolution of major distorted cognitions regarding body weight, body image, fear of fatness, pursuit of thinness, etc.
7. Resolution or initiation of management of significant medical complications
8. Improved family/interpersonal interaction
9. Formulation and resolution of central dynamic conflict
10. Development of age-appropriate identity
11. Aftercare plans for treatment
12. Relapse prevention plans and readmission criteria

healthy body weight, with rebuilding of body and organ tissue as well as organ functioning, not excessive fluid weight, as may occur with hyperalimentation. Restoration to a healthy body weight is a means, not an end, to comprehensive treatment. The conclusive work of treatment involves a fundamental and enduring change in distorted thinking concerning weight, shape, size, and appearance. Treatment is focused on decreasing the overinvestment in thinness as a means of dealing with crucial central issues in life, such as mood regulation, personal identity, or family stability.

The initial goal of inpatient care is medical stabilization. Medical stabilization is intended to differentiate between slowly produced symptoms of starvation that are part of the body's adaptive response to decreased energy intake and which will generally respond to simple nutritional rehabilitation versus those medical signs and symptoms that are life threatening or atypical. This distinction requires the clinician to thoroughly understand the adaptive responses of the body to starvation. Many of the social behaviors and psychological symptoms attributed to anorexia nervosa are, in fact, due to starvation and will normalize by restoration to a healthy body weight. The rapidity of weight loss, methods of weight loss, physical examination results, and laboratory tests are some of the factors that need to be understood in the acute medical stabilization of the patient. Some medical symptoms will improve with weight restoration alone (stable bradycardia in most cases) whereas others require acute intervention (prolonged QT interval). The key is to distinguish between adaptive responses to starvation, which will improve without specific intervention versus potentially life-threatening signs and symptoms.

The significance of nutritional rehabilitation cannot be stressed enough in any treatment setting. Patients are not able to perform the detailed psychological work of challenging and changing beliefs without also allowing their bodies, especially brain functioning, to recover physically as well. Placing the majority of the recovery and healing work in the beginning of treatment on psychotherapy alone without concurrently working on weight restoration is a questionable use of time and money.

In an inpatient or partial hospitalization setting, food is the patient's primary medicine. Sometimes it is the only medicine. At other times, it is one of several medications. The use of a treatment protocol that deals with all of the specifics related to management of the patient's weight restoration creates consistency. Nurses and nursing assistants initially remain with patients for 24-hour support and supervision, until a normal eating pattern is established and comprehensive assessment of the patient's psychological and physical state has been obtained. Nurses sit with patients at all meals and encourage them to eat. We emphasize psychological support and use the milieu for group encouragement while empathizing with the patient's fear of fatness. No discussion of weight or calories is permitted; rather, we emphasize self-understanding of the patient's feelings and thoughts. An empathic nursing-supervised weight restoration program using normal food in a milieu setting with group support results in patients' beginning to eat three meals a day with only moderate anxiety within 24 hours. Occasionally, very anxious patients receive a small amount of antianxiety agent (lorazepam, 0.5 mg 1 h before meals) for a week or two. Rarely, small doses of antipsychotic medications may be used. Using our approach a nasogastric tube is rare and in treating more than 900 patients, hyperalimentation has not been necessary in any case.

There are several approaches to setting the goal for desired weight gain. In general, we strive for a healthy normal weight. The three standards generally used are (a) the Metropolitan Life tables (35) for patients 18 and over; (b) the nomograms devised by Frisch and McArthur (36) for achieving the weight necessary for return of periods in females and for adolescent girls; or (c) a body mass index appropriate for age. A reasonable goal is the midrange of the weight on the Metropolitan Life chart for a given height (with appropriate age correction and, occasionally, frame correction) or a body mass index (BMI) between 20 and 25. For female patients younger than 18, with secondary amenorrhea, we use the weight identified by Frisch and McArthur (36) for a 50% chance of return of menstrual cycles. It should be noted that the weight for return of periods is about 10 pounds higher than the weight required to begin menstrual cycles during normal development. For patients below 14, 100% weight for height for age is used as the definition for 100% of expected weight in children and young adolescents, as available on the internet at http://www.cdc.gov/growthcharts/.

However, picking a number from a chart is not the whole answer. Some attention should be given to the weight at which the patient functioned well if she or he had a time of stable weight and height before the onset of illness. The average anorexic patient often begins dieting at 5–10% above the matched population ideal weight at the onset of dieting. There is a rationale for setting the goal weight of these patients at 5–15% above the "ideal" weight. Since many of these patients may be biologically normal only when above the ideal in weight. However, few patients accept this reasoning and few clinicians practice individualization of weight goals within the normal range.

Where practical considerations dictate a short inpatient treatment period, moderate weight gain to 85–90% of normal may have to be accepted. In this case, close follow-up is required in a partial hospitalization program or an outpatient clinic. A goal weight range, rather than a single point, should be set so that patients can fluctuate comfortably within a 4- to 5-pound (1.4 kg) range. The weight goal is not firmly set when the patient comes to the hospital but only after treatment has been underway for several weeks. The weight range is made as a decision among the team members if variation from protocol is needed. Not telling patients their goal weight range until they are in the middle of it allows changes to be made by staff without incurring the wrath or fear of patients perceiving that a promise is being broken about a given weight range.

The initial food prescribed begins with 1200–1500 calories per day, according to the patient's admission weight, low in fat, salt, and lactose. No diet foods of any kind are allowed. The dietitian has an essential role in relating to patients, families, and staff. They take a complete nutritional history from the patient upon admission. However, they do not discuss treatment directly with the patient until weight is in the maintenance range. Every day the dietitian is present at staff rounds to help make decisions about changes in dietary programs. If the dietitian and the patients interact directly during nutritional rehabilitation, patients may demand endless changes in menu. Patients name three specific foods to delete from their menu, but other than these three specific choices (e.g., artichoke, pork chops, scrambled eggs), they do not determine the foods prescribed. Vegetarianism is permitted only if part of an established religious or philosophical practice (for example, Seventh-Day Adventist) preceding the eating disorder. Most adolescent vegetarianism in eating-disordered patients represents an early phase of their eating disorder. Calories are increased by 500 every 4–5 days until a maximum of 3500–4500 calories per day is achieved. The exact number will depend on the individual rate of weight gain, the height of the patient, and the presence of gastrointestinal discomfort. Once nutritional rehabilitation has been underway for several weeks, most calories can be prescribed in fairly dense form, including a moderate amount of fats and sweets. A safe continuing weight restoration averaging 3 pounds a week in females and 4 pounds a week in males can be achieved without significant medical symptoms, except for occasional pedal edema (easily managed without diuretics by feet elevation, limitation of salt, and psychoeducation).

Although the initial emphasis of inpatient care is weight restoration and/or disrupting the chaotic binge–purge cycle, additional interventions, especially psychoeducation and cognitive–behavioral therapy (CBT) are soon added. These interventions include various theoretical models such as psychodynamic, systems, and cognitive–behavioral therapies using individual, group, family, occupational, and recreational therapy formats (15). Specific practice guidelines in the management of anorexia nervosa emphasize the use of individual and family therapy among other approaches during inpatient treatment (33). These guidelines suggest the use of cognitive therapy as a model for psychotherapy. CBT has been shown to be the most effective psychological method in the management of bulimia nervosa (37). CBT can be effectively applied to management of anorexia nervosa, although definitive demonstration of its effectiveness in anorexia nervosa has not been proven. Shared goals between the two disorders include decreased illness-driven eating and social patterns, and their replacement by healthy behaviors. Because anorexia nervosa and bulimia nervosa share symptoms (overemphasis on body shape and weight as sources of self-esteem and identity, relentless drive for thinness, phobic fear of normal weight, rigid dietary habits), CBT seems well suited for the management of a heterogeneous mix of eating disorders during inpatient treatment (37–39).

What is suggested as a model for inpatient treatment is a hospital unit with all psychological interventions based on the principles of CBT. CBT conceptualizes eating disorders in a developmental framework with primacy on cognition mediating distressed emotion and resulting abnormal behavior (40,41). However, this theory also accommodates factors from psychodynamic and biological paradigms. Cognitive theory in general, and especially theory of eating disorders, views biology as an important part of the disorder, similar to other disorders such as depression. The cognitive model also blends with more dynamic approaches, as it encompasses the idea that an individual's life does not occur in a vacuum. The model will acknowledge many interpersonal and intrapersonal factors that contribute to the etiologic progression and maintenance of the disorder. The cognitive model places a high value on developing alternate ways of seeing the world and coping with day-to-day events. Cognitive theory and therapy work with dynamic concepts by changing developmental templates, schemas, and core beliefs (42,43).

The cognitive model views an eating disorder as a final common pathway of multiple events or experiences (40). Through various life experiences interacting with personality features, specific distorted ideas regarding the self, the world, and the future are learned (schemas), which then create vulnerability to an eating disorder. Vulnerable individuals, who are often introverted, sensitive, persevering, fearful of the challenges of development, and socially isolated, develop the idea that weight loss will somehow alleviate psychological distress and dysphoria (40,44). Dieting, weight loss, and attaining thinness become factors these individuals manipulate in an attempt to exercise control over their internal and external environments (44,45). Continued weight loss, which has become a sign of control, leads to social praise at first; then, shortly after, social criticism that may be threatening to these patients' sense of internal and external control. This perceived criticism leads to increased social isolation that reinforces distorted cognitions and maladaptive behaviors of an eating disorder.

We use a design called the comprehensive model of cognitive therapy (46) to organize an inpatient unit. Unit leaders, primary therapists, and adjunctive therapists are all trained in cognitive therapy when using a comprehensive model. Each intervention is designed to blend with the other psychotherapies. The milieu (a) fully accommodates cognitive therapy; (b) supports individual, family, and group therapies with cognitive therapy interventions; and (c) integrates psychoeducational programs to complement and reinforce the learning of cognitive therapy principles. Beck's (47) original model, modifications of this model for inpatient settings (39,48), and adaptations by Garner et al. (44) for outpatient management of anorexia nervosa along with Fairburn's (49) approach to managing bulimia nervosa are the foundation of unit structure.

The cognitive therapy milieu operates on the premise that patients are affected by their environment and in turn influence that environment. The milieu is a microcosm of the patient's world providing the treatment staff and patient with an opportunity to understand their problems. Recreation of the patient's world assists the treatment team in identifying cognitive distortions, basic assumptions, schemas, and core beliefs as they occur, with recognition of transference relationships as conveying vital information about family and peer relationships. Through recognition, acknowledgment, and acceptance of their problems, patients can gain new insight that allows them to address and modify their distorted thinking patterns and beliefs.

PROGRAM SCHEDULING

Patients are involved in some form of treatment much of the day. A detailed weekly schedule is displayed in Table 3, which includes several

TABLE 3 Daily Patient Schedule

	Sun	Mon	Tue	Wed	Thu	Fri	Sat
	8:15–9:00 a.m. Breakfast	8:00–8:45 a.m. Breakfast	8:00–8:45 a.m. Breakfast	8:00–8:45 a.m. Breakfast	8:00–8:45 a.m. Breakfast	8:00–8:45 a.m. Breakfast	8:00–8:45 a.m. Breakfast
		8:45–9:30 a.m. Psychoeducation group	8:45–9:30 a.m. Psychoeducation group			8:45–9:30 a.m. Psychoeducation group	
	9:30–10:00 a.m. Religious Service	9:30–10:00 a.m. Activity	9:30–10:00 a.m. Activity	9:30–10:00 a.m. Activity	9:30–10:00 a.m. Activity	9:30–10:00 a.m. Activity	
		10:30–11:45 a.m. School	10:30–11:45 a.m. School	10:30–11:45 a.m. School	10:30–11:45 a.m. School	10:30–11:45 a.m. School	
			10:30–11:45 a.m. O.T. Meal preparation/ shopping	10:30–11:45 a.m. O.T. Meal preparation/ shopping			
	11:45–12:30 p.m. Lunch	11:45–12:30 p.m. Lunch	11:45–12:30 p.m. Lunch	11:45–12:30 p.m. Lunch	11:45–12:30 p.m. Lunch	11:45–12:30 p.m. Lunch	11:45–12:30 p.m. Lunch
		12:30–1:00 p.m. O.T. Meal plan preparation	12:30–1:00 p.m. O.T. Coping skills group		12:30–1:00 p.m. O.T. Coping skills group		

	2:00–3:00 p.m. Body perception group	1:30–3:00 p.m. Cognitive therapy group	2:00–3:00 p.m. Body perception group	2:00–3:00 p.m. Cognitive therapy group	2:00–3:00 p.m. Body perception group	2:00–3:00 p.m. Body perception group
2:30–3:00 p.m. Snack	2:30–3:00 p.m. Snack	2:30–3:00 p.m. Snack	2:30–3:00 p.m. Snack	2:30–3:00 p.m. Snack	2:30–3:00 p.m. Snack	2:30–3:00 p.m. Snack
	3:00–3:45 p.m. Activity	3:00–3:45 p.m. Activity	3:00–3:45 p.m. Activity	3:00–3:45 p.m. Activity	3:00–3:45 p.m. Activity	
5:00–5:45 p.m. Supper	5:00–5:45 p.m. Supper	5:00–5:45 p.m. Supper	5:00–5:45 p.m. Supper	5:00–5:45 p.m. Supper	5:00–5:45 p.m. Supper	5:00–5:45 p.m. Supper
	7:00–8:00 p.m. Activity	7:00–8:00 p.m. Activity	7:00–8:00 p.m. Activity	7:00–8:00 p.m. Activity	7:00–8:00 p.m. Activity	
			8:30–9:30 p.m. Psychoeducation group	8:30–9:30 p.m. Psychoeducation group		
8:30–9:00 p.m. Snack	8:30–9:00 p.m. Snack	8:30–9:00 p.m. Snack	8:30–9:00 p.m. Snack	8:30–9:00 p.m. Snack	8:30–9:00 p.m. Snack	8:30–9:00 p.m. Snack
11:30 p.m. Bedtime adolescents	11:30 p.m. Bedtime adolescents	11:30 p.m. Bedtime adolescents	11:30 p.m. Bedtime adolescents	11:30 p.m. Bedtime adolescents	11:30 p.m. Bedtime adolescents	11:30 p.m. Bedtime adolescents

types of group treatments. Typically they begin with a psychoeducational group, in which they learn about basic cognitive therapy principles, the effects of starvation, and principles of healthy social and psychological functioning. Patients participate in an activities therapy group three times per week with content focusing on building leisure time skills. An occupational therapy group meets twice a week. The first session focuses on meal planning and purchasing. The second session focuses on meal preparation and is followed by a structured group discussion of attitudes and emotions after the meal. Twice a week the patient participates in an additional occupational therapy group that focuses on coping skills and emphasizes role playing. Patients participate in a cognitive therapy group three times a week and that group alternates with a body perception group. Snacks are provided in the groups with a structured discussion time following the snack. Dinner is served with a structured observation and discussion time following the meal. Structured observation is divided into various levels with the most intense level being 24-h continuous observation by the unit staff. As a patient progresses through treatment, the amount of time under staff observation is changed (Table 4). Study time, if appropriate, is

TABLE 4 Inpatient Eating Disorder Observation Levels (EDO)

24-hour observation. Patient is under continuous observation by staff with
   bathroom locked.

Standard EDO on admission
   Standard EDO is from 8 a.m. until 10 p.m. for at least one week after admission.
Patients attend all unit activities provided their physical and mental health permit.

Eating Disorder Observation + 2
   Patient is observed by the unit staff for 2 h after each meal.

Eating Disorder Observation + 1
   Patient is observed by the unit staff for 1 h after each meal.

Eating Disorder Observation Meals Only
   Patient has not observation by unit staff after meals.

Indications for changing observation levels
   Unexplained weight fluctuations
   Strong impulse to behave inappropriately
   Staff suspicion that the patient is behaving inappropriately
   Abnormal of increase in serum amylase

scheduled before the evening meal, except on the weekends. A final social or recreational activity occurs from 7:00 p.m. until 8:30 p.m.

The interdisciplinary approach provides the patient with a comprehensive treatment program whereby each member of the team has a clear understanding of the unique and shared treatment goals of each discipline. Team members work closely together, meeting at least twice a week on these issues to provide the patients with the structure they need in treatment. This team focuses on the goal of changing illness behavior and thinking, not only in the protected environment of the inpatient unit but on an enduring basis after discharge. The treatment team consists of a staff psychiatrist, psychiatry resident, psychologist, advanced registered nurse practitioner (ARNP), primary nurse, social worker, occupational therapist, dietitian, and activities therapist. Some patients will also need a vocational rehabilitation therapist or, if the patient is a student, an educational consultant. This team works with the patient to understand his or her individual life history, including the cognitive conceptualization behind the eating disorder. The issues the team will work on in collaboration with the patient are multifaceted. These issues include self-esteem, body image, possible sexual abuse, addictions, family issues, marital relationships, parent–child relationships, and interpersonal dynamics. There is also a focus on coping skills for stress management, compulsive exercise, leisure time activities, nutrition and cooking, assertiveness, relaxation, mood, and perfectionism.

A comprehensive psychiatric evaluation is obtained by a detailed psychiatric interview. This time-honored process is supplemented by a standardized written assessment tool, such as the Eating Disorders Evaluation (50). This comprehensive, semistructured interview is designed to assess broad clinical features of an eating disorder, especially attitudes and behaviors related to the illness over the preceding 4 weeks. A part of the psychiatric case organization includes all features of the case, including a summary of pertinent features, diagnosis and differential diagnosis, etiological factors, treatment plans, and prognosis. Brief self-report measures such as the Eating Disorders Inventory (EDI; 51) and Eating Attitudes Test (EAT; 52) identify specific aspects of the disorder, including desire for thinness, binge–purge behavior, and restraint in eating. Because the EAT and EDI are valid, reliable, and easily administrated instruments, repeat administration of these tests can document severity of illness at admission as well as record improvements during treatment.

Often treatment of comorbid conditions is as challenging as the primary eating disorder itself. Personality functioning and the presence of axis I comorbid disorders such as depression and anxiety disorders are important to assess. Affective disorders are the most common associated axis I comorbidity, present in 50–80% of eating disorders with bulimic symptomology, and a substantial number of anorexic patients, with many having secondary but severe depressions. Intellectual functioning warrants assessment for a number of reasons. Many patients have expectations for academic or vocational performance beyond their ability based more on persevering traits than inherent giftedness. Evidence of actual level of intellectual functioning may be sympathetically used to change these expectations and therefore modify some of the cognitive distortions arising from such misperceptions. In addition, significant neuropsychological deficits are present in about 35% of starved patients.

Although supportive psychotherapy and psychoeducation are often used during the early phases of inpatient care, we are more aggressive in beginning a cognitive–behavioral psychotherapeutic approach from the earliest part of treatment. Individual and group therapy use Beck's model (46) with modifications specifically for an inpatient eating disorders unit (39,53). It must be recognized that this approach may be only partially effective until there is adequate weight restoration, but the basic concepts are familiar when patients are more effective in cognitive functioning. However, in our experience even patients who have difficulty with the more abstract concepts of cognitive therapy can benefit from the early behavioral components such as mood monitoring, problem solving, and graded task assignments. We also believe that early use of behavioral CBT methods establishes the groundwork for more cognitive interventions. With ongoing weight restoration through nutritional interventions early in therapy, there is a synergetic effect with the cognitive therapy. This work will be increasingly successful as weight restores a patient to 85–90% of a healthy goal weight and then to fully normal weight for age and height.

Individual cognitive therapy also places a high value on the articulate identification, expression, and understanding of emotions. Many times, "I feel fat" is the global and generic phrase for any dysphoria prior to cognitive therapy. Increased awareness, understanding, and expression of emotion are gradually achieved through the therapist's observation of inconsistencies, incongruities, and inappropriate emotional reactions from the patient's everyday events. Confirmation and reinforcement of emotions that are a genuine part of the patient's past and present experience are essential. The patient is encouraged to express all emotions, especially "unacceptable" emotions. With the therapist serving as a model for expression of emotion, the patient can learn that open expression of emotions does not lead to rejection (40) or out-of-control behavior. There is a consistent emphasis on separating "I feel" from "I think" statements, e.g., changing "I feel fat" to "I think I am fat and those thoughts make me anxious and depressed."

Cognitive therapy attempts to help the patient recognize and change the rigid standards employed to determine self-worth. The message communicated is that positive self-evaluation develops from success through mastery in small, stepwise, increasingly challenging personal activities. Exceptional or perfect performances are not necessary. Competence by way of reasonable standards (emphasizing adequacy, not perfection), as well as learning and accepting "in-betweens," is very important. Self-acceptance, despite personal shortcomings based on unrealistic standards, is a fundamental goal for the psychotherapist working with a patient with an eating disorder. Cognitive therapy can also address the lack of trust in and the fear of feelings or expression of emotions (40). To accomplish this, the therapist must confirm genuine expressions of inner feelings while labeling misconceptions and errors in the patient's thinking. Denial or absence of seemingly appropriate affect should be explored in greater detail. It is critical to progress slowly and let the patient learn to identify his or her emotions. Another crucial component of CBT is assisting patients in identifying their affective states and in promoting acceptance of these feelings as real and wholesome, with "no bad feelings, but responsible actions."

Group Therapy

Psychoeducational Group

All groups are ongoing and a patient will enter group immediately after admission to the unit. The psychoeducational group explores various aspects of cognitive therapy (i.e., cognitive distortions, automatic thoughts) in a didactic fashion and its relationship to an eating disorder. The purpose of this group is to teach patients the basic concepts of cognitive therapy and information about the effects of the disorder. After each group, assignments using these concepts are given to the patients to complete before the next group. Some of the objectives of this group are that the patient will:

> Define the basic cognitive therapy principles (i.e., cognitive triad, assumptions, automatic thoughts, cognitive distortions, schemas, core beliefs).
> Demonstrate the ability to rate his or her mood.
> Identify automatic thoughts that he or she experiences.
> Demonstrate application of the reframing technique for changing negative automatic thoughts.
> Demonstrate an ability to use the thought records.
> Define and then apply the problem solving to his or her own life experiences.
> Define or demonstrate at least one cognitive therapy intervention that is personally applicable (e.g., identifying automatic thoughts, chal-

lenging automatic thoughts, reattribution techniques, advantages/
disadvantages and homework).

The instructional methods used by the group leaders are didactic, role plays,
discussions, practice sessions, homework, peer feedback, and creative expression exercises (artwork, etc.). The psychoeducational groups run daily for 1
hour. Outcomes of the group are measured by satisfactory completion of
homework assignments, active participation in the group discussions, and
activities that reflect an understanding of the content being taught.

The materials and information given to each patient have been adapted
from various authors in the area of cognitive therapy. Ancillary areas covered
in this group include exploring self-identity and self-esteem, values clarification, feelings identification, and problem solving. Other psychoeducational
material has been integrated directly relating to eating disorders. Included is
information on the effects of starvation, how the disorder functions psychologically, and the social and media views of an individual's appearance (54).

Cognitive Group Therapy

Group cognitive therapy combines Beck's theory and interventions in a
process-oriented framework (15,55). Group therapy in the management of
eating disorders is increasingly recognized as an important, effective, and
economical psychotherapeutic tool (15). Group therapy may not only be
economical; it contains factors unique to effective groups, namely, peer
challenges, feedback, support, and empathic paralleling. As a basic approach,
a blend of process orientation (56) and cognitive–behavioral principles
(15,55) appears to be most effective. Blending of these two models gives the
group latitude to deal with personal and interpersonal issues. Using the
curative factors of group (56) and cognitive therapy principles creates a focus
on cognitive and developmental factors involved with eating disorders. The
group can also influence the perceptions of the patients and permit patients to
assist in each other's recovery from disorder through self-disclosure and
confrontation of symptomatic behavior, distorted ideas, and negative attitudes. An inpatient group may be more diagnostically heterogeneous (including anorexia nervosa and bulimia nervosa). However, the common themes of
both eating disorders blend the otherwise diverse population into a psychologically homogeneous group by emphasizing the common features.

In the groups that are run on the unit, such concepts as cognitive
distortions, automatic thoughts, schemas, and core beliefs are discussed in
a setting that uses situations that arose during the day or between groups. In
addition, material that comes from the group itself is available to show
how the ideas of cognitive therapy are ever present with patients. It is also
an opportunity for more skilled members of the group to assist newer group
members in first identifying automatic thoughts, schemas, and core beliefs.

A cognitive therapy group challenges the weight- and shape-centered view of the world that patients have established through their distorted cognitions. In our experience, much of the group work lends itself toward helping the patients understand how their cognitions affect their mood and consequent behaviors. Another healing factor is the ability of group members to easily identify in others the ramifications of their own eating disorder. As patients help others identify and change negative cognitions, they also improve their own, often coming to resolution of their issues as reflected in others.

Body Perception Group

Our body perception group focuses on helping patients understand their body distortions and how these distortions affect their lives and sustain the eating disorder. We have found this area to be one of the most difficult aspects of the illness. The group has been extremely valuable for adjusting distorted body images. The patients are supportive yet confrontive, helping each other face these distortions and bring their cognitions into the realm of reality. What we often see is that the distortion usually does not completely resolve, but through this work the patients learn to diminish the impact of these thoughts and begin to put them into proper perspective. The cognitive therapy model is effective in helping patients challenge their belief systems and realize their lack of validity, as well as establishing alternatives. When patients are challenged to provide a rationale to support these distortions, they are frequently surprised to find that they cannot offer any validation.

This group operates from two basic premises: (a) all patients in the group have the diagnosis of an eating disorder and (b) the diagnosis of an eating disorder usually includes a distorted body image. Therefore, the patients cannot trust their perceptions of how they appear to themselves and others. The format of the group is discussion based, with the patients sharing in each session how they are feeling about the changes their bodies are undergoing in the process of restoration. It is an accepted fact in the group that the patients' body sizes are changing and that is a frightening experience for them. The discussions within the group are twofold. First, patients are encouraged to openly and honestly express feelings and thoughts concerning body perceptions. Second, we move to fact-versus-fiction discussions regarding distorted body image. Patients need to discover that to feel positive about their bodies they must learn to rely on facts rather than distorted perceptions. By identifying, challenging, and reframing automatic thoughts, patients begin to feel different about their bodies.

Family Therapy

Family therapy maintains a cognitive framework designed to work with family communications and schemas (57). Family therapy is important to treatment outcome with this patient population and is an ongoing process in our program of care. Parents and siblings frequently exhibit a sense of hopelessness regarding the recovery of their family member, often intermixed with anger and anxiety, with fathers more often showing the former and mothers the latter. Many of the families we have worked with have been told that their family member will probably not survive. Family therapy sessions are held on a regular basis with the patient, family members, and/or a significant other. The content is determined by the patient's issues that have been pinpointed in the day-to-day treatment process. These families often have difficulty identifying feelings and expressing emotions, and not infrequently there are underlying family secrets and unspoken issues that impair open communication. The hopelessness and anger these individuals are feeling must also be addressed and assisted to resolution. The focus of the sessions is on the interactions between the patient and the family and resolution of the eating disorder. Our premise is that the eating disorder maybe a symptom of other unresolved underlying problems. However, families are assumed to be blameworthy for any aspect of the illness, and often need to be relieved of the belief that they could have prevented the illness, and that in fact this is an illness rather than a personal or family failing.

This work is always done within the CBT framework. The families are taught through the therapy sessions to identify feelings and automatic thoughts, to challenge automatic thoughts, and to reframe and examine the changes in their feelings before and after the challenge. Some of the parents have marital issues that need to be resolved, and such couples are referred to a therapist in their locale or within the facility of treatment where they can pursue these issues more intensely. Such issues may include triangulating, untreated mood disorders, waning marital bonding, and so forth.

Another form of family therapy is increasingly important while working with inpatients and partial hospitalization programs. A manual for psychotherapeutic interventions with families for adolescent AN has recently been developed (25) incorporating elements of the Maudsley treatment program that have been found effective for adolescent AN patients (58). This protocol underscores the central role of parents as a resource in the treatment of adolescent patients with AN. Unlike more traditional family therapy models in which the patient is seen as having developed a problem in response to external or internal factors (e.g., genetic, physiological, familial, or sociocultural), the Maudsley approach focuses on how the family can effectively promote healthy eating behavior per se. This treatment emphasizes the parents' ability to help the adolescent overcome the "intrusion" of AN in his or her normal development. The main focus of treatment is empowerment of the parents so that they can succeed in restoring their starving child. It is only after the eating disorder has been successfully addressed that the parents will hand control over eating back to the adolescent. It is at this point that the family will begin to discuss other issues.

The theoretical underpinning of the Maudsley approach is the view that the adolescent is imbedded in the family and that the parents are critical in the ultimate success of treatment. The eating disorder is seen to be interfering with regular adolescent development. Therefore, the parents should take an active role in their offspring's treatment while at the same time showing respect for the adolescent. This treatment pays close attention to adolescent development and guides the parents to assist their adolescent with developmental tasks once the eating disorder has been removed. In doing so, any meaningful work on other family conflicts or disagreements must be deferred until the eating disorder is out of the way. In some cases, effective parental guidance may prevent the hospitalization of even very starved adolescent patients.

Role of Medications in Treatment

The use of medicines to stimulate appetite is generally unhelpful and counter-productive for two reasons. First, appetite mechanisms in brain are normal even in starved individuals. Second, without psychotherapeutic improvement, increased appetite leads to increased anxiety and attempts to vomit or exercise. Antidepressants have been advocated for both anorexia and bulimia nervosa and may well have a role in management of comorbid depression in both (17). However, a suggested practice has been to prescribe antidepressants only after patients' body weights are normal, their eating patterns are normal, and after they have had experience with intensive psychotherapy. Antidepressants have been demonstrated to be generally ineffective in starved patients (16). After these three goals have been achieved, if the patient still meets criteria for major depressive illness, then antidepressants are prescribed. The current reports in the literature are not yet sufficiently convincing to suggest that antidepressants have a routine role during the low-weight phase of illness. Fluoxetine is approved for management of bulimia nervosa. We selectively, rather than generally, use selective serotonin reuptake inhibitors for management of the binge–purge subtype of anorexia nervosa since CBT alone is often effective. Obsessive-compulsive symptoms may also be improved with weight restoration and should be reevaluated after weight restoration before anti-OCD medications are used. Exceptions may of course occur. Occasionally patients benefit from prokinetic agents (Reglan) to decrease bloating, or H_2 blockers or proton pump inhibitors (Zantac or Prilosec) where reflux esophagitis is present.

THE DISCHARGE PROCESS

Aftercare planning begins as close as possible to the time of admission. Eating disorders severe enough to require inpatient treatment will require experienced long-term follow-up, preferably partial hospitalization followed by experienced outpatient treatment usually for one to several years. The data from follow-up studies encouragingly demonstrate that 76% of eating disorder symptoms in adolescents requiring inpatient treatment may be completely ameliorated after several years of relapse prevention (59). The characteristics of satisfactory aftercare include pre-discharge decision making concerning step-down to partial hospitalization versus outpatient treatment alone. We involve the aftercare team in the discharge process, transmitting information about the course of treatment, sharing both the philosophy and practice of treatment. Patients returning to rural areas or to areas without experienced professionals may soon experience worsening of their symptoms. This is particularly true in view of the increasingly common problem of managed care–driven discharge of patients before they have had a chance to establish adequate weight, healthy patterns of behavior, (eating and exercise), and decreased cognitive distortions. Data do not support the frequently practiced discharge of patients at very low weight, immediately after medical danger or self-harm danger has passed but well before a healthy body weight has been achieved.

Readmission to hospital for management of relapse will generally be more effective and shorter if it occurs sooner rather than later. Prompt readmission should occur when the patient falls below 85% of target weight but a higher threshold may be appropriate. In addition, maintenance of body weight in the metastable weight range of 85–90% of target without improvement after 6 months should also warrant readmission. Other proven reasons for admission to a hospital include return of severe depressive illness or serious medical complications of the eating disorder. Eating disorders are spectrum disorders with a variable course and severity. A subgroup of patients may require repeated admissions. There is a tendency to blame patients for return to illness, as if the eating disorder was entirely voluntary, and for some health professionals or families to take a negative or punitive view toward eating disorder patients requiring readmission. For those patients, a minority who do have a chronic, severe, and relapsing eating disorder, readmission is necessary whenever indicated by clinical symptomatology and should not be a source of stigma or rejection. Clinicians recognize the need for readmissions in other disorders, such as diabetes or cardiac disease, with comparable stigma.

PARTIAL HOSPITALIZATION/DAY TREATMENT

The goals of a partial/day hospitalization program in the management of anorexia nervosa are (a) restore patients weight to 95–100% of their target range; (b) develop effective personal application of cognitive therapy to defeat the core psychopathology of body image distortion, drive for thinness, and fear of fatness; (c) increase development of leisure skills—not a cultural nicety but an essential for patients turning to their eating disorder during unstructured time in place of driven activity or feeling "stuck" or bored; (d) develop healthy coping skills to deal with developmental and everyday challenges; (e) replace body image distortion, drive for thinness, and fear of fatness, with healthy, accurate beliefs and attitudes; (f) develop healthy family relationship; (g) develop and demonstrate accurate beliefs about nutrition, especially the role of a moderate amount of heart-healthy lipids in place of a fat-phobia; (h) stop all bingeing, purging, and restriction of caloric intake; and (i) develop healthy self-esteem and mood stabilization, especially through internal self-regulation.

For those patients who are having difficulty with weight restoration at the outpatient level, a partial/day hospitalization can also be of great value as a "step-up" in intensity. The structured program that monitors meals and activities can assist in positive weight restoration. Patients' nutritional intake can be systematically increased until they are taking in an adequate number of calories (approx. 3500/day) to sustain a weight increase of 2 pounds per week. Along with the monitoring of their weight restoration, a structured partial hospitalization program can also address the medical and psychological aspects of starvation that interfere with response to outpatient care. Often individuals with anorexia have difficulty with weight restoration despite the best of intention and desire. When this is the problem the use of a partial hospitalization program is beneficial. As mentioned earlier, without adequate restoration of weight much of what happens in therapy is hindered. The intensive structure in a partial program is similar to that in an inpatient program, with development of a milieu to enhance cognitive–behavioral principles.

The structure is different from inpatient care only in that part of the day is spent in this intensive milieu. The structure of the program ideally covers from 8 a.m. until 6 p.m. in order to accommodate three full meals and at least two snacks. One change during meals is that patients may have more access to the selection and preparation of their own meals. Also, patients may not have the constant observation during meals or just after meals, as these are gradually diminished.

Decision to admit a patient to a partial program is usually based on failure to make progress during outpatient treatment or as a step-down from inpatient care. Often progress is measured by weight restoration or weight stabilization, as well as by ability to challenge cognitive distortions, and improvement in comorbid symptoms, such as depression, obsessive-compulsive disorder, etc.

Third-party payers when working with inpatients with anorexia often request movement to partial hospitalization. A partial program as part of a continuum of treatment allows patients to move to less restrictive care. It would be prudent to move from inpatient to partial hospitalization when a patient is at least 80–85% of target weight range, but individuals may need more time in inpatient treatment based on empirical studies. Weight is not the only criteria for movement to a less restrictive level of treatment. The ability to engage in psychotherapy must also be taken into consideration. Also, there needs to be criteria for when to bring a patient back onto an inpatient treatment program if partial hospitalization is ineffective.

Treatment in a partial/day hospitalization program is primary handled in a group format, both for cost and effectiveness reasons. Group treatment can be varied for those patients who are more or less advanced in the use of cognitive therapy. Group approaches also offer more socialization in the context of the cognitive model, as well as more chances to practice the concepts during the day. A psychoeducation group functions much as in inpatient treatment, but it can be split into more or less advanced tracks. If a patient has begun the partial/day program after failure in outpatient treatment the psychoeducational group would focus on more basic principles of cognitive therapy. Groups would build on the principles of cognitive therapy with an emphasis on the use of mood ratings, mastery and pleasure, graded task assignments, identification of automatic thoughts, cognitive distortions, and use of thought records. In addition, information regarding the effects of starvation on the body and psychological processing would be introduced with an emphasis on how these affect the interaction of thoughts, feelings, and behavior.

Patients who are more advanced in the principles of cognitive therapy would have a different track for the psychoeducational group with a greater focus on the ideas of schemas and core beliefs. This group would also focus on the societal aspects of eating disorders and discuss how these unrealistic standards influence and perhaps contribute to their own cognitive distortions about weight, shape, and appearance. The main influence of this group would be on the identification of their own schemas in order to understand the developmental aspects of their disorder. Patients would be shown methods to spot their core distorted beliefs by monitoring their emotional shifts and situations in which they find themselves using their disorder as a method for coping with intense emotions. This group would also use other existing material to assist in changing schemas and core beliefs.

Cognitive group therapy is the main psychotherapeutic vehicle in the partial/day hospitalization program. This type of group (depending on availability of therapists) can be run daily but must occur at least twice a week. The length of the session also is dependent on the frequency of the meetings, ranging from four to five times each week to longer sessions twice a week. This group can have two possible formats. One format is based on the individual cognitive therapy session, with definite structure. At the beginning of the group an agenda is developed from topics presented by the group members. All members are encouraged to be a part of the group, but more often time is spent with an individual topic on an individual member. Other members of the group and the group leaders give feedback to the member(s) involved. In this format group leaders are more interactive and lead the discussion among the group members. The alternative format is to develop a more process-oriented group in the partial/day hospitalization program. This cognitive group therapy is similar to that discussed in the chapter on inpatient treatment, blending of process orientation (56), and cognitive–behavioral principles (15,55). These two models allows more group latitude to deal with various personal and interpersonal issues. The curative factors of group (56) and cognitive therapy principles create a focus on cognitive and developmental factors involved with eating disorders. This group format influences the perceptions of the patients and assists patients in recovering from their disorder through self-disclosure and confrontation of symptomatic behavior, distorted ideas, and schematic material. It also provides an environment that validates emotions and assists patients in tolerating uncomfortable feelings while facilitating self-understanding.

The body image group also parallels the group run in an inpatient setting with a focus on helping patients understand their body distortions and how these distortions affect their lives and sustain the eating disorder. Patients are supportive yet confrontive with one another, helping each other face their distortions and bring their cognitions into basis in fact.

Unlike inpatients, the patients in partial hospitalization spend part of the day outside of a formal treatment setting. This time may be very anxiety producing but represents an essential practical format for gaining mastery in an everyday unstructured setting. Urges to restrict, exercise, or purge can be strong. In order to prepare patients for these urges and for efficient use of free time, each day is ended with a planning group emphasizing a plan for healthy thinking and behavior when not in treatment. Format is structured around alternative healthy plans that each member needs to practice as an alternative to not engaging in the disorder. This may include alternatives to the urge to restrict, exercise/purge, or binge. Specific plans may include relaxation, journaling, use of thought records, distraction, contacting on-call staff, and using each other as supports during times of intense urges to engage in their disorder. Weekends also are very difficult for some patients in a partial/day hospitalization program. Again emphasis is placed on the patients using their own resources to not engage in the eating disorder and to prepare plans that offer a greater sense of control over the disorder, as well as increased pleasure in self-regulation and normal developmental social and recreational interactions. Occupational therapy can prepare patients for daily living experiences and work with them in meal preparation including choice of foods, purchasing food, and cooking meals. Groups of patients are exposed to meal planning, shopping, meal preparation, and the actual eating of the meal. This gives patients a chance to support each other in what may have been a very difficult and solitary task, i.e., grocery shopping. Food is purchased twice a week, and members of the group prepare and eat the meal together. Again, with the help of group support and leader assistance, the planning, preparation, and consumption of a meal is approached and the problems arising from this task are exposed and challenged. In addition, patients learn that food and meals can be a strong social "glue" that helps to create the social support that often has been lacking in an anorexic patient's life.

Activities therapy has an important role in assisting the inpatient to reduce potentially dangerous exercise patterns, especially important in patients with osteoporosis, and to increase healthy social, recreational, and leisure activities. Patients need to understand what "normal" exercise looks like. Patients will begin an exercise program while in the program, including basic aerobic exercise and weight training under supervision of the activities therapist. The group focuses on leisure activities and learns how to use time wisely and in healthy, relaxing ways. This is very important for patients who have engaged in overexercise. An exercise prescription is given in place of an all-or-none pattern of drivenness versus sedentary patterns.

Involuntary Patients

One subject that has important bearing on inpatient treatment and, to a lesser degree, on partial hospitalization is the use of involuntary treatment. Although a controversial subject, involuntary commitment to treatment, through a judiciously applied legal process, is at times a life-saving way to assist individuals who have a life-threatening disorder but refuse hospitalization. There is a very modest literature that looks at the usefulness of legal commitment, and suggestions have been made that in some cases eating disorder patients who desire not to be treated should be respected even if it may mean their death (60). We strongly disagree. The literature that exists is generally positive about the judicious use of involuntary treatment. Involuntary treatment clearly has benefit in the short term (61,62), with most patients expressing at the time of discharge recognition of their peril at the time of admission. Also civil commitment is a valuable treatment tool when life-threatening situations emerge in an individual with an eating disorder who lacks the competence to make treatment decisions (63). It is noted that involuntary treatment does not require more extreme measures, such as nasogastric tube feeding. In addition, there is little support that involuntary treatment damages the therapeutic relationship with the patient (62). The small literature that exists suggests that 10–15% of severely ill patients who refused treatment and were involuntarily committed have similar treatment results as those who were treated voluntarily (64). In addition, the majority of those treated involuntarily agreed retrospectively with the necessity of treatment and showed good will toward the treatment process. In summary, involuntary treatment must be considered at times, especially when the patient is in a life-threatening situation and in denial about the necessity of treatment.

REFERENCES

1. Dally P, Sargent W. Treatment and outcome of anorexia nervosa. Br Med J 1960; 1:1770–1773.
2. Silverman J. Anorexia nervosa: clinical observations in a successful treatment program. J Pediatrics 1974; 84.68–73.
3. Russell GFM. The present status of anorexia nervosa. Psychol Med 1977; 7:353–367.
4. Maloney MJ, Farrell MK. Treatment of severe weight loss in anorexia nervosa with hyperalimentation and psychotherapy. Am J Psychiatry 1980; 137:310–314.
5. Vandereycken W. The use of neuroleptics in the treatment of anorexia nervosa patients. In: Garfinkel PE, Garner DM, eds. The Role of Drug Treatment in Eating Disorders. New York: Brunner/Mazel, 1987.
6. Agras WS, Schneider JA, Arnow B, Rathburn SD, Telch CF. Cognitive-behavioral treatment with and without exposure plus response prevention in the treatment of bulimia nervosa: a reply to Leitenberg and Rosen. J Consult Clin Psychol 1989; 57:778–779.
7. Eckert ED, Goldberg SC, Halmi KA, Casper RC, Davis JM. Behavior therapy and anorexia nervosa. Br J Psychiatry 1979; 134:55–59.
8. Touyz SW, Beumont PJV, Glaun D, Philips T, Cowie I. A comparison of lenient and strict operant conditioning programs in refeeding patients with anorexia nervosa. Br J Psychiatry 1984; 144:517–520.
9. Vandereycken W. The place of behavior therapy in the inpatient treatment of anorexia nervosa. Br Rev Bulimia Anorexia Nervosa 1989; 3:55–60.
10. Andersen AE, Morse C, Santmyer K. Inpatient treatment of anorexia Nervosa. In: Garner DM, Garfinkel PE, eds. Handbook of Psychotherapy for Anorexia Nervosa and Bulimia. Guilford Press, 1985:311–343.
11. Andersen, A.E. New York:Inpatient and outpatient treatment of anorexia nervosa. In: Brownell KD, Foreyt J.P, eds., Handbook of Eating Disorders: Physiology, Psychology, and Treatment of Obesity, Anorexia and Bulimia.New York:Basic Books, 1986.
12. Garner DM, Garfinkel PE, Irvine MJ. Integration and sequencing of treatment approaches for eating disorders. Psychother Psychosom 1986; 67–75.
13. Vandereycken W. Inpatient treatment of anorexia nervosa: some research-guided changes. J Psychiatr Res 1985; 19:413–422.

14. Andersen AE, Bowers WA, Evans KK. Inpatient treatment of anorexia nervosa. In: Garner DM, Garfinkel PE, eds. Handbook of Treatment for Eating Disorders. 2d ed. New York: Guilford Press, 1997:327–353.

15. Bowers WA, Andersen AE. Inpatient treatment of anorexia nervosa: review and recommendations. Harvard Rev Psychiatry, 1994.

16. Strober M, Pataki C, Freeman R, DeAntonio M. No effect of adjunctive fluoxetine on eating behavior or weight phobia during the inpatient treatment of anorexia nervosa: an historical case-control study. J Child Adolesc Psychopharmacol 1999; 9:195–201.

17. Mitchell JE, Peterson CB, Myers T, Wonderlich S. Combining pharmacotherapy and psychotherapy in the treatment of patients with eating disorders. Psychiatr Clin North Am 24:315–324.

18. Kaye WH, Weltzin TE, Bulik CM. An open trial of fluoxetine in patients with anorexia nervosa. J Clin Psychiatry 1991; 52:464–471.

19. Keel PK, Mitchell JE, Davis TL, Crow SJ. Long-term impact of treatment in women diagnosed with bulimia nervosa. Int J Eating Disord 2002; 31:151–158.

20. Rosenblum J, Forman S. Evidenced-based treatment of eating disorders. Curr Opin Pediatrics 2002; 14:379–383.

21. Bowers WA, Ansher LS. Cognitions in anorexia nervosa: changes at discharge from a cognitive therapy milieu inpatient program. J Cognitive Psychother 2000; 14:393–401.

22. Wilson GT, Fairburn CC, Agras WS, Walsh BT, Kraemer H. Cognitive-behavioral therapy for bulimia nervosa: time course and mechanisms of change. J Consult Clin Psychol 2002; 70:267–274.

23. Nakash-Eisikovits O, Dierberger A, Westen D. A multidimensional meta-analysis of pharmacotherapy for bulimia nervosa: summarizing the range of outcome in controlled clinical trials. Harvard Rev Psychiatry 2002; 10:193–211.

24. Zhu AJ, Walsh BT. Pharmacologic treatment of eating disorders. Can J Psychiatry 2002; 47:227–234.

25. Lock J, Le Grange D, Agras WS, Dare C. Treatment Manual for Anorexia Nervosa: A Family-Based Approach. New York: Guilford Press, 2001.

26. Bezold H, MacDowell M, Kunkel R. Predicting psychiatric length of stay. Admin Policy Men Health 1996; 23:407–423.

27. Wiseman CV, Sunday SR, Klapper F, Harris WA, Halmi KA. Changing patterns of hospitalization in eating disorder patients. Int J Eating Disord 2001; 30:69–74.

28. Howard WT, Evan KK, Quintero-Howard CV, Bowers WA, Andersen AE. Predictors of success or failure of transition to day hospital treatment for in-patients with anorexia nervosa. Am J Psychiatry 1999; 156:1697–1702.

29. Anzai N, Lindsey-Dudley K, Bidwell RJ. Inpatient and partial hospital treatment for adolescent eating disorders. Child Adol Psychiatr Clin North Am 2002; 11:279–309.

30. Zipfel S, Reas DL, Thorton C, Olmsted MP, Williamson DA, Gerlinghoff M, Herzog W, Beumont PJ. Day hospitalization programs for eating disorders: a systematic review of the literature. Int J Eating Disord 2002; 31:105–107.

31. Thorton C, Beumont P, Touyz S. The Australian experience of day programs for patients with eating disorders. Int J Eating Disord 2002; 1–10.
32. Kaplan AS, Omlsted MP. Partial Hospitalization. In: Garner DM, Garfinkel PE, eds. Handbook of Treatment for Eating Disorders. 2nd ed. New York: Guilford Press, 1997:354–360.
33. American Psychiatric Association. Practice guideline for eating disorders (revised). Am J Psychiatry 157(suppl):1–39.
34. Yager J. Implementing the Revised American Psychiatric Association Practice Guidelines for the treatment of patients with eating disorders. Psychiatr Clin North Am 2001; 24:185–199.
35. Metropolitan Life Insurance Company. Metropolitan height and weight tables. New York, 1983.
36. Frisch RE, McArthur JW. Menstrual cycles: fatness as a determinant of minimum weight for height necessary for their maintenance or onset. Science 1974; 185:949–951.
37. Fairburn CG. Eating disorders. In: Clark DM, Fairburn CG, eds. Science and Practice of Cognitive Behavior Therapy. New York: Oxford University Press, 1997:209–242.
38. Eckert ED, Mitchell JE. An overview of the treatment of anorexia nervosa. Psychiatr Med 1989; 7:293–315.
39. Bowers WA. Cognitive therapy for eating disorders. In: Wright JH, Thase ME, Beck AT, Ludgate JW, eds. Cognitive Therapy with Inpatients: Developing a Cognitive Therapy Milieu. New York: Guilford Press, 1993.
40. Garfinkel PE, Garner DM. Anorexia Nervosa: A Multidimensional Perspective. New York: Brunner/Mazel, 1982.
41. Garner DM. Individual psychotherapy for anorexia nervosa. J Psychiatr Res 1985; 19:423–433.
42. Beck JS. Cognitive Therapy: Basics and Beyond. New York: Guilford Press, 1995.
43. Freeman A. A psychosocial approach to conceptualizing schematic development for cognitive therapy. In: Kuehlwein KT, Rosen H, eds. Cognitive Therapies in Action. New York: Jossey Bass, 1993:54–87.
44. Garner DM, Vitousek KM, Pike KM. Cognitive–behavioral therapy for Anorexia Nervosa. In: Garner DM, Garfinkel PE, eds. Handbook of Psychotherapy for Anorexia Nervosa and Bulimia. New York: Guilford Press, 1997:94–144.
45. Bowers WA. Cognitive model of eating disorders. J Cognitive Psychother An Int Quart 2001; 15:331–340.
46. Wright JH, Thase ME, Beck AT, Ludgate JW. Cognitive Therapy with Inpatients: Developing a Cognitive Therapy Milieu. New York: Guilford Press, 1993.
47. Beck AT, Rush J, Shaw BF, Emery G. Cognitive Therapy of Depression. New York: Guilford Press, 1979.
48. Bowers WA. Basic principles for applying cognitive–behavioral therapy to anorexia nervosa. Psychiatr Clin North Am 2001; 24:293–304.
49. Wilson GT, Fairburn CC, Agras WS. Cognitive–behavioral therapy for bulimia

nervosa. In: Garner DM, Garfinkel PE, eds. Handbook of Treatment for Eating Disorders. 2d ed. New York: Guilford Press, 1997:67–93.

50. Fairburn CG, Cooper PJ. The Eating Disorders Examination. 12th ed. In: Fairburn CG, Wilson GT, eds. Binge Eating: Nature, Assessment and Treatment. New York: Guilford Press, 1993:317–360.

51. Garner DM, Olmsted MP. Manual for the Eating Attitudes Test (EDI). Odessa, FL: Psychological Assessment Resources, Inc., 1993.

52. Garner DM, Garfinkel PE. The eating attitudes test. An index of the symptoms of anorexia nervosa. Psychol Med 1979; 9:273–279.

53. Garner DM, Garfinkel PE. Handbook of Treatment for Eating Disorders. 2d ed. New York: Guilford Press, 1997:145–177.

54. Garner DM. Psychoeducational principles in treatment. In: Garner DM, Garfinkel PE, eds. Handbook of Treatment for Eating Disorders. 2d ed. New York: Guilford Press, 1997:145–177.

55. Bowers WA. Eating disorders. In: White JR, Freeman AS, eds. Cognitive–Behavioral group therapy for specific problems and populations. Washington, DC: American Psychological Association, 2000:127–148.

56. Yalom I. The Theory and Practice of Group Psychotherapy. 4th ed. New York: Basic Books, 1995.

57. Dattilio FM. Families in crisis. In: Dattilio FM, Freeman A, eds. Cognitive–Behavioral Strategies in Crisis Intervention. New York: Guilford Press, 1994: 2789–3010.

58. Dare C, Eisler I. Family therapy for anorexia nervosa. In: Garner DM, Garfinkel PE, eds. Handbook of Treatment for Eating Disorders. 2d ed. New York: Guilford Press, 1997:307–326.

59. Strober M, Freeman R, Morrell W. The long-term course of severe anorexia nervosa in adolescents: survival analysis of recovery, relapse, and outcome predictors over 10-15 years in a prospective study. Int J Eating Disord 1997; 22:339–360.

60. Draper H. Anorexia nervosa and respecting a refusal of life-prolonging therapy: limited justification. Bioethics 2000; 14:120–133.

61. Ramsey R, Ward A, Treasure J, Russell GF. Compulsory treatment in anorexia nervosa. Short-term benefits and long-term mortality. Br J Psychiatry 1999; 175:147–153.

62. Russell GFM. Involuntary treatment in anorexia nervosa. Psychiat Clin North Am 2001; 24:337–350.

63. Appelbaum PS, Rumpf T. Civil commitment of the anorexic patient. Gen Hosp Psychiatry 1998; 20:225–230.

64. Watson TL, Bowers WA, Andersen AE. Involuntary treatment of eating disorders. Am J Psychiatry 2000; 157:1806–1810.

16

Nutrition Counseling for Anorexia Nervosa, Bulimia Nervosa, and Binge Eating Disorder

Jillian K. Croll
Eating Disorders Institute
St. Louis Park, Minnesota, U.S.A.

Dianne Neumark-Sztainer
University of Minnesota
Minneapolis, Minnesota, U.S.A.

Comprehensive care of patients with eating disorders involves a multidisciplinary treatment team with nutritional rehabilitation and stabilization as a significant cornerstone of treatment (1,2). Nutritional rehabilitation and counseling requires a skilled registered dietitian versed in eating disorder treatment approaches. The guiding principle in nutritional treatment of eating disorders is to help the patient become reacquainted with normal eating. Eating disorders rob sufferers of the practice of normal eating and frequently mask the body's natural hunger and satiety cues. This theft makes relearning how to honor the body's hunger and satiety signals, how to discern physiological urges to eat from emotional triggers, and how to view food and eating as a joyful, nourishing part of life rather than a frightening, threatening enemy, or a difficult and complex journey. Nutritional counseling involves guiding the patient through this process and helping him or her reestablish a healthy relationship with food.

NUTRITIONAL COUNSELING APPROACHES

The first step in nutritional management of an eating disorder, regardless of diagnosis, involves a thorough nutritional assessment (see Fig. 1 for a description of typical components of the initial eating disorder nutrition assessment). Information gathered from this assessment, along with pertinent medical, psychological, and psychiatric data, is used to determine appropriate level of treatment (i.e., inpatient, day, outpatient, residential, etc.) and to develop a nutritional treatment plan highlighting areas of focus for nutrition education, behavior modification plans, and expectations for weight restoration or stabilization, as appropriate. Nutritional approaches can vary across treatment settings and diagnoses, but typically involve nutritional rehabilitation, development of meal planning skills, normalization of eating patterns, and participation in experiential activities that allow for opportunities to practice new skills and stimulus control (2,3). Regular weight monitoring should be done by the dietitian or another medical provider.

Anorexia Nervosa

Nutritional Assessment

The initial nutritional assessment of a person suffering from anorexia nervosa should include a detailed history of the onset of the eating disorder, a thor-

Gather information from patient and family regarding:

- Detailed weight history, including high and low weight and ages at which these occurred
- Change in eating patterns with onset of the eating disorder
- Current typical eating behaviors
- 24 hour recall, either of previous day or typical day
- Current nutritional intake
- Past and present symptom use
- Food and eating "rules" dictated by the eating disorder
- Supplement Use
- Assessment of motivation to change eating behaviors
- Exercise patterns
- Treatment history
- Familial factors (familial dieting, comments or teasing about weight, use of diet products, etc.)

Review pertinent data:

- Growth charts (for children and adolescents)
- Electrolyte and hydration status, if available
- Weight, height, and vital signs
- Psychological and medical evaluation, if available

FIGURE 1   Components of an Initial Eating Disorders Nutritional Assessment.

ough recall of typical eating patterns and eating disorder symptom use, and questions regarding potential precipitating events (e.g., weight-related teasing, bodily changes associated with puberty, comments by family or friends, etc.). A detailed description of a typical day should include times of eating occasions, type and amount of food eaten, beverages consumed, and if and when bingeing and purging occurs. Research comparing reported intake to observed intake has shown that diet history given by patients with anorexia nervosa provides a quite reliable picture of nutritional intake (4). It is also important to assess the food rules dictated by anorexia. Typical food-related rules commonly seen with anorexia nervosa include the following: no eating after a certain time in the evening, no eating of specific foods (such as meat, sweets, fats, snacks), eating foods in a specific order, following certain caloric or fat gram daily limits, trying to go all day without eating, and isolating self from others while eating. Foods are often categorized as "good" or "bad" or "safe" or "scary," and these categorizations often determine eating behaviors (5). While these behaviors and rules are largely the result of semistarvation, they can perpetuate the eating disorder. Most tend to significantly decrease or abate with nutritional rehabilitation (6–8). A detailed exercise history, including type of exercise, duration, intensity, and compulsivity, is a necessary part of the evaluation to determine energy expended on physical activity. As with eating patterns, particular attention should be given to assessing exercise patterns in all settings: at home, at school, at health clubs, as part of clubs or teams, or in other settings. The physical activity level is often high in patients with anorexia nervosa and contributes significantly to energy balance (9,10). Thorough assessment is necessary, as anorexia imposes many rules and regulations. Clinicians may need to ask many questions, as patients may not readily volunteer information regarding eating disorder–related eating and exercise patterns and may have altered perceptions of these behaviors. Family members or friends, if present at the assessment, can often provide additional valuable historical data regarding the patient's eating habits and change in eating (e.g., onset of dieting; whether certain eating behaviors, like vegetarianism, predated the eating disorder or co-occurred with the eating disorder; etc.).

Nutritional Rehabilitation

In addition to weight restoration, nutritional interventions seek to correct any nutritional deficiencies resulting from the illness. Research has shown that patients with anorexia nervosa may have abnormal vitamin status, specifically indicators of low riboflavin and vitamin B_6, deficiencies in essential fatty acids, low serum albumin and other nutrients (11,12). Osteopenia is common among patients with anorexia nervosa (13–15), making dietary calcium intake a critical part of nutritional rehabilitation. Research suggests that weight restoration in conjunction with adequate dietary calcium and vitamin D is associated with improvement in bone mineralization (16,17).

Adequate nutrition rehabilitation can be a significant challenge. Many patients experience and are frustrated by delayed gastric emptying resulting from ongoing food restriction and complain of feeling excessively full in the early stages of treatment (18). Delayed gastric emptying and nutrient deficiencies typically resolve with ongoing treatment and normalization of dietary intake. A low-dose multivitamin, multimineral supplement is viewed as a low-risk component of nutritional rehabilitation (3). For patients who have had very minimal intake prior to initiation of treatment and need to restore considerable weight, edema frequently develops during the nutritional rehabilitation and refeeding process (19). The rapid weight gain associated with edema can be quite anxiety producing for patients, and they need ongoing reassurance that the rapid gain is primarily due to fluid accumulation and will resolve with continued treatment. Close medical monitoring, particularly in the beginning of inpatient treatment, is necessary to reduce the risk of refeeding syndrome, characterized by a sudden precipitous drop in phosphorus, magnesium, and potassium, and cardiac arrhythmias, particularly a prolonged QT interval (20–22). Slow progression of caloric intake and careful monitoring helps to prevent refeeding syndrome.

Weight Restoration Regimens

Weight restoration plans differ based on treatment setting and degree of weight restoration needed. In an inpatient setting, given the typically low caloric intake of patients prior to treatment, patients are generally started at a relatively low caloric level, approximately 1200–1500 kcal/day. Kilocalories are then increased incrementally by 200–300 per day over the course of 1–2 weeks to a caloric level that supports weight restoration of approximately 2–3 pounds (0.9–1.4 kg) per week (1,2). Similar expectations are common among residential treatment programs. In a day treatment setting, patients are typically started at a higher caloric level, approximately 1800 kcal/day, and increased incrementally 200–300 kcal/day to reach a level that supports adequate weight restoration. Weight restoration expectations are slightly lower in a day treatment setting, typically 1.5–2.0 pounds (0.68–0.90 kg) per week, since patients typically eat only one to two meals and one to two snacks during treatment hours and consume the rest of their meal plan outside of treatment. Because the majority of meals and snacks are eaten outside of treatment in an outpatient setting, caloric levels vary, depending on the severity of the weight loss and the progress the patient is able to make. Most outpatient settings have weight restoration guidelines of 1.0–2.0 pounds (0.45–0.90 kg) per week (1–3).

Energy needs increase as patients restore weight, due to both the restored body weight and increased metabolic rate (23–26), and become quite high (up to 3000–5000 kcal/day). Projected energy requirements for weight gain can be determined by adding estimated resting energy expenditure, requirements for activity, and kilocalories needed for weight restoration (see Fig. 2 for details regarding these calculations). It is important to note that this provides only an estimate, and patients will respond differently at different times in the process, as resting energy expenditure has been shown to increase and peak during refeeding (23–26). Kilocalorie levels may need frequent adjustment until the desired rate of weight restoration is achieved and weight restoration is adequate (1–3).

At high caloric levels, consuming adequate food may present a challenge to patients. Calorically dense foods, more frequent meals and snacks, or

Weight Restoration: Estimated Daily Kilocalorie Needs: REE + Activity Requirement + Weight Restoration Requirement

Weight Maintenance: Estimated Daily Kilocalorie Needs: REE + Activity Requirement

- Resting Energy Expenditure Estimate (REE)

  Harris-Benedict Equations:

  Women: REE=655 + (9.6 X weight in kilograms) + (1.8 X height in centimeters) –(4.7 X age in years)

  Men: REE=660 = (13.7 X weight in kilograms) + (5.0 X height in centimeters) –(6.8 X age in years)

- Activity Requirements Estimate

  REE X 1.2 to 1.3 for average energy requirements/moderate activity; 1.5-1.7 for high energy requirements/high activity

- Weight Restoration Requirements (approximately 3500 kilocalories per pound restored)

  2-3 pounds/week weight restoration goal: 7,000-10,500 kcals per week= 1,000-1,500 kcal per day

  1-2 pounds/week weight restoration goal: 3,500 –7,000 kcals per week= 500-1,000 kcal per day

  0.5 pounds/week weight restoration goal: 1,750 kcals per week= 250 kcal per day

FIGURE 2 Calculation of energy requirements. (From Harris JA, Benedict FG. (1919) Biometric studies of basal metabolism in man. Carnegie Institute of Washington: Publication No. 279.)

oral liquid supplements can be utilized to meet the high-energy needs of these patients. Some inpatient, partial, and residential programs use nasogastric tube feedings or total parenteral nutrition (TPN) to increase caloric consumption, but both require close medical monitoring, may increase the risk of refeeding syndrome, and may be unnecessarily overwhelming for some patients (1–3). Use of food rather than supplemental feedings or nutritional support approaches for weight restoration more effectively supports long-term recovery (2). Once patients restore weight and are able to remain in the clinician-established goal weight range, caloric intake may be gradually decreased to a maintenance range, typically 1800–2800 kcal/day (24).

Though it varies greatly by treatment program, in the early stages of inpatient and residential treatment patients typically have little choice in meal and snack foods and are asked to view the food they are being asked to eat as medicine. As patients are able to finish meals without refusing to eat or requiring any liquid supplements to replace uneaten foods, they progress to selecting meals and snacks based on their individualized meal plan. As patients progress in treatment, they gain independence with the meal plan and can participate in decisions regarding necessary meal plan changes. In day treatment and outpatient settings, patients have more flexibility in food choices, but initially may need to view food in the same way, as a medicinal type of treatment. In order to create an environment conducive to the changing of eating disorder behaviors, a number of rules must be enforced at mealtimes. Patients are typically allowed 30–60 min per meal and 15 min per snack; gum and mints, often used by patients to assuage denied hunger, are not allowed; caffeine intake is limited; and food-related behaviors, such as excessive cutting of food, taking tiny bites, hiding food, scraping off fat, and excessive use of condiments, are monitored and redirected. Across all settings, an individualized meal plan is created for each patient based on caloric and weight restoration needs, eating patterns, schedule, and special dietary needs (e.g., diabetes, lactose intolerance).

Meal Plans

The individualized meal plan serves many purposes. On a broad level, it can serve as the client's personalized road map to successful, normal eating. On a more detailed level, it provides the patient with a concrete presentation of what she or he needs to eat on a daily basis to progress in treatment. The meal plan is typically created with the client, taking into account true food likes and dislikes and the current prescribed caloric level. The meal plan encourages patients to challenge the eating disorder and themselves to reintroduce foods forbidden by the eating disorder. Meal plans, while calculated based on caloric needs, are usually presented in terms of servings from each food group, similar to the food guide pyramid recommendations (27), rather than calories. See Table 1 for examples of typical meal plans at different caloric

TABLE 1   Sample Meal Plans Across Increasing Kilocalorie Levels

Food group (approximate energy content per serving)	Kilocalorie level and servings per group[a]				
	1800	2400	3000	3600[b]	4200[b]
Protein (approximately 21 g protein, 200 kcal)	2	2	2	2	2
Dairy (approximately 100 kcal)	3	5	5	6	6
Grain (approximately 80–100 kcal)	6	9	11	12	12–14
Fruit (approximately 60–80 kcal)	3	5	6	8	10
Vegetable (approximately 25–40 kcal)	2	2	2	2	2
Fat (approximately 5–8 g fat, 45–70 kcal)	4	5	5	6	6
Dessert (approximately 200–300 kcal, minimum 5 g fat)	1	1	2	3	3–4

[a] Number of servings per groups varies; based on individualized meal plan created for patient.
[b] Liquid supplements may be used at higher calorie levels, if desired, to meet caloric needs. If liquid supplements are used, the number of grain and dessert servings may be reduced accordingly to meet required caloric level.

levels and Table 2 for recommended portion sizes of foods in each food group.

Detailed explanations of portion sizes, with food models, real food, or pictures, can help relieve some anxiety about forbidden foods and provide invaluable nutrition education for clients. Clear descriptions of portion sizes for each food group and typical examples of foods in each food group, with examples relevant to the client's culture, schedule, and habits, all help patients to challenge the eating disorder. Explanation of overall nutritional needs and discussion of specific nutrient needs and function help patients to understand the rationale behind the meal plan. The meal plan should include all the food groups, particularly challenging foods or food groups such as fats and desserts. Anorexia takes away a person's freedom with food, and the meal plan can be a powerful tool for allowing a person to reclaim the freedom of normal eating.

If patients are not able to eat challenging foods in the safe environment of treatment or with the support of their treatment team, it is unlikely that they will readily reincorporate those foods outside of treatment or when they are no longer engaged in treatment. Staff-supported experiential nutrition activities, such as eating in different types of restaurants, at food courts in shopping malls, and in other social settings, are often part of group treatment programs. Practice following the meal plan in a variety of settings in the

TABLE 2   Sample Portion Sizes for Each Food Group

Protein	3 ounces cooked meat, poultry, fish
	2 ounces of nuts
	2–3 ounces cheese
	3 eggs
	1/4 cup peanut butter
	8 ounces tofu
Dairy	1 cup milk
	1 cup yogurt
Grain	1 piece bread
	1 ounce dry cereal
	1 frozen waffle or pancake
	1/2 bagel or bun
	1/2 cup rice, pasta, or potato
	1 small tortilla
Fruit	Medium piece of fresh fruit
	1/2 cup canned or cooked fruit
	4 ounces of fruit juice
	1 cup fresh fruit
	1/4 cup dried fruit
Vegetable	1 cup raw vegetables
	1 cup mixed greens
	1/2 cup cooked vegetables
	6 ounces vegetable juice
Fat	1 teaspoon regular butter, margarine, oil
	1 tablespoon tub margarine or whipped butter
	1 tablespoon peanut butter, cream cheese, salad dressing
	2 tablespoons gravy or sour cream
	1–2 tablespoons guacamole
Dessert	Regular-size candy bar
	Medium brownie
	1/2 cup premium ice cream
	1 cup nonpremium ice cream or frozen yogurt
	1 large cookie, 2–3 homemade cookies, 4–6 sandwich-type cookies
	1 slice of pie or cake (1/8 or 1/9 of a pie or round cake)

Source: Adapted from Food Guide Pyramid http://www.nal.usda.gov/fnic/Epyr/pyramid.html) and Methodist Hospital Eating Disorders Institute meal planning materials.

context of treatment programming can help patients gain the necessary skills to navigate challenging and difficult situations they will likely face outside of the treatment setting. Given the exaggerated societal messages regarding limiting fat, sweets, sugar, and other foods, patients face a difficult task in overcoming those messages and incorporating challenging foods in their meal plan. Education regarding the concepts of normal eating is critical, including learning to eat when hungry, eating until full, including a wide variety of foods, not avoiding or fearing specific foods, eating with others, eating in a variety of settings, eating from all the food groups, not being obsessed with thoughts of food, not purging or exercising to counteract food eaten, etc. Normal eating includes having all kinds of foods, not categorizing foods as positive or negative, and incorporating variety and moderation as mainstays (28).

Ongoing Treatment

While many patients with anorexia nervosa experience inpatient or partial hospitalization treatment, most of the time spent in treatment is in an outpatient setting with a multidisciplinary team. Regular follow-up with the dietitian is necessary and generally occurs on a weekly basis, typically until weight restoration is complete and has been maintained for at least 2 weeks. Once the patient is within their goal weight range, visits with the dietitian may decrease in frequency to bimonthly or monthly. Visits often include taking the patient's weight. Weights should be taken with the patient wearing only a gown and undergarments, preferably with them facing away from the numbers on the scale. Weight changes are used as a guideline for meal plan changes and strategies and are an integral piece of medical monitoring. Because of the intense focus on weight associated with anorexia nervosa, discussions with the patient regarding current weight, weight change, and goal weights should focus on progress and strategies for change rather than be overly focused on numbers. As adequate weight restoration is achieved, energy needs decrease and the meal plan can be changed accordingly. Weight maintenance energy levels vary by individual based on age, gender, physical activity, and weight, but are typically in the range of 2000–2800 kcal/day. Figure 2 provides an equation for calculating weight restoration and weight maintenance needs.

Nutritional care in an outpatient setting incorporates a number of techniques to aid patients in the process of incorporating variety into their meal plan and regaining foods lost to the eating disorder. Usually clients will be asked to eat at structured, regular intervals and participate in self-monitoring, cognitive–behavioral therapy techniques (29,30) involving planning meals and snacks ahead of time, eating at set times, and keeping daily food records. Eating specific amounts and types of foods at appropriate set times throughout the day, even if not hungry, allows for relearning of hunger and satiety cues and normal eating patterns.

Food records include information about food and beverage intake, including time of meal or snack, location, whether alone or with others, what and how much was eaten, rating of hunger and satiety levels, as well as any thoughts or feelings associated with eating. If patients also struggle with bingeing and/or purging, urges or occurrences of the behaviors can be tracked on these forms as well. Review of the patient's food records provides an opportunity to discuss progress made with the meal plan and challenges faced with specific foods or situations. Self-monitoring can be challenging for some patients for a variety of reasons. It may be difficult for patients to write down what they are eating. It may seem overwhelming and anxiety provoking to see it all down on paper, or it may be difficult to record symptoms. For others, it may be another avenue for the perfectionism of anorexia to take hold, driving them to have perfectly written and detailed food records each week. Initially, patients often struggle with rating hunger and satiety levels because the eating disorder has resulted in loss of connection between hunger signals and eating behaviors. Reconnection to innate hunger and satiety signs may take considerable time. Clinicians should encourage patients to consider food records as another tool in the fight against anorexia and a way for them to remind themselves of their meal plan and their goals, rather than something to obsess about or feel like they have to do perfectly (see Fig. 3 for an example of a comprehensive food record form).

Family Involvement

With adolescent patients, parents need to be included in initial education sessions regarding the meal plan, portion sizes, expectations for the patient while in treatment, and ways family members can support the patient. While parents are often not present during ongoing follow-up sessions, they generally need to be regularly apprised of weight changes, progress with the meal plan, and strategies or goals for the week, as well as given the opportunity to ask questions regarding the meal plan. Parents also can provide insight regarding the patient's eating behaviors, successes, and difficulties at home that patients may not fully reveal to the clinician. For younger patients, there is evidence to suggest that the patient's family can be integrally involved in the reestablishment of normal eating patterns (31). This approach aids parents in supporting the recovery of their child by giving them primary jurisdiction over implementation of the meal plan and the patient's eating. Such approaches must be carefully implemented so as not to set up a power struggle between the patient and the parents, but rather should help parents to support their child in a constructive and productive manner. In this type of approach, parents would be more involved in ongoing nutrition sessions.

DAILY FOOD AND FEELINGS JOURNAL

Name: _____

Date _____

Circle Day: S M T W Th F S

extremely hungry		hungry		slightly hungry		balanced		slightly full		full		extremely full
0	1	2		3	4	5	6	7	8	9		10

Food or Drink (Description, Amount)	Time	Hunger Level	Where	With Whom	Feelings/Mood	Fullness after eating	Physical Activity	Binge/Purge or other symptoms

FIGURE 3 Example of a Food Record Form.

Regardless of their level of involvement in the meal plan, families often need assistance in knowing what to say to help patients have success with their meal plan. No one approach works well with all families, and families should be encouraged to ask the patient what they should and should not do or say to be supportive when it seems like the patient is struggling with the eating disorder during a meal or snack. To be most effective and productive, these conversations should take place outside of meal and snack times.

Overall, as part of a multifaceted approach to treatment of the whole person, carefully monitored nutritional rehabilitation is critical to recovery. Ongoing nutritional counseling helps patients with anorexia nervosa determine reasonable, achievable goals and to celebrate the successful accomplishment of those goals over time, and provides strategies for overcoming obstacles along the way.

Bulimia Nervosa

Nutritional Assessment

The initial nutritional assessment of a person suffering from bulimia nervosa is similar to that of anorexia nervosa (see Fig. 1 for typical assessment questions). A detailed description of a typical day should include all eating occasions, including binge and purge occurrences as well as nonbinge meals and snacks. A careful exploration of type and amount of food eaten and beverages consumed through the day can reveal an accurate picture of foods commonly eaten during a binge, triggers for binge and purge episodes, and those foods the patient is comfortable eating without feeling the need to purge. Typically, foods that are high in fat or sugar, such as fast food, bakery items, salty snack foods, candy, and ice cream, are foods considered "bad foods" or binge foods and are avoided unless purging is possible or planned (32). When purging is not planned or possible, patients with bulimia nervosa will usually restrict food intake or limit intake to foods considered to be healthy, such as fruit, vegetables, and other low-fat foods. Research has shown that when not engaging in binge eating, persons with bulimia nervosa exhibit significant dietary restraint, eat fewer meals and snacks, and take in significantly less energy and fat than controls (33,34). These findings, along with studies examining energy retained from binge eating after purging [approximately 1200 kcal/binge (35,36)], explain why many patients with bulimia nervosa have a relatively normal body weight despite characteristic restrictive eating alternating with binge eating and purging.

Nutritional Rehabilitation

Nutritional rehabilitation focuses on helping patients set goals around reducing binge–purge and restricting behaviors, increasing variety in food choices, practicing eating foods that are considered binge foods without purging, planning approaches for eating in challenging situations (e.g., restaurants, special occasions), and encouraging healthy, moderate exercise (1–3). Because individuals with bulimia nervosa typically maintain a normal or near-normal weight, weight restoration is not typically the focus of nutritional treatment. However, many patients desire a body weight that, while within a normal range, is unrealistically low for them given their genetic weight predisposition or set range (1,3). These patients need nutritional and therapeutic interventions and education to be able to accept a body shape and weight that may be different from than they desire, but ultimately where they are able to be emotionally and cognitively healthy.

The main focus of nutritional intervention and education for patients with bulimia nervosa is to establish a pattern of normal eating, with three meals and one to three snacks per day, in an effort to prevent the restrict–binge–purge cycle and allow the patient to become reacquainted with their hunger and satiety signals. Relearning normal eating patterns can be supported via a meal plan that provides a guide for the recommended meals and snacks and food records for self-monitoring. Meal plan structure is similar to those used with patients with anorexia nervosa, providing recommended servings from all food groups based on nutritional needs (refer to Tables 1 and 2 for details). Energy needs are dependent on current weight status, physical activity level, age, and gender. Typically, energy needs for people with bulimia nervosa are lower than those for people with anorexia nervosa needing to restore weight and as such remain more stable across treatment (3). While energy needs vary by individual, weight maintenance meal plans are typically in the range of 1800–2600 kilocalories (refer to Fig. 2 for energy requirement calculation equations).

Self-monitoring is a key element in the nutritional management of bulimia nervosa. Food records are also similar to those used with patients with anorexia nervosa, but often have a stronger emphasis on hunger and satiety levels, which can be useful in helping patients identify how periods of restriction result in binge episodes. In addition to periodic hunger and satiety ratings, food records should include food and beverage intake, time of meal or snack, location, whether alone or with others, what and how much was eaten, binge and purge urges or episodes, as well as any thoughts or feelings associated with eating. Patients may find it difficult and shameful to record binge and purge episodes or the amount of food eaten during binges, but regular documentation can help identify triggers and reduce binges (36). Patients may need to be encouraged to view food records and self-monitoring as objective data-gathering tools from which they can draw conclusions and identify solutions. Patients usually find that the food records help keep them on track with their meal plan and aid in planning eating on a day-to-day basis and for special events or occasions. Food records often provide direction to goal setting for the week. Weekly goals may include reincorporating one or more challenging foods into the diet (e.g., sharing a candy bar with a friend); eating in a challenging situation such as a restaurant, school cafeteria, or a friend's house (e.g., going to a fast-food restaurant); trying a difficult food-related task (e.g., grocery shopping); or participating in physical activity (e.g., walking for 30 minutes and stretching for 30 minutes 3 days that week).

Cognitive–Behavioral and Nutritional Therapies

It is well established that cognitive–behavioral therapy (CBT) is an effective intervention for the management of bulimia (29,37–41) and is a primary psychotheraputic approach. Inherent to CBT are a number of nutritional components, namely, nutrition education, meal planning, establishment of regular eating patterns, and discouragement of dieting (2,39). Studies have sought to examine the nutritional therapy components of CBT separately from the cognitive therapy components (38–40,42) and have found the nutritional counseling component to be an effective part of CBT. Hsu and colleagues support an approach including both components of CBT in which there exists overlap between the two approaches, but each component retains a primary distinctive focus, either cognitive or nutritional, during work with the patients to reduce symptom use and reestablish normal eating (39). Sundgot-Borgen and colleagues also support the integration of physical activity protocols into the treatment of these patients as a method of improving body image, promoting physical fitness, and reducing symptom use (38). The dietitian can have a key role in the nutritional components of CBT and physical activity recommendations and monitoring.

Nutrition Education and Counseling

The primary goals of nutritional intervention and education are to encourage development of normalized eating habits, improve nutrition knowledge, and support the development of skills related to grocery shopping, meal preparation, and situational stressors (e.g., restaurants, special occasions), so that the patients can follow the meal plan and prevent symptom re-occurrence (1,2,39,40). Education regarding principles of normal eating, psychological and physiological effects of starvation, nutritional requirements, and metabolism is critical (43). Nutrition education includes discussion of the benefits of the patient's self-imposed forbidden foods, such as fat or sweets, and the nutritional reasons for consuming adequate quantities of less forbidden but still challenging foods, such as dairy products for adequate calcium or meats for adequate protein intake (2). Patients may benefit from understanding the physiological effects of dieting, particularly the effects of diminished serotonin levels that occur with dieting (44). Restrictive food intake can result in decreased plasma tryptophan, the precursor of serotonin, and has been shown to be associated with alterations in mood, increased irritability, depressive symptoms, and weight and shape concerns (44–46). Skipping meals and restrictive eating can lead to increased use of binge-and-purge behaviors (33,34). Oftentimes patients need substantial education regarding the futility and riskiness of fad diets and need to be equipped with media literacy skills to sift through the innumerable messages regarding nutrition that are so readily available from the media. Once patients understand the concepts of metabolism as well as the effects of food restriction, weight maintenance, and normal eating, they are better equipped to focus on symptom reduction.

Patients may also need significant education regarding side effects of stopping binge–purge behavior. Cessation of laxative use or purging can result in fluid retention, weight shifts, and slow gastrointestinal function (2,3,47). Patients need to be informed that these uncomfortable changes are transitory and will resolve, but only if they continue to abstain from bingeing and purging. Adequate fluid intake, adequate dietary fiber from whole grains, fruits, and vegetables, and moderate exercise will aid in the reestablishment of body homeostasis (2,3). Some patients need high levels of support to manage the anxiety related to these side effects and may need an increased level of programming, such as a day treatment program, in order to stop binge–purge behaviors and effectively manage the side effects.

Ideas for Support of the Meal Plan

Patients typically have the most difficulty reintroducing forbidden foods into their regular eating patterns, for fear of weight gain or body composition changes, and need support and strategies to effectively reintegrate these foods (2,3). To facilitate reintroduction of challenging foods, patients may find that using single-serving food items or repackaging foods into smaller, portioned containers can help prevent the escalation of a binge when eating a challenging food (41).

Often patients find it easier to initially consume challenging foods in the company of family or friends, where they can find comfort in the distraction of social interaction and reassurance when others eat the same food. By asking support people to eat with them and engage in an activity after the meal, patients can receive support during the meal, as well as after the meal to help prevent them from being overly focused on the food that was just eaten. For patients who have experienced increased isolation or withdrawal from loved ones as a result of the eating disorder, asking support people to eat with them increases their social interaction and supports successful meal or snack completion. Families can help their loved ones by supporting the meal plan through planning, preparing, shopping, and eating with the patient, going to a variety of restaurants and social situations with the patient and supporting the patient's efforts to follow the meal plan in these challenging situations.

Nutritional intervention often focuses on helping patients to manage overwhelming situations that involve food by focusing on the component parts of the situation and making a plan for success using the meal plan as a guide. For example, if a patient has a great deal of difficulty going grocery shopping without it resulting in a binge–purge episode, the clinician can help the patient break down the task into manageable parts. First, together they can make a grocery list and determine what area of the store each food is in. Next they can determine what type and quantity of each food the patient needs to buy to meet his or her meal plan. At this point, it is important to explore what challenges may exist for particular foods and how those challenges can be overcome. For example, the meal plan discourages use of fat-free food items, but the patient feels compelled by the eating disorder to buy only fat-free cream cheese. So the patient takes a friend shopping and asks the friend to put regular cream cheese in the cart. Patients may need education regarding the nutritional benefits of challenging foods to understand that such foods generally provide more nutrients and satiety than fat-free or low-fat versions. After making the list and determining what needs to be purchased and where it is located, the dietitian may have the patient practice by going to the grocery store with the list, confirm the location of all the items, but not buy anything on this occasion. It is probably a good idea for the patient to take no money alone so as to help prevent a binge–purge episode. After this practice run, the patient may feel more assured of success because he or she is familiar with the location of items in the store. Then the patient would be asked to go to the grocery store, with a support person if necessary, to actually purchase the foods on the list in the specified quantities and report back to the clinician regarding success and challenges.

In addition to these techniques used in an outpatient setting, experiential nutritional activities are often part of partial day treatment or intensive outpatient treatment. Such activities typically include supported exposure to difficult foods or situations, such as meals out at restaurants, grocery shopping, or meal preparation for guests as a group. These experiential activities are commonly supervised by a dietitian and a psychologist or other clinician, and include a process group cofacilitated by both clinicians for the most effective utilization of the experience. Patients are often able to overcome challenging foods or situations in these types of experiential activities and recognize that they can complete food-related tasks that they thought were overwhelming.

Overall, as with anorexia nervosa, nutritional intervention and education is a critical part of a multifaceted approach to management of bulimia nervosa and seems most effective for patients when paired with cognitive–behavioral work with a psychologist or other clinician. Ongoing nutrition counseling helps patients with bulimia nervosa establish regular eating patterns and decrease symptom use, develop skills for use when reintroducing challenging foods, and have better understanding of nutritional needs and physiological effects of symptom use.

Binge Eating Disorder

Nutritional Assessment

Given that patients with binge eating disorder often seek treatment for obesity and that nutritional counseling is generally a service incorporated into obesity treatment, a nutrition professional may be the primary clinician discussing binge eating with the patient. Binge eating disorder research is in the relatively early stages and as such numerous assessment and treatment recommendations and protocols are under evaluation, many of which have nutritional therapy or nutrition education components. The initial nutritional assessment for binge eating disorder should include a detailed account of the onset of binge eating, a weight and dieting history, and any historical events the patient believes may be related to the binge eating (e.g., weight-related teasing; comments by parents, friends, significant other; etc.). In general, people experiencing binge eating are more likely to have had a history of being overweight since childhood, have a significant history of large weight fluctuations (20 pounds or more), and experience an increase in binge eating as weight increases (48–51). Because binge eating may develop during periods of dietary restriction, such as a very-low-calorie diet (52), a careful history of diet attempts and outcomes should be taken. Assessment should include a thorough recall of typical eating patterns and binge eating occurrence and duration, along with an assessment of the out-of-control nature of the reported binge eating episodes.

A detailed description of a typical day, including all eating occasions, can help identify patterns in eating and triggers for binge eating. As with bulimia nervosa, a careful exploration of type and amount of food eaten and beverages consumed through the day can reveal an accurate picture of foods commonly eaten during a binge, as well as those foods the patient eats outside of binge episodes. Typically, foods that are high in fat or carbohydrates and lower in protein, such as candy, baked goods, and ice cream, are foods included in binge episodes (49,52). Caloric contribution from binge eating to total daily intake varies greatly depending on the episode, ranging from a minor contribution of fewer than 100 kilocalories to a large contribution of several thousand kilocalories (49,53). Studies have shown an average caloric intake difference of approximately 1000 kilocalories between nonbinge eating days and binge days (54,55).

Nutrition Intervention and Education

Treatment for binge eating disorder to date has included CBT or interpersonal therapy with a mental health professional, often with the addition of a focus on weight regulation or loss with a nutrition professional. CBT treatment adapted from bulimia nervosa, focusing on normalizing eating habits, identifying triggers, and changing distorted attitudes regarding eating and weight in an effort to reduce or eliminate binge eating behaviors, is followed by a focus on realistic weight control. Research has shown that patients who are able to cease binge eating behaviors lose weight (49,56). Ongoing research involves examination of the most effective timing of the focus on weight control—either concurrently with CBT treatment or after the patient is able to demonstrate consistent, binge-free eating (36,57,58). When weight loss is discussed, it is critical that patients establish reasonable weight loss goals, such as a more modest 10–20% weight loss, rather than try to reach an "ideal weight." Moderate weight loss can result in improvements in blood pressure, lipid profile, and blood glucose control (59). Even if cessation of binge eating results in weight maintenance only, the typical ongoing weight gain associated with binge eating is avoided (60). In addition, regular physical activity can contribute to weight loss and at the same time help reduce binge eating. Research indicates the addition of exercise to CBT treatment results in significantly greater weight loss and abstinence from binge eating than CBT alone (61).

Nutritional counseling should include establishment of an individualized meal plan that incorporates three meals and one or more structured snacks per day, includes enjoyable foods, and encourages regular physical activity. The meal plan, based on a nondieting approach to eating, should focus on food groups and portions, not calories or calorie counting (62). (Refer to Tables 1 and 2 for sample meal plans and portion size guides.) The primary focus of the meal plan is on eating regular meals and snacks. While energy needs of patients with binge eating disorder may vary significantly based on weight, age, gender, and activity level, typical daily energy needs likely range from 1600 to 2200 kilocalories. Eating regularly scheduled meals and snacks throughout the day helps prevent physiological urges to binge resulting from overwhelming hunger (63). While patients are not required to eat particular foods at each meal and snack, the meal plan is designed to provide variety throughout the day and incorporate all food groups. When hunger identification or management is difficult, prepackaged single-serving food items or repackaging of foods into smaller, portioned containers can help provide guidance regarding serving size and prevent the escalation of a binge (63). The nondieting approach to weight management emphasizes that all foods can be included and has a strong focus on moderation. Rather than prescribing eating according to rigid diet rules, the nondieting approach encourages variety, moderation, and acceptance. It supports the establishment of normal eating and helps reduce binge eating, depression, anxiety, and body dissatisfaction (62,64). This approach may be challenging for a person who is used to implementing rigid diet rules in an effort to lose weight and/or decrease binge eating, but is ultimately liberating for patients.

Self-monitoring of eating habits via food records is an instrumental part of nutritional treatment. Food records should include food and beverage intake, time of meal or snack, location, whether alone or with others, what and how much was eaten, binge eating episodes, as well as any thoughts or feelings associated with eating (see Fig. 3 for a sample food record). It can be also be beneficial for patients to document physical activity on food records in order to track activity patterns in relation to eating habits and support behavior change efforts. Regular review of food records with the patient can identify patterns of eating and relationships between eating and situation, which provides direction for goal setting. While it may be difficult and shameful for patients to record the amount of food eaten during binges or their typical eating habits, the process can support healthful food choices, help identify triggers, and reduce binges (36). Attention must be given to the inundation of nutrition information and fad diets through the media and education provided regarding the misleading information associated with fad diets. Because enhanced self-acceptance seems to support recovery from binge eating disorder (65), patients must be equipped with appropriate media literacy skills to ward off conflicting societal messages regarding food, weight, and appearance and maintain positive attitudes about self-acceptance.

Patients also need nutrition education regarding appropriate portion sizes, menu planning, grocery shopping, dining out, variety and moderation with food choices to combat restrictive eating followed by binges, incorporating healthy eating into a busy lifestyle, and making positive food choices in stressful or triggering situations. Many patients have firmly held but unsubstantiated beliefs regarding nutrition or food and need sound nutrition information to dispel these myths. As patients learn more about normal eating and how to incorporate realistic principles of healthy eating into their lifestyle, they are better able to discern between sound nutrition information in the media and information with no factual basis.

On the whole, nutritional management of binge eating disorder focuses on cessation of binge eating and establishment of normal eating behaviors and regular physical activity, and is an integral part the overall therapeutic treatment for binge eating disorder. If necessary, focus on healthy, moderate weight loss or lifelong weight control can be incorporated as patients are able to reduce or cease binge eating behaviors.

SUMMARY OF NUTRITIONAL TREATMENT GOALS FOR ANOREXIA NERVOSA, BULIMIA NERVOSA, AND BINGE EATING DISORDER

Normalization of nutritional status and dietary habits is a primary goal in the management of eating disorders. Nutritional rehabilitation, education, and counseling are integral components of eating disorder treatment across all treatment settings and should be conducted by qualified nutritional personnel, typically a registered dietitian.

In summary, the main components and goals of nutritional treatment of anorexia nervosa include the following:

Adequate weight restoration through increased energy intake via food rather than enteral or parenteral nutrition products

Meal plan education and guidance focused on food groups, portion sizes, and variety to promote normalization of eating patterns

Supported reintroduction of foods eliminated from the diet to dispel fears related to these foods

Adequate nutrient intake to support nutritional recovery, possibly including a low-dose multivitamin and multimineral supplement

Nutrition education regarding normal, healthy eating; and normalization of dieting, restrictive eating, and excessive energy expenditure behaviors.

The guiding principles of nutritional management of bulimia nervosa include the following:

Normalization of eating patterns through establishment of regular meals and snacks

Adequate energy and nutrient intake to support weight maintenance or weight restoration, as necessary

Meal plan education and guidance emphasizing the importance of avoiding long periods without eating with a focus on hunger and satiety signals

Nutrition education regarding normal, healthy eating

Goal setting to achieve cessation of dieting or food restriction behaviors, excessive exercise, and binge–purge behaviors

Supported reintroduction of binge foods into the diet via stimulus control planning and experiential activities

Binge eating disorder nutritional treatment goals and components include the following, with particular attention to strategies for managing eating in high-risk or triggering situations and establishment of regular meals and snacks.

Normalization of eating patterns through establishment of regular meals and snacks

Meal plan education and guidance emphasizing the importance of avoiding long periods without eating, with a focus on hunger and satiety signals

Nutrition education regarding realistic healthy eating principles

Goal setting to achieve cessation of binge eating

Supported reintroduction of binge foods into the diet via stimulus control

When appropriate, introduction of a nondiet approach to weight control to facilitate lifelong weight management

Nutritional components of eating disorder treatment help patients to successfully overcome the eating disorder and maintain lifelong normal, healthy eating habits, through education, planning, skill development, and practice.

REFERENCES

1. American Psychiatric Association. Practice guideline for the treatment of patients with eating disorders. Am J Psychiatry 2000; 157(1):1–39.
2. American Dietetic Association. Nutrition intervention in the treatment of anorexia nervosa, bulimia nervosa, and eating disorder not otherwise specified (EDNOS). J Am Diet Assoc 2001; 101(7):810–819.
3. Rock CL, Curran-Celentano J. Nutritional management of eating disorders. Psychiat Clin North Am 1996; 19(4):701–713.
4. Hadigan CM, Anderson EJ, Miller KK, Hubbard JL, Herzog DB, Klibanski A, Grinspoon SK. Assessment of macronutrient and micronutrient intake in women with anorexia nervosa. Int J Eating Disord 2000; 28(3):284–292.
5. Sunday SR, Einhorn A, Halmi KA. Relationship of perceived macronutrient and caloric content to affective cognitions about food in eating-disordered, restrained, and unrestrained subjects. Am J Clin Nutr 1992; 55(2):362–371.
6. Garner DM. Pathogenesis of anorexia nervosa. Lancet 1993; 341:1631–1635.
7. Keys A, Brozek J, Henschel A, Mickelsen O, Taylor HL. The Biology of Human Starvation. Minneapolis: University of Minnesota Press, 1950.
8. Rock CL, Curran-Celentano J. Nutritional disorder of anorexia nervosa: a review. Int J Eating Disord 1994; 15(2):187–203.
9. Casper RC, Schoeller DA, Kushner R, Hnilicka J, Gold ST. Total daily energy

expenditure and activity level in anorexia nervosa. Am J Clin Nutr 1991; 53(5): 1143–1150.

10. Pirke KM, Trimborn P, Platte P, Fichter M. Average total energy expenditure in anorexia nervosa, bulimia nervosa, and healthy young women. Biol Psychiatry 1991; 30(7):711–718.

11. Rock CL, Vasantharajan S. Vitamin status of eating disorder patients: relationship to clinical indices and effect of treatment. Int J Eating Disord 1995; 18(3):257–262.

12. Holman RT, Adams CE, Nelson RA, Grater SJ, Jaskiewicz JA, Johnson SB, Erdman JW Jr. Patients with anorexia nervosa demonstrate deficiencies of selected essential fatty acids, compensatory changes in nonessential fatty acids and decreased fluidity of plasma lipids. J Nutr 1995; 125(4):901–907.

13. Bachrach LK, Katzman DK, Litt IF, Guido D, Marcus R. Recovery from osteopenia in adolescent girls with anorexia nervosa. J Clin Endocrinol Metab 1991; 72(3):602–606.

14. Rigotti NA, Neer RM, Skates SJ, Herzog DB, Nussbaum SR. The clinical course of osteoporosis in anorexia nervosa. A longitudinal study of cortical bone mass. JAMA 1991; 265(9):1133–1138.

15. Rigotti NA, Nussbaum SR, Herzog DB, Neer RM. Osteoporosis in women with anorexia nervosa. N Engl J Med 1984; 311(25):1601–1606.

16. Abrams SA, Silber TJ, Esteban NV, Vieira NE, Stuff JE, Meyers R, Majd M, Yergey AL. Mineral balance and bone turnover in adolescents with anorexia nervosa. J Pediatrics 1993; 123(2):326–331.

17. Hay PJ, Delahunt JW, Hall A, Mitchell AW, Harper G, Salmond C. Predictors of osteopenia in premenopausal women with anorexia nervosa. Calc Tissue Int 1992; 50(6):498–501.

18. Waldholtz BD, Andersen AE. Gastrointestinal symptoms in anorexia nervosa. A prospective study. Gastroenterology 1990; 98(6):1415–1419.

19. Vaisman N, Corey M, Rossi MF, Goldberg E, Pencharz P. Changes in body composition during refeeding of patients with anorexia nervosa. J Pediatrics 1988; 113(5):925–929.

20. Solomon SM, Kirby DF. The refeeding syndrome: a review. J Parent Ent Nutr 1990; 14:90–97.

21. Rock CL. Nutritional and medical assessment and management of eating disorders. Nutr Clin Care 1999; 2:332–343.

22. Fisher M, Simpser E, Schneider M. Hypophosphatemia secondary to oral refeeding in anorexia nervosa. Int J Eating Disord 2000; 28(2):181–187.

23. Obarzanek E, Lesem MD, Jimerson DC. Resting metabolic rate of anorexia nervosa patients during weight gain. Am J Clin Nutr 1994; 60(5):666–675.

24. Krahn DD, Rock C, Dechert RE, Nairn KK, Hasse SA. Changes in resting energy expenditure and body composition in anorexia nervosa patients during refeeding. J Am Diet Assoc 1993; 93(4):434–438.

25. Salisbury JJ, Levine AS, Crow SJ, Mitchell JE. Refeeding, metabolic rate, and weight gain in anorexia nervosa: a review. Int J Eating Disord 1995; 17(4):337–345.

26. Platte P, Pirke KM, Trimborn P, Pietsch K, Krieg JC, Fichter MM. Resting metabolic rate and total energy expenditure in acute and weight recovered patients with anorexia nervosa and in healthy young women. Int J Eating Disord 1994; 16(1):45–52.

27. Department of Health and Human Services and the United States Department of Agriculture. The food guide pyramid. 1996. http://www.nal.usda.gov/fnic/Fpyr/pyramid.html.

28. Satter E. How to Get Your Kid to Eat. . .But Not Too Much. Palo Alto, CA: Bull Publishing, 1987.

29. Wilson GT. Cognitive behavior therapy for eating disorders: progress and problems. Behav Res Ther 1991; 37(suppl 1):S79–S95.

30. Garner DM, Vitousek KM, Pike KM. Cognitive–behavioral therapy for anorexia nervosa. In: Garner DMG ed. Handbook of Treatment of Eating Disorders. New York: Guilford Press, 1997:94–144.

31. Lock J, LeGrange D, Agras WS, Dare C. Treatment Manual for Anorexia Nervosa: A Family-Based Approach. New York: Guilford Press, 2001.

32. Hetherington MM, Altemus M, Nelson ML, Bernat AS, Gold PW. Eating behavior in bulimia nervosa: multiple meal analyses. Am J Clin Nutr 1994; 60(6):864–873.

33. Hadigan CM, Kissileff HR, Walsh BT. Patterns of food selection during meals in women with bulimia. Am J Clin Nutr 1989; 50(4):566–759.

34. Weltzin TE, Hsu LK, Pollice C, Kaye WH. Feeding patterns in bulimia nervosa. Biol Psychiatry 1991; 30(11):1093–1110.

35. Kaye WH, Weltzin TE, Hsu LK, McConaha CW, Bolton B. Amount of calories retained after binge eating and vomiting. Am J Psychiatry 1993; 150(6):969–971.

36. Goldfein JA, Devlin MJ, Spitzer RL. Cognitive behavioral therapy for the treatment of binge eating disorder: what constitutes success? Am J Psychiatry 2000; 157(7):1051–1056.

37. Miller WR, Rollnick S. Motivational Interviewing: Preparing People to Change Addictive Behavior. New York: Guilford Press, 1991.

38. Sundgot-Borgen J, Rosenvinge JH, Bahr R, Schneider LS. The effect of exercise, cognitive therapy, and nutritional counseling in treating bulimia nervosa. Med Sci Sports Exercise 2002; 34(2):190–195.

39. Hsu LK, Rand W, Sullivan S, Liu DW, Mulliken B, McDonagh B, Kaye WH. Cognitive therapy, nutritional therapy and their combination in the treatment of bulimia nervosa. Psychol Med 2001; 31(5):871–879.

40. Hsu LK, Holben B, West S. Nutritional counseling in bulimia nervosa. Int J Eating Disord 1992; 11:55–62.

41. Fairburn CG, Agras WS, Wilson GT. The research on the treatment of bulimia nervosa: Practical and theoretical implications. In: Anderson GH, Kennedy SH, eds. The Biology of Feast and Famine: Relevance to Eating Disorders. San Diego: Academic Press, 1992:318–340.

42. Hsu LK, Santhouse R, Chesler BE. Individual cognitive behavioral therapy for bulimia nervosa: the description of a program. Int J Eating Disord 1991; 10:273–283.

43. Story M. Nutrition management and dietary treatment of bulimia. J Am Diet Assoc 1986; 86:517.
44. Cowen PJ, Smith KA. Serotonin, dieting, and bulimia nervosa. Adv Exp Med Biol 1999; 467:101–104.
45. Kaye WH, Gendall KA, Fernstrom MH, Fernstrom JD, McConaha CW, Weltzin TE. Effects of acute tryptophan depletion on mood in bulimia nervosa. Biol Psychiatry 2000; 47(2):151–157.
46. Smith KA, Fairburn CG, Cowen PJ. Symptomatic relapse in bulimia nervosa following acute tryptophan depletion. Arch Gen Psychiatry 1999; 56:171–176.
47. Mitchell JE, Specker SM, DeZwann M. Comorbidity and medical complications of bulimia nervosa. J Clin Psychiatry 1991; 52:13.
48. Telch CF, Agras WS, Rossiter EM. Binge eating increases with increasing adiposity. Int J Eating Disord 1992; 7:115–119.
49. Marcus MD. Binge eating in obesity. In: Fairburn CG, Wilson GT, eds. Binge Eating: Nature, Assessment, and Treatment. New York: Guilford Press, 1993: 77–96.
50. Wilfley DE, Grillo GM. Eating disorders: a women's health problem in primary care. Nurs Prac Forum 1993; 5:34–45.
51. Telch CF, Agras WS. The effects of a very low calorie diet on binge eating. Behav Ther 1993; 24:177–193.
52. Yanovski SZ, Leet M, Yanovski JA, Flood M, Gold PW, Kissileff HR, Walsh BT. Food selection and intake of obese women with binge-eating disorder. Am J Clin Nutr 1992; 56(6):975–980.
53. Rossiter EM, Agras WS, Telch CF, Bruce B. The eating patterns of non-purging bulimic subjects. Int J Eating Disord 1992; 11:111–120.
54. Timmerman GM. Caloric intake patterns of nonpurge binge-eating women. West J Nurs Res 1000; 20:103–118.
55. Yanovski SZ, Sebring NG. Recorded food intake of obese women with binge eating disorder before and after weight loss. Int J Eating Disord 1994; 15:135–150.
56. Wilson GT. Assessment of binge eating. In: Fairburn CG, Wilson GT, eds. Binge Eating: Nature, Assessment, and Treatment. New York: Guilford Press, 1999: 3227–3249.
57. Grillo GM. The assessment and treatment of binge eating disorder. J Pract Psychiatry Behav Health 1998; 4:191–200.
58. Williamson DA, Martin CK. Binge eating disorder: a review of the literature after publication of the DSM-IV. Eating Weight Disord: Stud Anorexia. Bulimia, and Obesity 1999; 4(3):103–114.
59. National Heart, Lung, and Blood Institute. Clinical guidelines on the identification, evaluation, and treatment of overweight and obesity in adults—The evidence report. Obesity Res 1998; 6(suppl 2):51S–209S.
60. Fairburn CG, Cooper Z, Doll HA, Norman P, O'Connor M. The natural course of bulimia nervosa and binge eating disorder in young women. Arch Gen Psychiatry 2000; 57(7):659–665.
61. Pendleton VR, Goodrick GK, Poston WS, Reeves RS, Foreyt JP. Exercise

augments the effects of cognitive-behavioral therapy in the treatment of binge eating. Int J Eating Disord 2002; 31(2):172–184.

62. Goodrick GK, Poston WS II, Kimball KT, Reeves RS, Foreyt JP. Nondieting versus dieting treatment for overweight binge-eating women. J Consult Clin Psychol 1998; 66(2):363–368.

63. Fariburn CG, Marcus MD, Wilson GT. Cognitive-behavioral treatment of binge eating and bulimia nervosa. In: Fairburn CG, Wilson GT, eds. Binge Eating: Nature, Assessment, and Treatment. New York: Guilford Press, 1993:361–404.

64. Tanco S, Linden W, Earle T. Well-being and morbid obesity in women: a controlled therapy evaluation. Int J Eating Disord 1998; 23(3):325–339.

65. Devlin MJ. Binge-eating disorder and obesity. A combined treatment approach. Psychiatr Clin North Am 2001; 24(2):325–335.

17

An Overview of Cognitive–Behavioral Approaches to Eating Disorders

Stephen A. Wonderlich, James E. Mitchell, and Lorraine Swan-Kremier

University of North Dakota School of Medicine and Health
   Sciences and the Neuropsychiatric Research Institute
Fargo, North Dakota, U.S.A.

Carol B. Peterson and Scott J. Crow

University of Minnesota
Minneapolis, Minneapolis, U.S.A.

Cognitive–behavioral therapy (CBT) is the most thoroughly studied form of treatment for the eating disorders. Consistent with other behavior therapy interventions, CBT generally avoids the modification of underlying psychological conflicts in favor of the direct change of cognitions and behavior that comprise the eating disorders. Furthermore, CBT attempts to modify those cognitive and behavioral processes, which are thought to maintain the disorder, or be proximal causal variables, while not addressing more distal factors that may have causal significance (e.g., early relationships). Like the CBT techniques used to manage mood and anxiety disorders (1,2), CBT for bulimia nervosa is generally a short-term treatment in which the clinician is encouraged to actively focus and direct the process of change.

Most of the empirical studies of CBT for eating disorders have examined the efficacy of this technique in the management of bulimia nervosa (BN), although its extrapolation to binge eating disorder (BED) has gained increased attention in recent years. While descriptions of treatments for anorexia nervosa (AN) often include key elements of CBT, controlled treatment trials for this disorder have been limited.

COGNITIVE BEHAVIORAL THERAPY IN THE MANAGEMENT OF BULIMIA NERVOSA

CBT for BN is designed to reduce the frequency of binge eating and purging behaviors while simultaneously reducing restrictive eating patterns (3). CBT for BN generally targets the modification of several key bulimic behaviors. First, there is an explicit emphasis on decreasing restrictive dieting and increasing the consumption of calories through eating meals and snacks. Second, dysfunctional thoughts about shape and weight are directly confronted and alternative thought patterns encouraged. Third, bulimic individuals are encouraged to identify the triggers or precipitants of bulimic behavior and develop alternatives to high-risk binge eating situations. Finally, through the moderation of extreme thought processes and enhancement of behavioral control, CBT is posited to indirectly enhance self-esteem. These goals are pursued in the context of a collaborative treatment relationship through the implementation of several clinical techniques (4,5): (a) daily self-monitoring of food consumption patterns, maladaptive cognitions, and binge/purge behaviors; (b) learning to identify the presence of problematic thoughts and questioning the logic associated with such thoughts; (c) the development of active and systematic approaches to identifying problems in living, constructing and testing solutions to these problems; and (d) identifying healthy lifestyle patterns that facilitate the prevention of relapse of bulimic symptoms.

COGNITIVE BEHAVIORAL THERAPY IN THE TREATMENT OF BULIMIA NERVOSA

Table 1 delineates more than 20 controlled trials of CBT for BN (7,35). As can be seen, whether provided in an individual or group therapy format, CBT has been shown to be superior to minimal or waiting-list control intervention in terms of reducing the frequency of binge eating and purging behaviors. These findings have been discussed in a number of detailed reviews of studies of psychotherapy outcomes in BN (3,6), but it is important to note that a significant fraction of bulimic individuals remain symptomatic at the end of these short-term structured treatments or relapse after completing treatment. Furthermore, Table 1 reveals that CBT has generally been superior to other interventions including behavior therapy, psychodynamically oriented psychotherapy, supportive psychotherapy, and pharmacotherapy. Interestingly, however, studies comparing CBT to interpersonal therapy (IPT), an approach originally developed for the management of depression with no explicit focus on bulimic symptoms, have revealed essentially no difference in efficacy at long-term follow-up (21,31). These findings have resulted in debate about what factors are most significant for the etiology and maintenance of BN, as well as the most appropriate treatment for BN (36). However, the wealth of evidence documenting the efficacy and rapid action of CBT for BN leads most to continue to consider CBT as the treatment of choice for this condition (37).

COGNITIVE BEHAVIORAL THERAPY IN THE TREATMENT OF BINGE EATING DISORDER

Many of the techniques that have been used in the management of BN have been adapted and slightly modified for the management of BED. Generally speaking, CBT has been effective in reducing the frequency of binge eating episodes in subjects with BED (38,39). Interestingly, and similar to the BN treatment literature, interpersonal therapy (IPT) has been shown to be as effective as CBT in binge reduction in subjects with BED (39). Furthermore, follow-up assessments of BED subjects with both types of treatment reveal slight increases in binge eating over time, but a general persistence of the treatment effect (40). A common finding in the management of BED is that currently available psychological treatments are reasonably effective in reducing binge frequency but seem to have little effect on short-term weight loss. This is a significant finding for the participants, who oftentimes are overweight or obese and desire a more potent effect for their weight. A recent large-scale follow-up study suggested that treated BED individuals lost approximately 5% or more of their body weight and furthermore that those who were abstinent from binge eating were most likely to maintain these losses (40). This is significant in that BED subjects often follow a trajectory of continued weight gain over time, and the ability to preempt such weight gain and even obtain small degrees of weight loss may be clinically significant. Furthermore, even a 5% weight loss for this population may confer significant health benefits and should not be considered trivial.

COGNITIVE BEHAVIORAL THERAPY IN THE MANAGEMENT OF ANOREXIA NERVOSA

CBT for AN shares numerous features with CBT for BN. For example, CBT for both conditions emphasizes psychoeducation about medical and dietary factors, cognitive restructuring approaches, and behavioral interventions surrounding increased food consumption through meals and snacks (41). However, there are also differences between CBT for AN and BN. Some of the differences may be attributable to symptomatic differences between AN and BN, particularly the need for weight gain in AN, as well as the greater degree of symptom egosyntonicity in AN. Furthermore, the motivation for treat-

TABLE 1 Controlled Trials for Cognitive–Behavioral Therapy for Bulimia Nervosa

Author, Year	Format	Treatment	N	Completers (%)	Reduction in BE (%)	Abstinent at end of treatment %
Lacey, 1983 (7)	Individual + group	Individual + group	30	100	95	90
Connors et al., 1984 (8)	Group	Psychoeducation	26	77	70	
Yates and Sambrailo, 1984 (9)	Group	CBT + BT	24	67		13
		CBT				0
Kirkley et al., 1985 (10)	Group	CBT	14	93	97	0
		Nondirective	14	64	64	0
Ordman and Kirschenbaum, 1985 (11)	Individual	Full	10	100		20
		Brief	10	100		20
Lee and Rush, 1986 (12)	Individual + group	CBT	15	73	70	29
Wolchik et al., 1986 (13)	Individual + group	Psychoeducation	13	85	58	0
Wilson et al., 1986 (14)	Group	Cognitive restructuring + ERP	9	85	82	71
		Cognitive restructuring				
Fairburn et al., 1986 (15)	Individual	CBT	8	67	51	33
		Short-term focal	12	92	87	0
Laessle et al., 1987 (16)	Group	ET	12	92	80	0
			8	100		38
Leitenberg et al., 1988 (17)	Group	CBT + ERP (ss)	11	91	73	36
		CBT + ERP (ms)	12	92	67	33
Freeman et al., 1988 (18)	Individual + group	Individual CBT	32	66	79	
		Individual BT	30	83	87	
		Group	30	63	87	

Study	Setting	Treatment				
Agras et al., 1989 (19)	Individual	Self-monitor	19	84	63	24
		CBT	22	77	75	56
		CBT + ERP	17	94	52	31
Mitchell et al., 1990 (20)	Group	CBT + placebo	33	88	89	45
		CBT + imip	40	83	92	56
		Imip	45	74	49	16
Fairburn et al., 1991 (21)	Individual	CBT	25	84	97	71
		IPT	25	88	89	62
		BT	25	76	91	62
Fichter et al., 1991 (22)	Individual	Fluoxetine + BT	20	100	46.7	
		Placebo + BT	20	100	25.4	
Wilson et al., 1991 (23)	Individual	CBT + ERP	11	82	91	67
		CBT	11	73	95	88
Laessle et al., 1991 (24)	Group	Nutrition management	27	81	70	50
		Stress management	28	93	70	27
Garner et al., 1993 (25)	Individual	Psychodynamic	30	83	69	
		CBT	30	83	73	
Agras et al., 1992 (26)	Individual	Desip 16 wk	12		33	
		Desip 24 wk	12		54	
		CBT + desip 16 wk	12		72	
		CBT + desip 24 wk	12		75	
		CBT – 24 wk	12		68	
Mitchell et al., 1993 (27)	Group	CBT High emphasis on abstinence/high intensity	33	88	77	70
		High/low	41	88	78	73
		Low/high	35	86	88	71
		Low/low	34	82	32	32
Thackwray et al., 1993 (28)	Individual	Self-monitoring	47	83	82	69
		Behavioral			100	100
		CBT			89	92

TABLE 1 Continued

Author, Year	Format	Treatment	N	Completers (%)	Reduction in BE (%)	Abstinent at end of treatment %
Goldbloom et al., 1997 (29)	Individual	Fluoxetine	23	61	70	17
		CBT	24	67	80	43
		Fluoxetine + CBT	29	44	87	25
Walsh et al., 1997 (30)	Individual	CBT + medication	23	65	87	52
		CBT + placebo	25	64	65	24
		SPT + medication	22	73	55	18
		SPT + placebo	22	73	46	18
		Medication	28	57	69	29
Bulik et al., 1998 (31)	Individual	CBT + ERP – B	135	79	89	66
		CBT+ ERP – P			81	45
		Relax			79	47
Agras et al., 2000 (32)	Individual	CBT	110	71	86	29
		IPT	110	76	51	33
Agras et al., 2000 (33)	Individual	CBT	194	72		41
Hsu et al., 2001 (34)	Individual	CBT	100	85		35
		CBT + NT		89		52
		NT		17		17
		Support group		24		24
Jacobi et al., 2002 (35)	Group	CBT	53	58	34	
		CBT + fluoxetine		67	61	
		Fluoxetine		75	42	

CBT, cognitive behavioral therapy; BT, behavioral therapy; ERP, exposure and response preventions; ss, single site; ms, multiple sites; IPT, interpersonal psychotherapy; SPT, supportive therapy; Imip, imipramine; Desip, desipramine; NT, nutritional counseling.

ment in AN may be different than in BN, which can influence the style and timing of the interventions (42).

There is limited evidence supporting the efficacy of CBT in treating patients with AN. One study found CBT to be as effective as behavior therapy (43), and a more recent investigation suggested that CBT was useful in preventing relapse among weight-recovered anorexic individuals (44). However, there is a clear need for a rigorous empirical trial of CBT for AN. Difficulties associated with all treatment trials for AN (e.g., low base rate disorder, marked treatment resistance, high dropout rates) make such a study difficult. Large multicenter research strategies are likely to be needed to successfully complete such a study. Currently, CBT for AN is best conceptualized as one component of a multifaceted treatment plan that includes other modalities, such as family therapy, drug therapy, nutritional rehabilitation, and the use of hospital-based treatments. Such a multidisciplinary approach is consistent with recent practice guidelines for AN (45).

GUIDELINES FOR COGNITIVE BEHAVIORAL TREATMENT OF THE EATING DISORDERS

As noted previously, CBT is intended to be a symptom-focused, short-term treatment that attempts to directly modify eating disorder symptoms and associated behaviors. An emphasis is placed on proximal causal or maintaining factors for the disorders, and distal, historical, and causal factors are deemphasized. Furthermore, interventions are generally oriented around active patient participation, self-monitoring of ongoing behavior, completion of homework, active efforts to confront and modify thinking, and other behaviorally oriented approaches, while more psychodynamic interventions, focusing on treatment resistance, transference, countertransference, and unconscious cognitive thought processes, are not utilized.

CBT is also a structured treatment, which generally follows a predetermined sequence of strategies. For example, Table 2 outlines a general sequencing of treatment phases from CBT for BN, which may be modified somewhat for application with AN or BED. Phase I is quite behavioral in nature with an emphasis on teaching the patient essential medical and dietary concepts as well as to identify when problem behaviors are occurring and environmental stimuli that precipitate or prevent eating disorder symptoms. Furthermore, the patient is directly encouraged to diversify their meal plan with a particular emphasis on inclusion of feared foods. Phase II takes a decidedly more cognitive approach with an emphasis on identifying maladaptive cognitions and subjecting them to careful examination and empirical testing to determine their accuracy and objectivity. Also, patients are encouraged to monitor sequences of their behavior in the form of eliciting cues and

TABLE 2   Phases of Cognitive–Behavioral Therapy

Phase One: Normalization of Eating Behavior
   1. Self-monitoring
   2. Psychoeducation (risks of semistarvation, restraint theory)
   3. Stimulus control
   4. Contingency management
   5. Exposure to high-risk foods and situations
Phase Two: Cognitive Interventions
   1. Identifying maladaptive cognitions
   2. Cognitive restructuring
   3. Addressing underlying beliefs
   4. Cues and chains of cognitions and behaviors
   5. Psychoeducation (problem solving, body image, assertiveness,
      stress management)
Phase Three: Relapse Prevention
   1. Psychoeducation ("lapse" vs. "relapse")
   2. Exposure and response prevention
   3. Specific plan for lapse and relapse scenarios

---

mediating behaviors and cognitions and, ultimately, eating disorder behaviors. Finally, in phase III patients who have made substantial behavioral change are encouraged to develop plans to prevent relapse and maintain a healthier lifestyle.

Initiating CBT

The initial sessions of CBT must take into account the patient's likely ambivalence about making a change and emphasize the development of therapeutic rapport. In particular, eating-disordered individuals with highly obsessional, paranoid, or avoidant cognitive styles may enter treatment with considerable hesitation. Several authors (37,40) have discussed approaches to managing such ambivalence that are consistent with CBT. These interventions typically include recognizing the adaptive functions of the disorder for the patient, accepting the patient's thought processes as genuine, and a demonstration by the clinician of a clear knowledge of both general psychopathology and also eating disorders.

Self-Monitoring

Early in CBT, the patient is provided with some type of self-monitoring form, which may include information about time of day, environmental situations, food and liquid consumed, presence of eating disorder symptoms, and associated maladaptive thoughts and feelings. Such a self-monitoring approach is a clinically useful way to gather a considerable amount of information about the patient's day-to-day "ecological niche" surrounding their eating disorder symptoms. Patients should be instructed about the importance of self-monitoring, which is designed to provide them with a greater sense of control over and knowledge about their eating disorder symptoms.

Early in treatment, patients may be encouraged to record the consumption of meals, snacks, and bulimic symptoms (binges) in their self-monitoring records. This allows the clinician to see the presence or absence of well-structured schedules of eating that are reasonably dispersed throughout the day. Obviously, anorexic individuals' food records will reveal the absence of healthy and diversified eating, while the record of a bulimic individual may reveal a more chaotic and unpredictable pattern of eating. Self-monitoring may ultimately include an identification of environmental cues for particular types of eating behaviors, including binge eating, skipping meals, and purging. Eventually, the patient may also include data on particular thoughts and feelings in the face of specific environmental events or cues. Thus, the self-monitoring may help the clinician and patient to identify a pattern of particular environmental stimuli, associated intrapsychic activity in the form of cognitions and feelings, and overt behavioral activity such exercising, binge eating, or purging.

Cues and Consequences

One important aspect of self-monitoring is to help the patient identify stimuli that elicit problematic eating behaviors. For example, self-monitoring may reveal that periods of significant food restriction precede binge eating or that interpersonal conflict precedes periods of significant starvation. It is important for the individual to begin to identify those stimuli—whether cognitive, behavioral, or environmental—that increase the likelihood of specific eating disorder behaviors. Once these stimuli are identified, patients need to learn to respond to these stimuli in an alternative fashion. For example, if driving by a grocery store is a trigger to stop, buy binge food, and binge-eat, the patient may simply attempt to identify an alternative route that does not include exposure to the grocery store. Another useful strategy for dealing with triggers for problematic behaviors is distraction. For example, the experience of seeing ones body shape in a mirror may be a trigger for purging behavior or excessive exercise. However, if the patient can learn to create a "pause" between the stimulus and the problematical behavior, there may be time to develop alternatives and modify thought processes. Also, it may be useful for patients to learn to use certain stimuli to elicit positive healthy behaviors, which are part of their recovery. For example, patients may be encouraged to eat all of their meals at scheduled times and at a particular place in their home. These changes help to link positive eating behaviors to particular stimuli and avoid the association of eating and random or unpredictable stimuli.

Treatment should also focus on the consequences of eating behavior. First, patients need to be educated about the potential negative consequences of eating disorder symptomatology. Typically, these include medical, social, and financial consequences of their eating disorder behavior. However, patients should also be encouraged to identify the positive consequences of their eating disorder behavior. For example, for the extremely shy and inhibited individual, the solitary lifestyle of AN with extreme eating behaviors and individual exercise regimes may assist them in managing social anxiety. Alternatively, binge eating and purging behaviors may help the bulimic individual to avoid negative emotions associated with critical self-evaluation and negative social comparison. It is often useful to discuss with patients how the eating disorder is helpful to them and begin to identify alternative means of meeting similar needs. Recently, some clinicians have utilized strategies in which patients identify the positive and negative aspects of their eating disorder behaviors, and are also asked to identify what the consequences of their eating disorder behaviors will be 5 or 10 years from now (41,44). Furthermore, they might be asked how their lives might change if they continue to engage in their eating disorder as opposed to achieving recovery. Such strategies help the patient to identify more clearly the potential destructive consequences of their symptoms in the future but also fully acknowledge the benefits they obtained from these symptoms currently.

Cognitive Restructuring

Figure 1 depicts a basic cognitive model underlying CBT. This model emphasizes the close relationship between thoughts, feelings, and behaviors. In CBT, cognitions or thoughts are a central operational construct. It is not stressful environmental stimuli that are ultimately thought to result in eating disorder symptoms but the cognitive appraisal of those stimuli. For example, an eating-disordered individual may see her body in the mirror (stimulus) and have the thought "Oh no, I can't believe how fat I've become." Such a thought is associated with a negative emotional response, and in combination this thought and feeling may increase the likelihood of some self-destructive behavior (i.e., dieting, purging). Thus, eating-disordered individuals are encouraged to examine their cognitions carefully, identify instances of maladaptive thinking, and attempt to identify a more adaptive response to the cue.

Typically, patients are able to identify problematic thinking patterns through self-monitoring. At this point in the treatment, self-monitoring logs

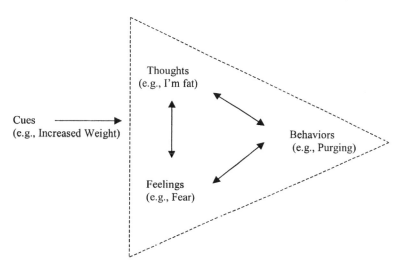

FIGURE 1 Model underlying cognitive–behavioral therapy.

may begin to include areas in which cognitions and feelings can be recorded. Patients are encouraged to simply describe their thoughts or feelings without censorship as they occur. This may be difficult at first and patients must be encouraged to practice identifying their thoughts. Often, eating-disordered individuals, like persons with other forms of psychopathology, display specific types of maladaptive thinking. Beck et al. (2) catalogued many of these cognitions in depressed individuals and found recurring themes and categories that have been described in eating disorder patients as well (37). These include dichotomous thinking (e.g., if I am not beautiful, I am ugly), overgeneralization (e.g., I wasn't able to follow a meal plan today so I will never be able to follow one), emotional reasoning (e.g., I know I am fat because I feel fat), catastrophizing (e.g., I have gained 3 pounds in 2 weeks, I know that I am becoming obese), and others. Patients should be taught about various forms of maladaptive thinking so that they can begin to monitor for the presence of such thinking in their daily activities. Once the patient has identified such negative thinking patterns, they can begin to work toward modification. Two general strategies are frequently employed in CBT for the eating disorders: (a) behavioral experimentation and (b) testing the validity of the thought-through questions.

Behavioral experimentation refers to identifying a negative thought and the logical or predicted consequence or outcome associated with that thought. Then, the individual intentionally creates a behavioral situation, that should result in the predicted outcome if the thought is accurate. Typically, because of the high degree of distortion in the maladaptive thought, the behavioral prediction is not confirmed through the experiment. For example, if an individual has the thought "eating three meals a day will make me fat," the patient and clinician can devise an experiment to test this thought. For example, the patient may agree that if she was able to eat three meals a day for at least 5 days, this would provide a good test of whether or not she would gain weight, as oppose to staying the same or perhaps even losing weight. If the patient were willing to try this on a trial basis for 5 days, she could actually weigh herself before starting and again 5 days later. Of course, the patient would have to agree to engage in the experiment and be willing to report on the outcome. Most likely, at least in BN, there would be little change in weight because calories may be ingested through meals rather than traditional binge eating patterns. The patient should be encouraged to identify the inference that can be drawn from the experiment and whether or not it conflicts with the prediction associated with the eating disorder.

The second means of restructuring thought patterns is to assist the patient in questioning the actual thought. For example, if a patient had the thought "I will be happy when I am below 100 pounds," the therapist may ask a series of questions to test the validity of this idea. For example, the patient may be asked if she had ever been below 100 pounds previously and whether or not she was happy then. If not, the therapist may ask what it means that she weighed less than 100 pounds and was not happy. If she states that she was happy, the therapist may ask if she was happy all the time. It would be expected that she was not happy all the time, and that could lead to a discussion of what other factors must have influenced her mood besides weight, given that she was under a 100 pounds but still had periods of unhappiness. Also, the patient may be asked if she knew any other people who weighed less than a 100 pounds and whether or not they were happy. In general, the therapist should take the approach of asking the patient what evidence there is to support the thought that weighing less than 100 pounds will make her happy and, alternatively, what evidence there is that fails to support the thought. Ideally, the therapist and patient collaboratively examine the evidence for the thought, examine its validity, and begin to develop more adaptive and accurate alternative thought patterns.

Early in treatment, cognitive restructuring tends to focus on issues surrounding food, weight, and shape. However, as the individual gains greater control of symptoms, cognitive restructuring may move to other associated problems. Issues regarding interpersonal relationships, intimacy, academic or vocational success, and broader issues associated with personality functioning may also be targeted. However, these issues are unlikely to be a central theme for the therapy, especially in short-term treatment.

Recently, cognitive approaches to the management of AN have placed a greater emphasis on interpersonal functioning and deeper cognitive structures, particularly self-schemas and interpersonal schemas (41). As the therapist listens to descriptions of maladaptive or automatic thoughts, recurrent themes of cognition about self or others may be identified. Particularly with anorexic individuals, working with these more generalized and stable attitudes about the self and the behavior of others may be useful. For example, the individual who believes that she must be loved by everyone, *and* that other people tend to be extremely critical and rejecting, displays schemas about self and others that are highly maladaptive and may promote further entrenchment in eating disorder symptoms as a means of avoiding frightening interpersonal scenarios. Helping such patients to recognize the thoughts about self and others and possibly the origins of such thinking is important, but the fundamental approach to cognitive restructuring remains intact. Individuals must subject such schemas to empirical tests to evaluate their accuracy. However, it is important to remember that attempts to modify these types of deeper cognitive structures may be arduous and time consuming, and will probably not be included in short-term treatments.

Problem Solving and Social Skills Training

Other strategies may be included in CBT for eating disorders. Often, patients will suggest that their eating disorder symptoms have become coping strategies for a wide variety of problems. In this situation, it is important that the therapy focus on the more productive problem-solving strategies. In some fashion, the following problem-solving steps should be introduced to the patient: (a) recognize that problems cannot be avoided and are a normal part of living; (b) specify in a detailed fashion the nature of the problem; (c) once the problem is clearly understood, brainstorm solutions to the problem without worrying about the adequacy of the solutions; (d) after carefully considering the pros and cons of each option, choose one of the solutions and try it out; (e) after trying one of the solutions, evaluate it to see if the problem has been resolved. This series of steps, originally outlined by D'zurilla and Goldfried (46), may with practice help the individual to identify solutions to problems that are outside the realm of eating disorder symptoms.

One specific type of problem solving lies in the area of interpersonal relationships. Many problems in living involve relationships to other people. When this is the situation, patients should be encouraged to carefully identify the nature of the problem they are having with the other person. Assertiveness training is a helpful approach to several types of interpersonal problems, including difficulty in expressing negative emotions, problems setting limits, and problems expressing positive feelings. In therapy, role playing may greatly facilitate the patient's ability to effectively deal with problematic interpersonal situations. Seeing the clinician model appropriate social responses in a role play with the patient may facilitate imitation. The old teaching axiom of "see one, do one, teach one," is an appropriate way to think about improving social skills.

Case Study

Cindy was a 28-year-old, married mother of a 6-year-old son and 3-year-old daughter at the time of presentation to the outpatient eating disorders clinic. She had recently relocated to the area after her husband took a managerial position with a local manufacturing company. The impetus to her seeking treatment was the distress and shame she'd been experiencing since her daughter walked into the bathroom and observed her mother vomiting.

Cindy was seen for an initial evaluation, which included a detailed review of the onset of eating disorder symptoms, current eating patterns and compensatory behaviors, thoughts and feelings associated with weight and shape, weight and menstrual history, as well as assessment of comorbid psychopathology, chemical use, medical status, and psychosocial history.

Cindy reported the onset of eating disordered behavior at the age of 15 when she entered a new high school following her family's relocated. She recalls her volleyball teammates ridiculing others' appearance and feared that she would also be the subject of ridicule. Cindy began skipping breakfast and lunch (a practice common to her peer group) and consuming only low-calorie and low-fat foods at the evening meal with her family. She was motivated to continue dieting by the attention she received from peers. Cindy recalled first self-inducing vomiting after she ate pizza and sweets at a postgame celebration. Vomiting behavior quickly escalated, and Cindy also began to binge-eat. She indicated that because she could vomit she would "make it worth my while" and consume "forbidden foods" she enjoyed. Binge eating and vomiting continued at a rate of two or three times a week throughout high school and her early college years. Although she continued to be extremely concerned about her weight and shape, Cindy maintained a 6-year abstinence from binge eating and vomiting after she left college, married, had a child, and breast-fed.

Cindy described a gradual relapse in eating disorder symptoms in the year before her relocation. Anticipating loneliness in a new town, frustrated that she had not met her goal of completing her degree, and increasingly disparaging of her body and abilities, Cindy attempted to lose weight through dietary restriction believing she would feel more confident and better about herself in general. Binge eating and vomiting quickly returned and escalated. At the time of presentation to the outpatient eating disorder clinic, Cindy weighed 145 pounds at a height of 5 foot 4 inches (body mass index = 24.9).

She reported extreme dissatisfaction with her shape, feeling extremely fat and unworthy as a result of her weight. Cindy reported her ideal weight as 110 pounds, believing she would be more confident, a better mother, and more acceptable to others.

In attempts to achieve her ideal weight, Cindy had a daily plan to avoid dietary fat, restrict calories to 1000 kcal/day, and exercise for 60 min. Cindy described "losing the battle" to follow her strict plan and admitted to binge eating and purging daily. Each day began with attempting to avoid eating, only to be preoccupied with food, often distracting her from tasks at hand and time with her children. She typically nibbled on food she prepared for her daughter's snack and midday meal. Chastising herself, concluding she had already "blown it" for the day, and vowing to begin anew the next day, Cindy reported binge eating on her children's uneaten meals, 12 ounces of chips, and 6 cups of ice cream in the early afternoon during the children's nap time.

Cindy denied use of laxatives, enemas, diuretics, syrup of ipecac, chewing and spitting, or rumination of food. She denied exercising in an excessive manner, in fact berated herself for not achieving her plan of daily exercise. Cindy had been on an antidepressant for 15 months; however, she continued to struggle with dysphoric mood, amotivation, low energy, poor concentration, and low self-esteem. Based on evaluation results, it was recommended that Cindy participate in individual CBT for bulimia. She was referred to her primary physician for review of medications and serum electrolytes.

Cindy's treatment began with a detailed description of the cognitive model of the maintenance of bulimia with particular emphasis on the cyclic relationship between strict dieting (avoidance of eating, restriction of intake, and food avoidance), binge eating, and purging. Cindy agreed that insecurity and low self-esteem precipitated and exacerbated concerns about her weight and shape, and she believed that her eating disorder had become a way to cope with these negative mood states. Self-monitoring was presented as the initial treatment assignment. Cindy was instructed to record the time and place of eating episodes; type and amount of food eaten; whether the episode was considered a meal, snack, or binge; whether vomiting occurred; and thoughts, feelings, and circumstances surrounding the episode of eating (Fig. 2). She was informed of the importance of accurate self-monitoring and its part in providing vital information on triggers for eating disorder behaviors as well as guiding treatment sessions. Despite anticipating embarrassment about the therapist being aware of the intimate details of her eating disorder, Cindy left the session stating an understanding of and commitment to the CBT plan.

Despite her stated commitment, Cindy arrived at her second scheduled appointment having not self-monitored. Time was taken to explore with Cindy what had interfered with her completing this crucial first assignment,

INITIALS _____ DAY _____ DATE _____

Time	Food & Liquid Consumed	Place	B	V/L	Context (CUES)

FIGURE 2 Food and liquid daily monitoring form.

and the discussion gave way to identifying the advantages and disadvantages of addressing her eating disorder. Cindy expressed significant ambivalence regarding treatment, embarrassment and shame about her symptoms, and fear of becoming fat were she to change her behavior. Cindy was provided with reassurance that most normal-weight patients do not gain weight as a result of CBT.

Cindy presented to her third session having completed self-monitoring, which was reviewed in great detail with particular emphasis on potential cues of binge eating and vomiting. A pattern of dietary restriction, avoiding foods thought to be "fattening," and avoiding eating in general were highlighted as examples of strict dieting which left Cindy vulnerable to binge eating. The importance of eating consistently throughout the day was stressed, and Cindy collaborated on developing a plan for having regular meals and snacks consisting of food and portion sizes that she was prepared to consume without vomiting. Cindy was easily able to adapt her eating to the scheduled eating pattern she provided for her young children and found that three meals and three snacks could be consumed in the presence of others, which would further decrease the risk of binge eating and vomiting.

The next several sessions focused on implementing Cindy's plan for consistent eating while continuing to monitor her weight through weekly weighing. Cindy was surprised by an improvement in energy and mood as well as renewed interest in spending time with her children. Given her significant fear of weight gain and subsequent food avoidance, Cindy was instructed to develop a hierarchy of feared foods. Each day, Cindy developed a plan for introducing a food from the bottom of the hierarchy that may trigger binge eating and engaging in an alternative behavior immediately following the consumption until the urge to vomit subsided. Weekly weighing provided Cindy with valuable evidence that these foods could be consumed without weight gain, which in turn provided motivation for continuing to add previously avoided foods.

As episodes of binge eating and vomiting decreased and became intermittent, Cindy's treatment began to focus on those factors that had been maintaining her eating disorder, in particular distorted thoughts and beliefs about food, eating, weight and shape, and the use of dietary restricting, binge eating, and vomiting as a means of managing life stress and negative mood. The presence of maladaptive thoughts as cues for eating disorder behaviors was identified using self-monitoring forms where Cindy had also been monitoring her thoughts associated with eating episodes. These thoughts were then challenged using cognitive restructuring. For example, Cindy identified her belief that "eating fat will make me fat" and more specifically indicated a belief that she would gain 5 pounds if she consumed a food containing more than 5 grams of dietary fat per serving. Cindy was challenged to test this belief by setting up an experiment in which she consumed ice cream without vomiting and later in the week monitored her weight. She was instructed to consume the ice cream in the presence of her husband, utilize alternative behaviors for a specified period of time and/or spend time out of the house should the urge to vomit occur. This process of challenging maladaptive thoughts through empirical testing and evidence gathering was repeated as Cindy worked through her list of feared foods, exposed herself to high-risk situations, and confronted negative thoughts about her weight and shape.

Cindy's participation in CBT also revealed a longstanding pattern of engaging in binge eating and vomiting in response to a variety of negative mood states, including loneliness, frustration, interpersonal conflict, and self-disparagement. Cindy was increasingly able to implement cognitive restructuring and alternative behaviors at such times, but struggled with extreme negative self-appraisal, which continued to place her at risk for binge eating and vomiting. Not completing her educational degree and the lack of social contacts since relocating were identified as cues for self-disparagement and subsequent eating disorder behavior. Problem solving was applied wherein Cindy clearly identified why social isolation was problematic, generated options for solving the problem, including joining a parents-of-preschoolers group, taking courses to finish her degree, attending community functions, and joining a church. A similar process of problem solving was applied to Cindy's struggle with not completing her degree, as well as a variety of problems of daily life.

After 4 months of treatment, Cindy achieved abstinence from binge eating and purging, was consistently eating a variety of foods, and reported increasing confidence as she tackled what had previously been viewed as insurmountable environmental stressors. The final stage of treatment focused on maintaining the changes that Cindy had made in treatment and developing a relapse prevention plan. Cindy considered what situations may place her at risk for relapse (e.g., another relocation, her daughter's transition into school) and developed a plan for managing eating disorder symptoms should they arise. She was informed of the possibility of a reemergence of symptoms in times of stress or transition and was reassured that utilizing the skills she developed in treatment would likely curtail a relapse. Cindy reviewed the techniques she had learned and devised a plan for returning to self-monitoring, making sure she was utilizing alternative behaviors and remaining connected with her social supports. Cindy agreed that three consecutive weeks of binge eating and vomiting should signal the need to return to treatment; however, she felt confident that she would be able to interrupt the cycle of binge eating and vomiting.

CONCLUSION

CBT is a treatment for a wide variety of eating disorder symptoms that has received considerable empirical support and continues to be the modality of choice for a variety of eating disorder clinical presentations. CBT may evolve and be modified in future studies; already applications in telemedicine, CD-ROM, and Palm Pilot applications have emerged. Furthermore, variations of CBT have been developed with a greater emphasis on interpersonal functioning, emotional responding, and alternative cognitive structures. There continues to be a need for enhanced approaches to educating mental health professionals about the applications of CBT to eating-disordered patients, and a lack of dissemination of these treatments remains a limiting factor for eating-disordered individuals.

ACKNOWLEDGMENTS

Supported by research grants from the McKnight Foundation and the National Institute of Mental Health (R01-MH59234) and the National Institute of Diabetes, Digestive and Kidney Diseases (R01-DK61912; R01-DK60432; P30-DK50456), and the Neuropsychiatric Research Institute.

REFERENCES

1. Beck AT, Emery G. Anxiety Disorders and Phobias. New York: Basic Books, 1985.
2. Beck AT, Rush AJ, Shaw BF, Emery G. Cognitive Therapy of Depression. New York: Guilford Press, 1979.
3. Peterson CP, Mitchell JE. Cognitive behavior therapy. In: Gabbard GO, ed. Treatment of Psychiatric Disorders. 2d ed. Washington, DC: APA Press, 1995.
4. Fairburn CG, Marcus MD, Wilson GT. Cognitive behavioral therapy for binge eating and bulimia nervosa: a comprehensive treatment manual. In: Fairburn CG, Wilson GT, eds. Binge Eating: Nature Assessment and Treatment. New York: Guilford Press, 1993:361–404.
5. Mitchell JE, Peterson CB. Cognitive–behavioral treatment of eating disorders. Dickstein LD, Riba MB, Oldham JM, eds. Review of Psychiatry. Vol. 16:. Washington, DC: APA Press, 1995:I-107–I-134.
6. Crow S, Mitchell JE. Bulimia nervosa. In: Mitchell JE, ed. The Outpatient Treatment of Eating Disorders: A Guide for Therapists Dietitians and Physicians. Minneapolis: University of Minnesota Press, 2001:26–59.
7. Lacey JH. An outpatient treatment program for bulimia nervosa. Int J Eat Disord 1983; 286:1609–1613.
8. Connors ME, Johnson CL, Stuckey MK. Treatment of bulimia with brief psychoeducational group therapy. Am J Psychiatry 1984; 141:1512–1516.

9.   Yates AJ, Sambrailo F. Bulimia nervosa: a descriptive and therapeutic study. Behav Res Ther 1984; 5:505–517.

10. Kirkley BG, Schneider JA, Agras WS, Bachman JA. Comparison of two group treatments for bulimia. J Consult Clin Psychol 1985; 53:43–48.

11. Ordman AM, Kirschenbaum DS. Cognitive behavioral therapy for bulimia: an initial outcome study. J Consult Clin Psychol 1985; 53:305–313.

12. Lee NF, Rush AJ. Cognitive–behavioral group therapy for bulimia. Int J Eat Disord 1986; 5:599–615.

13. Wolchik SA, Weiss L, Katzman MA. An empirically validated short-term psychoeducational group treatment program for bulimia. Int J Eat Disord 1986; 5:21–34.

14. Wilson GT, Rossiter E, Kleifeld EI, Lindholm L. Cognitive behavioral treatment of bulimia nervosa: a controlled evaluation. Behav Res Ther 1986; 24:227–238.

15. Fairburn CG, Kirk J, O'Connor M, Cooper PJ. A comparison of two psychological treatments for bulimia nervosa. Behav Res Ther 1986; 24:629–643.

16. Laessle RG, Waadt S, Pirke KM. A structured behaviorally oriented treatment for bulimia nervosa. Psychother Psychosom 1987; 48:141–145.

17. Leitenberg H, Rosen JC, Gross J, Nudelman S, Vara LS. Exposure plus response prevention treatment of bulimia nervosa. J Consult Clin Psychol 1988; 56:535–541.

18. Freeman CPL, Barry F, Dunkeld-Turnbull J, Henderson A. Controlled trial of psychotherapy for bulimia nervosa. Br Med J; 296:521–525.

19. Agras WS, Schneider JA, Arnow B, Raeburn SD, Telch CF. Cognitive behavioral and response prevention treatments for bulimia nervosa. J Consult Clin Psychol 1989; 57:215–221.

20. Mitchell JE, Pyle RL, Eckert ED, Hatsukami D, Pomeroy C, Zimmerman R. A comparison study of antidepressants and structured intensive group psychotherapy in the treatment of bulimia nervosa. Arch Gen Psychiatry 1990; 47:149–157.

21. Fairburn CG, Jones RT, Peveler RC, Carr SJ, Solomon RA, O'Connor ME, Burran J, Hope RA. Three psychological treatments for bulimia nervosa. Arch Gen Psychiatry 1991; 48:463–469.

22. Fichter MM, Leibl K, Rief W, Brunner E, Schmidt-Auberger S, Engel RR. Fluoxetine versus placebo: a double-blind study with bulimic inpatients undergoing intensive psychotherapy. Pharmacopsychiatry 1991; 24:1–7.

23. Wilson GT, Eldredge KL, Smith D, Niles B. Cognitive behavioral treatment with and without response prevention for bulimia. Behav Res Ther 1991; 29:575–583.

24. Laessle RG, Beumont PJV, Butow P, Lennerts W, O'Connor M, Pirke KM, Touyz SW, Waadt S. A comparison of nutritional management with stress management in the treatment of bulimia nervosa. Br J Psychiatry 1991; 159:250–261.

25. Garner DM, Rockert W, Davis R, Garner MV, Olmsted MP, Engle M. Comparison of cognitive behavioral and supportive expressive therapy for bulimia nervosa. Am J Psychiatry 1993; 150:37–46.

26. Agras WS, Rossiter EM, Arnow B, Schneider JA, Telch CG, Raeburn SD, Bruce

B, Perl M, Koran LM. Pharmacologic and cognitive behavioral treatment for bulimia nervosa: a controlled clinical comparison. Am J Psychiatry 1992; 149: 82–87.

27. Mitchell JE, Pyle RL, Pomeroy C, Zollman M, Crosby R, Seim H, Eckert ED, Zimmerman R. Cognitive behavioral group psychotherapy for bulimia nervosa: the importance of logistical variables. Int J Eat Disord 1993; 14:277–288.
28. Thackwray DE, Smith MC, Bodfish JW, Meyers AW. A comparison of behavioral and cognitive behavioral interventions for bulimia nervosa. J Consult Clin Psychol 1993; 61:639–645.
29. Goldbloom DS, Olmsted M, Davis R, Clews J, Heinmaa M, Rockert W, Shaw B. A randomized controlled trial of fluoxetine and cognitive behavioral therapy for bulimia nervosa. Behav Res Ther 1997; 35:803–811.
30. Walsh BT, Wilson GT, Loeb KL, Devlin MJ, Pike KM, Roose SP, Fleiss J, Waternaux C. Medication and psychotherapy in the treatment of bulimia nervosa. Am J Psychiatry 1997; 154:523–531.
31. Agras WS, Walsh BT, Fairburn CG, Wilson GT, Kraemer HC. Multicenter comparison of cognitive behavioral therapy and interpersonal therapy for bulimia nervosa. Arch Gen Psychiatry 2000; 57:459 468.
32. Hsu LK, Rand W, Sullivan S, Liu DW, Milliken B, McDonagh B, Kaye WH. Cognitive therapy, nutritional therapy and their combination in the treatment of bulimia nervosa. Psychol Med 2001; 32:871–879.
33. Bulik CM, Sullivan PF, Carter FA, McIntosh VV, Joyce PR. The role of exposure with response prevention in the cognitive–behavioural therapy for bulimia nervosa. Psychol Med 1998; 28:611–623.
34. Agras WS, Crow SJ, Halmi KA, Mitchell JE, Wilson CT, Kraemer HC. Outcome predictors for the cognitive behavior treatment of bulimia nervosa: data from a multisite study. Am J Psychiatry 2000; 157:1302–1308.
35. Jacobi C, Dahme B, Dittmann R. Cognitive–behavioural, fluoxetine and combined treatment for bulimia nervosa: short-and long-term results. Eur Eat Disord Rev 2002; 10:179–198.
36. Agras WS, Rossiter EM, Arnow B, Telch CF, Raeburn SD, Bruce B, Koran L. One year follow up of psychosocial and pharmacologic treatments for bulimia nervosa. J Clin Psychiatry 1991; 52:29–33.
37. Peterson CB, Mitchell JE. Cognitive behavioral therapy for eating disorders. In: Mitchell JE, ed. The Outpatient Treatment of Eating Disorders: A Guide for Therapists, Dietitians, and Physicians. Minneapolis: University of Minnesota Press, 2001:145–167.
38. Smith DE, Marcus MD, Kaye W. Cognitive behavioral treatment of obese binge eaters. Int J Eat Disord 1992; 12:257 262.
39. Wilfley DE, Agras WS, Telch CF, Rossiter EM, Schneider JA, Cole AG, Sifford L, Raeburn SD. Group cognitive behavioral therapy and group interpersonal therapy for the nonpurging bulimic: a controlled comparison. J Consult Clin Psychol 1993; 61:296–305.
40. Wilfley DE, Welch RR, Stein RI, Spurrell EB, Cohen LR, Saelens BE, Dounchis JZ, Frank MA, Wiseman CV, Matt GE. A randomized comparison of group

cognitive behavioral therapy and group interpersonal psychotherapy for the treatment of overweight individuals with binge eating disorder. Arch Gen Psychiatry 2002; 59:713–721.

41. Garner DM, Vitousek KM, Pike KM. Cognitive behavioral therapy for anorexia nervosa. In: Garner DM, Garfinkel PE, eds. Handbook of Treatment for Eating Disorders. 2nd ed. New York: Guilford Press, 1997:94–144.

42. Serpell L, Treasure J. Bulimia nervosa: Friend or foe? The pros and cons of bulimia nervosa. Int J Eat Disord 2002; 32:164–170.

43. Channon S, De Silva P, Hemsley D, Perkins R. A controlled trial of cognitive–behavioural and behavioural treatment of anorexia nervosa. Behav Res Ther 1989; 27:529–535.

44. Pike KM. Relapse prevention for anorexia nervosa. Paper presented at the Seventh New York International Conference on Eating Disorders, New York, 1996.

45. American Psychiatric Association. Practice guideline for the treatment of patients with eating disorders (revision). Am J Psychiatry 2000; 157(Suppl):1–39.

46. D'zurilla TJ, Goldfried MR. Problem solving and behavior modification. J Abnorm Psychol 1971; 78:197–226.

18

An Overview of Family Evaluation and Therapy for Anorexia Nervosa, Bulimia Nervosa, and Binge Eating Disorder

Deborah Marcontell Michel and Susan G. Willard
Tulane University School of Medicine
New Orleans, Louisiana, U.S.A.

Family therapy encompasses a group of psychotherapies that focus on the entire family unit in terms of interaction and change, instead of focusing on any individual member. Although the specific theories, treatment approaches, and goals of particular schools vary, most strive to facilitate change within the family in order to reduce or eliminate problematic interactions and behaviors.

The roots of family therapy can be traced back to the 1950s when Gregory Bateson conducted his seminal research with schizophrenics and their families on levels of communication. His research, along with many notable others such as Nathan Ackerman, Murray Bowen, Salvador Minuchin, Jay Haley, and Virginia Satir, led to the family movement. This movement represented more than just a new approach to therapy. Instead, it was a different way of looking at behavior that emphasized the examination of communication between individuals in relationships (1).

In this chapter, we begin by identifying and explaining some of the basic concepts of family therapy, and by linking these principles to how family therapists work to facilitate change. Next, we provide a brief historical perspective on the family treatment of those with eating disorders and descriptions of common family characteristics. Major models of family therapy used

425

to treat persons with eating disorders are then presented, along with the empirical evidence to support their use. We also provide guidelines for clinical practice of family therapy including important areas of inquiry in family evaluation, common issues in family therapy, and potential obstacles to assessment and treatment.

BASIC CONCEPTS AND PRINCIPLES OF FAMILY THERAPY

To appreciate the family therapist's perspective of a given individual's behavior, a synopsis of the basic concepts and principles of family therapy is in order. Foley (2) described the family unit as an open system. A *system* comprises sets of different parts that are interconnected with all parts affecting the other parts. Furthermore, each part has a relationship to the other parts in a stable manner. The family system is considered open because it has a continuous flow of elements entering and leaving the system. Open systems are further characterized by wholeness, relationship, and equifinality. *Wholeness* is the interdependence between the parts of the system. This principle emphasizes not only the individuals in the family but also the relationships among them. *Relationship*, then, examines the interactions between the parts of the family and focuses on what is happening, not *why* it is happening. The family therapist therefore carefully analyzes interactions among all family members. Finally, *equifinality* refers to the tenet that open systems are not dictated by their initial conditions; thus, difficulties can be eliminated if changes are made at any point in time within the system. Consequently, a family therapist focuses on the present, not the past, with the idea that an intervention can be made at any time to change the system.

According to Foley (2), family relationships are made up of interlocking *triangles* that lend stability to the system and function to reduce or increase its emotional intensity. Thus, whenever the emotional balance between two family members becomes too distant or too close, a third family member can restore equilibrium and stability. One of the tasks of the family therapist is to analyze the existing triangles in the family system and intervene to change the system. The process by which the system adjusts itself is termed *feedback*. When *negative feedback* is given in response to deviation from the existing system, the deviation is corrected and balance is restored. By contrast, *positive feedback* prevents the system from returning to its original state, forces it to change, and thereby destroys the former system. Instead of attempting to directly correct a problematic behavior, the family therapist may use this principle to exaggerate a symptom to the point at which it causes the original dysfunctional system to collapse.

HISTORY OF FAMILY THERAPY IN TREATMENT OF EATING DISORDERS

Today the need for family therapy in treating eating disorders from a bio-psychosocial approach is widely accepted (3). References have been made, however, to the importance of the role of the family in the development and maintenance of anorexia nervosa (AN) ever since its appearance in medical literature during the 1800s. Early writers believed that the families were harmful and should be excluded from the patient's treatment (4,5). It was not until the early 1970s that the family dynamics involved in AN were more fully appreciated through the observations and writings of Hilde Bruch (6). She noted the association between eating disorders and difficulty with individuation and emotional separation from the family of origin. In the mid to late 1970s, Mara Selvini-Palazzoli (7) and Salvador Minuchin and colleagues (8,9) pioneered the systematic application of family therapy to the treatment of AN with their schools of systems therapy and structural therapy, respectively. More recently, a group of clinicians at the Maudsley Hospital in London have developed the Maudsley model of family therapy for AN (10).

Obviously, the history of family therapy in the treatment of eating disorders has focused on the development of methods to treat individuals with AN. These approaches have also been applied to the family treatment of bulimia nervosa (BN) and will be discussed later. For a more detailed account of the history and development of family therapies in the treatment of eating disorders, see Dare and Eisler (10).

FAMILY CHARACTERISTICS OF INDIVIDUALS WITH AN EATING DISORDER

Minuchin and his cohorts at the Philadelphia Child Guidance Center presented family characteristics they found typical of families having a child with AN (8,9). The attributes included enmeshment, rigidity, overprotectiveness, lack of conflict resolution, and involvement of the child in parental discord. Enmeshment referred to the diffusion of boundaries resulting in emotional overinvolvement. Rigidity in the family organization reflected a lack of flexibility in the face of developmental stages requiring change. The observed overprotectiveness often was not limited to the identified patient or the eating disorder, yet it served to constrain the child's autonomy and independence. The rigidity and overprotectiveness of the families left little room for conflict negotiation. Consequently, problems were usually left unresolved. Involvement of the ill child in parental conflict (a detrimental triangle) resulted in the child playing an important role in the family pattern of conflict avoidance. As a result, the child received powerful reinforcement for remaining ill.

In families having a child with BN, Schwartz et al. (11) observed the same interaction patterns described by the Philadelphia group in addition to social isolation, appearance consciousness, and a special meaning attached to food and eating. In a study of family therapy, these researchers found that the particular issues around which the attributes were displayed depended on the degree of "Americanization," or drive to achieve dominant cultural values, versus ethnic identity of the family in question. From this research, the authors identified three family typologies that are very similar to the ones described below.

As cited in Michel and Willard (12), three types of family organizations commonly seen in families who have a daughter with BN have been described by Root et al. (13). The authors did not observe differences based on subtype and, although their focus was on a bulimic population, our experience is that these characteristics may also be seen in families who have a daughter with AN. One type of organization is the "perfect family." Appearance is of utmost importance, as this family strives to appear perfect to outside observers and the family reputation is sacred. Family members are therefore expected to think, act, and feel the "right" way. The family is governed by rigid rules and the identified patient tends to be a very high achiever relative to family standards. An eating disorder in this family may represent any or all of the following: (a) passive rebellion, (b) creation of a separate identity, (c) suppression of or distraction from feelings by focusing on food, and (d) assertion of personal control in the midst of familial control.

A second family organization, as described by Root and her colleagues (13), is the "overprotective family." This family encourages dependence and refuses to acknowledge needs for independence. Anger is seldom openly displayed, so that passive-aggressive behaviors develop, thereby hindering direct expressions of rebellion. Eating disorder symptoms may reflect a means of passive rebellion and indirect expression of anger while simultaneously reaffirming dependence on family members.

The last family organization discussed by Root et al. (13) is the "chaotic family," which has virtually no rules, organization, or consistency. The availability and expression of love is unpredictable, and conflicts are usually resolved by physical aggression and/or psychological intimidation. Physical and/or sexual abuse is often present. Consequently, eating disorder symptoms may function as a safe way to express anger, provide a means of separation from the abusive situation, and/or assert consistency in one's life. It can, however, also represent a form of self-destructive behavior.

There are other family characteristics commonly found among families of an individual with an eating disorder (12). Weight is often a family issue. One or more family members may be overweight or excessively thin, and there may be an overconcern with food and food-related issues in the household. In this case, it is not uncommon to see one or both parents engaged in chronic dieting and/or rigid exercise regimens. Adolescents in these families may be especially vulnerable to the use of dieting and exercising as a means of bonding with parents who are obviously preoccupied with such issues themselves. In addition, some parents of children with eating disorders have vicariously experienced their children's successes and accomplishments. As signs of puberty ensue, the parents often get depressed or frightened about what the future will hold when the children are grown and gone. The unconscious pressure on these youngsters, then, is to maintain the child role and to not grow up. Family loyalty to retain homeostasis is often chosen over normal development, which would lead to separation and independence. Other characteristics that may be observed include a highly critical parent, parental depression, or marital problems. In the latter case, the child may receive the spoken or unspoken message that independence, autonomy, and leaving home will cause the family system to fall apart.

We are aware of only one study describing the family characteristics of individuals with binge eating disorder (BED). Hodges et al. (14) compared the families of those with BED, AN-restricting type (AN-R), AN-binge/eating purging type (AN−B + P), BN, and normal controls. The investigators found that those with BED endorsed less family cohesion and less encouragement to express honest feelings than the other eating disorder groups. They also described their families as more isolated, more sedentary, and limited in terms of emphasis on independence. Furthermore, the BED group rated their families lower on achievement orientation, intellectual-cultural orientation, and moral religious emphasis. Finally, they described their families as having less structure, fewer rules, and less predictability than the other eating disorder groups. When compared to individuals with AN-R and AN-B + P, the BED group reported more conflict that was similar to the group with BN.

Compared to subjects without an eating disorder, individuals with BED in the Hodges et al. (14) study reported more familial conflict and described their families as more rigid in terms of rules and procedures used to regulate family life. The BED group also endorsed less independence, cohesiveness, and expressiveness in addition to less focus on pursuit of political, social, cultural, and intellectual endeavors or participation in social or recreational activities. The authors caution that data were gathered via self-report and no other means of corroboration obtained, yet the patients' accounts may provide useful information for treatment.

FAMILY EVALUATION

In order to determine the needs of the family and to decide what therapeutic interventions are appropriate, an evaluation of the family is in order. This is in accordance with the APA Practice Guidelines for the Treatment of Eating Disorders (15). The evaluation should include all members living within the home and, at times, the clinician may bring in other family members who do not live in the home but have been identified as family members having significant relationships with the identified patient. The purpose of the assessment is to ascertain what role, if any, the family environment played in the development and maintenance of the eating disorder and to what degree those issues, if present, remain (16).

Evaluation of the family includes basic psychosocial information about members such as demographic data, present and past living arrangements, psychiatric history, medical history, educational and occupational history, and social history. Inquiry into significant family events is also important as is the assessment of family traditions. Gathering background information on each parent's family of origin is helpful so that multigenerational patterns of relating and behaving can be identified. Regarding the evaluation of physical or sexual abuse, our family and individual assessments are conducted separately by different therapists. Although we acknowledge that not all clinicians are in a position to practice in this manner, it is our opinion that this arrangement makes it comparatively easier for the identified patient to disclose such sensitive information. Our experience in most cases of ongoing abuse, however, is that it will not be disclosed until a stronger therapeutic relationship has been established with the individual psychotherapist. Though we are unaware of any published data to directly support this clinical observation in a psychotherapy setting, it is consistent with research demonstrating significant delay in child and adolescent disclosure of sexual abuse, if the abuse is disclosed at all (17).

In addition to conducting a standard psychosocial interview of the family, Andersen (18) compiled a list of areas which should be investigated including (a) interactional patterns, (b) flexibility, (c) sensitivity, (d) family supports and stresses, (e) performance of stage-appropriate tasks, and (f) family knowledge of the illness. Examination of interactional patterns includes such topics as quality of the marital relationship, spousal agreement on parenting behavior, family satisfaction and companionship, communication patterns, and the general affective atmosphere of the family. Flexibility refers to how easily the family system allows members to change in terms of communication and roles they play in response to situations and stressors. In evaluating the sensitivity component, the practitioner assesses whether family members demonstrate emotional hypersensitivity and overreactivity, or uninvolvement and insensitivity, to one another. Evaluation of family supports and stresses includes the degree of support, or lack thereof, that family members provide to one another as well as any sources of significant strength and stress within the family. In addition, evaluation of outside supports and stressors is important. Regarding the performance of stage-appropriate tasks, the clinician assesses the age appropriateness of rules and responsibilities that are assigned to family members, particularly children. Finally, the clinician needs to know family members' understanding of the illness in terms of etiology, treatment, and recovery as well as their thoughts, feelings, and behaviors associated with it. In particular, knowledge of family attitudes and behaviors that may hinder the patient's ability to recover is critical so that they may be quickly examined and resolved (16). Similarly, family members' preoccupation with weight and appearance, which may sabotage the identified patient's efforts at recovery, must be addressed early on (19).

Vanderlinden and Vandereycken (20) stress that family assessment is a continuous process throughout family treatment. They recommend performing a functional analysis of the eating disorder within the family system. The goal is to formulate hypotheses about how the eating disorder functions within the family. The following questions, then, are important to remember throughout the process: (a) How does the symptom serve to stabilize the family? (b) What role does the family play in stabilizing the symptom? (c) Around what central theme is the problem organized? (d) What consequences will follow change in the family? (e) What is the therapeutic dilemma?

Standardized, self-report instruments that the practitioner may find helpful in assessing quality of familial relationships and interactions from an individual family member's point of view are available. A selection of these include the Leuven Family Questionnaire (21), the Family Evaluation Scale (FES; 22), the Family Adaptation and Cohesion Evaluation Scale (FACES; 23), and the Family Assessment Measure (FAM; 24). Of course, it is incumbent on the linician to be familiar with the purposes, strengths, and limitations of any questionnaire chosen for use as explained by the test developer.

FAMILY THERAPY IN THE TREATMENT OF ANOREXIA NERVOSA

As mentioned earlier, Minuchin, Selvini-Palazzoli, and their coworkers were among the first to develop specific family treatments for AN. Minuchin's group described a psychosomatic family model of AN (8,9), in which certain factors combine to produce children with severe psychosomatic illnesses. The factors include a physical vulnerability in the child, dysfunctional family characteristics (described above), and an adaptive role that the sick child plays in the family's pattern of conflict avoidance. Their approach to treatment was coined *structural family therapy*, the goal of which was to alter the dysfunctional family interactions by limiting certain family interactions and encouraging others. By doing so, the need for the symptomatic behavior (i.e., anorexic behavior) would be reduced or eliminated. For example, the therapist determines that a mother is enmeshed with her ill daughter, preventing the daughter from having meaningful relationships with her father and brother. The structural therapist would attempt to increase the emotional distance between the mother and daughter, while simultaneously encouraging closer relationships between the daughter and her father, between the siblings, and between the parents. Minuchin's group also advocated that the parents take charge of their anorexic child's eating by instituting "family meal sessions." During these sessions, it was the job of the parents to unite in taking control over their child's eating behavior while the therapist monitored family interactions, intervening when necessary.

Evidence in support of the structural approach, as reported by Minuchin et al. (9), consists of a detailed study spanning 7 years. During that time, assessment, treatment, and follow-up data were collected on 50 families having a child with AN. Six of the identified patients were males. The median age was 14.5 years with a range from 9 to 21 years. All patients received treatment less than 3 years after the onset of illness. The average length of treatment was 6 months with a range of 2–16 months. Family therapy was typically conducted on a weekly basis.

Therapists in the study (9) described three trends in treatment that emerged based on the identified patient's age. Preadolescents were not seen individually. Instead, conjoint therapy (identified patient seen with family) was conducted initially with a shift to marital therapy later. Familial issues centered on increasing parental control and effectiveness as well as improving the parental coalition. For the adolescent group, conjoint family therapy and marital therapy were conducted along with individual sessions. Siblings were seen alone with the identified patient when judged appropriate. Issues centered on increasing autonomy and independence in the adolescent. In the young adult sample, the primary therapeutic issue was separation from the family of origin. Conjoint family sessions alone were therefore done in the beginning, with a quick shift to separate individual plus nonconjoint family sessions.

Of the original sample, 80% were followed for 2 years or more. The total follow-up time ranged from 1.5 to 7 years. Results of the investigation showed that 86% of the patients achieved full recovery from anorexic symptoms and correlated psychosocial deficits. Four percent improved somewhat in both areas, 6% did not improve, and 4% relapsed (9). Martin (as cited in Dare and Eisler, 10) demonstrated similar findings with a related model of therapy.

Though considered a landmark in family treatment of anorexia nervosa, Minuchin's study has been criticized for various methodological weaknesses, including inadequate sample sizes, overlapping meanings of constructs, a focus on pathological polarities regarding familial interactions, and a lack of empirical measures to assess outcome (25,26).

To address some of the criticisms of Minuchin's psychosomatic model, authors of a Flemish study operationally defined and measured the concepts by behavioral methods and self-report (26). The concepts were behaviorally redefined as follows: "intensity of intrafamilial boundaries" for enmeshment, "degree of family adaptability" for rigidity, "the family's way of handling conflict" for lack of conflict resolution, and "degree of avoidance/recognition of intrafamilial tension" for overprotectiveness. The study included families having a child with AN, BN, or eating disorder–not otherwise specified. Evidence of convergent and discriminant validity for intensity of intrafamilial boundaries, degree of family adaptability, and the family's way of handling conflict was found using the behavioral methods. Self-report showed only convergent validity for the family's way of handling conflict. The findings did not support the concept of overprotectiveness. The authors concluded that it is important for clinicians to keep in mind the difference in conceptualizations of the family climate between professional observers and family members when conducting family therapy.

The *Milan systems model* developed by Selvini-Palazzoli and her colleagues in Italy (7,27) emphasized the role of the eating disorder in maintaining homeostasis in the family system. *Homeostasis* refers to the balance that occurs when all family members adhere to their given, often unspoken, rules of behavior. The Milan group believed that these rules had become overly rigid in families of anorexic patients and interactions were therefore limited to those that kept the status quo. According to Dare and Eisler (10), therapy was designed to introduce a new way of conceptualizing the problematic interactions and symptomatic behavior, noting their adaptive functions in the family. To accomplish this task, an end-of-session intervention in the form of a "message to the family" may be given. In addition to remaining neutral in relation to the family, the Milan group also believed that it was important to remain neutral as to whether or not change in the family should occur and, if so, in what form. Consequently, the Milan family systems therapist gleans information from the family via interview, encourages them to examine their interactions, and leads them to ultimately challenge problematic beliefs and interactions. The Milan group's studies have been criticized for a lack of systematic study of interaction, matched control groups, and methodologically appropriate assessment procedures (28).

Additional support for the Milan approach has been documented by Stierlin and Weber (as cited in Dare and Eisler, 10) in a study of families having a child with AN or BN. Family therapy tended to be brief with an average of six sessions per family. Upon termination, treatment gains in regard to eating disorder symptoms were limited but at follow-up, which ranged from 2 to 9 years, approximately two-thirds of the subjects had attained a normal weight and were menstruating. Similar improvements were noted in family and peer relationships. The study was limited, however, by the fact that it was not conducted under controlled conditions.

The *Maudsley model* of family therapy for adolescents with AN incorporates structural components but differs from the two aforementioned approaches in that these practitioners do not assume that the family is dysfunctional (10). Instead, this London-based group posited that a significant amount of the "dysfunction" reported in families with a child with AN may be the result of the development of a life-threatening illness, changes in the child's mood and behavior, potential blaming by professionals, and failure of initial therapeutic efforts (10). Nevertheless, the Maudsley clinicians observed many of the same family characteristics as described by Minuchin and Palazzoli (29). Le Grange (30) explains that therapy is time limited and typically proceeds through three clearly defined phases: (a) refeeding the person with anorexia nervosa, (b) negotiating new patterns of relationships, and (c) termination. During the refeeding phase, the focus is on eating disorder symptoms. Like the structural family therapists, the Maudsley group advocates that the parents take charge of the child's eating and a family meal session may be included in this phase. Once the child begins to cooperate with increased food intake and there is a discernible change of mood within the family, patterns of relationships and other family issues can be discussed. Such discussion takes place around how these problems affect the parents in their efforts to ensure that the child's weight increases steadily. Following weight restoration, the termination phase begins with an emphasis on the child establishing a healthy adolescent or young adult relationship with the parents that does not include the eating disorder. Some clinicians also see the patient individually (10).

In adult patients with AN, the approach is modified so that attempts are made to remove the eating disorder from its central and controlling role in the relationships between the identified patient and other family members. Furthermore, there is not typically a push for the parents to take charge of the adult child's eating (31).

Recently, the Maudsley approach was used to develop a professional, family-based treatment manual targeting adolescents with AN (32,33). Favorable results were reported for weight restoration and associated psychological features at 6-month follow-up. The authors caution, however, that the results are preliminary, short term, and include only 19 cases. A larger, longer term treatment trial is underway at this writing.

The Maudsley group has conducted a number of controlled trials comparing different forms of therapy for adolescents with AN in an effort to shape their own approach (10). In addition, they have shown that adolescents under age 19 with anorexia nervosa for less than 3 years respond very well to the Maudsley model of family therapy in the short term (34,35) and at 5-year follow-up (36). In adults with AN, an early study tentatively demonstrated that adult patients derive greater benefit from individual supportive therapy than from the Maudsley model of family therapy for adults (34). A more recent study (31) found that adult patients benefited from 1 year of family therapy, but not significantly more so than from 1 year of focal psychoanalytic psychotherapy or 7 months of cognitive–analytical therapy. In addition, benefits were limited in that some patients were substantially malnourished at follow-up. It was noted that this particular group carried a poor prognosis as defined by late onset of illness, a chronic course of illness, and unsuccessful previous treatments, all of which may have negatively affected the outcome.

The Maudsley group has also been interested in how expressed emotion of family members affects family treatment for both AN and BN. *Expressed emotion* is a pattern of hostile, critical, and intrusive interactions first studied in families of schizophrenics with high rates of such associated with poor prognosis (37). One study from the Maudsley researchers found that high maternal expressed emotion predicted early dropout from family treatment but not from individual treatment (38). Criticism from either parent at the beginning of treatment predicted a poor outcome, leading researchers to conclude that for highly critical families, separate parent counseling may be of more benefit than conjoint family therapy (39). Similarly, a Dutch study using a variety of family therapies/counseling approaches to manage adolescent AN and BN found that a critical maternal attitude was predictive of a poorer outcome at termination and at 1-year follow-up (40).

A fourth model of family therapy for treating adolescents with AN is *behavioral family systems therapy* (41,42). It closely resembles the Maudsley approach with conjoint family sessions and three phases of treatment. In the first phase, the parents are encouraged to take control of the youngster's eating with coaching from the therapist, much as they would if she were a young child unwilling to take medicine for a disease. Once successful, the second phase focuses on family structure, the role of the eating disorder symptoms in the family system, and cognitive distortions about food, body weight, and family life. Once the identified patient's target weight is reached, the third phase starts by gradually returning control of eating back to the adolescent. Issues of individuation and communication between the parents and adolescent are also addressed.

Robin et al. (42) describe an investigation comparing behavioral family systems therapy to ego oriented individual psychotherapy (41), in which the adolescent receives weekly individual sessions and the parents attend bimonthly family sessions alone. They found that the systems approach produced greater weight gain upon termination. By 1-year follow-up, however, this effect had diminished. Regarding eating attitudes, depression, and interoceptive awareness (awareness and identification of internal bodily sensations such as hunger), the two forms of therapy were equally effective at termination, 1-year follow-up, and in a limited sample of subjects at 4-year follow-up. With respect to general family conflict, both groups improved comparably, based on the researchers' judgments of videotaped interactions. Interestingly, no significant reports of this type of conflict were reported by family members before or after treatment. Both groups reported a high level of eating-related conflict prior to treatment, which improved for both groups following treatment. Thus, because both groups included family interventions, Dare and Eisler (10) concluded that the findings tend to underscore the value of family therapy in the treatment of AN.

Much has been written about the families of those with AN, and overall, the literature on family treatment, particularly in adolescents, clearly warrants its use in clinical practice. Despite variations in approaches, all are concerned with the family's role in food and weight issues as well as individual concerns, familial issues, and psychosocial functioning. Our experience, too, corroborates the necessity for family treatment of AN. More specifically, it is through family therapy that vital, core issues that may be determined to underlie the eating disorder symptoms (such as separation and individuation) can be identified and resolved.

FAMILY THERAPY IN THE TREATMENT OF BULIMIA NERVOSA

The literature on family treatment for BN is sparse compared to that for AN. Several reasons for this discrepancy have been postulated (42). First, it is a comparatively new disorder, having been given a distinct identity in 1980. Second, those affected tend to be older and may no longer be living with their families of origin at the time they seek treatment. Nevertheless, in the following section we present two systemic treatment models developed for a bulimic population as well as a synopsis of studies examining the effectiveness of family therapy in the treatment of BN from the structural, Milan, and Maudsley approaches.

Root et al. (13) developed a systemic–feminist approach to treatment based on their theoretical descriptions of family types described earlier, although they did not perform studies to test the efficacy of the therapy. The therapeutic model incorporated aspects of the structural, Milan, and strategic schools of family therapy. In their experience, this family population did not always present with all of the characteristics that Minuchin and his colleagues described. Instead, they observed the family typologies outlined earlier (perfect, overprotective, and chaotic). Their model of family therapy centered around systemic, developmental, and life cycle issues as they played out in the families they encountered. The issues included individuation and separation, boundaries, organization, and difficulties expressing and resolving feelings. Enmeshment and difficulty leaving home often characterized the individuation and separation issues. The boundary problems encompassed physical space and privacy, rules about respect for boundaries, and tolerance of emotional distance. Boundaries were sometimes lacking or impermeable. Regarding organization, systems need rules or organization to regulate actions or expressions. Thus, a system can be too rigidly organized or it can be disorganized. In the experience of Root and her coworkers, all the families they treated had difficulty expressing and resolving feelings, particularly anger, resentment, jealousy, grief, depression, anxiety, and insecurity. The clinicians argued that difficulties in this arena resulted in the actual bulimic symptoms; they postulated that a system that disallows certain feelings and cannot adapt encourages either an explosive discharge of feelings or development of psychosomatic illnesses. Thus, a child in this type of system subsequently learns that directly expressing certain emotions causes a parent to become explosive or ill.

Another purely theoretical approach to family treatment for BN has been described by Jack Brandes (43) of the University of Toronto. He asserted that families having a child with BN have difficulties with attachment and loss. In his practice, many families related accounts of actual loss and abandonment through illness, death, change in socioeconomic status, and immigration followed by social isolation. He hypothesized that the concerns these families have with appearance, demeanor, and performance may represent worries about being unacceptable and unappealing to society. Symptomatic behavior, i.e., bulimic behavior, may therefore be a means of coping with social isolation, separation, and loss. The treatment model Brandes (43) proposed to treat families having a child with BN consisted of four phases that embraced structural, cognitive, and psychoeducational components. He noted that the family may be seen exclusively, or individual and/or marital sessions may be added as clinically appropriate. The first phase of treatment is assessment in which the therapist "joins" with the family (establishes a therapeutic alliance), performs a family history, works to reduce shame and blame, and educates the family about BN. The second phase, early treatment, focuses on dietary reeducation and encouraging the identified patient to own the bulimic symptoms. There is also an emphasis on loss and abandonment themes, self-sacrifice of the identified patient, and individual identity in the family. The third stage of treatment addresses individual concerns, marital issues, separation, and integration into the community. Termination, the final phase of treatment, focuses on feelings of loss and abandonment regarding treatment. To ease the difficulty of termination, the therapist contracts for future contacts with the family.

An investigation by Schwartz et al. (11) involved 30 families having an adolescent or adult child with BN treated from a structural–systemic approach. The treatment model focused on patient differentiation from the family of origin, with work in this area initiated prior to directly targeting bulimic symptoms so that symptoms would not be reactivated by family dynamics. Treatment occurred in the following stages: (a) motivating the patient and family for differentiation, (b) guiding the differentiation process, (c) targeting the symptoms with specific interventions, and (d) relapse prevention. In this study, the mean frequency of bulimic episodes was 19 per week, ranging from 5 to 63. Individual sessions were often alternated with family sessions, and treatment lasted an average of 27 sessions over 9 months with a range of 2–90 sessions. The average length of illness was 6.8 years with a range of 1–23. Follow-up spanned from 1 to 42 months with a mean of 16 months. At follow-up, 66% of the identified patients were either abstinent or had 1 bulimic episode per month, 10% had 2 episodes per month up to 1 per week, 10% reported 2–4 episodes per week, and 14% suffered from more than 5 episodes per week. Of the 7 patients functioning at the bottom two levels, 4 dropped out of treatment with fewer than 8 sessions. Thus, overall, the majority had a good outcome with a structural–systemic approach even though the severity level was high and the identified patients had a chronic course of illness. The study is limited by its relatively small sample size and lack of controlled experimental conditions.

Further support for the structural model as it relates to BN is seen in the work of Kog et al. (26). As previously discussed in the section on AN, evidence for three concepts of the psychosomatic model from which the structural approach stems was found.

German investigators tested the Milan model in a bulimic population by comparing a 2-month trial of inpatient psychoanalytical group therapy to 1 year of systemic outpatient therapy (44). Outcome was measured at 14, 26, and 38 months after treatment initiation. Results indicated that both therapies were effective in reducing symptoms of BN and correlated features, with only a slight advantage for the inpatient treatment regimen despite the other therapies associated with it. Nevertheless, the researchers were unable to differentiate the effects of the two treatment regimens.

An early study by the Maudsley group (34) compared response to family therapy and to individual supportive psychotherapy in young adult women with BN. No substantial differences were found between the groups, and both had a poor outcome. The authors speculated that the sole use of the given interventions was not sufficient to produce a more positive outcome. A later study by the group investigated the Maudsley model in eight female adolescents with BN (45). As in treatment for AN, the parents are charged with the task of normalizing the child's eating and reducing binge–purge episodes with the guidance of the therapist. After eating patterns have been regulated, control over eating behavior is given back to the adolescent. Other issues are then addressed, as outlined earlier in the section on AN. Results indicated that one subject had a good outcome, five had an intermediate outcome, and one had a poor outcome. Overall, average outcome scores significantly improved following treatment, although the study was limited by a small sample and lack of a control group.

Despite the relative dearth of empirical information on the effectiveness of family treatment in BN, family therapy is clinically accepted as an important component in the comprehensive treatment of BN, particularly in younger patients. Our experience has shown family therapy to be quite helpful in resolving issues that may contribute to the development and maintenance of the eating disorder. It is particularly useful when used in conjunction with individual psychotherapy focused on individuation and identity formation combined with the use of cognitive–behavioral techniques to address symptom reduction.

BINGE EATING DISORDER

BED is a newly described phenomenon that is currently diagnosable only with the eating disorder–not otherwise specified category of the *Diagnostic and Statistical Manual of Mental Disorders*, 4th ed, (46). It was also proposed as an area for further study. Subsequently, much research has begun in this area on clinical correlates, etiology, and treatment. As of this date, we are unaware of any case descriptions or controlled trials on the use of family therapy for this disorder.

Although there are no investigations on the use of family therapy in BED, one study examined the effectiveness of spousal involvement in treatment. Gorin et al. (47) conducted a study of 94 females comparing the use of manualized, standard group cognitive–behavioral treatment (CBT) of BED, group CBT with spouse involvement, and a wait-list control group. The average age of participants was 45 years and subjects were randomly assigned to the treatment conditions. Spouses were asked to attend all sessions and assist in setting goals to help with binge eating cessation and weight stabilization. Frequency of binge eating, body mass index (BMI), eating psychopathology, general psychopathology, and marital satisfaction were evaluated pre- and posttreatment as well as at 6-month follow-up. Although both CBT groups significantly improved in terms of binge eating, BMI, eating psychopathology, and general psychopathology when compared to controls, spousal involvement did not result in superior results compared to standard CBT. The authors speculated that the type of spousal intervention may not have been effective or that there may be something about the nature of BED that limits spousal influence on treatment. They also hypothesized that spousal involvement may have served as a catalyst for binge eating in some subjects if the spouses were perceived to be critical or unsupportive. The study was limited by attrition across the experimental conditions (34%) and by the lack of a specialized measure to diagnosis BED.

We have approached family treatment for BED based on need as judged through clinical assessment of the patient. As with the other eating disorders, if it is determined that the family plays a major role in the origin and maintenance of the disorder, family therapy is recommended. Given that patients presenting with BED tend to be older, family therapy may not necessarily include the family of origin. Instead, the patient's current family unit is a more likely candidate. Nevertheless, any family members may be asked to participate if such is clinically expected to be useful.

FAMILY THERAPY IN CLINICAL PRACTICE

Our own approach to family therapy with those afflicted with an eating disorder stems from a combined structural and Milan systems conceptualization. We have stated elsewhere (12) that the family system is typically the context out of which an eating disorder has developed and therefore requires some degree of change if the affected adolescent is to overcome her eating disorder in that environment. For patients who are in a relatively older age range and no longer live with their families of origin, family therapy may not be necessary. In some cases, patients do well in treatment without family participation. When a patient still lives with her family, however, family therapy is often very helpful for recovery. It is also indicated if the family is living separately but is obviously functioning as a stimulating factor in the illness. If the patient is married, marital therapy may be suggested as an adjunctive treatment.

Perednia et al. (48) described a pyramid model of family treatment in which there are different levels of intervention based on familial need. All parents receive guidance and education counseling, a subset participate in family therapy (which may evolve into marital therapy for some couples), and, finally, a few parents are referred for individual psychotherapy. This model allows for maximum flexibility in treatment from a family-oriented position, with the authors asserting that not all families are "disturbed."

Instead, they posit that some suffer from a temporary, situational crisis, whereas others exhibit more basic psychopathology.

From a structural–systemic perspective, family therapy is typically geared to understanding the role that the individual with an eating disorder has characteristically held within the family system and how the illness has contributed to maintaining whatever homeostasis has been achieved. Table 1 lists common therapeutic issues. Like Perednia et al. (48), we have noted (12) that family therapy sometimes evolves into marital therapy for the parents or individual therapy for one or both parents, particularly as the child gets better. In our experience, it is not unusual for a parent to be referred for individual therapy at the outset of treatment, if it is clear that the primary family problem lies within that particular parent–child relationship.

Whether or not dysfunctional family characteristics are part of the cause of eating disorders in offspring or if these observed problems are a result of the stress associated with having a child with an eating disorder is controversial (3). In fact, there is a great deal of information accumulating on the genetic transmission of eating disorders (see Chapter 7), though experts recognize that it is likely to be the interaction between genetics and environment, including sociocultural influence, that is responsible for the development of these disorders (49). Regardless, it is never helpful or appropriate to place blame on family members for the development of the illness (12). Explaining the biological propensity that an individual may have toward an eating disorder can provide the practitioner with a nonblaming means of joining with the family, and any stigma which may be felt is likely to be reduced. By edu-

---

TABLE 1 Common Issues in Family Therapy of AN and BN

---

1. Communication problems such as lack of communication, miscommunication, direct or indirect failure to allow open expression of feelings (for instance, the message that it is not okay be angry or upset), mixed, or double messages
2. Lack of appropriate parent–child boundaries (such as failure to respect privacy), enmeshment (emotional overinvolvement), disengagement (emotional distance)
3. Fears around patient growing up and becoming independent
4. Roles that family members play which contribute to the development and maintenance of the eating disorder (for example, the child may be the mediator between parents in an unstable marriage)
5. Control and power within the family
6. Unrealistic family expectations of individual members, and of the family as a unit

---

Source: Ref. 12.

cating the family about eating disorders in this manner and enlisting their support in therapeutic endeavors, any potential defensiveness may be reduced or avoided. Consequently, the family's insight and esteem can be enhanced, facilitating full engagement in the therapeutic process. Most families experience strong emotional responses in reaction to a child's development of an eating disorder. These responses may include feelings of fear, frustration, guilt, demoralization, desperation, and anger, and many parents blame themselves or others (50). Family therapy may therefore serve as a much-needed forum for parents and siblings to identify, express, and resolve their thoughts, feelings, and beliefs as well as receive education about the nature of eating disorders and recovery.

In our practices, family therapy is conducted in conjunction with individual psychotherapy using separate therapists. It has been acknowledged that the use of family therapy with individual psychotherapy greatly improves the chance of a full recovery (19), and this combination of treatment has been recommended in the Practice Guideline for the Treatment of Eating Disorders (15). We believe that having separate therapists facilitates the individuation–separation process. More specifically, this method allows the patient to have a person, i.e., psychotherapist, of his or her own with whom to work on individuation, separation, and identity issues. Simultaneously, the family works with a therapist of their own, with whom they can address their concerns and find support and guidance. In addition, we argue that this arrangement makes it is easier for the individual therapist to manage confidentiality issues between the identified patient and other family members. It also eases the therapeutic burden of treating such complicated and challenging illnesses by having two therapists dividing the labor (43). Finally, we believe, like others (51), that this combination of treatment addresses family dysfunction (if it is present) on two levels, namely, the individual level where it has been introjected, as well as in the current family system. As part of this team approach, the family therapist does not see the identified patient individually, but may see (a) all family members, (b) the identified patient with the parents, (c) the identified patient with the siblings, (d) the parents alone, or (e) the siblings alone. In other words, different combinations of individuals may be seen at any given time depending on the therapeutic issues at hand. Of course, regular communication between the individual psychotherapist and family therapist is essential to avoid splitting and to ensure that everyone is headed in the same direction with mutual goals (12).

Again, we recognize that not all practitioners are in a practical or theoretical position to utilize separate individual and family therapists. Positive aspects of one psychotherapist treating the identified patient and the family include immediate knowledge of individual and family issues, efficiency, and cost containment. Thus, successful treatment is certainly possible with one psychotherapist, although the sole clinician may have a greater number of therapeutic issues to process simultaneously.

Goldner and Birmingham (35) noted that while some schools of family therapy advocate parental control over the child's eating, most clinicians do not follow this approach. Their belief is that the family can be most helpful by relinquishing the battles around food and weight, and strengthening their relationships in other areas. They encourage families to transfer the responsibility of food and weight concerns to the identified patient and the treatment team. Their experience with families using this approach has been positive, with families reporting the diminishing of long-standing battles therefore allowing them to work on communication skills and improved relationships. We, too, subscribe to this approach, with food issues handled by an experienced registered dietician who is a critical member of our treatment team. Our experience has been similarly positive.

FAMILY OBSTACLES TO ASSESSMENT AND TREATMENT

Although many families welcome help for themselves and the identified patient, some may present obstacles to assessment and treatment (52). Denial of an eating disorder, minimization of the problem, and/or denial of the psychological underpinnings may be present (15,53,54). For some families, according to Michel (37), education about eating disorders may remove these obstacles altogether, or at least help diminish them. For others, the psychological origins of the disorder may be too disturbing for family members to deal with directly. Consequently, therapeutic efforts may be resisted as the family struggles to maintain homeostasis. Treatment resistance, as well as a lack of familial motivation to change, may be related to denial and/or a need to maintain the identified patient's role in the family system. Regardless of the etiology of the defensiveness or resistance, these issues must be resolved before a therapeutic alliance can be established, thereby increasing the likelihood of achieving a positive outcome (12,55).

SUMMARY

The family therapy movement began in the 1950s and represented a change in the way in which behavior was viewed, emphasizing present interactions and relationships between family members. The majority of family treatment models and studies on the efficacy of family therapy in treating eating disorders have focused on AN. Nevertheless, it is widely accepted in clinical practice that family therapy is required in comprehensive treatment for both AN and BN, particularly in younger patients still living at home. Empirical support for family treatment of AN and BN exists, but well-controlled outcome investigations are somewhat limited (3). In the case of BED, a recently defined problem, family treatment has not been studied. However, there may be a role for family therapy in treatment if the clinician determines that family members have a role in the origin or maintenance of the illness.

Dysfunctional family characteristics of those with eating disorders have been identified and, for those with AN or BN, clinicians have described family typologies. Whether or not these attributes are part of a dysfunctional system that produces an individual with an eating disorder is debatable, as some experts believe that it may be the result of the stress associated with having a child with AN or BN. In addition, the importance of biological factors in the development of AN and BN is becoming more evident, along with environmental influences. Regarding the environmental factors, we have previously noted (12) that the family may contribute to the development of, or exacerbate, an eating disorder by providing an environment that can hinder an adolescent in establishing an identity, practicing effective communication skills, and/or learning adaptive coping skills. Within the context of the family, his or her eating disorder may function to establish an identity separate from the family, to cope with stressors, to distract from negative feelings, and to provide what the patient considers to be a means of "safe" self-expression of feelings.

With regard to clinical practice, it is usually essential for patients living with their families of origin to participate in family therapy, as everyone in the family is affected by these disorders. For those no longer living at home, family therapy may be limited to couples therapy, marital therapy, or the current family system. If, however, members of the family of origin are found to still stimulate the eating disorder, it will be necessary to include them in family treatment. In very critical or abusive families, family therapy may need to take the form of parent counseling or nonconjoint family therapy. A thorough evaluation of the family and family dynamics at the outset will assist the clinician in sorting out these issues and in conducting effective family therapy. In addition, the combination of family therapy and individual therapy appears to be quite prevalent as each form of treatment can provide a useful and complementary function, which facilitates recovery. Finally, some families present obstacles to assessment and treatment, including denial of the eating disorder, minimization of the problem, and/or denial of the psychological underpinnings. These issues must be resolved and the family engaged in a therapeutic alliance in order to increase the likelihood of achieving a successful outcome.

REFERENCES

1. Hoffman L. Foundation of Family Therapy: A Conceptual Framework for Systems Change. New York: Basic Books, 1981:16–19.
2. Foley VD. Family therapy. In: Corsini RJ, ed. Current Psychotherapies. 3rd ed. Itasca, IL: F. E. Peacock, 1984:447–490.
3. Lemmon CR, Josephson AM. Family therapy for eating disorders. Child Adol Psychiatry Clin of North Am 2001; 10:519–542.
4. Gull WW. Anorexia nervosa (apepsia hysterica, anorexia hysterica). Trans Clin Soc London 1874; 7:22–28.
5. Lasegue C. De l'anorexie hysterique. Arch Gen Med 1873; 1:384–403.
6. Bruch H. Eating Disorders: Obesity, Anorexia Nervosa, and the Person Within. New York: Basic Books, 1973.
7. Selvini-Palazzoli M. Self-Starvation. New York: Jason Aronson, 1974.
8. Minuchin S, Baker L, Rosman BL, Liebman R, Milman L, Todd TC. A conceptual model of psychosomatic illness in children. Arch Gen Psychiatry 1975; 32:1031–1038.
9. Minuchin S, Rosman BL, Baker L. Psychosomatic Families: Anorexia Nervosa in Context. Cambridge, MA: Harvard University Press, 1978.
10. Dare C, Eisler I. In: Garner DM, Garfinkel PE, eds. Handbook of Treatment for Eating Disorders. New York: Guilford Press, 1997:307–324.
11. Schwartz RC, Barrett MJ, Saba G. Family therapy for bulimia. In: Garner DM, Garfinkel PE, eds. Handbook of Psychotherapy for Anorexia Nervosa and Bulimia. New York: Guilford Press, 1985:280–307.
12. Michel DM, Willard SG. When Dieting Becomes Dangerous: Understanding and Treating Anorexia and Bulimia. New Haven, CT: Yale University Press, 2003.
13. Root MPP, Fallon P, Friedrich WN. Bulimia: A Systems Approach to Treatment. New York: W.W. Norton and Co., 1986.
14. Hodges EL, Cochrane CE, Brewerton TD. Family characteristics of binge-eating disorder patients. Int J of Eat Disord 1998; 23:145–151.
15. American Psychiatric Association Work Group on Eating Disorders. Practice guideline for the treatment of patients with eating disorders. Rev Am J Psychiatry 2000; 57(suppl 1):1–39.
16. Woodside DB, Shekter-Wolfson LF, Garfinkel PE, Olmsted MP. Family interactions in bulimia nervosa II: complex intrafamily comparisons and clinical significance. Int J Eat Disord 1999; 17:117–126.
17. Paine ML, Hansen DJ. Factors influencing children to self-disclose sexual abuse. Clin Psychol Rev 2002; 22:271–295.
18. Andersen AE. Practical Comprehensive Treatment of Anorexia Nervosa and Bulimia. Baltimore, MD: The Johns Hopkins University Press, 1985:135–148.
19. Pelch BL. Eating disordered families: Issues between the generations. In: Lemberg R, Cohn L, eds. Eating Disorders: A Reference Sourcebook. Phoenix: Oryx Press, 1999:121–123.
20. Vanderlinden J, Vandereycken W. Family therapy within the psychiatric hos-

pital: Indications, pitfalls, and specific interventions. In: Vandereycken W, Kog E, Vanderlinden J, eds. The Family Approach to Eating Disorders: Assessment and Treatment of Anorexia Nervosa and Bulimia. New York: PMA Publishing, 1989:263–310.

21. Kog E, Vertommen H, DeGroote T. Family interaction research in anorexia nervosa: the use and misuse of a self-report questionnaire. International Journal of Family Psychiatry 1985; 6:227–243.

22. Moos RH, Moos BS. Family Environment Scale Manual. 2d ed. Palo Alto, CA: Consulting Psychologists Press, 1986.

23. Waller G, Slade P, Calam R. Family adaptability and cohesion: relation to eating attitudes and disorders. Int J Eat Disord 1990; 9:225–228.

24. Skinner H, Santa-Barbara J, Steinhaur P. The family assesment measure. Can J Commun Ment Health 1983; 2:91–105.

25. Kog E, Vandereycken W, Vertommen H. Multimethod investigation of eating disorder families. In: Vandereycken W, Kog E, Vanderlinden J, eds. The Family Approach to Eating Disorders: Assessment and Treatment of Anorexia Nervosa and Bulimia. New York: PMA Publishing, 1989:81–106.

26. Kog E, Vertommen H, Vandereycken W. Minuchin's psychosomatic family model revised: a concept-validation study using a multitrait-multimethod approach. Fam Proc 1987; 26:235–253.

27. Selvini-Palazzoli M, Boscolo L, Cecchin G, Prata G. Paradox and Counterparadox. New York: Jason Aronson, 1978.

28. Kog E, Vandereycken W. The facts: a review of research data on eating disorder families. In: Vandereycken W, Kog E, Vanderlinden J, eds. The Family Approach to Eating Disorders: Assessment and Treatment of Anorexia Nervosa and Bulimia. New York: PMA Publishing, 1989:25–68.

29. Dare C, Le Grange D, Eisler I, Rutherford J. Redefining the psychosomatic family: Family process of 26 eating disorder families. Int J Eat Disord 1994; 16: 211–226.

30. Le Grange D. Family therapy for adolescent anorexia nervosa. 1999; 55:727–739.

31. Dare C, Eisler I, Russell G, Treasure J, Dodge L. Psychological therapies for adults with anorexia nervosa: randomised controlled trial of out-patient treatments. Br J Psychiatry 2001; 178:216–221.

32. Lock J, Le Grange D. Can family-based treatment of anorexia nervosa be manualized? J Psychother Pract Res 2001; 10:253–261.

33. Lock J, Le Grange D, Agras WS, Dare C. Treatment Manual for Anorexia Nervosa: A Family Based Approach. New York: Guilford, 2002.

34. Russell GFM, Szmukler GI, Dare C, Eisler I. An evaluation of family therapy in anorexia nervosa and bulimia nervosa. Arch Gen Psychiatry 1987; 44:1047–1056.

35. Dare C, Eisler I, Russell GFM, Szmukler GI. Family therapy for anorexia nervosa: implications from the results of a controlled trial of family and individual therapy. J Marital Fam Ther 1990; 16:39–57.

36. Eisler I, Dare C, Russell GFM, Szmukler GI, Le Grange D, Dodge E. Family

and individual therapy in anorexia nervosa: a five-year follow-up. Arch Gen Psychiatry 1997; 54:1025–1030.

37. Kaplan HI, Sadock BJ. Contributions of the psychosocial sciences to human behavior. In: Synopsis of Psychiatry: Behavioral Sciences Clinical Psychiatry. 6th ed. Baltimore, MD: Williams & Wilkins, 1991:104–154.

38. Szmukler GI, Eisler I, Russell GF, Dare C. Anorexia nervosa, parental "expressed emotion" and dropping out of treatment. Br J Psychiatry 1985; 147:265–271.

39. Le Grange D, Eisler I, Dare C, Hodes M. Family criticism and self-starvation: A study of expressed emotion. J Fam Ther 1992; 14:177–192.

40. Van Furth EF, Van Strien DC, Martina LM, Van Son MJ, Hendrickx JJ, Van Engeland H. Expressed emotion and the prediction of outcome in adolescent eating disorders. Int J Eat Disord 1996; 20:19–31.

41. Robin AL, Siegal PT, Koepke T, Moye AW, Tice S. Family therapy versus individual therapy for adolescent females with anorexia nervosa. J Dev Behav Pediat 1994; 15:111–116.

42. Robin AL, Gilroy M, Dennis AB. Treatment of eating disorders in children and adolescents. Clin Psychol Rev 1998; 18:421 446.

43. Brandes J. Outpatient family therapy for bulimia nervosa. In: Woodside DB, Shekter-Wolfson L, eds. Family Approaches in Treatment of Eating Disorders. Washington, DC: American Psychiatric Press, 49–66.

44. Jager B, Liedtke R, Kunsebeck HW, Lempa W, Kersting A, Seide L. Psychotherapy and bulimia nervosa: evaluation and long-term follow-up of two conflict-orientated treatment conditions. Acta Psychiatr Scand 1996; 93:268–278.

45. Dodge E, Hodes M, Eisler I, Dare C. Family therapy for bulimia nervosa in adolescents: an exploratory study. J Fam Ther 1995; 17:59–77.

46. American Psychiatric Association. Diagnostic and Statistical Manual of Mental Disorders. 4th ed. Washington, DC, 1994.

47. Gorin AA, Le Grange D, Stone AA. Effectiveness of spouse involvement in cognitive behavioral therapy for binge eating disorder. Int J Eat Disord 2003: 421–433.

48. Perednia C, Van Vreckem F, Vandereycken W. Parent counseling: From guidance to treatment. In: Vandereycken W, Kog E, Vanderlinden J, eds. The Family Approach to Eating Disorders: Assessment and Treament of Anorexia Nervosa and Bulimia. New York: PMA Publishing, 1989:249–261.

49. Klump K. A genetic link to anorexia. In: DeAngelis T, ed. Monitor on Psychology. March 2002; 33(3):34–36.

50. Goldner EM, Birminghan CL. Anorexia nervosa: methods of treatment. In: Alexander-Mott L, Lumsden DB, eds. Understanding Eating Disorders: Anorexia Nervosa, Bulimia Nervosa, and Obesity. Washington, DC: Taylor & Francis, 1994:135–157.

51. Gowers S, Norton K, Halek C, Crisp AH. Outcome of outpatient psychotherapy in a random allocation treatment study of anorexia nervosa. Int J Eat Disord 1994; 15:165–177.

52. Michel DM. Psychological assessment as a therapeutic intervention in hospital-
     ized patients with eating disorders. Prof Psychol Res Pract. In press.
53. Casper RC, Troiani M. Family functioning in anorexia nervosa differs by sub-
     type. Int J Eat Disord 2001; 30:338–342.
54. Powers P. Management of patients with comorbid medical conditions. In:
     Garner DM, Garfinkel PE, eds. Handbook of Treatment for Eating Disorders.
     2d ed. New York: Guilford Press, 1997:424–436.
55. Willard SG. Anorexia and Bulimia: The Potential Devastation of Dieting.
     Plainfield, NJ: Patient Education Press, 1990.

19

Interpersonal Psychotherapy for Anorexia Nervosa, Bulimia Nervosa, and Binge Eating Disorder

M. Joy Jacobs

San Diego State University/University of California San Diego
Joint Doctoral Program in Clinical Psychology
San Diego, California, U.S.A.

R. Robinson Welch and Denise E. Wilfley

Washington University School of Medicine
St. Louis, Missouri, U.S.A.

INTRODUCTION

Originally developed by Gerald Klerman and colleagues (1) for the management of unipolar depression, interpersonal psychotherapy (IPT) is a brief, time-limited therapy that has been successfully adapted for the management of eating disorders. First successfully adapted for the management of bulimia nervosa (BN) (2,3), IPT has since proven effective, via an innovative group format, for binge eating disorder (BED). Currently, the role of IPT in the management of anorexia nervosa remains unclear.

THEORETICAL FOUNDATIONS OF INTERPERSONAL PSYCHOTHERAPY

IPT was initially developed not as a novel therapy, but as an attempt to reflect interpersonally focused treatment for depression already in practice in the 1970s and 1980s (4,5). IPT is theoretically rooted in theories developed by Adolf Meyer, Henry Stack Sullivan, and John Bowlby. In the 1950s, Meyer postulated that psychopathology was rooted in maladjustment to one's social environment (6). During the same time period, Henry Stack Sullivan (who was responsible for popularizing the term "interpersonal") theorized that a patient's interpersonal relationships, rather than intrapsychic processes alone, constituted the relevant focus of therapeutic attention. Sullivan believed that individuals could not be understood in isolation from their interpersonal relationships and posited that enduring patterns in these relationships could either encourage self-esteem or result in anxiety, hopelessness, and psychopathology (7). The work of John Bowlby, specifically his attachment theory, is also associated with IPT. Bowlby emphasized the importance of early attachment in the later development of interpersonal relationships and emotional well-being (8). According to Bowlby, failures in attachment resulted in psychopathology. Incorporating aspects of the theories posited by Meyer, Sullivan, and Bowlby, IPT acknowledges a two-way relationship between social functioning and psychopathology; interpersonal dysfunction results in psychopathology and psychopathology results in a deterioration in interpersonal functioning.

INTERPERSONAL FUNCTIONING AND EATING DISORDERS: EMPIRICAL BASIS

IPT for eating disorders is based on compelling evidence that interpersonal factors have a significant role in the etiology and maintenance of these disorders. Eating-disordered individuals typically have a history of more frequently difficult social experiences, including problematic family histories and specific interpersonal stressors, than non-eating-disordered individuals (9–12). These individuals also experience a wide range of social problems, including loneliness, lack of perceived social support, low self-esteem, low social adjustment, and poor social problem–solving skills (13–20); this combination of factors may inhibit their ability to cope with interpersonal stressors (21–24). Furthermore, interpersonal difficulties, low self-esteem, and negative affect (25–28) may be interconnected and associated with dysfunctional eating patterns (29). These related factors may then create a vicious cycle, each exacerbating the other and combining to precipitate and/or maintain eating disorder symptoms. IPT aims to improve interpersonal functioning, self-esteem, and negative affect as they relate to each other and to eating disorder symptoms.

INTERPERSONAL PSYCHOTHERAPY FOR EATING DISORDERS

Ideally, in each session of IPT for eating disorders, symptoms should be explicitly and repeatedly linked to problems in interpersonal functioning. Research versions of IPT for eating disorders to date have avoided an explicit symptom focus in order to clearly distinguish IPT from cognitive–behavioral therapy (CBT) in comparison studies. Because of this, research studies investigating the use of IPT for eating disorders have typically not adequately addressed specific eating disorder symptoms. In clinical settings, however, consistent attention to the relationship between eating disorder symptoms and problems in interpersonal functioning is recommended for maximal therapeutic impact.

The fundamental structure and techniques of IPT are similar for all three eating disorders. The essentials concepts of IPT and the specific tasks of each phase of treatment are described in detail below.

Basic Interpersonal Psychotherapy Concepts

Interpersonal Problem Areas

IPT is designed to help patients identify and address *current* interpersonal problems. Treatment focuses on the resolution of problems within four social domains that are associated with the onset and/or maintenance of the eating disorder, namely, interpersonal deficits, interpersonal role disputes, role transitions, and grief (Table 1). *Interpersonal deficits* apply to those patients who are socially isolated or who are in chronically unfulfilling relationships. For patients with this problem area, unsatisfying relationships and/or inadequate social support are frequently the result of poor social skills. *Interpersonal role disputes* are conflicts with a significant other (e.g., a partner, other family member, coworker, or close friend) that emerge from differences in expectations about the relationship. *Role transitions* include difficulties associated with a change in life status (e.g., graduation, leaving a job, moving, marriage/divorce, retirement, change in health status). *Grief* is identified as the problem area when the onset of the patient's symptoms is associated with the loss of a person or a relationship, either recent or past. IPT for eating disorders focuses on identifying and changing the maladaptive interpersonal context in which the eating problem has been developed and maintained.

Percentages of problem areas were obtained from psychotherapy studies for BN and BED (30,31) and from an interview-based study for AN (32). For all three disorders, grief was uncommon whereas role disputes were fairly common. The notable differences among the disorders were that inter-

TABLE 1 Interpersonal Problem Areas: Description, Goals, and Strategies (Klerman et al., 1984; Weissman et al., 2000)

Interpersonal problem area	Description	Goals	Strategies
Interpersonal deficits	A history of social isolation, inadequate, and/or unsatisfying interpersonal relationships	• Reduce social isolation • Enhance quality of existing relationships • Encourage formation of new relationships	• Review and evaluate past significant relationships • Explore recurrent patterns in relationships • Identify interpersonal patterns in session and relate them to similar patterns in the patient's life
Interpersonal role disputes	Conflicts with a significant other (i.e., spouse, family member, coworker, close friend)	• Identify nature of the dispute • Explore options for resolution • Modify expectations and rectify faulty communication to facilitate a satisfactory resolution • If no resolution is possible, encourage patient to reassess relationship (i.e., modify expectations, consider dissolution)	• Determine stage of the dispute • Explore how differing role expectations relate to the dispute • Identify available resources to bring about change

Role transitions	Significant changes in life status (i.e., leaving a job, moving, marriage/divorce, retirement, illness)	• Accept loss of old role • Recognize positive and negative aspects of both the old role and new roles • Restore patient's self-esteem by developing a sense of mastery in the new role	• Explore patient's feelings regarding the role change • Encourage development of new skills and social support for the new role
Grief	Complicated bereavement following loss of a loved one	• Facilitate mourning process • Help patient identify new relationships and activities	• Educate patient about the grieving process • Reconstruct the patient's relationship with the deceased • Explore associated feelings (positive and negative) • Encourage establishment of new interests and relationships

Source: Adapted from Wilfley DE, Stein RI, Welch RR. Interpersonal psychotherapy for the treatment of eating disorders. In: Treasure, J, Schmidt U, Dare C, Van Furth E, eds. Handbook of Eating Disorders, 2nd ed. Sussex: John Wiley & Sons, (in press).

personal deficits were more likely to be found among BED and AN patients, and role transitions were more common among BN patients.

Treatment Structure

IPT for eating disorders typically lasts 15–20 sessions over a 4- to 5-month period (33,34). The treatment is demarcated by three phases. The *initial phase* is dedicated to identifying the problem area that will be the target for treatment. The *intermediate phase* is devoted to working on the target problem area(s). The *termination phase* is devoted to consolidating gains made during treatment and preparing patients for future work on their own. Each phase of treatment for eating disorder patients, along with clinical vignettes illustrating implementation of the treatment, will be described in detail below.

Therapeutic Stance

Similar to other therapies, IPT places importance on establishing a positive therapeutic alliance between therapist and patient. Specifically, the IPT therapeutic stance is one of warmth, support, and empathy. The therapist is active and advocates for the patient rather than remaining neutral. By phrasing things positively, the therapist helps the patient feel comfortable and aims to foster a safe and supportive working environment. Confrontations and clarifications are offered in a gentle and timely manner, and the therapist is careful to encourage the patient's positive expectations of the therapeutic relationship. In addition, the therapist conveys a hopeful stance and optimistic attitude about the patient's ability to recover.

Implementing Interpersonal Psychotherapy for Eating Disorders

Tasks of the Treatment Phases (Table 2)

The Initial Phase. Sessions 1–5 typically constitute the initial phase of IPT for eating disorders. After assessing the patient's current eating disorder symptoms and obtaining a history of these symptoms, the therapist gives the patient a formal diagnosis. Therapist and patient then discuss the diagnosis as well as what might be expected from treatment. As described below, assignment of the sick role during this phase serves the dual function of granting the patient the permission to recover, as well as the responsibility to recover. The therapist explains the rationale of IPT, underscoring that therapy will focus on the identifying and altering dysfunctional interpersonal patterns related to eating disorder symptomatology. As discussed below, in order to determine the precise focus of treatment, the therapist conducts an interpersonal inventory with the patient and develops an interpersonal formulation based on this. In the interpersonal formulation, the therapist links

TABLE 2 Therapist Tasks for Interpersonal Psychotherapy

Initial Phase: Sessions 1–5
- Assess eating disorder symptoms, current and past
- Make formal diagnosis
- Assign the sick role
- Explain rationale and nature of IPT
- Conduct the interpersonal inventory
    Review significant relationships, past and present
    Identify interpersonal catalysts of binge eating, extreme dietary restraint, etc.
- Using consensus, define problem area and develop treatment plan

Intermediate Phase: Sessions 6–16
- Implement treatment plan
- Use strategies and techniques specific to the identified problem area
- Make connections between interpersonal events and eating problems
- Illuminate relationship between interpersonal problem area and eating, weight, and shape issues

Termination Phase: Sessions 17–20
- Reflect on progress made to date
    Work to foster feelings of accomplishment and competence
- Educate patient about the end of treatment and associated emotions (i.e., grief)
- Set goals for future work
- Identify early warning signs of future difficulty and potential plans of action

---

Source: Adapted from Wilfley DE, Stein RI, Welch RR. Interpersonal psychotherapy for the treatment of eating disorders. In: Treasure, J, Schmidt U, Dare C, Van Furth E, eds. Handbook of Eating Disorders, 2nd ed. Sussex: John Wiley & Sons, 2003; 253–270.

the patient's eating disorder to one of the four interpersonal problem areas. The patient's concurrence with the therapist's identification of the problem area and agreement to work on this area are essential before beginning the intermediate treatment phase.

DIAGNOSIS AND ASSIGNING THE SICK ROLE.   After a thorough psychiatric review has been conducted, the patient is formally diagnosed with an eating disorder and assigned the "sick role." The purposes of assigning the sick role are both theoretical and practical. Consistent with the medical model, receiving a formal diagnosis reinforces the idea that the patient has a known condition that can be managed. Accurate diagnosis is essential to effective treatment. The giving of a diagnosis also explicitly identifies the patient as in need of help. The sick role is assigned not to condescend to the patient but rather to temporarily exempt the individual from other responsibilities in order to devote full attention to recovery. This is particularly important for eating-disordered patients, many of whom tend to set aside their own needs and desires in order to care for and please others. If this applies in a particular case, the therapist may explicitly highlight the patient's excessive caretaking tendencies and encourage the patient to redirect this energy from others to her own recovery. In doing so, the therapist clarifies the rationale behind IPT—that by improving the patient's patterns of interpersonal functioning, the patient's eating disorder symptoms are expected to improve as well.

THE INTERPERSONAL INVENTORY.   At the beginning of IPT, an interpersonal inventory examining the patient's interpersonal history is conducted. The interpersonal inventory may take 1–3 sessions to complete. A thorough interpersonal inventory is essential for adequate case formulation and development of an optimal treatment plan. The clinical importance of investing the time involved in conducting a comprehensive interpersonal inventory cannot be overemphasized; accurate identification of the patient's primary problem area can be difficult and is key to success in therapy.

Included in the interpersonal inventory is a review of the patient's current close relationships, current social functioning, relationship patterns, and expectations. Changes in interpersonal relationships are explored and discussed with reference to the onset and maintenance of eating disorder symptoms. For each person who is important in the patient's life, the following information is assessed: frequency of contact, activities shared, satisfactory and unsatisfactory aspects of the relationship, and ways that the patient would like to change the relationship. The therapist obtains a chronological history of significant life events, fluctuations in mood and self-esteem, interpersonal relationships, and eating disorder symptoms. From this review, the therapist can work with the patient to make connections between certain life experiences and eating disorder symptoms. Thorough exploration of this interrelationship typically helps patients to more clearly understand the rationale behind IPT. Upon completion of the interpersonal inventory, the therapist should have helped the patient identify a primary interpersonal problem area(s).

THE INTERPERSONAL FORMULATION.   Upon completion of the interpersonal inventory, the therapist should have developed an individualized interpersonal formulation, including identification of the patient's primary problem area. Although some patients may present for treatment with difficulties in several problem areas, the time-limited nature of the treatment necessitates a focused approach. The therapist, with the agreement of the patient, should assign one, or at most two, problem area(s) upon which to develop a treatment plan. The goals developed at this stage will be referenced at each future session and will guide the day-to-day work of the treatment. For examples of individual case formulations, the reader is referred to (35). If more than one problem area is identified, the patient may choose to work simultaneously on both or may decide to first address the problem area that seems most likely to be responsive to treatment. For example, when a patient has role disputes and interpersonal deficits, clinical attention might first be focused on role disputes, since interpersonal deficits reflect long-term patterns that may require considerably more time and effort to change. Once the role dispute has been resolved, therapist and patient would then decide how to best address the more entrenched interpersonal deficits.

The Intermediate Phase. Once the patient and therapist have agreed on the primary problem area and have set treatment goals, the intermediate phase of treatment begins. An essential task throughout the intermediate phase is to strengthen the connections patients make between difficulties in their interpersonal lives and eating problems. The intermediate phase typically lasts a total of 8–10 sessions and constitutes the "work" of the therapy. The strategies and goals of the intermediate phase are shaped by the primary problem area targeted in the treatment.

THERAPEUTIC GOALS AND STRATEGIES BY PROBLEM AREA. The eating disorders therapist should also implement specific treatment strategies based on the identified problem area. These are discussed below.

Interpersonal Deficits. If interpersonal deficits is the primary problem area, as is frequently the case with BED and AN patients, treatment strategies should be utilized in order to reduce the patient's social isolation, to enhance the quality of existing relationships, and to encourage the formation of new relationships. It is crucial to determine why the patient is having difficulty forming and/or maintaining relationships. Conducting a review of past significant relationships will be particularly useful in making this assessment. During this review, attention should be given to both the positive and negative aspects of the relationships, as well as an investigation of potentially recurrent patterns in these relationships. If appropriate, the therapist should then relate the problematic patterns occurring in the patient's present relationships to relationship patterns already known to be problematic. Use of the therapeutic relationship (discussed in greater detail in "General Therapeutic Techniques," below) is also helpful in the treatment of patients with interpersonal deficits. Use of this technique provides an illustration of interpersonal patterns that may be the source of difficulties in other relationships and provides the patient helpful feedback on his or her interactive style.

Interpersonal Role Disputes. Interpersonal role disputes occur frequently in eating disorder patients and may be especially common among BN patients (11). Patients who are particularly affected by this problem area are typically involved in conflicts with a significant other (i.e., spouse, other family member, close friend, or coworker). The goals of treatment include clearly identifying the nature of the dispute and exploring options for its resolution. Important in this will be making a determination regarding the stage of the dispute. Once the stage of the dispute becomes clear, it may be important to modify the patient's expectations and remedy faulty communication in order to bring about adequate resolution. Particularly helpful in leading to a resolution may be an exploration of how nonreciprocal role expectations relate to the dispute. If resolution is not possible, it will be important to encourage the patient to either reassess expectations of the relationship or to consider dissolving the relationship and mourning its loss.

Role Transitions. Role transitions typically involve major life cycle changes that effect an important aspect of the patient's self-identification. Common role transitions include a career change (i.e., promotion, firing, retirement), a family change (marriage, divorce, birth of a child), the beginning or end of an important relationship, a move, graduation, or diagnosis of a medical illness. The goals of therapy include mourning and accepting loss of the old role, recognizing the positive and negative aspects of both the old and new roles, and restoring the patient's self-esteem by having him or her develop a sense of mastery in the new role. Key strategies in achieving these goals include a thorough exploration of the patient's feelings related to the role change and encouraging the patient to develop new skills and adequate social support for the new role.

Grief. Grief is the least common primary problem area among eating disorder patients. Grief is most obviously identified as the problem area when the onset of the patient's symptoms is associated with the death of a loved one, recent or past. However, grief may not be limited to the physical death of a loved one. Grief can also result from the loss of a significant relationship or the loss of an important aspect of one's identity. Compared to the other problem areas, grief can be resolved relatively quickly. Goals for managing a complicated bereavement include facilitating the mourning process and helping the patient to identify new relationships and activities to compensate for the loss. Patients must be educated about the grieving process and be encouraged to explore all feelings that arise. As well as profound sadness, grief may evoke feelings of anger toward the deceased and subsequent guilt for this anger; patients must be encouraged to explore these emotions as well. During the grieving process, patients frequently idealize what has been lost; a thorough reconstruction of both the positive and negative aspects of what has been lost may help the patient to develop a more balanced view. As patients become less focused on the past, they should be encouraged to consider new ways of increasing their involvement with others and to establish new interests.

Therapeutic Techniques.

FOCUSING ON GOALS. IPT is a directed, goal-oriented therapy. Thus, it is important that the therapist maintain a focus each week on how the patient is working on his or her goals between sessions. Phrases such as "moving forward on your goals" and "making important changes" are used to encourage patients to be responsible for their treatment while reminding them that altering interpersonal patterns requires attention and persistence. In session, unfocused discussions are redirected to the key interpersonal issues. By explicitly addressing goals each week, the patient can begin working toward necessary changes. This goal-oriented focus has been supported by research on IPT maintenance treatment for recurrent depression, which has demonstrated that the therapist's ability to maintain focus on interpersonal themes is associated with better outcomes (36).

In the following vignette, note how the therapist initiates the discussion about goals and helps a patient in treatment for BN with interpersonal deficits work on her goals[*]:

Therapist: Victoria, now that we have just started this middle phase of therapy, I wanted to check in with you to see how your work is coming on your goals. You mentioned last week that you are starting to become more aware of interpersonal triggers of bingeing and purging.

Victoria: This week I started paying more attention to what is happening as I'm having the urge to binge. It's a little overwhelming, since so much seems to be going on—a fight with my mother, missing my boyfriend, feeling stressed out about school. I'm starting to get a better sense of what's happening with me when I get the urge to binge, but I don't know what to do with that information once I have it!

Therapist: That's a great start in identifying feelings that become triggers, Victoria. Clearly a lot of things are playing into your desire to binge. How were you able to become more aware of what was happening with you when you felt the urge to binge?

Victoria: Well, I'm used to just reacting, to just giving in to the urge to binge as soon as I feel it—just like we talked about in our first ses-

---

[*] Please note that in order to most clearly illustrate the therapeutic principles discussed in the text, this and the other clinical vignettes included below appear to offer more rapid results than may typically be expected clinically.

sions. Now I'm aware that a switch seems to go off inside of me when I have the urge to binge. Stopping and checking in with myself about what I'm feeling slowed down the frenzy that usually characterizes my binges. Although I didn't avoid binge episodes completely this week, I can identify at least one or two occasions where I lost the desire to binge once I took a breather and checked in with myself.

Therapist: What specifically did you notice was happening with you?

Victoria: I noticed how difficult it is for me to confront my mother and how dependent I feel on my boyfriend being around to compliment me for my self-esteem. I realized that sometimes I'm not communicating what I want or need from these relationships. I don't feel like I know how to do this and end up expressing—or is it suppressing?—my frustration through food.

Therapist: Good work, Victoria. You've discovered some really important clues to your interpersonal triggers. Now that you're becoming more aware of the circumstances surrounding your urge to binge, we can begin to work on helping you find more effective ways to manage your feelings and relationships. As we discussed earlier, this will help you eliminate your binge eating.

Victoria: That sounds great.

As the above vignette illustrates, critical to IPT for eating disorders is helping to facilitate and strengthen the connections patients make between their problematic eating and difficulties in their interpersonal lives. Focusing on specific goals provides a structure in which to do this.

MAKING CONNECTIONS.   A crucial task of the intermediate phase is helping patients recognize the connections between eating difficulties and interpersonal events during the week. As patients learn to make these connections and develop strategies to alter the interpersonal context in which the eating behavior occurs, the cycle of the eating disorder is interrupted. In the following vignette, also in the intermediate phase, the therapist encourages a patient with interpersonal role disputes in treatment for AN to talk about the connections she has made between her desire to restrict her food intake and difficulties she has with her alcoholic father:

Therapist: How has the week gone with your goals, Anna?

Anna: What I've noticed is that whenever my dad is drinking, I just want to starve myself. I get busy making sure his bills are paid and that his other things get done, and then I want to restrict more than ever! I sense that this is my way of shutting down—focusing on not eating is a way for me to block out all the stuff that's happening with my dad. I never realized that connection until recently. I just focused on wanting to be thin.

Therapist: This is great work, Anna! One of the things we've been working on is getting you to become more aware of what's happening around you when you feel the desire to restrict most intensely. You've just made an important connection between your stress and fear related to your father's behavior and your wanting to restrict. Now that you can more clearly see that connection, how would you like to start working on your relationship with your father?

REDIRECTING ISSUES RELATED TO EATING, SHAPE, AND/OR WEIGHT. Eating disorder patients may frequently bring up issues in session relating to distressing eating behavior (e.g., binge episodes) or may want to engage in extended discussion relating to eating, shape, and weight. Although these issues are relevant insofar as they reflect the clinical status of the patient's eating disorder, the therapist must be attentive to keep the session "on track," i.e, focused on the patient's treatment goals. In such situations, the therapist should gently but firmly redirect the patient back to work on the treatment goals. As discussed above, dialogue related to eating disorder symptomatology must be repeatedly linked to its functional role in the interpersonal domain. The following example illustrates how a therapist can redirect discussion and help the patient focus on the treatment goals:

Therapist: What did you want to work on today, Jim?

Jim: I've been really stressed out lately. I have two exams this week and a research paper due. I didn't have much time to eat, which was good, but I had a huge binge on Saturday night. I found myself in the kitchen gorging on chips, cookies, pizza, basically anything that didn't move. I was so embarrassed when my roommate walked in and saw what I was doing. I probably would still be eating if he hadn't walked in.

Therapist: One of the things you shared with me last week was that eating is a way for you to relieve stress, to unwind. Instead of allowing yourself a break or sharing your feelings with friends, you'll turn to food.

Jim: I definitely did that. You wouldn't believe how I was shoving food in by the mouthful, I couldn't eat fast enough, I wanted...

Therapist: Jim, let me refocus you for a moment, back to your goals. How have your efforts to reach out to other students been coming?

Jim: Pretty good. I've started studying in the library, so that I can hang out in the student lounge when I need a break. I've met a few people that way. It's hard for me though because I always feel insecure in social situations. I feel like other people may be judging me or don't like me.

Therapist: As we discussed last week, for a long time you've been sheltering yourself from that insecurity by avoiding others and using food to cope with stress. I wonder if as you practice being more social and build up your support system, you'll start to feel more comfortable socially. You'll have more friends to turn to when you're stressed and be less likely to turn to food. In the short time we've been working together, you've already met several new people. Not surprisingly, you only had one overeating episode this past week. You said earlier that you were bingeing nightly during similarly stressful times in the past.

The above discussed therapeutic techniques (i.e., focusing on goals; connecting eating symptoms and interpersonal problems; redirecting eating, weight, or shape issues) are utilized with patients in all four problem areas.

By the end of the intermediate phase, patients are often acutely aware that treatment will soon be ending. The therapist should begin to discuss termination explicitly and address any anxiety the patient may be experiencing regarding it. The therapist should begin to prepare the patient for emotions that may arise with termination, including grief related to the ending of treatment.

The Termination Phase. The termination phase typically lasts four to five sessions. During this phase, the therapist should encourage the patient to reflect on progress made during therapy and to outline goals for remaining work. Patients are encouraged to identify early warning signs of relapse (e.g., overeating, restricting, negative mood) and to identify potential plans of action. Patients are reminded that eating disorder symptoms tend to arise in times of difficulty and are encouraged to view such symptoms as important early warning signals. Identifying potential plans of action in such situations will serve to increase the patient's sense of competence and security. Nevertheless, it is also essential to assist patients in identifying warning signs and symptoms that may indicate a need for professional intervention in the future.

General Therapeutic Techniques

Throughout therapy, the therapist should maintain a consistent focus on the interpersonal context of the patient's life. Eating disorder symptoms should thus be analyzed in light of the interpersonal difficulties constituting the backdrop of those symptoms. Although this approach is unique to IPT, some of the therapeutic techniques utilized in IPT are similar to techniques used in other therapies. In addition to the therapeutic techniques described above, other helpful techniques include exploratory questions, encouragement of affect, clarification, communication analysis, and use of the therapeutic relationship [for a more detailed description of these and other techniques, please see (1)].

Exploratory Questions. Use of general, open-ended questions can facilitate the free discussion of material. This is particularly true in the initial phases of a session. For example, the therapist might say, "Tell me about your relationship with your husband." Once this has generated discussion, progressively more specific questioning would ensue.

Encouraging Affect. IPT's focus on affect evocation and exploration is especially relevant for eating disorder patients, given that problematic eating often functions as a way to regulate negative affect. Specifically, the IPT therapist helps patients: (a) acknowledge and accept painful affects, (b) use affective experiences to bring about desired interpersonal changes, and (c) experience suppressed affects.

Frequently, eating-disordered patients are emotionally constricted in situations when others would typically experience strong emotions. For example, sometimes patients will deny feeling upset when it is clear that an upsetting interaction has just occurred. In this situation, the therapist might say, "Although you said you were not upset, it appears to me that you have shut down since mentioning the situation with your husband." By explicitly noting the discrepancy, the therapist will attempt to draw out affect that has been suppressed.

Clarification. This technique is useful in calling attention to contradictions that may have occurred in the patient's presentation of material and increases the patient's awareness about what she or he has actually communicated. For example, contradictions between the patient's affect and speech may be noteworthy (i.e., "While you were telling me how upset you are about your father, you had a smile on your face. What do you think that's about?").

Communication Analysis. This technique is used to identify any communication difficulties that the patient may be experiencing and to help the patient alter ineffective communication patterns. Typically, the therapist will ask the patient to recall in great detail a recent interaction or argument with a significant other. Together, patient and therapist work to identify any communication difficulties and to find more effective communication strategies.

Use of the Therapeutic Relationship. The premise behind this technique is that people have characteristic patterns of interacting with others.

The technique is utilized by exploring the patient's thoughts, feelings, expectations, and behavior in the therapeutic relationship and relating these to the patient's characteristic way of behaving and/or feeling in other relationships. This technique is particularly relevant and useful for patients with interpersonal deficits and interpersonal role disputes. Use of this technique offers the patient the opportunity to understand the nature of his or her difficulties in interacting with others and provides the patient with helpful feedback on his or her interaction style.

REVIEW OF OUTCOME STUDIES

IPT has been adapted for the treatment of BN, BED, and AN, respectively. Although IPT as tested for major depression includes a consistent focus on depressive symptomatology, research applications of IPT for eating disorders have not included a strong focus on eating disorder symptoms. This focus has been avoided in order to minimize procedural overlap with cognitive–behavioral therapy (CBT). However, clinical experience strongly suggests that significant therapeutic benefit is derived from consistent attention to the role of specific eating disorder symptoms as "red flags," signaling interpersonal difficulties in need of clinical attention.

Interpersonal Psychotherapy for Bulimia Nervosa

CBT is currently the most researched, best established treatment for BN (37). To date, IPT is the only psychological treatment for BN that has demonstrated long-term outcomes comparable to those of CBT. Thus far, all controlled studies of IPT have been comparison studies with CBT. Early studies indicated similar short- and long-term outcomes for binge eating between CBT and IPT (3,38). A more recent multisite study (39) comparing CBT and IPT as treatments for BN found that in the short term (posttreatment) patients receiving CBT demonstrated higher rates of abstinence from binge eating and lower rates of purging. By long-term follow-up (8 months and 1 year following treatment), these rates were equivalent. The more rapid effects of CBT compared to IPT may be at least partially explained by the relative lack of focus on eating disorder symptomatology in the research version of IPT. Despite relatively slower response rates, however, IPT patients rated their treatment as more suitable and expected greater success than did CBT patients. This finding suggests that BN patients may perceive the interpersonal focus of IPT as more relevant to their disorder and to their treatment needs than a more cognitive–behavioral focus on distortions related to weight and shape.

When choosing between IPT and CBT for an individual patient, the therapist and patient should together evaluate the advantages and disadvantages of each treatment. To date, more data support the efficacy of CBT. CBT has been shown to produce more rapid effects for BN, although IPT produces equivalent outcomes over the long term. IPT may be particularly well suited to patients presenting with interpersonal difficulties or for patients who express a distaste for elements of CBT (i.e., keeping food diaries, thought recording). Finally, therapist expertise is relevant to the choice of treatment; both IPT and CBT are specialty treatments and should be administered only by trained practitioners.

IPT for Binge Eating Disorder

The use of IPT for BED was based on the earlier success of IPT in BN (40). Wilfley and colleagues first adapted IPT to a group format for BED patients (41,42). New strategies were developed to specifically address interpersonal deficits, an interpersonal problem area that occurs more frequently in BED patients than BN patients. In IPT for BED, group members with interpersonal deficits are encouraged to use the group as a "live" social network. This social milieu is designed to decrease social isolation, support the formation of new social relationships, and serve as a model for initiating and sustaining social relationships outside of the therapeutic context (33). Self-stigmatization is common among BED patients; this stigmatization contributes to the maintenance of the disorder. Group therapy thus offers a radically altered social environment for BED patients, who typically endeavor to keep shameful eating behaviors hidden from others.

Similar to BN, CBT has been shown to have specific and robust treatment effects in BED (42–49). Two studies have compared IPT with CBT and found that IPT has comparable effects to CBT in the management of BED. The first study, comparing group CBT and IPT, revealed that both treatments were more effective than a wait-list control group at reducing binge eating and had equivalent significant reductions in binge eating in both the short and long term (42). In a second study, which included a substantially larger sample size, both CBT and IPT demonstrated equivalent short- and long-term efficacy in reducing binge eating and associated specific and general psychopathology, with approximately 60% of patients remaining abstinent from binge eating at 1-year follow-up (31). The time course of almost all outcomes with IPT was identical to that of CBT. The one treatment-specific difference was a significantly greater reduction in dietary restraint among CBT patients at posttreatment and 4-month follow-up; however, IPT demonstrated parity with CBT by the 8- and 12-month follow-ups. Findings from the two aforementioned studies indicate that IPT represents an efficacious treatment alternative for BED. Similar to BN, considerations relevant to the choice among treatment options for a given BED patient include the individual patient's symptom profile and preferences, as well as therapist expertise.

Interpersonal Psychotherapy for Anorexia Nervosa

Given the dearth of randomized controlled treatment trials studying AN, some have argued that it may be impossible to generate empirically based recommendations regarding treatment (37). To date, family therapy has been the most studied treatment for AN (37). Specifically, family therapy has been found to be efficacious for adolescents with a short duration of illness (50,51). However, the often chronic nature of AN, particularly in adult patients, limits the generalizability of these findings.

No controlled studies have yet demonstrated the efficacy of IPT for AN. In the first trial to compare IPT, CBT, and nonspecific supportive clinical management (NSCM) for AN, McIntosh and colleagues (52) found that NSCM was superior to both IPT and CBT for improving the core features of AN. As developed and manualized for this study, NSCM was delivered by highly trained eating disorder specialists; the treatment focused on the patient's presenting eating disorder symptoms. Similar to other treatment trials using IPT for eating disorders, the IPT condition in this study did not include a focus on eating disorder symptomatology. However, McIntosh and colleagues (32) advise, that optimal delivery of IPT with anorexic patients in clinical settings should include an ongoing review of the connections between the interpersonal problem areas of interest and core anorexic symptoms. Given the ego syntonic nature of AN, the relative lack of focus on eating disorder symptoms in this research trial may have blunted IPT's effect and avoided the essential work of therapy (52). Alternatively, it may be that the supportive, nondirective approach offered in NSCM is superior to a specialized psychotherapy (52), particularly in the weight regain phase of AN treatment.

Nevertheless, given the importance of interpersonal functioning in etiological theories of AN (32), it makes sense to continue to explore IPT's utility in treatment of the disorder. Specifically, investigation of the clinical effectiveness of IPT for AN that includes a focus on eating disorder symptoms as they relate to interpersonal problems is warranted. It may be that IPT for AN is optimally delivered in the context of other adjunctive treatments (e.g., pharmacological, nutritional) rather than as a "stand-alone" treatment. Staging of treatment may also be important; perhaps IPT is more suitable for the maintenance and relapse prevention stages of treatment than for the weight regain phase. Alternatively, a combination therapy including components of both IPT and CBT may provide a more efficacious treatment than IPT or

CBT alone. Given the state of current research, however, no definitive clinical recommendations regarding IPT for AN can be made.

SUMMARY AND FUTURE DIRECTIONS

IPT for eating disorders is a focused, time-limited treatment that targets interpersonal problem(s) associated with the onset and/or maintenance of the eating disorder. The interpersonal focus is highly relevant to eating disorder patients, many of whom experience difficulties in interpersonal functioning. Depending on the patient's primary problem area, specific treatment strategies and goals are incorporated into the treatment plan. The primary problem area is determined by conducting a thorough interpersonal inventory and devising an individualized interpersonal formulation for each patient. IPT has resulted in significant and well-maintained improvements for the management of BN and BED; its role in the management of AN has yet to be determined.

The interpersonal focus of IPT has traditionally been more readily embraced by clinicians than CBT; IPT may also be an easier therapy in which to become proficient. In the future, the efficacy of IPT in eating-disordered populations may be further enhanced by including a specific focus on eating disorder symptomatology in the treatment. In addition, further adaptations of the group format, which has demonstrated promise with BED patients, may be usefully extended to other patient subpopulations who would likely benefit from the support of a group modality (i.e., adolescents). Additional research is needed regarding the mechanisms by which IPT achieves its effects, predictors of treatment outcome, and the effectiveness of IPT for eating disorders in clinical settings. Finally, advances in neuroscience, specifically increased sophistication in neuroimaging techniques, offer the potential to investigate the impact of IPT on brain function in eating disorder patients. Such studies have revealed changes in brain function in depressed patients treated with IPT (53,54); similar studies of IPT for eating disorders may provide useful information regarding physiological mechanisms influencing treatment response. Such empirically based refinements of the content and delivery of IPT may thus further enhance its clinical utility in the management of eating disorders.

REFERENCES

1. Klerman GL, Weissman MM, Rounsaville BJ, Chevron ES. Interpersonal Psychotherapy of Depression. New York: Basic Books, 1984.
2. Fairburn CG, Jones R, Peveler RC, Carr SJ, Solomon RA, O'Connor ME,

Burton J, Hope A. Three psychological treatments for bulimia nervosa: a comparative trial. Arch Gen Psychiatry 1991; 48:463–469.

3. Fairburn CG, Peveler RC, Jones R, Hope RA, O'Connor ME. Predictors of 12-month outcome in bulimia nervosa and the influence of attitudes to shape and weight. J Consult Clinical Psychol 1993; 61:696–698.

4. Klerman GL, Weissman MM. Interpersonal psychotherapy for depression: background and concepts. In: Klerman GL, Weissman MM, eds. New Applications of Interpersonal Psychotherapy. Washington, DC: American Psychiatric Association, 1993:3–26.

5. Frank E, Spanier C. Interpersonal psychotherapy for depression: overview, clinical efficacy, and future directions. Clin Psychol Sci Pract 1995; 2:349–369.

6. Meyer A. Psychobiology: A Science of Man. Springfield, IL: Charles C Thomas, 1957.

7. Sullivan HS. The Interpersonal Theory of Psychiatry. New York: WW Norton, 1953.

8. Bowlby J. Attachment and Loss. Vol. 1. Attachment. New York: Basic Books, 1982.

9. Schmidt U, Tiller J, Blanchard M, Andrews B, Treasure JL. Is there a specific trauma precipitating anorexia nervosa? Psychol Med 1997; 27:523–530.

10. Fairburn CG, Doll HA, Welch SL, Hay PJ, Davies BA, O'Connor ME. Risk factors for binge eating disorder: a community-based, case-control study. Arch Gen Psychiatry 1998; 55:425–432.

11. Fairburn CG, Welch SA, Doll HA, Davies BA, O'Connor ME. Risk factors for bulimia nervosa. Arch Gen Psychiatry 1997; 54:509–517.

12. Segrin C. Interpersonal Processes in Psychological Problems. New York: Guilford Press, 2001.

13. Gual P, Perez-Gaspar M, Martinez-Gonzalez MA, Lahortiga F, Irala-Estevez J, Cervera-Enguix. Self-esteem, personality, and eating disorders: baseline assessment of a prospective population-based cohort. Int J Eat Disord 2002; 31:261–273.

14. Herzog DB, Keller MB, Lavori PW, Ott IL. Social impairment in bulimia. Int J Eat Disord 1987; 6:741–747.

15. O'Mahony JF, Hollwey S. The correlates of binge eating in two nonpatient samples. Addict Behav 1995; 20:471–480.

16. Ghaderi A, Scott B. Prevalence and psychological correlates of eating disorders among females aged 18–30 years in the general population. Acta Psychiatr Scand 1999; 99:261–266.

17. Rorty M, Yager J, Buckwalter JG, Rossotto E. Social support, social adjustment, and recovery status in bulimia nervosa. Int J Eat Disord 1999; 26:1–12.

18. Troop NA, Holbrey A, Trowler R, Treasure JL. Ways of coping in women with eating disorders. J Nerv Ment Dis 1994; 182:535–540.

19. Grissett NL, Norvell NK. Perceived social support, social skills, and quality of relationships in bulimic women. J Consult Clin Psychol 1992; 60:293–299.

20. Tiller JM, Sloane G, Schmidt U, Troop N, Power M, Treasure JL. Social sup-

port in patients with anorexia nervosa and bulimia nervosa. Int J Eat Disord 1997; 21:31–38.

21. Tanofsky-Kraff M, Wilfley DE, Spurell E. Impact of interpersonal and ego-related stress on restrained eaters. Int J Eat Disord 2000; 27:411–418.

22. Tuschen-Caffier B, Vogele C. Psychological and physiological reactivity to stress: an experimental study on bulimic patients, restrained eaters and controls. Psychother Psychosom 1999; 68:333–340.

23. Telch CF, Agras WS. Obesity, binge eating and psychopathology: are they related? Int J Eat Disord 1994; 15:53–61.

24. Garner DM, Vitousek KM, Pike KM. Cognitive–behavioral therapy for anorexia nervosa. In: Garner DM, Garfinkel PE, eds. Handbook of Treatment for Eating Disorders. 2nd ed. New York: Guilfor Press, 1997:94–144.

25. Stice E, Akutagawa D, Gaggar A, Agras WS. Negative affect moderates the relation between dieting and binge eating. Int J Eating Disord 2000; 27:218–229.

26. Telch CF, Agras WS. Do emotional states influence binge eating in the obese? Int J Eat Disord 1996; 20:271–279.

27. Powell AL, Thelen MH. Emotions and cognitions associated with bingeing and weight control behavior in bulimia. J Psychosom Res 1996; 40:317–328.

28. Schupak-Neuberg E, Nemeroff CJ. Disturbances in identity and self-regulation in bulimia nervosa: implications for a metaphorical perspective of "body as self." Int J Eat Disord 1993; 13:335–347.

29. Steiger H, Gauvin L, Jabalpurwala S, Seguin JR, Stotland S. Hypersensitivity to social interactions in bulimic syndromes: relationship to binge eating. J Consult Clin Psychol 1999; 67:765–775.

30. Fairburn CG, Peveler RC, Jones R, Hope RA, O'Connor ME. Predictors of 12-month outcome in bulimia nervosa and the influence of attitudes to shape and weight. J Consult Clinical Psychol 1993; 61:696–698.

31. Wilfley DE, Welch RR, Stein RI, Spurrell EB, Cohen LR, Saelens BE, Dounchis JZ, Frank MA, Wiseman CV, Matt GE. The psychological treatment of binge eating disorder (BED): a comparison group of cognitive behavioral therapy and interpersonal psychotherapy. Arch Gen Psychiatry 2002; 59:713–721.

32. McIntosh VV, Bulik CM, McKenzie JM, Luty SE, Jordan J. Interpersonal psychotherapy for anorexia nervosa. Int J Eat Disord 2000; 27:125–139.

33. Wilfley DE, Frank MA, Welch R, Spurrell EB, Rounseville BJ. Adapting interpersonal psychotherapy to a group format (IPT-G) for binge eating disorder: toward a model for adapting empirically supported treatments. Psychother Res 1998; 8:379–391.

34. Fairburn CG, Doll HA, Welch SL, Hay PJ, Davies BA, O'Connor ME. Risk factors for binge eating disorder: a community-based, case-control study. Arch Gen Psychiatry 1998; 55:425–432.

35. Wilfley DE, Stein RI, Welch RR. Interpersonal psychotherapy for the treatment of eating disorders. In: Treasure J, Schmidt U, Dare C, Van Furth E, eds. Handbook of Eating Disorders. 2d ed. Sussex: John Wiley & Sons, 2003; 253–270.

36. Frank E, Kupfer DJ, Wagner EF, McEachran AB, Cornes C. Efficacy of interpersonal psychotherapy as a maintenance treatment of recurrent depression: contributing factors. Arch Gen Psychiatry 1991; 48:1053–1059.
37. Wilson GT, Fairburn CG Eating disorders. In: Nathan PE, Gorman JM, eds. Treatments That Work. 2d ed. New York: Oxford University Press, 2002.
38. Fairburn CG, Norman PA, Welch SL, O'Connor ME, Doll HA, Peveler RC. A prospective study of outcome in bulimia nervosa and the long-term effects of three psychological treatments. Arch Gen Psychiatry 1995; 52:304–312.
39. Agras WS, Walsh BT, Fairburn CG, Wilson GT, Kraemer HC. A multicenter comparison of cognitive–behavioral therapy and interpersonal psychotherapy for bulimia nervosa. Arch Gen Psychiatry 2000; 57:459–466.
40. Fairburn CG, Jones R, Peveler RC, Carr SJ, Solomon RA, O'Connor ME, Burton J, Hope A. Three psychological treatments for bulimia nervosa: a comparative trial. Arch Gen Psychiatry 1991; 48:463–469.
41. Wilfley DE, MacKenzie KR, Welch RR, Ayres VE, Weissman MM. Interpersonal Psychotherapy for Group. New York: Basic Books, 2000.
42. Wilfley DE, Agras WS, Telch CF, Rossiter EM, Schneider JA, Cole AG, Sifford L, Raeburn SD. Group cognitive–behavioral therapy and group interpersonal psychotherapy for the nonpurging bulimic individual: a controlled comparison. J Consult Clin Psychol 1993; 61:296–305.
43. Grilo CM, Masheb RM, Heninger G, Wilson GT. Controlled comparison of cognitive behavior therapy and fluoxetine for binge eating disorder. Paper presented at the Academy for Eating Disorders International Conference on Eating Disorders, Boston, MA, April 2002.
44. Devlin MJ. Psychotherapy and medication for binge eating disorder. Paper presented at the Academy for Eating Disorders International Conference on Eating Disorders, Boston, MA, April 2002.
45. Ricca V, Mannucci E, Mezzani B, et al. Fluoxetine and fluvoxamine combined with individual cognitive-behavior therapy in binge eating disorder: a one-year follow-up study. Psychother Psychosom 2001; 70:298–306.
46. Nauta H, Hospers H, Kok G, Jansen A. A comparison between a cognitive and a behavioral treatment for obese binge eaters and obese non-binge eaters. Behavior Therapy 2000; 21:441–461.
47. Kenardy J, Mensch M, Bowen K, Green B, Walton J. Group therapy for binge eating in type 2 diabetes: A randomized trial. Diabet Med March 2002; 19(3):234–239.
48. Marcus MD, Wing RR, Fairburn CG. Cognitive behavioral treatment of binge eating vs. behavioral weigh control on the treatment of binge eating disorder. Ann Behav Med 1995; 17:SO90.
49. Telch CF, Agras WS, Rossiter EM, Wilfley DE, Kenardy J. Group cognitive–behavioral treatment for the non-purging bulimic: an initial evaluation. J Consult Clin Psychol 1990; 58:629–635.
50. Eisler I, Dare C, Russell GF, Szmukler GI, Le Grange D, Dodge E. Family and individual therapy in anorexia nervosa: a 5-year follow-up. Arch Gen Psychiatry 1997; 54:1025–1030.

51. Eisler I, Dare C, Hodes M, Dodge E, Russell G, Le Grange D. Family therapy for adolescent anorexia nervosa: the results of a controlled comparison of two family interventions. J Child Psychol Psychiatry 2000; 41:727–736.

52. McIntosh VV, Jordan J, Carter FA, Luty SE, McKenzie JM, Bulik CM, Joyce PR. Three psychotherapies for anorexia nervosa: a randomized controlled trial. Paper presented at the Academy for Eating Disorders International Conference on Eating Disorders, Boston, MA, April 2002.

53. Brody AL, Saxena S, Stoessel P, et al. Regional brain metabolic changes in patients with major depression treated with either paroxetine or interpersonal therapy. Arch Gen Psychiatry 2001; 58:631–640.

54. Martin SD, Martin E, Rai SR, et al. Brain blood flow changes in depressed patients treated with interpersonal psychotherapy or venlafaxine hydrochloride. Arch Gen Psychiatry 2001; 58:641–648.

20

Use of Dialectical Behavior Therapy in the Eating Disorders

Marsha D. Marcus and Michele D. Levine

Western Psychiatric Institute and Clinic,
   University of Pittsburgh School of Medicine
Pittsburgh, Pennsylvania, U.S.A.

Dialectical behavior therapy (DBT), developed by Marsha Linehan, is a comprehensive treatment program based on cognitive and behavioral principles that are complemented by acceptance-based strategies derived primarily from Zen Buddhism. Originally designed for individuals with borderline personality disorder (BPD) and self-injurious behaviors, DBT has been shown to significantly improve the outcome in this population. Because of its efficacy in treating BPD, clinicians and researchers have become interested in the application of DBT to other difficult, refractory, or chronic conditions, including eating disorders. Moreover, comorbid BPD is common among eating disorder patients, and self-injurious and suicidal behaviors also are common (see Chapter 9). One recent report found that approximately 20% of women with an eating disorder diagnosis endorsed an episode of self-harm in the previous 6 months, and one-third of these indicated self-injuring at least several times per month (1).

However, it is important to note that our use of DBT in the treatment of patients with eating disorders is not limited to individuals with comorbid BPD or parasuicidal behavior. We have found DBT to be useful in the treatment of any chronic eating disorder, including restricting anorexia nervosa, because of its acceptance of and tolerance for refractory symptoms and matter-of-fact emphasis on the need for change. DBT may have particular utility for anorexia nervosa (2) because chronically restricting patients often find it excruciatingly difficult to modify symptoms, and consequently avoid or resist treatment. DBT incorporates specific techniques for working with patients who are ambivalent about change, and specific strategies for maintaining commitment to treatment. Similarly, chronic anorexia patients often have limited ability to negotiate emotionally or interpersonally difficult situations. DBT emphasizes the need for acquisition of life skills to promote effective functioning and recovery. Finally, DBT provides an effective methodology for dealing with therapists' responses to patients, which is often helpful when treating numbers of chronically ill patients with anorexia nervosa. Accordingly, we have used DBT as an outpatient treatment for eating disorder patients, irrespective of eating disorder diagnosis, who have not responded to front-line treatments, and have incorporated DBT principles in the treatment of patients in our inpatient and partial hospitalization programs.

In this chapter, we first provide a brief overview of the philosophy and assumptions of DBT and a description of the treatment with comments regarding the applicability of DBT to the management of eating disorders. Next, we present information on the efficacy of DBT in BPD and other disorders, along with evidence bearing on its utility in managing disordered eating. Finally, we discuss additional aspects of the implementation of DBT and its principles in our program. Although we describe the basics of DBT, a detailed presentation of its principles and procedures is beyond the scope of this chapter. These are explicated in full in Dr. Linehan's text, *Cognitive–Behavioral Treatment of Borderline Personality Disorder* (3), and skills manual, *Skills Training Manual for Treating Borderline Personality Disorder* (4). Information about DBT training and resources also can be found on the web site of the Behavioral Technology Transfer Group (http://www.behavioraltech.com).

PHILOSOPHY AND ASSUMPTIONS OF DIALECTICAL BEHAVIOR THERAPY

A dialectical world view is at the core of DBT. In its broadest sense, dialecticism refers to the philosophy that reality comprises opposing forces, "thesis" and "antithesis," and when these polarities are balanced or integrated, the resulting "synthesis" immediately creates a new set of opposing forces. Thus, reality is by its nature complex and dynamic with the important corollary that there is not one correct point of view or understanding. The implications of a dialectical world view are manifold and permeate DBT. They include a responsibility on the part of the therapist to identify the "truth" in the patient's behavior, validate it, and accept responsibility to make use of persuasion to encourage the development of synthesis and a new and more adaptive reality for patients. A dialectical world view has important implications for patients as well. For example, patients are helped to accept that truth is not an absolute and that apparently opposing beliefs or emotions can exist simultaneously in the same individual.

The adoption of a dialectical world view has profound advantages in the management of refractory eating disorder behaviors. Symptoms of eating disorders are perplexing, confounding, and often repugnant to patients' friends, family members, some health care professionals, and even the patients themselves. Thus, the conscious and deliberate attempt on the part of clinicians who work with these individuals to understand the validity of eating disorder symptoms as efforts to cope with aversive circumstances is a critical tool in the establishment and maintenance of an effective working relationship. Similarly, a dialectical world view recognizes and accepts the difficulty of change and the ambivalence that eating disorder patients have about modifying or relinquishing their symptoms. The deliberate balance between acceptance and pulling for change also serves to reduce ambivalence about the therapist, who may be perceived as intrusive or controlling.

ETIOLOGY OF BORDERLINE PERSONALITY DISORDER

Linehan's model of the etiology of BPD also is dialectical in nature. The biosocial model (3) posits that the development of a borderline personality is the result of a transaction between a biological vulnerability to emotional dysfunction and an invalidating environment that creates and maintains borderline behavior patterns over time. Emotional dysfunction is defined as difficulty in modulating emotions and increased vulnerability to intense emotional experiences, which can be summarized in three ways. First, an individual may be highly sensitive to emotional experience, having a low threshold for emotions and developing immediate, intense reactions. Second, dysregulated emotional processing may mean that an individual has a heightened reactivity, or a stronger than average response, to some emotional cues. Finally, emotion dysregulation may take the form of a slow return to a baseline level of emotion. This slow return can be problematic because new events are more likely to rekindle an intense emotion during the period in which the individual is regaining emotional equilibrium.

The second idea in the biosocial model is the invalidating environment, which refers to any environment that continually communicates that an individual's reactions are faulty, exaggerated, or inappropriate. Examples of environmental invalidation include failing to validate an individual's private experience, oversimplifying the ease of problem solving, or punishing an emotional display. In the context of an invalidating environment, an individual with a vulnerable emotional processing system fails to learn to tolerate or trust her private emotional and cognitive experiences. Some environments are obviously invalidating, e.g., an environment where physical or sexual abuse occurs. It is important to note, however, that invalidation need not be intentional or dramatic, but occurs when the environment consistently is unresponsive to the needs of a particular vulnerable individual.

The ongoing interaction of vulnerability and invalidation results in emotion dysregulation, which in turn leads to the emotional, cognitive, and behavioral symptoms that serve a regulating function. Within this framework, chronic suicidal urges and parasuicidal behaviors are understood as legitimate, if ultimately dysfunctional, attempts to solve problems in an individual who experiences intense suffering in a life that often seems unbearable. Thus, although the overarching goal of DBT is to help the patient develop a life that is worth living, a more proximal goal of treatment is to reduce maladaptive problem solving and enhance adaptive functioning in response to emotional dysregulation.

The biosocial model of the etiology of BPD overlaps neatly with the affect regulation model of eating disorder symptoms. In the affect regulation model, eating-disordered behaviors, such as binge eating, food or calorie restriction, overexercising, and purging, are seen as efforts to modulate strong negative or aversive affective experiences. Because DBT is specifically designed to address the core problem of emotion regulation, it provides a clear framework for addressing problem behaviors in eating disorders. Furthermore, a growing body of research evidence has documented that eating disorders aggregate in families, and there is increasing consensus that biological vulnerability is involved in the pathogenesis of eating disorders. Thus, a biosocial framework of etiology provides a meaningful heuristic to understand the complex cascade of factors that lead to the expression of eating disorder syndromes.

DIALECTICAL BEHAVIOR THERAPY

DBT makes a series of assumptions about patients that are critical to the successful implementation of treatment and that inform all intervention strategies. Two DBT assumptions, that "Patients are doing the best that they can" and that "Patients want to improve," are the core of a successful therapeutic stance. These seemingly simple assumptions are critically important in work with chronic or refractory patients, where therapists may feel at times that patients do not want to get better or are not trying hard enough. However, assuming that a patient does not want to recover or is not trying is a prototype of invalidation for the patient who is likely to feel misunderstood, which in turn leads to frustration, anger, or shame. Importantly, the adoption of these assumptions by the therapists does not mean that patients consistently feel that they want to recover or are always trying their best; rather, the therapist adopts the assumptions until fact finding in session with the patient leads to a different conclusion.

The next assumptions, which seem paradoxical, and thus embody a dialectical world view, are that "Patients need to do better, try harder, and be more motivated" and that "Patients may not have caused all of their own problems, but must solve them anyway." That patients need to do better to have a worthwhile life usually is self-evident, and they require substantial help to reduce barriers to change, increase motivation, and enhance skills. Similarly, although the patient requires help from the therapist (and usually from others in her life), the business of change is hard work, and the patient, by necessity, carries the burden of changing. Finally, DBT makes the assumption that "Patients cannot fail in therapy." The treatment may fail, but not the patient. This assumption reflects an imperfect knowledge regarding how to help and a profound awareness of the difficulty of change.

The dialectic between the assumptions that patients are doing the best that they can, and that they need to try harder and carry the responsibility for change has clear applicability to the treatment of eating disorders, where there often is the unfortunate assumption that patients do not want to relinquish their symptoms. In some instances, the fear of a life without the eating disorder is overwhelming, but patients invariably express a longing for a life free of eating disorder–related debility.

In summary, the philosophy and assumptions of DBT reflect a basic understanding of the nature of reality, the etiology of psychiatric disorder, and the role and meaning of psychiatric symptoms. Like other cognitive–behavioral treatments, DBT systematically utilizes the complete arsenal of change strategies but balances the focus on change with respect for the truth in patient symptom behaviors and acceptance of the difficulty of change. We have found this framework to be eminently suitable for work with eating disorder patients who have not responded to initial treatment or who have had multiple recurrences of disorder.

MODES OF TREATMENT IN DIALECTICAL BEHAVIOR THERAPY

Standard outpatient DBT includes four treatment modes, all of which are important to the progress of therapy: (a) weekly individual therapy, (b) weekly group-based skills sessions, (c) telephone consultations, and (d) regular consultation meetings for the therapists. Individual treatment focuses on three primary targets: life-threatening behaviors, therapy-interfering behaviors, and quality-of-life–interfering behaviors. A fourth target area, increasing behavioral skills, is addressed primarily in the context of the weekly skills group. The sanctioned use of the telephone is designed to provide patients with the opportunity to obtain coaching in real-life situations to promote the generalization of skills outside of the therapy setting. Finally, DBT involves a regular consultation with a team that provides support for therapists working with difficult patients.

DBT progresses in stages. In the pretreatment phase patients are oriented to treatment, and the patient and therapist agree on the overall goals of the work. One cannot overemphasize that nothing in DBT is done without directly involving, educating, and obtaining agreement from patients before the initiation of a treatment strategy or treatment plan. The first stage of treatment, which generally lasts about one year, focuses on reducing acute symptoms and increasing behavioral skills. DBT research has focused predominantly on the outcome of the first stage of treatment, and the content of the current chapter also focuses on the initial year of DBT.

The target of the second stage of DBT is decreasing posttraumatic stress if present. The reasoning behind deferring a focus on these symptoms is based on the assumption that patients have to acquire the basic abilities and external supports to tolerate the painful work involved in dealing with trauma. The final stage of DBT focuses on increasing self-respect and achieving individual goals, which in the DBT framework are possible only after the patient has developed some ability to trust herself and the therapist.

Commitment Strategies in Dialectical Behavior Therapy

Because the treatment process is acknowledged to be difficult, the notion of commitment is critical in DBT. Commitment to participating in DBT for a specified period of time and working on the overall goal of building a life worth living and reducing life-threatening behaviors are regarded as necessary to initiate effective treatment. The patient also is asked to commit to collaborating in the treatment procedures within a given session. In addition to these general commitments, commitment occurs at a more specific level, as commitment is sought to carry out the behavior changes agreed on by the patient and therapist. The therapist directly elicits a patient's agreement to try new behaviors or work on specific problem areas. Conversely, the therapist also highlights the patient's freedom to make her own choices while clearly presenting the realistic consequences of those choices.

There are specific DBT strategies for eliciting and maintaining commitment to treatment. These strategies include highlighting and discussing the pros and cons of a commitment to change, playing the devil's advocate (i.e., questioning the wisdom of change) to strengthen commitment and heighten a sense of self-control, or use of the "foot in the door, door in the face" technique (i.e., getting a small commitment, then requesting a major change) to pull for patient commitment to specific goals and procedures. Throughout treatment the therapist highlights previous commitments made by the patient in an effort to clarify and strengthen current commitments. The DBT conceptualization of commitment as a dynamic process that occurs over time is helpful in working with chronic eating disorder patients, whose commitment to change is often uncertain and wavering.

Individual Therapy in Dialectical Behavior Therapy

Individual therapy occurs once a week, and the individual therapist assumes primary responsibility for patient care. Individual sessions are active and structured, with the therapist and patient agreeing to focus work on the hierarchy of treatment targets in the service of the overall goal of building a worthwhile life. This hierarchy serves to organize the work of the therapist and patient both within and across sessions. As noted above, DBT specifies three treatment areas that are targeted in the order of importance. The first goal of treatment is to decrease suicidal and other life-threatening behaviors. This goal addresses self-injurious behaviors as well as suicidal ideation, threats, and plans. Because staying alive is the *sine qua non* for building a life worth living, the occurrence of parasuicidal ideation or behavior takes precedence over other agenda items each week.

Next on the treatment hierarchy are behaviors that interfere with the therapeutic process. Examples of therapy-interfering behaviors by a patient include noncompliance with agreements made with the therapist or failing to attend sessions. The importance accorded to therapy-interfering behaviors is an acknowledgment that the continuity of treatment must be preserved if improvements are to be made, and reflects an ongoing emphasis on maintaining the therapeutic relationship. The third target in the treatment hierarchy includes behaviors related to the patient's quality of life. This domain includes most symptoms and also focuses on areas of general dysfunction, such as financial difficulties, interpersonal problems, or problems related to school or employment.

For the most part, eating disorder behaviors, such as calorie restriction and binge purge behaviors, are targeted as quality-of-life issues. One exception is that significant calorie restriction in a low-weight patient is considered therapy interfering for two reasons. First, starvation and weight loss frequently lead to an inpatient hospitalization, which interferes with outpatient DBT. Second, patients who are actively anorexic are often cognitively unable to benefit from psychotherapy. Similarly, there are times when symptoms can be considered therapy interfering and thus assume a higher priority in treatment. For example, if a patient is restricting liquids to the extent that she requires rehydration and misses treatment, then this behavior can be construed as therapy interfering. Specific eating disorder behavior targets are summarized in Table 1.

The focus of any individual therapy session is determined by a review of the patient's diary card. The diary card is a weekly record of the patient's daily actions, including drug and alcohol use, parasuicidal acts, feelings of misery, suicidal ideation, and urges to self-harm. We have modified the standard DBT diary card to include eating disorder behaviors as shown in Figure 1. Therapy begins each week with a review of this card, which is then used to set the session agenda. Failure to complete the card is considered therapy-interfering behavior, and the first order of business is to complete the card or recreate it.

Next, a specific problem behavior gleaned from a review of the diary card is selected according to the hierarchy of treatment targets, and a detailed functional analysis of the problem behavior is conducted. This analysis, called a behavior chain analysis, begins with a clear definition of the problem behavior, and a review of general and situation-specific precipitants of the behavior. Together, the therapist and client determine and list the thoughts, feelings, and circumstances that link a precipitating event to the problem behavior. Equal emphasis is placed on identifying points in the behavior chain at which an alternative, adaptive response could have been initiated. Therapy then proceeds with a solution analysis, which includes identification of the skills needed and analysis of any factors that prevented the client from utilizing these skills in the specific situation. The focus on specific problems and the use of cognitive and behavioral strategies in DBT is similar to that in other evidenced-based treatments.

However, in contrast to other cognitive–behavioral treatments, DBT requires that the strategies that focus on change (i.e., problem solving) and those based on acceptance (i.e., validation) are of equal importance, and the therapist continually seeks to balance problem solving and validation in each session. Validation strategies are those that clearly communicate to the pa-

TABLE 1   DBT Treatment Hierarchy in Standard DBT for Eating Disorders

Eating disorder behavior	Intervening factors	Placement in DBT hierarchy
Restricting food intake	Low weight AN	Therapy Interfering
	Weight-restored AN	Quality of life interfering
Purging	Low medical risk	Quality of life interfering
	High medical risk	Therapy interfering
Weight below target		Therapy interfering
Binge eating		Quality of life interfering
Excessive exercise		Quality of life interfering

Dialectical Behavior Therapy
DIARY CARD

Name _____
Date Started _____

		Eating Disorder Behaviors						Other		Self-Harm					
		# Vomiting	# Binges	#Laxatives	# Diet Pills	# Minutes Exercise	# Meals + Snacks Restricted*			Suicidal Ideation (0-5)	Misery (0 5)	Urges (0-5)	Action (Yes/No)	Used Skills (0-7)	
Sunday															
Monday															
Tuesday															
Wednesday															
Thursday															
Friday															
Saturday															
TOTAL															

*Restricting means not eating all prescribed exchanges for that meal/snack according to current meal plan.

Used Skills Ratings:

0 = Not though about or used
1 = thought about, not used, didn't want to use
2 = Thought about, not used, wanted to use
3 = Tried, but couldn't use them

4 = Tried, could do them, but they didn't help
5 = Tried, could use them, helped
6 = Didn't try, used them, they didn't help
7 = didn't try, used them, helped

FIGURE 1   DBT diary card adapted for eating disorder behaviors.

tient that her behavior can be understood and makes sense in the context of her experience. Therapists are required to actively observe patients, effectively utilize reflection skills, and work to identify the truth (even if it is only a small part of a largely ineffective or dysfunctional reaction) in the patient's responses to her environment. There are numerous emotional, behavioral, and cognitive validation strategies that are described briefly below.

Emotional validation strategies include providing opportunities for emotional expression, helping the patient to observe and label her emotions, and communicating in a nonjudgmental fashion that feelings are valid and understandable. The DBT therapist also employs behavioral validation strategies that involve identification of patient's self-imposed behavioral demands and working to modify negative judgments by helping patients to accept that all behavior is understandable given the circumstances. There is, though, an important distinction between understanding and approving of a given behavior, specifically, bad behavior is understandable but not desirable, and usually ineffective. For example, self-injurious behavior is understandable as a strategy to avoid overwhelmingly negative affect, but it has deleterious consequences for the health of the individual and often has negative effects on an individual and her social milieu as well. Finally, cognitive behavior strategies focus on helping patients to identify dysfunctional thoughts and values, and to differentiate between facts and an individual's interpretation of the facts.

Although a discussion of the full range of the dozens of DBT strategies is not feasible here, we have presented several important strategies to illustrate the deliberate and active role of the therapist in pulling for change and validating the wisdom in the patient's choices, and the ways in which DBT strategies are adapted for use with eating disorder patients.

Dialectical Behavior Therapy Skills

DBT requires that patients participate in weekly skills training sessions as well as individual psychotherapy based on the assumption that patients with chronic or refractory difficulties lack the behavioral skills to make and sustain life changes. Specifically, patients often display what Linehan terms *apparent competence*. That is, an individual may be accomplished and intelligent, yet lack basic skills to regulate mood, tolerate distress, and assertively negotiate interpersonal relationships. The discrepancy between apparent competence and lack of ability to effectively and accurately communicate feelings is clearly evident in eating disorder patients. An effective, competent demeanor often masks the reality of inner conflict, turmoil, and insecurity.

Four specific skill areas related to the problems of dysregulated emotions and ineffective problem solving are targeted (4). The four skill modules are (a) mindfulness, (b) interpersonal effectiveness, (c) emotion regulation, and (d) distress tolerance. The practice and application of the skills is reinforced continually during individual therapy and are a specific focus of telephone consultations with a patient. An overview of the content in each of these skill areas follows.

Mindfulness practice is rooted in the Zen tradition of acceptance and nonjudgmental attitude. The skills taught in this module involve learning to observe, identify, and participate in a range of experiences with awareness. The module begins by describing the idea of "wise mind," a term used to refer to the synthesis, of "emotion mind," which includes feelings, wishes, and impressions, and "rational mind," which consists of thoughts, logic, and facts. Patients cultivate the ability to focus attention on one thing at a time, and the concept of focusing on what is effective or doing what works in a given situation is reinforced.

Distress tolerance skills focus on coping with unpleasant and painful emotions and situations. DBT provides concrete crisis survival strategies to increase the ability to tolerate distress and accept life as it is in the moment. There are several classes of distress tolerance strategies, including distraction strategies, self-soothing strategies (we utilize all of the self-soothing strategies with eating disorder patients except for self-soothing with food), strategies to improve the moment, and thinking of pros and cons. Acceptance skills include cultivation of radical acceptance and willingness. Radical acceptance involves acknowledging and accepting current emotions, thoughts, and environmental situations and developing a capacity to accept painful emotions as a part of life. Willingness describes the development of a capacity to be fully alive at every moment.

Emotion regulation skills involve identifying and labeling emotions, and effectively managing extreme emotional states. The module includes lessons on the function of emotions, as well as skills to decrease emotional vulnerability and increase positive emotional experiences. With eating disorder patients, the emphasis on identifying and labeling emotions is particularly important because severe calorie restriction and other eating disorders symptoms may serve to numb feelings, with the result that patients have a significantly narrowed affective range. Thus, it is often necessary to help the eating disorder patient to recognize feelings so as to learn how to regulate them.

Interpersonal effectiveness skills include assertiveness and interpersonal problem solving. Effective strategies for identifying a goal and developing a plan to obtain the changes an individual wants without sabotaging important relationships or losing self-respect in an interpersonal situation are taught. Within the group setting, ways of asking for what one needs, saying no, and coping with interpersonal conflict also are modeled and practiced.

In summary, the incorporation of skills training in DBT reflects the assumption that patients who must change to have a life worth living need the tools to achieve that goal. Some patients may lack even the most basic emotional, cognitive, or behavioral skills, whereas others have the needed skills but lack the capacity to implement them in real-life situations. Overall, the aim in DBT is to eliminate dysfunctional or ineffective behaviors and replace them with skillful ones.

Use of the Telephone in Dialectical Behavior Therapy

The purposes of telephone contact in DBT are to encourage the generalization of DBT skill use in daily life and to provide patients with a between-session opportunity to clarify or repair relationship problems with the therapist. Telephone contacts between a therapist and client are encouraged, but DBT specifies that phone conversations be brief and focused. Problem resolution is accomplished during the individual therapy session. As always is the case in DBT, rules on the use of the telephone are discussed and agreed on prior to their initiation.

An important aspect of telephone use in DBT is the "24-hour rule." Based on the idea that telephone contact with a primary therapist may be reinforcing and that the first treatment target is the elimination of self-harm, patients commit to the idea that they may not speak to their therapist on the telephone for a full day following an episode of self-injury. The 24-hour rule is discussed in detail prior to the onset of the treatment, and specific plans are made for how and where the patient will receive medical care after self-injury should it occur. In our experience, patients readily understand the rationale for 24-hour rule. Specifically, since the patient and therapist have agreed to work on eliminating this problem behavior, the time in which the therapist can be helpful is *before* self-injury occurs.

The Dialectical Behavior Therapy Consultation Team

The final DBT treatment mode is the consultation or supervision team. Difficult patients frequently evoke strong feelings from therapists (and others who care about them). Competent, successful treatment requires that therapists maintain an awareness of responses that may interfere with treatment and develop effective tools to manage them. Thus, therapists participate in a consultation team (composed of at least one other DBT therapist) that provides ongoing support and coaching to therapists working with difficult patients. The consultation team meets weekly to discuss cases with the goal of encouraging therapists' motivation, enhancing their skills, and promoting a dialectical view of the patient and her problems.

In summary, DBT requires a considerable commitment of time and energy on the part of the patient and the treatment team, as individual therapy, skills training, telephone use, and a therapist consultation team are standard. However, in the context of the considerable morbidity of BPD and other difficult-to-treat psychiatric disorders, such as chronic eating disorders, the investment required for DBT is regarded as cost effective.

DIALECTICAL BEHAVIOR THERAPY EFFICACY

Because it was developed to manage self-injurious behaviors in individuals with BPD, the initial DBT treatment outcome research was conducted with this population and several studies have documented the efficacy of DBT. Specifically, compared to women who received treatment as usual in the community, those treated with DBT reported reductions in both the number and severity of parasuidal acts (5). DBT also resulted in reductions in the number of hospitalizations, lower rates of treatment attrition, and improved global functioning compared to treatment as usual (5,6). Moreover, one year posttreatment, psychological adjustment was improved and distress lower in those who had received DBT compared to usual treatment (6).

DBT also has been adapted and tested in the management of other chronic behavior problems, particularly substance abuse and eating disorders. In DBT for substance abuse, the primary behavioral targets are expanded to include the cessation of drug use and the continuity of therapy. Additional treatment strategies designed to enhance the attachment of the patient to the therapist also are incorporated (7,8). To date, all of the research on the use of DBT for substance abuse has been conducted with women who have been diagnosed with both substance dependence and BPD. In general, these studies have demonstrated the utility of DBT. Compared to women who received treatment as usual in the community, women who received DBT engaged in less drug use and reported better global and social adjustment and less anger at the end of 1 year of treatment and at 4-month follow-up (8).

Recently, Linehan and colleagues (9) reported results of an investigation that compared standard DBT to an intensive, standardized treatment program, termed comprehensive validation therapy, which utilized only a subset of DBT strategies, i.e., acceptance and validation. Results of this trial indicated that in both treatment programs, women decreased drug use during treatment and over a 4-month follow-up period, although the women who received standard DBT maintained treatment gains better than those who received comprehensive validation therapy. Furthermore, although both treatments were effective in reducing levels of psychopathology, women were significantly less likely to drop out of the comprehensive validation treatent than DBT. These data suggest that the acceptance strategies of DBT, even in the absence of the behaviorally focused change strategies, may be effective, as both DBT and comprehensive validation therapy, a treatment involving acceptance-based DBT strategies, appear to be effective in decreasing substance use in women with BPD.

Telch and colleagues have adapted and tested a group-based version of DBT designed for individuals with binge eating disorder (BED) (10–12). This program has been effective in decreasing binge eating behavior and maladaptive attitudes about eating, shape, and weight. In one study (11), 89% of the women with BED who completed the 20-week DBT group treatment were abstinent from binge eating compared to only 13% of those in the waitlist group, and more than half of the women who received DBT maintained their binge eating abstinence in the 6 months following the end of treatment. Similarly, group-based DBT was related to significant decreases in binge eating among women who met modified criteria for bulimia nervosa (criteria were modified to decrease the required binge/purge frequency to once per week) (13). Although women who received DBT did not report improvements in mood or depressive symptoms compared to those on a waiting list, none of the patients dropped out of the DBT treatment. In summary, initial evidence has suggested that a group-based version of DBT is useful in the management of BED and bulimia nervosa.

In summary, there is evidence that DBT is useful in the treatment of individuals with BPD, substance abuse, and eating disorders. Longer term randomized controlled trials are needed to document its efficacy, but initial studies have provided encouraging results.

DIALECTICAL BEHAVIOR THERAPY ACROSS THE EATING DISORDERS CONTINUUM OF CARE

Our Eating Disorders Program at Western Psychiatric Institute and Clinic offers a full continuum of services, and patients move across levels of care as indicated by clinical status. We have a dedicated 11-bed inpatient unit that provides care primarily to low-weight patients who require medical monitoring and refeeding. Occasionally, normal-weight patients with intractable vomiting or other purge behaviors that have led to medical sequelae are more briefly hospitalized, as are other eating disorder patients with psychiatric exacerbations (e.g., suicidal patients). The average length of stay on the inpatient unit is approximately 4 weeks. The Partial Hospital Program is provides a 5-day-per-week program for patients who require close monitoring and meal supervision. The schedule comprises three longer days (noon to 8 p.m.) with lunch and dinner, and two shorter days (9 a.m. to 1 p.m.) with breakfast and lunch. The average length of stay in Partial Hospital is 3 weeks. The Intensive Outpatient Program provides 9 hours of program over three evenings from 5 p.m. to 8 p.m., and includes dinner. This provides a step-down level of care for patients who have been in Partial Hospital, or a step up for patients who are not benefiting from regular outpatient treatment. Standard DBT, as described above, is offered to appropriate patients as part of our outpatient clinic that provides psychotherapy, family therapy, nutrition counseling, and medical monitoring for patients with the full spectrum of eating disorders.

We have incorporated DBT principles in each level of care in our program. Some of the strengths of DBT are that it provides an overall philosophy for understanding refractory symptoms, encourages a compassionate and nonjudgmental stance for all treaters, and offers nonpejorative, easily understood language to describe patient behaviors and staff responses to patients. Although it is not feasible or appropriate to provide formal DBT training to all of the professional and paraprofessional staff that work with patients, we have disseminated the assumptions of DBT and provided training on the use of consultation to help staff deal with feelings they have about working with patients. We also have provided training to ensure that staff members temper cognitive–behavioral strategies for change with balancing doses of validation and acceptance. DBT language is used across the program, and patients as well as staff members understand the meaning of terms used in DBT skills training. The use of common terminology promotes the development of cohesion and sense of purpose in the therapeutic milieu.

In the inpatient unit, patients are exposed to the DBT skills modules, particularly mindfulness and distress tolerance as well as to the use of behavior chain analyses. Exposure to DBT skills is intensified in the Partial Hospital Program, and patients are encouraged to make use of DBT skills throughout acute treatment. Patients in the partial program also must commit to working on recovery and not to engage in symptom behavior on the premises. Thus, eating-disordered behaviors that occur on the premises, such as food restriction or purging, are considered therapy interfering regardless of the patient's degree of medical risk. If patients engage in problem behaviors they are asked to do behavior chain analyses, which are then reviewed with the therapist. The therapist and patient then agree on a plan to repair any negative consequences of the problem behavior.

SUMMARY

We have successfully utilized DBT in the management of chronic eating disorders as it provides a treatment context in which change not only is possible but also is explicitly nurtured and reinforced in the context of respect for and acceptance of patients' struggles and ambivalence. DBT principles can be disseminated to ancillary staff who work with patients and to families to promote positive and constructive means for understanding difficult behavior.

Although research is needed to determine if DBT confers benefits for chronic eating disorder patients over and above care as usual, our clinical experience suggests that DBT benefits patients and the staff who work with them.

REFERENCES

1. Paul T, Schroeter K, Dahme B, Nutzinger DO. Self-injurious behavior in women with eating disorders. Am J Psychiatry 2002; 159:408–411.
2. McCabe EB, Marcus MD. Is dialectical behavior therapy useful in the management of anorexia nervosa? Eat Disorders J Treat Prevent 2002; 10:335–337.
3. Linehan MM. Cognitive Behavioral Treatment of Borderline Personality Disorder. New York: Guilford Press, 1993.
4. Linehan MM. Skills Training Manual for Treating Borderline Personality Disorder. New York: Guilford Press, 1993.
5. Linehan MM, Armstrong HE, Suarez A, Allmon D, Heard HL. Cognitive-behavioral treatment of chronically parasuicidal borderline patients. Arch Gen Psychiatry 1991; 48:1060–1064.
6. Linehan MM, Heard HL, Armstrong HE. Naturalistic follow-up of a behavioral treatment for chronically parasuicidal borderline patients. Arch Gen Psychiatry 1993; 50:971–974.
7. Dimeff L, Rizvi SL, Brown M, Linehan MM. Dialectical behavior therapy for substance abuse: a pilot application to methamphetamine-dependent women with borderline personality disorder. Cogn Behav Prac 2000; 7:457–468.
8. Linehan MM, Schmidt H, Dimeff LA, Craft JC, Kanter J, Comtois KA. Dialectical behavior therapy for patients with borderline personality disorder and drug-dependence. Am J Addict 1999; 8:279–292.
9. Linehan MM, Dimeff LA, Reynolds SK, Comtois KA, Welch SS, Heagerty P, Kivlahan DR. Dialectical behavior therapy versus comprehensive validation therapy plus 12-step for the treatment of opioid dependent women meeting criteria for borderline personality disorder. Drug Alcohol Depend 2002; 67:13–26.
10. Telch CF, Agras WS, Linehan MM. Group dialectical behavior therapy for binge-eating disorder: a preliminary, uncontrolled trial. Behav Ther 2000; 31:569–582.
11. Telch CF, Agras WS, Linehan MM. Dialectical behavior therapy for binge eating disorder. J Consult Clin Psychol 2001; 69:1061–1065.
12. Wiser S, Telch CF. Dialectical behavior therapy for binge-eating disorder. J Clin Psychol 1999; 55:755–768.
13. Safer DL, Telch CF, Agras WS. Dialectical behavior therapy for bulimia nervosa. Am J Psychiatry 2001; 158:632–634.

21

Psychopharmacology of Anorexia Nervosa, Bulimia Nervosa, and Binge Eating Disorder

Joanna E. Steinglass and B. Timothy Walsh
New York State Psychiatric Institute, Columbia University
New York, New York, U.S.A.

As the fundamental causes of eating disorders remain unknown, it is no surprise that development of successful treatments has not come easily. Nonetheless, much progress has been made. The current mainstays of treatment of eating disorders are psychological interventions, including cognitive therapy, behavioral therapy, family therapy, and nutritional counseling (1). Clinicians have generally looked to medication to augment the effects of psychological intervention, or as a primary intervention when such treatment is unavailable or ineffective.

The role of psychopharmacology in eating disorders has been greatly clarified in the last decade. But, as in the case of other psychiatric disorders, the limited understanding of the basic pathophysiology handicaps the ability to design psychopharmacological treatments. In the absence of a specific biological model, a range of differing perspectives has prompted attempts to identify medication treatments for anorexia nervosa (AN), bulimia nervosa (BN), and binge eating disorder (BED). In general, studies of medications in AN have been disappointing. In contrast, in BN, antidepressants are clearly effective at reducing binge eating and purging behaviors. Studies of BED are at an earlier stage but have already yielded promising findings. A consistent observation across the eating disorders is the need for double-blind, placebo-controlled studies to assess efficacy, as a medication often looks promising in case studies or open trial but fails to show superiority to placebo in a rigorously controlled trial.

This chapter will review the current data on the use of medications in the management of AN, BN, and BED with the intention of providing the clinician with information needed to make decisions about pharmacological treatment. The data will be reviewed according to what has been shown to be useful on the basis of controlled trials. Each illness—and stage of illness in the case of AN—will be considered separately and different outcome measures will be discussed when available.

ANOREXIA NERVOSA

Anorexia nervosa is characterized by a relentless pursuit of thinness and fear of becoming fat: patients starve themselves to extremes of low weight, resulting in amenorrhea and risk of death. Treatment must target multiple aspects of the disorder as patients need to gain weight, extinguish eating-disordered behaviors, and alter cognitions that foster these behaviors. Current recommendations focus on a multidisciplinary approach to treatment, including psychotherapies with cognitive–behavioral components. Inpatient treatment for patients at very low weight focuses on behavioral interventions and nutritional counseling to encourage eating and weight gain in conjunction with beginning to challenge cognitive disturbances. Nonetheless, AN has been difficult to treat and has a high relapse rate. Thus medications are under investigation both to facilitate initial treatment and to prevent relapse.

Study of the management of AN lends itself to multiple possible outcome measures. The major initial concern is weight restoration, which can be readily assessed by the amount and the rate of weight gain. In the long term, rate of relapse is an important outcome, defined as significant weight loss or reemergence of restrictive or binge–purge behaviors. Interwoven through both phases of treatment (weight gain and relapse prevention) is the complex problem of body image dissatisfaction.

Many psychopharmacological interventions have been tried, beginning with the work of Dally and Sargant on antipsychotics in the 1960s. Due to the limited understanding of the biological basis of AN, medication trials have been driven by unproven theoretical models and/or by an interest in taking advantage of medication side effects. While anecdotal reports of successful treatments have been published, only a small number of randomized controlled trials have been conducted, and definitive psychopharmacological treatment has not been identified.

Antidepressants

Antidepressant treatment for AN is a reasonable notion given the common concomitant symptoms of anxiety and depression. Many patients with AN describe low mood, low energy, poor concentration, loss of interest, and social isolation. The ritualized behaviors around eating and the obsessive preoccupation with shape and weight can be conceptualized as on the spectrum of obsessive-compulsive disorder (OCD), a syndrome that is also responsive to antidepressant medication.

Controlled trials of several different medications to promote weight gain have been generally discouraging. Initial studies involved tricyclic antidepressants (TCAs), with the hope that the side effect of weight gain would add to the benefits of treating mood disturbance. There have been three randomized controlled trials of TCAs. In one, clomipramine was associated with a slower rate of weight gain than placebo despite increased appetite, and there were no long-term effects at 1 and 4 years (2). In a study of amitriptyline versus placebo, there was no significant difference in weight gain (3). A second study of amitriptyline, which also had a third arm in which subjects received the serotonin (5-HT) antagonist cyproheptadine, showed no major benefit of amitriptyline (4). TCAs are known to prolong the QTc interval, which is also affected by AN. These observations, coupled with concerns that TCAs in children and adolescents may be linked to sudden death (5), suggest that TCAs should be rarely used for patients with AN at low weight.

In light of their benign side effect profile and efficacy in many other disorders, selective serotonin reuptake inhibitors (SSRIs) would appear promising in the management of in AN. Initial anecdotal evidence that fluoxetine might be beneficial for weight gain and mood symptoms (6) was supported in an open trial (7). However, the single randomized placebo-controlled trial of fluoxetine did not support these results. Attia et al. (8) conducted this trial of 33 patients with AN at low weight. All patients received inpatient care in addition to either fluoxetime (60 mg/day) or placebo for 7 weeks or until they reached 90% of ideal body weight and maintained it for a week. Fluoxetine conferred no benefit on weight gain, irrespective of subtype (restricting versus binge–purge). This finding is consistent with an open trial of Strober et al. (9) who administered fluoxetine to 33 inpatients.

While the studies of medication treatment in the acute phase focused on weight gain, some studies also included measures of other dimensions of AN. Mood symptoms have been found to improve with weight gain, with no added benefit from medication (8,34). The open trial of Strober et al. described above (9) examined severity of weight phobia and abnormal eating behaviors and found no evidence that fluoxetine treatment was of benefit. Attia and colleagues (8) assessed the effect of medication on body image dissatisfaction, a core component of AN, and noted significant improvement with weight gain in scores on Body Satisfaction Questionnaire (BSQ) in both placebo and fluoxetine groups, although not to within the normal range in either group.

Somewhat more promising results have been found in the relapse prevention phase, but there is just one randomized controlled trial. Thirty-five women with AN, restricting subtype, entered a double-blind, randomized, controlled trial after inpatient weight restoration and received either fluoxetine (10–60 mg/day) or placebo for 11 months (10). Subjects receiving medication were significantly more likely than those who received placebo to maintain near-normal weight for one year. Interpretation of data from the randomized trial is limited in that dosage of fluoxetine was not controlled for, nor was additional treatment (i.e., psychotherapy) restricted. Subjects were limited to those with restricting subtype, and there is no information on the effect of medication on parameters other than weight. In addition, a naturalistic study of Strober et al. (11) comparing relapse among patients receiving open fluoxetine treatment to relapse among a group of matched, historical controls failed to detect evidence of a benefit from fluoxetine. Nonetheless, the study of Kaye et al. (10) is virtually the only placebo-controlled examination of medication in AN that found a statistically and clinically significant impact of medication compared to placebo. Further study is needed to determine replicate and extend this finding.

In summary, there is little reason to think that antidepressants add substantially to the standard inpatient management of AN. Given the widespread benefits of antidepressant medication in other, seemingly related psychiatric disorders, the lack of impact of antidepressants is surprising. Kaye et al. (12) have shown that patients at low weight have low levels of 5-hydroxyindole-acetic acid (5-HIAA), the major metabolite of serotonin, which improve with weight gain. Low levels of 5-HIAA suggest that patients have low levels of brain serotonin, which is consistent with the finding that dieting in non-eating-disordered women reduces tryptophan levels (the amino acid that is the substrate for serotonin) and reduces serotonin production (13). Thus, it may be that antidepressants are ineffective at low weight because they have insufficient substrate (14). This is supported by the finding that tryptophan depletion has been shown to reverse the effects of SSRIs in depressed patients (13).

Notably, virtually all studies of patients at low weight have been conducted in an inpatient setting, where nonpharmacological interventions are effective in producing weight gain. At least theoretically, there is potential for benefit from medication in an outpatient setting, where weight gain tends to be slower.

Antipsychotics

Pharmacological treatment in AN began with antipsychotics. The theoretical rationale for the use of this class of medication derives from the near-delusional quality of beliefs about shape and weight held by some patients with AN. Dally and Sargant (15) studied chlorpromazine (1600 mg/day) and found that while the rate of weight gain was enhanced compared to historical controls, there were significant negative effects including seizures and the emergence of binge–purge behavior. Furthermore, benefits were not sustained over long-term follow-up. Pimozide was studied subsequently in a randomized, controlled trial of hospitalized patients (16). The authors found a trend toward slightly higher daily weights while on pimozide, but effects on psychological symptoms were inconsistent. In a study of sulpiride among hospitalized patients receiving either medication or placebo for 3 weeks, there was no significant effect of medication on weight gain (17). Due to the known long-term side effects of the older antipsychotics and the side effects noted in some of the early studies, these medications are not generally recommended for management of AN.

    With the advent of the new generation of antipsychotics, which have a lower incidence of tardive dyskinisia, extrapyramidal symptoms, and decreased likelihood of seizures, the possible usefulness of this class of medications has again been raised. Olanzapine would appear particularly promising as the prominent side effect of weight gain might be advantageous in AN. There have been several case reports of the use of olanzapine (5–10 mg/ day) comprising about 10 hospitalized patients who had been refractory to other treatments (18–20). The patients described in these reports held near-delusional beliefs about their bodies, with no other psychotic symptoms. Mehler et al. (20) reported that while there was no dramatic improvement in the rate of weight gain after initiation of medication, there was a marked improvement in patient's cognitive style. One patient with a history of restricting developed binge–purge behavior while taking olanzapine (19). Olanzapine is a potentially promising intervention for AN, but its efficacy has not yet been established. In light of the research on antidepressants, where promising case reports and open studies were not born out in randomized controlled trials, further study of olanzapine and other second-generation antipsychotics is needed before definitive conclusions can be drawn. In addition, an important clinical consideration is whether patients will agree to a medication so clearly associated with weight gain.

Other Agents

A number of other medication classes have been tried, targeting primarily the weight gain phase of AN. Cyproheptadine, an antihistaminic agent that acts centrally to decrease serotonin activity, has been studied in several controlled trials after it was noted to cause weight gain in other conditions. Results have been mixed. In the first placebo-controlled trial (21), cyproheptadine did not improve weight gain. A second study found that cyproheptadine was associated with improved weight gain in a subgroup of severely ill patients (22). In a trial comparing amitriptyline, cyproheptadine, and placebo (mentioned above) (4), the authors noted no significant weight gain in the cyproheptadine group. However, they did note a difference between subtypes such that individuals with the restricting subtype showed an increased rate of weight gain with cyproheptadine whereas individuals with the binge–purge subtype showed an increased rate of weight gain with amitriptyline.

Consistent with patients' complaints about feelings of fullness and early satiety, patients with AN have been found to have slowed gastric emptying (23). Open trials of motility agents have been conducted using metoclopramide, bethanacol, cisapride, and domperidone (14). Few agents have been subjected to randomized controlled trials. Metaclopramide was found to decrease gastric emptying time (24), but a randomized controlled trial could not be completed because of the emergence of depression likely related to the CNS effects of the drug (25). Cisapride is a motility agent with mixed agonist/antagonist properties. It is an antagonist at the serotonin 5-HT$_3$ receptor and an agonist at the 5-HT$_4$ receptor. Cisapride was shown to improve gastric emptying time in a small, randomized, placebo-controlled study ($N = 12$) (26), but improvements in weight gain were not noted . In a larger study, Szmukler et al. (27) described improvement in gastrointestinal symptoms but no difference between medication and placebo groups with respect to gastric emptying or weight gain. Thus, the clinical benefits of cisapride in AN are uncertain. Furthermore, it was recently withdrawn from the market in the United States due to cardiac conduction effects, including prolonged QT interval and reports of sudden death.

Patients often describe their eating disorder symptoms as overwhelmingly strong urges to eat or to diet in a manner that bears some similarity to descriptions of drug cravings. Several studies have been conducted to examine the potential utility of opiate antagonists. Open trials of intravenous naloxone and oral naltrexone in underweight patients suggested improved weight gain (28). One placebo-controlled trial of naltrexone (200 mg daily) using a crossover design was conducted in patients with AN and BN (29). While the authors did not report results on weight gain in AN, they found that binge eating and purging rates diminished.

Zinc deficiency has notable similarities to AN. It is associated with weight loss, dysphoria, appetite and taste changes, and amenorrhea. Zinc deficiencies have been noted in low-weight AN populations (30), an unsurprising finding given the level of overall malnutrition. In contrast to most studies of AN, a number of the studies of zinc supplementation were conducted in children and adolescents. Three randomized controlled trials (30–32) and one open trial (33) of zinc supplementation (50–100 mg elemental zinc/day) have been reported. In a randomized controlled trial in children (31), there was no significant weight effect in the zinc-treated group. In adolescents, Katz et al. (30) found improvement in depression and anxiety in the adolescents who received zinc, but no effect on weight gain. In contrast, Birmingham et al. (32) found that zinc supplementation was associated with an increased rate of weight gain, even without evidence of zinc deficiency. In light of these mixed results, the utility of zinc supplementation is uncertain.

Other novel approaches to improving weight gain have included lithium, for its weight gain and mood stabilizing properties, and tetrahydrocannabinol (THC) for its appetite-enhancing effect. Lithium was associated with a small weight increase in one small, short-duration placebo-controlled trial (34). THC was compared to diazepam in a small randomized, double-blind trial using a crossover design (35). There was no benefit from THC with respect to food intake or weight gain, and THC was associated with significant side effects, including paranoia, sleep disturbance, and interpersonal sensitivity.

A major medical complication of AN is osteoporosis/osteopenia. Estrogen replacement therapy has been used to treat osteoporosis in postmenopausal women and therefore has been explored as an adjunctive treatment in AN. However, a randomized controlled trial assessing the bone densities of subjects receiving estrogen and progestin versus no medication found no significant changes in the hormone-treated group (36). Those patients who resumed menses showed improvement in bone density. These data suggest that, at present, the best documented intervention to arrest bone loss in AN is weight gain sufficient to restore regular menstruation.

BULIMIA NERVOSA

Bulimia nervosa is characterized by recurrent binge eating followed by inappropriate compensatory behaviors, such as vomiting. Because in DSM-IV, AN has diagnostic precedence over BN, patients with AN who meet criteria for BN are considered as having the binge–purge subtype of AN. Thus, most patients with BN are of normal weight. Like patients with AN, those with BN have a disturbance of body image and unduly value their shape and weight when evaluating their self-esteem. Bulimia nervosa is more common than AN, with a prevalence of 1–5% in adolescent and young adult women (37). BN tends to be managed in the outpatient setting, making clinical trials less complicated and costly than with AN and, presumably for these reasons, more numerous. In addition, studies of medications in the management of BN have yielded more promising results, most notably with antidepressants.

Antidepressants

The study of antidepressant medications resulted from the observation that patients with BN, like those with AN, often describe depressive symptoms. Over the past 20 years, many antidepressants have been found to be more effective than placebo in reducing binge–purge episodes in normal-weight women with BN (38,39). While TCAs (40–45), monoamine oxidase inhibitors (46–48) and SSRIs (49–51) have all been shown to be effective, there are no direct comparisons to suggest superiority of one drug over another. SSRIs have come into favor due to their overall acceptable side-effect profile. Open trials of sertraline (52) and fluvoxamine (53,54) have reported good results, but only fluoxetine, at a dose of 60 mg daily, has been shown to be effective in randomized, controlled trials (49,50). Antidepressants consistently decrease eating-disordered behaviors and improve mood in patients with BN, regardless of the presence of major depressive episode (49). In addition, two randomized controlled trials have suggested efficacy of SSRIs in prevention of relapse (55,56).

While studies of antidepressants have generally been favorable, the study of bupropion must be mentioned for its significant side effects. In this trial of 55 women with BN (57), bupropion (up to 450 mg/day) was effective at reducing binge–purge behavior. The study was terminated prematurely, however, because four women experienced grand mal seizures. Because of this association, bupropion is specifically not recommended in management of BN, and the package insert indicates that bupropion is contraindicated in the treatment of patients with a current or past diagnosis of BN or AN.

The clinical significance of the difference between antidepressant medication and placebo is complicated by the broad range of effect between studies. The improvement in binge frequency reported in controlled trials ranges from 31% to 91% decrease (58,59). Remission rate (cessation of binge–purge behavior) was often not reported and when reported, ranged from 4% to 34% (58). The improvement in BN with antidepressant medication is clear, but the low remission rate suggests that there are limitations to this treatment.

Medication trials have generally focused on binge–purge behaviors as the primary outcome, but a few studies have also assessed body image dissatisfaction. Most use the BSQ or the Eating Disorders Inventory Body Dissatisfaction Scale (EDI-BD), which are self-report measures that address how patients feel about body parts or their whole body. While these measures do not address all of the dimensions of body dissatisfaction, they may serve as a crude measure of this important variable. Interestingly, some, (45,49) but not all, (60–62) studies suggest that it is possible to see change in body dissatisfaction with medication treatment alone. Thus, the impact of antidepressants on body dissatisfaction remains unclear.

Overall, the use of antidepressant medications in the management of BN is well supported but there remain some gaps in the knowledge base. The current data are mostly derived from short-term studies that range from 6 to 8 weeks duration. Most trials have been conducted with normal weight women who use self-induced vomiting to purge. Thus, it is unknown if these results can be generalized to apply to other patients, such as men, adolescents, and those who compensate for binge eating through other behaviors, e.g., excessive exercise. Areas for further study include the optimal duration of treatment and the long-term efficacy of antidepressants.

Anticonvulsants

An early clinical model conceptualized BN as a seizure disorder, with binge–purge episodes thought to represent paroxysmal events. Small trials with the anticonvulsants phenytoin (63) and carbamazepine (64) did not suggest a robust response to medication. A recent case report (65) of a woman with epilepsy and BN who was treated with topiramate and showed improvement in binge–purge behaviors and in attitude about shape and weight raised the possibility that topiramate may have benefit in the management of BN. Results from a randomized, double-blind, placebo-controlled trial of topiramate (25–400 mg/day) have been presented, showing reduction in binge and purge duration and frequency (66). Although preliminary, these results are encouraging.

Other Agents

Some agents have been studied based on biological models, as opposed to clinical models, of BN. These models have focused mainly on the potential role of serotonin, which has been shown to impact various aspects of feeding. As increased serotonergic function tends to decrease food intake, it was hypothesized that medications that increase serotonin would decrease binge eating behavior (67). L-Tryptophan, the amino acid precursor of serotonin, was examined in a randomized, placebo-controlled trial ($N = 13$), but no drug–placebo difference was detected (68). Fenfluramine, a serotonergic agent that both blocks reuptake and increases release, was studied with mixed results. In a randomized, placebo-controlled trial using a crossover design, fenfluramine was shown to decrease binge–purge frequency (69). However, in two subsequent placebo-controlled trials, the medication showed no benefit (70,71). Fenfluramine was withdrawn from the market in 1997 due to an association with cardiac valve abnormalities.

Another model for treatment of BN focuses on the feeding behaviors of patients, specifically their difficulty in identifying satiety. This model postulates that binge eating and purging might lead to desensitization of the vagal nerve afferents, which have a key role in signaling satiety. Subjects with BN were found to have an increased somatosensory pain threshold, which may indirectly reflect altered vagal nerve activity (72). Based on these observations, Faris and colleagues (73) conducted a 4-week randomized, placebo-controlled trial in BN and found that ondansetron (24 mg/day), a medication that blocks $5-HT_3$ receptors involved in visceral stimulation of the vagal nerve, was associated with a significant decrease in binge–purge behaviors.

One clinical model of BN focused on the similarities between binge–purge behaviors and addictive behaviors, drawing on the evidence that endogenous opiates may be involved in appetite changes. In a small, open trial of naltrexone, an opiate antagonist, 7 of 10 patients with BN improved with complete or partial remission (74). One randomized, controlled trial including AN and BN patients found a decrease in binge–purge behaviors with naltrexone (100–200 mg/day) (29), whereas a randomized, controlled trial using a lower dose (50 mg/day) showed no benefit (75).

Lithium has also been studied. Hsu et al. (60) conducted a randomized, placebo-controlled, 8-week trial of lithium (mean lithium level = 0.62) in patients with BN. Both placebo and medication groups improved, and there was no significant difference between the groups.

Combination Treatment

While the above data clearly support the efficacy of antidepressants in BN, controlled trials have also shown the efficacy of psychotherapy alone (see Chapters 17, 19, and 20). Seven randomized controlled trials have, in different ways, compared treatments in an attempt to assess the benefits of psychotherapy versus pharmacotherapy versus a combination of the two. Overall, the studies suggest that cognitive–behavioral therapy (CBT) alone is probably more effective in reducing binge eating and purging behaviors, but that the addition of medication provides some additional benefit.

The first study, conducted by Mitchell and colleagues (62), randomized subjects to one of four treatment arms for 10 weeks: imipramine alone, placebo alone, intensive group therapy alone, or imipramine with intensive group therapy. The psychotherapy intervention provided was an unusually intensive group therapy, which included joint meals with the therapist on five occasions during the first week of treatment. Outcome measures assessed eating behaviors, affective symptoms, and attitudinal measures. The reduction in eating-disordered behaviors in response to intensive group therapy was impressive, and no added benefit from imipramine could be detected. On the other hand, combination treatment significantly improved affective symptoms more than either treatment alone. In a follow-up study, Keel et al. (76) found that 10 years posttreatment, all three active treatment groups showed significant improvement in social functioning as compared with placebo. There were no significant differences on measures of depression, body image, or eating disorder behavior.

A study of the combination of individual CBT with desipramine reached broadly similar conclusions. Agras and colleagues (77) randomly assigned patients to one of five treatment arms: desipramine for 16 weeks, desipramine for 24 weeks, CBT only for 16 weeks, CBT and desipramine for 16 weeks, and CBT for 16 weeks and desipramine for 24 weeks. Response to CBT was clearly superior to that for desipramine alone. There were some indications that patients receiving CBT combined with 24 weeks of desipramine had the best outcome, but these results were not statistically robust.

The finding of Mitchell et al. (62) that medication may add to the benefits of psychological treatment was also noted in a study by our own group (78). Patients were randomly assigned to one of five treatment arms for 16 weeks: medication alone, CBT and medication, CBT and placebo, supportive psychotherapy (SPT) and medication, SPT and placebo. The design allowed for a change in medication from the TCA desipramine to the SSRI fluoxetine under double-blind conditions. Patients assigned to receive active medication were given desipramine, but if response was not satisfactory or if significant side effects developed, patients were switched to fluoxetine. It was clear that CBT was more effective than SPT in reducing disturbed eating behaviors. In addition, active medication augmented the improvement in both behavioral and attitudinal measures associated with psychological treatment.

Goldbloom et al. (79) conducted a study of combination treatment with three treatment arms: fluoxetine alone, CBT alone, and fluoxetine and CBT combined. This study was limited by a significant dropout rate (43%), which contributed to an inability to detect statistically significant differences between treatments on most measures. There was a significant difference in subjective reports of binge episodes, which were most improved with combination treatment.

In another study of fluoxetine, medication or placebo was combined with 8 weeks of nutritional counseling (80). The nutritional intervention had components similar to CBT, but with a psychoeducational focus replacing cognitive restructuring. While the authors report on this as an assessment of combined treatment, the psychotherapy intervention is sufficiently different from CBT that it is difficult to compare findings. Nonetheless, there was a rapid and significant improvement in both groups in binge eating and purging. There were few differences between fluoxetine and placebo groups, but some indications that fluoxetine augmented improvement in some psychological spheres, such as concerns with shape and weight. Bacaltchuk et al. (81) performed a meta-analysis of the studies of psychotherapy plus pharmacotherapy in BN. While their conclusions are subject to the usual limitations of meta-analyses, in the short term remission was more likely with combination of medication and psychotherapy than with either treatment alone.

Conclusions drawn from the above studies must be considered with caution. One major problem is that the largest studies were conducted before the widespread use of SSRIs, making it difficult to extrapolate from these data to current clinical practice. The limited information available suggests that CBT is likely to be more effective and more acceptable to patients than is a course of antidepressant medication. However, the data are reasonably consistent in indicating that the addition of an antidepressant to psychotherapy modestly augments improvement in psychological symptoms and, perhaps, in disturbance of eating behavior. The effectiveness of medication in reducing relapse is uncertain.

BINGE EATING DISORDER

The more recently recognized syndrome of binge eating disorder is characterized by episodes of binge eating without compensatory behaviors. Although not required for the diagnosis, BED is usually associated with obesity. As is the case with AN and BN, several clinical features of BED can be appropriately viewed as outcome measures. The ideal intervention would reduce the binge eating behavior, improve psychological disturbances such as depression and overconcern with body image, and promote weight loss. To date, most treatment studies have focused on the behavioral and psychological components, leaving weight loss as a secondary goal. As this disorder is relatively newly codified in the DSM-IV, only a small number of controlled medication studies have been published.

Antidepressants

Based on the efficacy of antidepressants in the management of BN and the similarities between these two disorders, most research has focused on antidepressants. An early placebo-controlled trial of "nonpurging BN" found that desipramine was effective in the short-term reduction of binge eating (82). However, symptoms reemerged 4 weeks after medication discontinuation. A randomized, controlled trial has also shown imipramine to be effective (83). More recently, two studies have found benefits from SSRIs. In one randomized controlled trial of fluvoxamine (50–300 mg/day) (84) and one randomized controlled trial of sertraline (50–200 mg/day) (85), the authors reported a significant reduction in binge eating behavior as well as a decrease in BMI in the medication groups as compared with placebo. As with most of the medication trials in eating disorders, these short-term results do not provide information as to sustained benefit of medications.

Other Agents

As with AN and BN, a number of other classes of medication have received some attention as being of possible use in the management of BED. Topiramate is the latest to show promise. In one open label-study of 13 patients with BED, topiramate was associated with weight loss (86). Appolinario et al. (87) reported a case study of a patient who responded to topiramate after other treatments had been unsuccessful. McElroy et al. (88) conducted a placebo-controlled, double-blind trial of topiramate in 61 patients with BED. Topiramate-treated subjects showed significantly greater reductions in binge frequency, binge day frequency, and other measures of symptom severity, as well as significant reduction in BMI.

Trials of dexfenfluramine yielded some promising results. Dexfenfluramine was associated with a decrease in binge eating, and when used in combination with phentermine, with weight loss, as well (89,90). However, dexfenfluramine has since been withdrawn from the market due to its association with cardiac valve abnormalities. An open trial of sibutramine, an appetite suppressant approved for the management of obesity, suggested that use of this agent was associated with improvement in both binge eating and weight loss (91). A controlled trial has been conducted, but results are not yet available. The opiate antagonist naltrexone was studied in a randomized placebo-controlled trial which also included an imipramine arm (89). While both medication groups showed improvement, there was no difference from placebo.

Combination Treatment

Antidepressant medications appear to provide short-term benefit in the management of BED, but the benefits do not appear to be sustained beyond the discontinuation of the medication. Several studies have examined the benefits of combined treatment, but, at present, the data are insufficient to support clear conclusions (83,92–95).

CONCLUSIONS AND TREATMENT RECOMMENDATIONS

Anorexia Nervosa

Psychopharmacological interventions have not been shown to provide significant benefit to underweight patients with AN. The mainstays of treatment are nonpharmacological, and focus on nutritional rehabilitation and relapse prevention. There is preliminary evidence that fluoxetine may be of benefit for relapse prevention after patients have regained to a normal or near-normal weight.

Bulimia Nervosa

The data on the use of antidepressants in the treatment of BN are convincing in indicating that that fluoxetine is safe and beneficial. While it is likely that other SSRIs would be effective, only fluoxetine has been examined in placebo-controlled trials, and should be used in a dose of 60 mg/day. Most patients can be rapidly titrated to this dose over the course of a week. There are no available data to guide treatment for relapse prevention or to suggest recommended length of treatment. Bupropion is not recommended in the management of BN because of the risk of seizure. There are consistent indications that medications modestly enhance the benefits of psychological treatment.

Binge Eating Disorder

While emerging data suggest that SSRIs and, perhaps, antiobesity agents may provide some benefits, at present there is insufficient information to make firm treatment recommendations regarding the use of medication for BED.

REFERENCES

1. American Psychiatric Association. Practice guidelines for the treatment of patients with eating disorders (Revision). Am J Psychiatry (Supplement) 2000; 157(1):1–39.
2. Lacey J, Crisp AH. Hunger, food intake and weight: the impact of clomipramine on a refeeding anorexia nervosa population. Postgrad J Med 1980; 56(suppl 1): 79–95.
3. Biederman J, Herzog D, Rivinus T, et al. Amitriptyline in the treatment of anorexia nervosa: a double-blind, placebo-controlled study. J Clin Psychopharmacol 1985; 5, 10–16.
4. Halmi K, Eckert E, LaDu T, Cohen J. Anorexia nervosa: treatment efficacy of cyproheptadine and amitriptyline. Arch Gen Psychiatry 1986; 43:177–181.

5. Wilens T, Biederman J, Baldessarini R, et al. Cardiovascular effects of therapeutic doses of tricyclic antidepressants in children and adolescents. J Am Acad Child Adolesc Psychiatry 1996; 35:1491–1501.

6. Ferguson J. Treatment of an anorexia nervosa patient with flouxetine. Am J Psychiatry 1987; 144:1239.

7. Gwirtsman H, Guze B, Yager J, Gainsley B. Fluoxetine treatment of anorexia nervosa: an open clinical trial. J Clin Psychiatry 1990; 51:1378–1382.

8. Attia E, Haiman C, Walsh T, Flater S. Does fluoxetine augment the inpatient treatment of anorexia nervosa? Am J Psychiatry April 1998; 155(4):548–551.

9. Strober M, Pataki C, Freeman R, DeAntonio M. No effect of adjunctive fluoxetine on eating behavior or weight phobia during the inpatient treatment of anorexia nervosa: an historical case-control study. J Child Adol Psychopharmacol 1999; 9(3):195–201.

10. Kaye W, Nagata T, Weltzin T, et al. Double-blind placebo-controlled administration of fluoxetine in restricting and restricting-purging-type anorexia nervosa. Biol Psychiatry 2001; 49:644–652.

11. Strober M, Freeman R, DeAntonio M, Lampert C, Diamond J. Does adjunctive fluoxetine influence the post-hospital course of anorexia nervosa? A 24-month prospective, longitudinal follow-up and comparison with historical controls. Psychopharmacol Bull 1997; 33:425–431.

12. Kaye W, Ebert M, Raleigh Mea. Abnormalities in CNS monoamine metabolism in anorexia nervosa. Arch Gen Psychiatry 1984; 41:350–355.

13. Kaye W, Gendall K, Strober M. Serotonin neuronal function and selective serotonin reuptake inhibitor treatment in anorexia and bulimia nervosa. Biol Psychiatry 1998; 44:825–838.

14. Attia E, Mayer L, Killory E. Medication response in the treatment of patients with anorexia nervosa. J Psychiat Pract 2001; 7:157–162.

15. Dally P, Sargant W. A new treatment of anorexia nervosa. British Medical Journal 1960; 1:1770–1773.

16. Vandereycken W, Pierloot R. Pimozide combined with behavior therapy in the short term treatment of anorexia nervosa. Acta Psychiatr Scand 1982; 66:445–450.

17. Vandereycken W. Neuroleptics in the short-term treatment of anoreixia nervosa: a double-blind placebo-controlled study with sulpiride. Br J Psychiatry 1984; 144:288–292.

18. Jensen V, Mejlhede A. Anorexia nervosa: treatment with olanzapine. Br J Psychiatry July 2000; 177:87.

19. La Via M, Gray N, Kaye W. Case reports of olanzapine treatment of anorexia nervosa. Intl J Eat Disord 2000; 27:363–366.

20. Mehler C, Wewetzer C, Schulze U, Warnke A, Theisen F, Dittmann R. Olanzapine in children and adolescents with chronic anorexia nervosa: a study of five cases. Eur Child Adol Psychiatry 2001; 10:151–157.

21. Vigersky R, Loriaux D. The effect of cyproheptadine in anorexia nervosa: a double-blind trial. In: Vigersky R, ed. Anorexia Nervosa. New York: Raven Press, 1977:349–356.

22. Goldberg S, Halmi K, Eckert E, Casper R, Dacis J. Cyproheptadine in anorexia nervosa. Br J Psychiatry 1979; 134:67–70.
23. Stacher G, Kiss A, Wiesnagrotzki S, et al. Oesophageal and gastric motility disorders in patients categorized as having primary anorexia nervosa. Gut 1986; 27:1120–1126.
24. Domstad P, Shis W, Humphries L, DeLand F, Digenis G. Radionuclide gastric emptying studies in patients with anorexia nervosa. J Nucl Med 1987; 28:816–819.
25. Modolsfsky H, Jeuniewic N. Preliminary report of metoclopramine in anorexia nervosa. In: Vigersky R, ed. Anorexia Nervosa. New York: Raven Press, 1977: 373–375.
26. Stacher G, Abatzi-Wenzel T, Wiesnagrotzki S, Bergmann H, Schneider C, Gaupmann G. Gastric emptying, body weight and symptoms in primary anorexia nervosa: long term effects of cisapride. Br J Psychiatry 1993; 162:398–402.
27. Szmukler G, Young G, Miller G, Lichtenstein M, Binns D. A controlled trial of cisapride in anorexia nervosa. Int J Eat Disord 1995; 17:345–357.
28. Kaye W. Opioid antagonist drugs in the treatment of anorexia nervosa. In: Garfinkel P, Garner D, eds. The Role of Drug Treatments for Eating Disorders. New York: Brunner/Mazel, 1987:150–160.
29. Marrazi M, Bacon J, Kinzie J, et al. Naltrexone use in the treatment of anorexia nervosa and bulimia nervosa. Int J Clin Psychopharmacol 1995; 10:163–172.
30. Katz R, Keen C, Litt I, Hurley L, Kellams-Harrison K, Glader L. Zinc deficiency in anorexia nervosa. J Adol Health Care 1987; 8:400–406.
31. Lask B, Fosson A, Rolfe U, Thomas S. Zinc deficiency and childhood-onset anorexia nervosa. J Clin Psychiatry 1993; 54:63–66.
32. Birmingham C, Goldner E, Bakan R. Controlled trial of zinc supplementaion in anorexia nervosa. Int J Eat Disord 1994; 15:251–255.
33. Safai-Kutti S. Oral zinc supplementation in anorexia nervosa. Acta Psychiatr Scand 1990; 361:S14–S17.
34. Gross H, Ebert M, Faden V, Goldberg S, Nee L, Kaye W. A double-blind controlled trial of lithium carbonate in primary anorexia nervosa. J Clin Psychopharmacol 1981; 1:376–381.
35. Gross H, Ebert M, Faden V, et al. A double-blind trial of delta9-tetrahydrocannacinol in primary anorexia nervosa. J Clin Psychopharmacol 1983; 3:165–171.
36. Kiblanski A, Biller B, Schoenfeld D, Herzog D, Saxe V. The effects of estrogen administration on trabecular bone loss in young women with anorexia nervosa. J Clin Endocrinol Metab 1995; 80:898–904.
37. Kotler L, Devlin M, Walsh BT. Eating disorders and related disturbances. 2002; 410–430.
38. Walsh B, Devlin M. The pharmacologic treatment of eating disorders. Psychiatr Clin North Am 1992; 15:149–160.
39. Mitchell J, Raymond N, Specke S. A review of the controlled trials of pharmacotherapy and psychotherapy in the treatment of bulimia nervosa. Int J Eat Disord 1993; 14:229–247.

40. Agras W, Dorian B, Kirkley B, et al. Imipramine in the treatment of bulimia: a double-blind controlled study. Int J Eat Disord 1987; 6:29–38.
41. Barlow J, Bloluin J, Blouin A, Perez E. Treatment of bulimia with desipramine: a double-blind crossover study. Can J Psychiatry 1988; 33:129–133.
42. Hughes P, Wells L, Cunningham C, et al. Treating bulimia with desipramine: a double-blind, placebo-controlled trial. Arch Gen Psychiatry 1986; 43:182–186.
43. Mitchell J, Groat R. A placebo-controlled, double-blind trial of amitriptyline in bulimia. J Clin Psychopharmacol 1984; 4:186–193.
44. Pope HJ, Hudson J, Jonas Jea. Bulimia treated with imipramine: a placebo-controlled, double-blind study. Am J Psychiatry 1983; 140:554–558.
45. Walsh B, Hadigan C, Devlin M, Gladis M, Roose S. Long-term outcome of antidepressant treatment for bulimia nervosa. Am J Psychiatry 1991; 148:1206–1212.
46. Kennedy S, Piran N, Warsh J, et al. A trial of isocarbozacid in the treatment of bulimia nervosa. J Clin Psychopharmacol 1988; 8:391–396.
47. Walsh B, Stewart J, Roose S, Gladis M, Glassman A. Treatment of bulimia with phenelzine: a double-blind placcbo controlled study. Arch Gen Psychiatry 1984; 41:1105–1109.
48. Walsh B, Gladis M, Roose Sea. Phenelzine vs placebo in 50 patients with bulimia. Arch Gen Psychiatry 1988; 45:471–475.
49. Fluoxetine Bulima Nervosa Collaborative (FBNC) Study Group. Fluoxetine in the treatment of bulimia nervosa: a multi-center, double-blind, placebo-controlled trial. Arch Gen Psychiatry 1992; 49:139–147.
50. Goldstein D, Wilson M, Thompson Vea. Fluoxetine Bulimia Nervosa Collaborative Study Group. Long term fluoxetine treatment of bulimia nervosa. Br J Psychiatry 1995; 166:660–666.
51. Pope HJ, Keck PE Jr, McElroy S, et al. A placebo-controlled study of trazodone in bulimia nervosa. J Clin Psychopharmacol 1989; 9:159–254.
52. Roberts J, Lydiard R. Sertraline in the treament of bulimia nervosa [letter]. Am J Psychiatry 1993; 150:1753.
53. Ayuso-Guttierrez J, Palazon M, Ayuso-Mateos J. Open trial of fluvoxamine in the treatment of bulimia nervosa. Int J Eat Disord 1994; 15:245–249.
54. Spigset O, Pleym H. Case report of successful treatment of bulimia nervosa with fluvoxamine [letter]. Pharmacopsychiatry 1991; 24:180.
55. Fichter M, Kruger R, Rief W, Hollan R, Dohne J. Fluvoxamine in prevention of relapse in bulimia nervosa: effects of eating specific psychophathology. J Clin Psychopharmacol 1996; 16:9–18.
56. Romano S, Halmi K, Sarkar N, Koke S, Lee J. A placebo-controlled study of fluoxetine in continued treatment of bulimia nervosa after successful acute fluoxetine treatment. Am J Psychiatry 2002; 159:96–102.
57. Horne R, Ferguson J, Pope HJ, et al. Treatment of bulimia with buproprion: a multicenter controlled trial. J Clin Psychiatry 1988; 49:262–266.
58. Walsh B. Psychopharmacologic treatment of bulimia nervosa. J Clin Psychiatry 1991; 52(10, suppl):34–48.

59. Bacaltchuk J, Hay P, Mari J. Antidepressants versus placebo for the treatment of bulimia nervosa: a systematic review. Aust N Z J Psychiatry 2000; 34:310–317.

60. Hsu L, Clement L, Santhuse R, Ju E. Treatment of bulimia nervosa with lithium carbonate, a controlled study. J Nerv Ment Dis 1991; 179:351–355.

61. Leitenberg H, Rosen J, Wolf J, Vara L, Detzwwer M, Srebnik D. Comparison of cognitive-behavior therapy and desipramine in the treatment of bulimia nervosa. Behav Res Ther 1994; 32:37–45.

62. Mitchell J, Pyle R, Hatsukami D, Pomeroy C, Zimmerman R. A comparison study of antidepressants and structured group therapy in the treatment of bulimia nervosa. Arch Gen Psychiatry 1990; 47:149–157.

63. Wermuth B, Davis K, Hollister L, Stunkard A. Phenytoin treatment of the binge-eating syndrome. Am J Psychiatry 1977; 134:1249–1253.

64. Kaplan A, Garfinkel P, Darby P, Garner D. Carbamazepine in the treatment of bulimia. Am J Psychiatry 1983; 140:1225–1226.

65. Knable M. Topiramate for bulimia nervosa in epilepsy. Am J Psychiatry 2001; 158:322–323.

66. Hoopes S, Reimherr F, Kamin M, Karvois D, Rosenthal N, Karim R. Topiramate treatment of bulimia nervosa. Scientific and Clinical Report Session 2: Eating Disorders. Philadelphia, PA: American Psychiatric Association, May 2002 (Annual meeting).

67. Liebowitz S. The role of serotonin in eating disorders. Drugs 1990; 39(suppl 3): 33–48.

68. Krahn D, Mitchell J. Use of L-tryptophan in treating bulimia (letter). Am J Psychiatry 1985; 142, 1130.

69. Blouin A, Blouin J, Bushnik T, Zuro C, Mulder E. Treatment of bulimia with fenfluramine and desipramine. J Clin Psychopharmacol 1988; 8:261–269.

70. Fahy T, Eisler I, Russell G. A placebo-controlled trial of d-fenfluramine in bulimia nervosa. Br J Psychiatry 1993; 162:597–603.

71. Russel G, Checkley S, Feldman J, Eisler I. A controlled trial of d-fenfluramine in bulimia nervosa. Clin Neuropharmacol 1988; 11:S146–S159.

72. Faris P, Kim S, Meller W, et al. Effect of ondansetron, a 5-HT$_3$ receptor antagonist, on the dynamic association between bulimic behaviors and pain thresholds. Pain 1998; 77:297–303.

73. Faris P, Kim S, Meller W, et al. Effect of decreasing afferent vagal activity with ondansetron on symptoms of bulimia nervosa: a randomised, double-blind trial. Lancet 2000; 355:792–797.

74. Jonas J, Gold M. Treatment of antidepressant-resistant bulimia with naltrexone. In J Psychiatry Med 1987; 16:305–309.

75. Mitchell J, Christenson G, Jennings J, et al. A placebo-controlled, double-blind crossover study of naltrexone hydrochloride in outpatients with normal-weight bulimia. J Clin Psychopharmacol 1989; 9:94–97.

76. Keel PK, Mitchell J, Davis T, Crow S. Long-term impact of treatment in women diagnosed with bulimia nervosa. Int J Eat Disord 2000; 31:151–158.

77. Agras W, Arnow B, Schneider J, et al. Pharmacologic and cognitive-behavioral

treatment for bulimia nervosa: a controlled comparison. Am J Psychiatry 1992; 49:82–87.

78. Walsh B, Wilson G, Loeb K, et al. Medication and psychotherapy in the treatment of bulimia nervosa. Am J Psychiatry 1997; 154:523–531.

79. Goldbloom D, Olmstead M, Davis R, et al. A randomized controlled trial of fluoxetine and cognitive behavioral therapy for bulimia nervosa: short term outcome. Behav Res Ther 1997; 35:803–811.

80. Beumont P, Russell J, Touyz S, et al. Intensive nutritional counseling in bulimia nervosa: a role for supplementation with fluoxetine? Aust N Z J Psychiatry 1997; 31:514–524.

81. Bacaltchuk J, Trefiglio R, Oliveira I, Hay P, Lima M, Mari J. Combination of antidepressants and psychological treatments for bulimia nervosa: a systematic review. Acta Psychiatr Scand June 26 1999; 101:256–267.

82. McCann U, Agras W. Successful treatment of nonpurging bulimia nervosa with desipramine: a double-blind, placebo-controlled study. Am J Psychiatry 1990; 147:1509–1513.

83. Laederach-Hofman K, Graf C, Lippuner K, Lederer S, Michel R, Schneider M. Imipramine and diet counseling with psychological support in the treatment of obese binge-eaters: a randomized, placebo-controlled double-blind study. Int J Eat Disord 1999; 26:231–244.

84. Hudson J, McElroy S, Raymond N, et al. Fluvoxamine in the treatment of binge-eating disorder: a multicenter placebo-controlled, double-blind trial. Am J Psychiatry 1998; 155:1756–1762.

85. McElroy S, Casuto L, Nelson E, et al. Placebo-controlled trial of sertraline in the treatment of binge eating disorder. Am J Psychiatry 2000; 157:1004–1006.

86. Shapira N, Goldsmith T, McElroy S. Treatment of binge-eating disorder with topiramate: a clinical case series. J Clin Psychiatry 2000; 61:368–372.

87. Appolinario J, Coutinho W, Fontenelle L. Topiramate for binge-eating disorder. Am J Psychiatry 2001; 158:967–968.

88. McElroy S, Arnold L, Shapira N, et al. Topiramate in the treatment of binge eating disorder associated with obesity: a randomized, placebo-controlled trial. Am J Psychiatry February 2003; 160(2):255–261.

89. Alger S, Schwalberg M, Bigaouette J, et al. Effect of a tricyclic antidepressant and opiate antagonist on binge-eating in normal weight bulimic and obese binge-eating subjects. Am J Clin Nutr 1991; 53:865–871.

90. Stunkard A, Berkowits R, Tanrikut C, Reiss E, Young L. d-Fenfluramine treatment of binge eating disorder. Am J Psychiatry 1996; 153:1455–1459.

91. Appolonario JC, Godoy-Matos A, Fontenelle LF, et al. An open trial of sibutramine in obese patients with binge eating disorder. J Clin Psychiatry 2002; 63:28–30.

92. Agras W, Telch C, Arnow B, et al. Weight loss, cognitive–behavioral, and desipramine treatments in binge eating disorder. An additive design. Behav Ther 1994; 25:225–238.

93. Devlin M, Goldfein J, Carino J, Wolk S. Open treatment of overweight binge

eaters with phentermine and fluoxetine as an adjunct to cognitive–behavioral therapy. Int J Eat Disord 2000; 28:325–332.

94.   Marcus M, Wing R, Ewing L, Kern E, Gooding W, McDermott M. A double-blind, placebo controlled trial of fluoxetine plus behavior modification in the treatment of obese binge eaters and non-binge eaters. Am J Psychiatry 1990; 147:876–881.

95.   Grilo C, Masheb R, Heninger G, Wilson G. Controlled comparison of cognitive behavorial therapy and fluoxetine for binge eating disorder. In: Mitchell J, ed. Scientific II Session. International Conference on Eating Disorders. BED and Obesity. Boston: Academy for Eating Disorders, April 28, 2002.

22

Eating Disorders, Victimization, and Comorbidity: Principles of Treatment

Timothy D. Brewerton
Medical University of South Carolina
Charleston, South Carolina, U.S.A.

Comorbidity is the rule rather than the exception when it comes to eating disorders (EDs), particularly bulimia nervosa (BN). The common types of comorbid psychiatric disorders (on axes I and II) and comorbid medical disorders (on axis III) are reviewed in Chapters 8, 9, and 10, respectively. Comorbidity is simply the coexistence of one disorder with another disorder in the same person. When one disorder, e.g., major depressive disorder (MDD), occurs with another in the present time this constitutes *current* prevalence or history, whereas when another disorder occurs at any point during the lifetime of the individual it constitutes *lifetime* prevalence or previous history of that comorbid disorder. While current comorbidity is more strongly the purview of clinicians managing acute EDs, particularly in an inpatient setting, obtaining the lifetime history of all forms of comorbidity is extremely important in order for the clinician to see the "big picture," the "forest" *and* the "trees," and the wholistic, developmental, and biopsychosocial perspective.

The themes of this chapter are that (a) a cluster of comorbid disorders and their symptoms co-occur together more often than chance would dictate, and that this link is highly associated with a history of victimization and subsequent PTSD; and (b) the victimization and PTSD must be specifically and adequately addressed in order to optimize *full* recovery from not only the ED but all associated comorbid disorders. Victimization usually refers specifically to major physical boundary violations, such as rape, molestation, and aggravated assault. All of these common events are crimes in all developed countries, and there may be important legal ramifications for these patients to process in therapy. Of course, victimization may also involve other traumatic experiences, such as witnessing a homicide, severe emotional abuse, and neglect (physical and emotional).

Just as there is a spectrum of trauma and victimization, there is also a spectrum of trauma-related disorders (1–4). The disorders that group together within this trauma-related spectrum include eating (especially BN), affective (especially MDD), anxiety (especially post-traumatic stress disorder, PTSD), substance use, dissociative, somatoform, impulse control, and disruptive disorders on axis I and cluster B disorders, especially borderline personality disorder (BPD), on axis II. On axis III, most of the major leading illnesses that cause significant mortality and morbidity in the United States, including obesity, have been linked to major childhood abuse and adversity (5,6). Mounting evidence attests to the powerful psychobiological underpinnings of trauma on multiple developing and evolving systems, notably the central nervous system (CNS), the autonomic nervous system (ANS), as well as the immune, endocrine, and cardiovascular systems (4,7).

Axis II (personality) disorders are not reliably diagnosed quickly, or in the face of significant axis I psychopathology, or prolonged semistarvation. This has been evident since the famous Minnesota semistarvation experiments in the 1940s by Keys and colleagues (see Chapter 8) (8). Taken together, the scientific literature strongly supports an aggressive focus on axis I disorders first, which then often leads to improvement or even disappearance in apparent axis II disorders. A more prolonged evaluation allows the clinician to collect and clarify further information not only from the patient but from family members, previous treatment providers, and other potential sources, e.g., teachers, coaches, friends, extended family. It is only after an extended evaluation has been completed and after improvement in axis I psychopathology has occurred that a reliable and accurate axis II diagnosis can be made with any certainty.

Some of the best data regarding prevalence rates of common comorbid psychiatric disorders in the United States come from the National Comorbidity Study (9). In a large representative sample of more than 8000 U.S. residents interviewed, lifetime prevalence of any axis I psychiatric disorder (not including EDs) was 48%. The lifetime prevalence for having any type of anxiety disorder was 24.9%, for having any affective disorder was 19.3%, and for having any substance abuse and/or dependence was 26.6%. The lifetime prevalence of PTSD was 7.8% (10% in women, 5% in men).

In the National Women's Study (NWS), there were similar findings in a random sample of more than 4000 women who agreed to take part in a highly structured interview. The lifetime prevalence of PTSD was found to be 12.5% in this representative sample of U.S. women (10). The anonymity of this telephone survey may have actually allowed for more open and honest disclosure than a "face-to-face" interview.

A central and common finding of both the National Comorbidity Study and the NWS was that psychiatric comorbidity was highly associated with a history of serious victimization and especially a lifetime history of PTSD. In the National Comorbidity Study the odds ratios for major axis I disorders ranged from 2.4 to 4.5, and similarly increased rates were found in the NWS (1,11). In another large, well-controlled study of 1411 female twins, childhood sexual abuse, especially genital rape, predicted an odds ratio of 5.62 for the development of BN and 5.05 for the development of two or more psychiatric disorders (12). This was an especially important and powerful study given that it controlled for genetic influences.

RELATIONSHIP OF EATING DISORDERS TO TRAUMA HISTORY AND PTSD

It is well established that the role of trauma or victimization is a significant risk factor for BN in association with comorbid axis I psychopathology (13). In this study, two centers (University of North Dakota and Medical University of South Carolina) reviewed all available studies to date using strict a priori inclusion and exclusion criteria. Six hypotheses were tested, four of which were supported by the data. These included the following:

1. Childhood sexual abuse (CSA) is associated with BN, which was supported by 8 of 12 studies.
2. CSA is more common in BN than AN, which was supported by 4 of 6 studies.
3. CSA is a specific risk factor for EDs, which was not at all supported.
4. CSA is associated with greater severity, which was not supported by the data (but only three studies were included).
5. Particular features of CSA are associated with ED symptoms, which was supported by 4 of 5 studies; these included decreased social competence; poor maternal relationship; unreliable parenting; severity of CSA, and presence of lifetime PTSD, which was a finding from the NWS (14).
6. CSA is associated with comorbidity in ED subjects, which was supported by 5 of 6 studies.

One of the studies included in this review was the NWS (14), which remains the most comprehensive study of the relationship of trauma history and PTSD to EDs and comorbidity in a large national sample. Structured telephone interviews of a representative sample of over 4000 U.S. women from four stratified geographical areas assessed detailed histories of crime victimization experiences (rape, molestation, attempted sexual assault, and aggravated assault), PTSD, MDD, EDs and substance abuse/dependence using DSM-IIIR and DSM-IV (binge eating disorder, BED) criteria. The lifetime prevalence rates for the EDs were as follows: BN = 2.4%, BED = 1.0%; AN = 0.23%. In comparing BN and non-BN/BED subjects who completed the survey, the following lifetime prevalence rates were obtained: completed rape: 26.6% v. 3.3% ($p < 0.01$); contact sexual molestation: 22.0% v. 12.0% ($p < 0.05$); attempted assault: 26.8% v. 8.4%, $p < 0.001$; any direct crime victimization (one or more of the above): 54.4% v. 31.0% ($p < 0.001$); lifetime PTSD: 37% v. 12% ($p < 0.001$); current PTSD: 21% v. 4% ($p < 0.001$). In comparing BED versus non-BN/BED subjects, there were no significant differences except for lifetime PTSD: 22% v. 12% ($p < 0.01$). In the AN group there were no reports of rape, molestation, aggravated assault, or PTSD at all. The age of first rape occurred *before* the age of first binge in 84% of all BN cases. The corresponding numbers for only adolescent rapes (12–17 years) and only child rapes (≤11 years) were 96% and 100%, respectively. These data provide substantial validity to the notion that victimization is a causative risk factor for BN, albeit a nonspecific one. In addition, the age of first binge for BN subjects was significantly earlier in cases of rape resulting in PTSD compared to those with rape without PTSD or no rape. Interestingly, the prevalence rates for BN were significantly higher in those subjects with histories of rape with PTSD (10.4%) compared to those with rape without PTSD (2.0%) or those with no rape (2.0%), which strongly suggests that PTSD rather than prior abuse per se best predicts the development of BN. In the NWS links between trauma, dissociative symptoms, and BN were also found (15). BN subjects had significantly more "forgetting" or psychogenic amnesia of traumatic events (27%) than BED subjects (12%) or non-ED subjects. This was defined as an endorsement by subjects that they forgot all or part of traumatic events. Multiple linear regression using psychogenic amnesia as the dependent variable identified the following significant variables (in decreasing order of significance): lifetime PTSD, childhood rape, lifetime major depression, molestation, emotional problems in the family, laxative abuse, total number of victimization experiences, age, and vomiting (15). Based on these and other data, it was hypothesized that purging behaviors, such as vomiting and laxative abuse, rather than binge eating per se, are maladaptive behaviors linked to

PTSD and MDD that facilitate avoiding, numbing, and forgetting traumatic memories.

Since the publication of the review by Wonderlich and colleagues, there have been two large reviews on sexual abuse and EDs, both of which support the importance of this link in at least a subgroup of ED patients (16,17).

Of course, not all patients with EDs have been victimized. However, the index of suspicion rises substantially as the number of comorbid psychiatric disorders rises. In the NWS there were clear links between trauma, PTSD, and comorbidity with affective, anxiety, and substance use disorders (SUDs). A very robust linear relationship exists between the number of comorbid axis I diagnoses and the percentage of subjects with histories of child rape, rape at any age, and any direct victimization experience (unpublished data). 100% of the subjects with all four diagnoses (BN, MDD, PTSD, SUD) had experienced at least one major direct victimization experience in their life (rape, molestation, aggravated assault). Fifty percent of these same subjects with all four diagnoses reported a childhood rape (≤ 17 years old).

There have been a number of more recent studies on EDs, victimization, and comorbidity, all of which lend further support to this relationship. Some of these studies will be reviewed below.

Kenardy showed links between past sexual and/or physical abuse and weight dissatisfaction and/or disordered eating in young and middle-aged women (18), while Romans reported higher rates of EDs in women who have experienced CSA (19). In this study, the factors that increased the risk of developing an ED in women who had experienced CSA were belonging to a younger age cohort, experiencing menarche at an early age, and experiencing high paternal overcontrol. Low maternal care was specifically associated with the development of AN, whereas early age of menarche differentiated women with BN. Younger age and early age of menarche also differentiated the CSA + ED women from the psychiatric comparison group.

In a clinical study that supports the link between PTSD and EDs, Gleaves and colleagues stated that 74% of 293 women admitted to a residential treatment center who completed a PTSD symptom scale reported a traumatic experience and 52% reported symptoms consistent with a diagnosis of PTSD (20). Of 112 AN patients, 47% met PTSD criteria, and of 103 BN patients 62% met PTSD criteria. In a clinical sample of recovered BN patients, abused subjects showed a trend toward more frequent lifetime diagnoses of PTSD and substance dependence compared with nonabused subjects (21). These results suggest that abusive experiences may be associated with some of the psychopathology of BN, particularly that which is related to anxiety, substance abuse, and more severe core ED pathology. In another study, women comorbid for BN and substance dependence were found to have the highest frequency and the most severe histories of sexual abuse compared to bulimic women without substance dependence (22).

In an Australian sample of hospitalized patients, nearly one-half of ED patients reported a history of child sexual abuse and one-quarter reported child physical abuse, and these rates were significantly higher than those for the control group (23). In addition, dissociative experiences were found to be common and strongly associated with history of abuse and self-mutilation (24).

In a Japanese study of ED patients and controls, physical punishment histories tended to be more prevalent among patients with AN-BP or BN than among AN-R or controls. AN-BP and BN patients with physical punishment histories had twofold higher scores on the Dissociative Experiences Scale (DES) and significantly more frequent histories of self-mutilation (67% v. 33%) compared with patients without such histories (25). Multi-impulsivity in Japanese ED patients was associated with suicide attempts, self-mutilation, BPD, and parental loss (26). In a study of Italian ED patients and controls, self-destructive behavior appeared to be the most important predictor of a history of sexual and/or physical abuse in ED patients (27).

Some interesting data have emerged that support the association between EDs, victimization, and comorbidity in males, both men and boys. In a sample of more than 24,000 U.S. veterans, Striegel-Moore and colleagues found that women and men with EDs had significant comorbidity with substance abuse and mood disorders (28). In addition, women with EDs had higher rates of anxiety disorders and BPD. Lipschitz and colleagues reported that hospitalized adolescent males with PTSD were more likely to have comorbid EDs as well as other anxiety disorders and somatization (29). In a survey of a statewide representative sample of 9943 students in grades 7, 9, and 11 in Connecticut, Neumark-Sztainer and coworkers reported increased disordered eating among those who reported sexual or physical abuse, as well as low levels of family communication and parental caring and expectations (30). The links between abuse and disordered eating persisted even after controlling for differences in familial and psychosocial factors. The odds ratio for the development of disordered eating following sexual abuse was 1.99 for girls and 4.88 for boys, whereas the odds ratio following physical abuse was 2.0 for girls and 1.95 for boys.

Other data in children and adolescents lend further strength to these interrelationships (31–35). In one well-controlled study, Wonderlich and colleagues compared 20 sexually abused girls with 20 age-matched nonabused control girls aged 10–15 years who completed psychometric instruments, including the Kids' Eating Disorders Survey, the McKnight Risk Factor Survey, and the Body Rating Scale for Adolescents (31). Abused children, in comparison with control children: (a) had significantly higher rates of weight dissatisfaction, purging, and dieting behavior; (b) ate significantly less when emotionally upset; and (c) were less likely to exhibit perfectionistic tendencies but more likely to desire thinner body types. This was the first controlled study to support similar findings in adults.

In a study of three samples of ninth through twelfth graders including over 5000 students, sexual victimization (independent of physical victimization) was associated with weight regulation in adolescent girls, and it was also associated with more extreme forms as well as multiple forms of weight regulation. Urban girls with sexual victimization had significantly higher rates of purging than urban girls without such experiences (32).

Other studies in children and adolescents have been published demonstrating significant associations between binge–purge behavior and sexual or physical abuse. This has been shown in large national samples of adolescents in both the United States (33) and Sweden (34). These links have also been shown to persist in sexually abused children long past the time of abuse (35).

Data supporting a role for various forms of abuse as a risk factor for BED have also emerged in the literature over the last several years. Grilo and colleagues showed higher rates of childhood psychological, physical, and sexual maltreatment in outpatients with BED (36). A total of 83% of BED patients reported some form of childhood maltreatment, including 59% reporting emotional abuse, 36% physical abuse, 30% sexual abuse, 69% emotional neglect, and 49% physical neglect. There were no differences in the distribution of any form of childhood maltreatment by gender, obesity status, body mass index, binge eating, or attitudinal features. Only physical neglect was associated with dietary restraint in women, whereas emotional abuse was associated with greater body dissatisfaction, higher depression, and lower self-esteem in men and women, and sexual abuse was associated with greater body dissatisfaction in men. Another study also identified other forms of victimization besides abuse, like bullying and discrimination, as risk factors for BED (37). Unfortunately, these studies did not report on rates of PTSD in these patients.

Other investigators have also expanded the spectrum of abuse that may contribute to the development of EDs, including neglect (38), childhood emotional abuse (39,40), adverse family background (41), and extreme food deprivation (42).

In terms of studies of mediating variables between prior child abuse and BN, research have shown that impulsivity and core beliefs involving shame, self-esteem, and perceived control are significant mediating variables to consider in terms not only of etiology but of treatment planning as well (43–48).

RELATIONSHIP OF COMORBID DISORDERS TO TRAUMA HISTORY AND PTSD

The most common axis I disorders that are comorbid with each of the major EDs have been extensively reviewed in Chapter 8. These include affective and anxiety disorders for AN, BN, and BED, as well as SUDs for BN, AN-BP, perhaps BED, but not AN-R. Other data support associations between BN and dissociative disorders (DDs) or symptoms, somatoform disorders (SDs), impulse control disorders (ICDs), and disruptive behavior disorders (DBDs). Each of these types of disorder has been strongly linked to history of victimization and PTSD in the scientific literature, which has been reviewed elsewhere (46).

Trauma may therefore serve as an "organizing principle" when thinking about etiology from a biopsychosocial perspective in many (but not all) comorbid ED patients. However, the greater the degree of comorbidity, the greater are the chances of a trauma history having played a significant role in precipitating the onset of the overall course of mental illness. Trauma-related disorders may share common underlying factors that account for such interrelationship, e.g., dysregulation in neuropsychobiological mechanisms, such as serotonin and other neurotransmitter disturbances (see Chapter 11), as well as common cognitive schema involving issues of self-esteem, control, guilt, and shame.

Affective Disorders

A lifetime prevalence of major depressive disorder (MDD) has been found in association with AN and BN in 24–88% of reported cases, depending on the study (see Chapter 8). To a much lesser extent, this pattern of higher affective disorders in ED patients runs true for dysthymia (19–20%) and bipolar disorder (4–13%) as well, particularly BPD type II with a seasonal pattern. Depressive symptoms that do not meet full criteria for an affective disorder are also common in ED patients (depression NOS).

Each of these affective disorders has been reported to have higher than expected rates of a history of trauma or victimization, and more often than not the trauma occurred during childhood or adolescence. It is important for the clinician to realize that fully two-thirds of all rapes of women in the United States occur before the age of 18 (NWS). The frequency of rape in decreasing order is in girls aged 12–17 years, then in girls at or below 11 years old, then in women ages 18–24 years. After this age period, the frequency of rape decreases with age precipitously. Childhood sexual and physical abuse has been found to be highly associated with MDD and affective disturbances in general (7,49–55), and Gladstone reported that depressed patients with childhood abuse histories were more likely associated with BPD (see "Axis II Comorbidity" below) (54).

In addition, a history of physical or sexual abuse in childhood has been found to be particularly associated with MDD with reversed neurovegetative features, e.g., hyperphagia and hypersomnia, whether or not manic subjects are included (55). A significant relationship between mania and childhood physical abuse was also found. Across analyses there was a significant main effect of female gender on risk of early sexual abuse, which has been a consistent finding in the literature. These results suggest an association between early traumatic experiences and particular symptom clusters of depression, mania, or both in adults.

Anxiety Disorders

Just about all of the anxiety disorders, with the possible exception of panic disorder, also occur in ED patients (23–75%) at higher than expected rates when compared to rates in the general population. These data have been much more extensively reviewed in Chapter 8 and will not be discussed at length. However, the general ranges reported are as follows: PTSD (37–62%), obsessive-compulsive disorder (OCD) (3–66%), social phobia (16–55%), panic disorder (5–10%), generalized anxiety disorder (GND) (12%), simple phobia (13%). Taken together, it is evident from this research that one of the most common anxiety disorders presenting in the ED population is PTSD, a finding from the NWS (14). Although there are many studies of the rates of child abuse and other victimization experiences in ED samples (13,14,16,17,56), a paucity of reliable data exists on the prevalence of PTSD in subjects with EDs.

An important and consistent finding is that anxiety disorders are usually primary and the ED is usually secondary. Much has been published on this particular comorbid dyad in the last few years, as noted in Chapters 6 and 8. It appears that anxiety symptoms, particularly those involving behavioral inhibition and obsessionality, are important risk factors for the development of EDs. Anxiety typically persists and often worsens following the onset of an ED. In the NWS, sexual assault and PTSD symptoms began before the first binge ever occurred in 84% of all rapes and nearly 100% of rapes occurring during childhood (≤17 years old) (in subjects with BN only).

A diagnostic *sine qua non* for PTSD is of course the occurrence of a traumatic event. However, all of the other anxiety disorders have been reported to have high rates of victimization, including OCD, panic disorder, GAD, social phobia, simple phobia, as well as separation anxiety disorder and overanxious disorder in kids (29,51–53,57–62).

Substance Use Disorders

Affective and anxiety disorders are seen at higher frequencies in all of the EDs, but when it comes to SUDs there is a striking difference between AN and BN, with BED falling somewhere in the middle. Rates in the EDs range from 0% to 37%, with restricting AN having less than expected rates of SUDs and BN patients having much greater rates than expected (see Chapter 8). Some form of substance abuse may be a compensatory strategy inherent to BN, e.g., abuse of laxatives, diuretics, CNS stimulants (ranging from cocaine to ephedra-containing over-the-counter preparations) (63). Some BN patients use alcohol, opiates, and/or nicotine as appetite suppressants and anabolic steroids to build muscle. Alcohol and other CNS depressants may also serve to depress inhibitory influences so as to facilitate vomiting. The use of marijuana and other psychedelics may complicate the clinical picture, causing further body image distortion, anxiety, and mood alterations (64). SUDs have been linked not only to bulimic disorders but to previous traumas as well (49,65,66). Dansky and colleagues demonstrated in the NWS that the major reason alcohol abuse so commonly coexists with BN is because they share comorbid PTSD (66).

Dissociative Disorders

Next to PTSD, which requires an identified traumatic event, the DDs as a group are most closely linked to trauma. This link between trauma and dissociative phenomena has been well described in the literature (4,67,68). DDs and their symptoms have been described all over the world and are commonly related to severely overwhelming traumatic experiences, particularly when occurring during childhood, and include derealization, depersonalization, time distortions, cognitive and memory alterations (including amnesia), identity alterations, and somatic sensations. Dissociative disorders (particularly dissociative identity disorder, DID) are very real disorders of memory, consciousness, and identity that represent the devastating effects of unusually severe and often chronic violent abuse during childhood. Axis I comorbidity is quite common, and several investigators have reported high frequencies of EDs and behaviors in DID patients (69–71). Conversely, high frequencies of dissociative symptoms have been reported in ED patients, particularly BN (72–85), and in nonclinical samples with ED pathology (86,87). Previously, there were no detailed studies of both dissociative symptoms, such as psychogenic amnesia (PA), and victimization experiences, such as rape, in a representative group of women with and without EDs. Data generated as part of the NWS provided an opportunity for a more controlled examination of these relationships.

As part of the PTSD screening, respondents were designated as having PA if they endorsed ever "forgetting" all or part of a significant traumatic event, a question that was part of the PTSD module. Respondents with BN endorsed PA 2.5 times more often than non-BN/non-BED respondents (27% v. 11%, $p < 0.000033$, χ^2square), and there was a trend for a similar difference between BN and BED (11%, $p < 0.09$). These results imply that purging, rather than bingeing per se, is more closely associated with an endorsement of PA. It is likely that bulimic behaviors are maladaptive mechanisms with psychobiological underpinnings linked to PTSD and depression that facilitate avoiding, numbing and forgetting traumatic memories (15).

Somatoform Disorders

Disturbances in body perception and overt body distortion are somatoform symptoms inherent to the EDs, especially AN. Links between somatoform disorders (SDs) and EDs have also been reported in the literature (88–91). A recent family study showed clustering of OCD with EDs and SDs (89), particularly body dysmorphic disorder (BDD). BDD and EDs are similarly characterized by obsessive and compulsive phenomenology targeted on the body despicable. Other investigators have noted the connection between EDs and BDD (90,91).

Links between SDs and prior victimization, especially CSA, are well known (92–97). Among adult females, child abuse contributes not only to general somatic preoccupation but to specific somatic symptoms in the chest and throat areas as well (97). Interestingly, these body areas are those that are involved in vomiting behavior. SDs are intimately linked to DDs as well as to other axis I comorbidity. Somatoform dissociation is a unique construct that is highly characteristic of DD patients, a core feature in many patients with SDs, and an important symptom cluster in a subgroup of patients with EDs (88). Other studies report that measures of somatization are significantly positively correlated with measures of dissociation.

Impulse Control Disorders

The ICDs, such as trichotillomania, kleptomania, compulsive buying, as well as self-mutilation, have been associated with the EDs, particularly BN (45,98–104) and to some extent BED (94). As noted in Chapter 9, impulsivity is a common comorbid personality trait in the EDs, particularly BN. Patients with ICD and other impulsive behaviors have high rates of traumatic histories (105,106).

ICDs have been hypothesized to exist on an obsessive-compulsive spectrum (107–109). In a study designed to characterize impulsive versus compulsive self-injurious behavior in patients with EDs, CSA and anxiety were found to significantly predict impulsive self-injury, whereas obsessionality and age predicted compulsive self-injury (102). Wonderlich and colleagues tested a number of mediational pathways between CSA and subsequent eating disturbance and found that behavioral impulsivity was the most significant mediating factor (44).

From a clinical and preventive perspective, it is important to note that individuals who have been sexually abused as children are at a higher risk for being revictimized as adults, possibly in part due to the increased rates of impulsivity that follow abuse (110,111) and perhaps due to repetition compulsion. Revictimization serves to amplify the impact of childhood sexual trauma on selective attention to trauma-related stimuli, contributing to increased defenses and hence psychopathology, as well as more self-blame and refractoriness to treatment (112,113).

Attention Deficit–Hyperactivity Disorder and Disruptive Behavior Disorders

Attention deficit–hyperactivity disorder (ADHD) and the EDs do co-occur with each other although not at an increased rate. Stimulants not only can be used in patients with BN or BED to manage the ADHD, they may also be helpful for the binge eating as well (114–116). However, a major danger in this area is misdiagnosis. Common comorbid disorders that can be associated with alterations in attention, concentration, and/or arousal, such as MDD, PTSD, and DDs, can be misdiagnosed as ADHD, particularly in children who were abused at an early age. Dykman has demonstrated higher rates of externalizing symptoms in sexually and physically abused children (62), and Gold and Teicher reported higher activity levels in abused prepubertal children as measured by computerized activity monitors (117). Nevertheless, the combined type of ADHD has been found to be associated with child abuse in girls meeting ADHD criteria compared to controls (118). Physical abuse in particular has been found to drastically increase the diagnosis of ADHD (119). In contrast, ADHD, and perhaps DBDs, may also increase the risk of being physically abused by caretakers, probably as a result of increased activity and impulsivity (120).

In terms of DBDs, Thompson and colleagues reported higher rates of aggressive behavior in adolescent girls with binge eating, purging, and dietary restriction, and opine that this is a neglected area in the field (121). Geist and coworkers reported that oppositional defiant disorder (ODD) occurs more commonly in adolescents with EDs associated with binge–purge symptoms (122). ODD has been reported to be associated with a history of physical or sexual maltreatment as well as PTSD symptoms (123,124). DBDs are often precursors to the development of antisocial personality disorder, which has also been linked to child abuse and neglect as discussed below.

Axis II Comorbidity

The most common personality disorders (PDs) associated with the EDs have been extensively reviewed in Chapter 9. In short, cluster C disorders [obsessive-compulsive personality disorder (OCPD), avoidant personality disorder (APD), and dependent personality disorder (DPD)] are common to both AN and BN. In particular, OCPD and its traits are the best studied of this cluster and have been shown to be important risk factors in the development of EDs (125).

Although there are no clear links between cluster C disorders and victimization or PTSD, childhood emotional neglect has been associated with an increased risk for APD during adolescence and early adulthood (126). It is important to note that the presence of APD may contribute more avoidance to that already inherent to PTSD and therefore make it even harder for the traumatized ED patient to disclose abuse and face the exposure work required.

Childhood emotional neglect has also been associated with increased risk for paranoid and cluster A PD symptom levels during adolescence and early adulthood, and childhood physical neglect has been associated with an increased risk for schizotypal PD and with cluster A PD symptom levels (126).

It is also noted in Chapter 9 that cluster B disorders, and their associated trait of impulsivity, decidedly occur more frequently in the BN and AN binge–purge type than in the AN restricting type of ED. Data show strong links not only between BPD and patients with binge–purge symptomatology, but also between BPD and histories of victimization, PTSD, affective disorders, other anxiety disorders, SUDs, DDs, SDs, ICDs, DBDs, and ADHD (127–130). BPD is also highly associated with multiple comorbid axis I disorders (131–133) as well as with prior abuse and neglect. Other cluster B personality disorders, such as narcissistic personality disorder (NPD) and antisocial personality disorder (APD), have also been associated with child abuse and neglect (134).

Course and Outcome

The effects of trauma history on the clinical course and treatment outcome of EDs and their comorbidity is unknown. Few or no data exist on this important topic because it has not been a commonly identified variable in treatment studies. However, clinical experience suggests that trauma history and especially subsequent PTSD history carries a worse prognosis. PTSD itself is a chronic disorder with one-third of cases followed up 10 years later still meeting full criteria (1). Bell examined the question of whether concurrent psychopathology at presentation influences response to treatment for BN and found no consistent relationship between outcome and any axis I disorder (135). However, Bell also noted that most of the studies assessing axis II dysfunction show that borderline symptom severity or cluster B personality disorder, which is linked to prior victimization, can impair outcome. Similarly, multi-impulsivity, which is also linked to abusive histories, is associated with poor long-term prognosis following treatment (136,137). Anderson reported that abused BN patients treated in an inpatient setting were more likely to be rehospitalized in the 3-month postdischarge period than non-abused BN patients, which lends support to the notion that trauma may retard the recovery process from an ED (138).

PRINCIPLES OF TREATMENT FOR THE COMORBID ED PATIENT WITH VICTIMIZATION

How does the clinician approach treatment of the ED patient with significant trauma-related psychiatric comorbidity? What should the clinician do first besides be respectful of the patient's struggle? What are the general principles in the management of comorbidity with EDs? As was noted by Brown, "there is a dearth of treatment suggestions to deal with the comorbid problems of the patient with an ED and a history of abuse" (56). The general principles in the management of comorbidity with EDs are outlined in Table 1, but will be elaborated here. The most tried-and-true initial approach for any patient with or without complex symptomatology is to perform a complete psychiatric evaluation, which substantially reduces the chances of misdiagnosis. Such a comprehensive evaluation must include histories of all forms of abuse and neglect, major life events or stressors, as well as natural disasters and witnessing of violence. Many patients are not comfortable revealing major traumatic events during an initial interview, so evaluation must be seen as an ongoing process that blends into the treatment process and continues to shape it. Any number of screening and diagnostic instruments may be used in the course of a complete evaluation, and this is extensively discussed in Chapter 2 as well as in available practice guidelines, which will be discussed below.

Of course, the formation and maintenance of a therapeutic alliance is not only the starting point for but also the subsequent foundation of future work and progress. Comorbidity has been reported to be a significant factor related to ED treatment dropout (139). All involved staff and clinicians, especially the primary therapist and/or psychiatrist, must work extra hard to convey a sense of trustworthiness, honesty, straightforwardness, knowledge, and nonjudgmental positive regard, which are essential ingredients for any

TABLE 1 General Principles in the Management of Comorbidity with Eating Disorders

A. Complete Psychiatric Evaluation/Diagnosis
 1. Identify relative chronology: primary v. secondary status v. concurrent
 2. Identify functional links between disorders, e.g., avoidance of trauma-related memories, affects, behaviors, cognitions, and their cues (e.g., self-medication hypothesis)
 3. Treat concurrently whenever possible: it is a matter of emphasis or focus.
 4. Emphasis is determined by the level of danger, risk, and/or brain–body impairment.
B. Normalizing Brain Function Is Necessary for Effective Psychotherapy and Antidepressant Efficacy
 1. Nutritional education/stabilization/rehabilitation
  "First we eat, then we talk."—Walter Vandereycken (144)
  Stages/phases of treatment—Garner and Garfinkel (143)
  a. Starvation effects: *The Biology of Human Starvation*, Keys et al., 1950: dieting, restricting, and weight loss induce mental and physical symptoms in otherwise healthy individuals (8).
  b. Tryptophan depletion studies: dieting depletes neurotransmitters in the CNS
  c. Nutritional rehabilitation greatly helps to normalize brain function in ED patients.
  c. Refeeding significantly alleviates mood and anxiety dysregulation
  d. Refeeding allows antidepressants to work.
  e. Refeeding allows psychological issues to "rise" and become clarified (allows psychotherapy to work)
 2. Treat withdrawal/achieve abstinence ("Say no, then go"): concurrently with no. 1, as required
 3. Requirements for effective psychotherapy include grossly intact brain function, ability to attend, ability to learn, motivation, willingness to change and supportive relationship(s). Starved and/or intoxicated brains can't learn well.
C. Intensive Psychotherapy
 1. Cognitive–behavioral therapy (CBT) (see Chapter 17): is the most scientifically supported psychotherapy for ED's and most forms of trauma-related comorbidity. Thus CBT has almost universal application in the comorbid population. The inclusion of prolonged exposure with cognitive reprocessing appears to be essential in the successful treatment of PTSD (149–154). EMDR appears to include both of these components and readily facilitates the CBT of trauma work (155).
 2. Interpersonal therapy (IPT) (see Chapter 19): is an established second line treatment approach instead of or in addition to CBT. IPT and CBT are theoretically compatible if not complementary.

TABLE 1 Continued

   3. Family therapy (see Chapter 18): is mandatory in all children and
      adolescents unless circumstances do not permit, and it should be
      considered in all cases.
   4. Dialectical behavior therapy (see Chapter 20): is particularly useful in
      comorbid BPD, multi-impulsivity, ICD's.
   5. Experiential psychotherapies, e.g., gestalt, "body work," movement
      therapy, psychodrama, etc., can be important for working on body image/
      trauma issues and for accessing emotional states.
   6. Psychodynamic psychotherapy: should be adjunctive only.
D. Psychopharmacology (see Chapter 21)
   1. Antidepressants (see Table 3)
   2. Other psychotropic agents
      a. *Ondansetron*: consider in refractory BN after at least two adequate
         antidepressant trials.
      b. *Olanzapine*: consider in low weight AN, especially R-AN, comorbid
         with affective and/or anxiety disorder(s).
      c. *Naltrexone*: consider in refractory cases, comorbid alcohol abuse/
         dependence, and/or self-mutilation.
E. Use Available Practice Guidelines and Treatment Manuals
   1. Use American Psychiatric Association (APA) Practice Guidelines for the
      Treatment of Eating Disorders: www.psych.org/clin_res/guide.bk.cfm.
   2. Use PTSD/Child Abuse Practice Guidelines:
      a. Expert Consensus Guidelines for the Treatment of PTSD: www.psy-
         ch.org/clin_res/guide.bk.cfm.
      b. American Academy of Child and Adolescent Psychiatry (AACAP):
         www.aacap.org; has practice guidelines as well as Facts For
         Families.
      c. Child Sexual and Physical Abuse: Guidelines for Treatment was
         codeveloped by the National Crime Victims Research and Treatment
         Center and the Center on Sexual Assault and is an excellent source of
         guidance, including references for treatment manuals (www.musc.e-
         du/cvc/) (167).
   3. Use Other Practice Guidelines as Needed
      a. www.psychguides.com for obsessive-compulsive disorder (OCD),
         bipolar disorder, schizophrenia, attention deficit hyperactivity disorder
         (ADHD), depression in women, and mental retardation.
      b. www.issd.org for dissociative disorders.
      c. www.psych.org/clin_res/prac_guide.cfm for APA Practice Guidelines
         for MDD, bipolar disorder, SUD's, PD, schizophrenia, BPD.
      d. www.aacap.org for other AACAP practice guidelines.

successful course of therapy, but especially for comorbid ED patients with trauma histories and related disorders. In addition, it is important that countertransference feelings be monitored closely and kept in check. In my experience, sometimes traumatized patients do not even realize that they have been victimized until someone explains to them the detailed definitions of the abuse in question, e.g., rape, assault, aggravated assault, bullying, etc. This is especially true for patients who were abused during early childhood. Only later, after a significant degree of cognitive development has occurred, do some victims of CSA realize that they were victims. In this sense the therapist serves as someone who offers a more objective perspective and who assists the traumatized patient in reframing her experiences in the context of consensual reality. All too often denial, avoidance, self-blame, and shame cloud the view of the meanings of prior traumatic events. It must also be remembered that ED patients are as a group highly suggestible or hypnotizable (140). The clinician treating traumatized ED patients must take every precaution to elicit his or her patients' histories without being suggestive that these events did or did not occur. Whenever traumatic events that occurred during childhood or adolescence are reported, the clinician should be sure to understand and obey all reporting laws mandated by the local state and/or country government.

As a complete list of disorders is being determined it is essential for comprehensive treatment planning that clinicians determine the chronological order in which the disorders first occurred or appeared. Which disorder came first in relation to the other identified comorbid disorders? What disorders are concurrent? What are the traumas and when did they happen in relation to the disorders identified? It is useful over time to work with the patient to construct a phenomenological, cause-and-effect–based time line and schema in which the development and evolution of their problems makes overall sense to them. It is likely that this information will evolve gradually and be referred to in therapy again and again. Identifying the functional links of meaning between comorbid disorders and life events can be very informative and instructive for patient, family, and therapist in terms of identifying and challenging cognitive distortions. One very common theme underlying the link between EDs and trauma-related comorbidity is that maladaptive coping mechanisms, such as bingeing, purging, dieting, substance abuse, dissociation, self-mutilation, compulsive behavior, etc., are ways to avoid trauma-related states, i.e., memories, affects, behaviors, and thoughts, which are often triggered by any number of cues. This phenomenon is another type of "compensatory behavior" and is essentially another variation of the self-medication hypothesis (141). Self-punishment also has a lot of cognitive explanatory power for many traumatized ED patients.

What disorder is primary and what disorder is secondary, tertiary, etc.? If the onset of the ED came before the onset of the MDD, then the ED is the primary disorder and MDD is the secondary disorder, which may in part be due to the ED. If the ED came after the MDD, then the ED is secondary and may in part be due to the MDD. In other words, as discussed in Chapter 6, primary disorders may be risk factors for the development of secondary disorders. There has been a long tradition in medicine to ascertain this type of information, to develop a chronology of events and their subsequent sequelae, as a way to guide treatment and "go to the source" of a patient's problems. A secondary depression may be more likely to respond to weight restoration and successful management of the ED, whereas a primary depression may more likely linger on or be an impediment to the ED recovery process unless it is managed more aggressively. Interestingly, research shows that most episodes of MDD are secondary, and they tend to be more persistent and severe than primary MDD episodes (142). Similar to the above example, to the extent that an ED is secondary to victimization and the posttraumatic stress process, it is important to eventually and adequately address this primary problem.

Whenever possible, comorbid disorders should be managed concurrently, but again, it is a matter of emphasis and prioritization. Which disorder or problem should the clinician focus on first? A useful guideline that should determine the clinician's initial emphasis, for both ethical and medicolegal reasons, is the current level of danger, risk, and/or brain/body impairment. It is necessary to normalize or stabilize brain function in order for the psychotherapeutic enterprise to "take hold" and succeed. The idea that the nutritional instability common to all ED patients must be addressed before more intensive psychotherapy can be effectively utilized is common knowledge among experts in the field. Garner and Garfinkel noted that the typical stages or phases of treatment start with refeeding, nutritional stabilization, and rehabilitation, which sometimes require a structured setting and program (143). Walter Vandereycken put it succinctly when he said, "First we eat, then we talk" (144). In short, all patients should receive nutritional education and counseling as reviewed in Chapter 16, and these messages must be in sync with the primary psychotherapeutic process.

The body of knowledge that must be conveyed includes several key points, including (a) the powerful semistarvation effects in conscientious objectors reported by Keys (8) and discussed in Chapter 8, and which lead to the conclusion that dieting induces mental and physical symptoms de novo, and (b) the implications of the tryptophan depletion studies to EDs as noted in Chapters 11 and 16, which basically indicate that dieting depletes neurotransmitters and this in turn has significant and rapid clinical effects (145). It is also important to explain to patients and families that refeeding alone may alleviate mood and anxiety dysregulation to some degree, but that it is also not going to "fix everything." In some ways certain symptoms of the traumatized ED comorbid patient may get worse before they get better, and this is useful to predict. Refeeding may allow patients to start "feeling their feelings" again and to therefore begin to process them, usually with increasing intensity. Their eating-disordered brains slowly but surely start to function better and better as neurotransmitter and neurohormone levels move toward normalization (see Chapters 11, 12, and 13). For this reason, nutritional rehabilitation, especially weight gain in AN, not only *allows antidepressants to work* but also *allows psychotherapy to work*. In effect, once patients begin to think and feel more clearly as a result of refeeding, the real psychological issues can "rise" to awareness and become clarified, processed, and "digested." Nevertheless, the alexithymia that is characteristic of ED patients and other psychosomatic conditions may be an important clinical issue to address (146).

When substance abuse complicates the picture, one should always manage withdrawal and dependence aggressively and as much as possible achieve abstinence ("Say no, then go"). Just as starved brains can't learn very well, intoxicated brains can't either. Basic requirements for effective psychotherapy include grossly intact brain function, including the ability to attend and the ability to learn–unlearn. In addition, sufficient motivation, the willingness to change, and the presence of supportive relationship(s) are important ingredients for progress. If necessary, motivational enhancement therapy (MET) may be beneficial in highly resistant patients (147).

Once brain function has been stabilized and the process of normalization is well on its way, more intensive psychotherapy can begin or intensify. The phases of nutritional rehabilitation and intensive psychotherapy are not absolutely distinct, but instead tend to overlap and merge into one another. The major forms of psychotherapy that have been shown to have empirical evidence for their effectiveness in the EDs are cognitive–behavioral therapy (CBT), interpersonal therapy (IPT), family therapy (FT), and dialectical behavior therapy (DBT), all of which are reviewed in Chapters 17, 18, 19, and 20, respectively. Experiential psychotherapies have not been rigorously studied, but may have important roles in the recovery of comorbid ED patients, particularly in dealing with body image concerns, accessing emotional states, and being exposed to one's own self, so to speak. Likewise, elements of psychodynamically oriented psychotherapy may be useful adjuncts in treatment, but this should never be the only or primary modality used.

It is imperative that the clinician who wants to effectively manage EDs and their comorbid psychiatric disorders familiarize themselves not only with the American Psychiatric Association's Practice Guidelines for the Treatment of Eating Disorders (www.psych.org/clin_res/guide.bk.cfm), but with other practice guidelines and treatment manuals as well on an as-needed basis (www.psychguides.com; www.issd.org; www.psych.org) (148,149). Therapeutic techniques adequate for the non-comorbid ED are not likely to address other problems and disorders, so the clinician must rely on his or her own resources, creativity, and ability to integrate a multitude of approaches in order to tailor the best treatment to match the uniqueness of each patient. Specific aspects and approaches regarding specific comorbid combinations are outlined in Table 2.

Lest it seem too overwhelming or daunting, it is important to realize that there are a number of commonalities inherent to the treatment of ED patients with comorbid trauma-related disorders, including psychoeducation, CBT, and pharmacotherapy. When using general relaxation techniques it is, in my opinion, better to avoid progressive muscle relaxation in ED patients. This inadvertently focuses attention on specific body parts that are "emotionally loaded" for ED patients, which often serves to heighten anxiety rather than lower it. Techniques that focus on the breath with or without the use of visualization appear to work best in my view. When anxiety disorders enter the clinical picture, the addition of prolonged exposure to CBT is clearly indicated (149–154). Adequate time needs to be spent educating the patient about the rationale for in vivo exposure using lay explanations for extinction, conditioned cues, experiential learning, and why anxiety is a necessary component for exposure to work. Hence, medicating away anxiety with benzodiazepines should be avoided and can be countertherapeutic to the management of PTSD. In explaining the rationale for prolonged exposure, most patients can understand the concepts of classical conditioning, or perhaps the notion of finishing "unfinished business," decreasing the "power" of the memories, or "tying up loose ends." They can usually embrace the goal of being able to remember traumatic events and even talk about them without feeling the intense negative feelings that have become so familiar, and which have driven them in part to ED "solutions." In addition, eye movement desensitization and reprocessing is an effective strategy for PTSD and may be a useful adjunct to trauma work (www.emdr.org) (155). In my experience, it complements CBT and exposure work quite well.

IPT techniques can be added for comorbid patients who do not respond to CBT or who reach an impasse in treatment (see Chapter 19). DBT may be useful for a variety of self-destructive behaviors, particularly in the patient with comorbid ICD, BPD, and/or multi-impulsivity (see Chapter 20). Appropriate family therapy consisting of specific goals jointly identified by the patient and the therapist should be carefully considered for all patients (see Chapter 18).

Psychopharmacological interventions tend to be the rule rather than the exception when dealing with comorbid problems associated with the EDs, particularly comorbid affective and anxiety disorders, and this is generally

TABLE 2   Treatment Caveats for Specific Comorbid Combinations

I. Treating PTSD and ED's
1. Use general relaxation techniques, but avoid progressive muscle relaxation.
2. Educate about both Dx's. Establish chronology/sequence of events.
3. Educate about bingeing, purging and starvation effects as possible avoidance/numbing, emotional regulation strategies.
4. Focus on ED first and assess change. Predict possible initial worsening (less numbing, more reexperiencing and hyperarousal).
5. Use Expert Consensus Guidelines on the Treatment of PTSD (see www.psychguides.com) and other available practice guidelines and treatment manuals (149–154).
6. EMDR appears to be as effective for PTSD as CBT with exposure, but can readily be used together.
7. Explain the rationale for in vivo exposure: Extinction; conditioned cues; experiential learning; anxiety necessary.
8. Explain the rationale for prolonged exposure: classical conditioning; "unfinished business"; decreasing the "power" of the memories; goal is to remember the event, even talk about it, without feeling the intense negative feelings.
9. Common therapeutic approaches include psychoeducation, CBT, and pharmacotherapy. Include prolonged exposure in the CBT for PTSD and other anxiety disorders. In addition to the usual areas of focus in cognitive therapy for ED's, the themes of guilt, shame, control, trust, intimacy, and safety are also extremely salient.

II. Treating Comorbid Depression and AN
1. Emphasis on refeeding/nutritional rehabilitation (and abstinence if SUD) first.
2. Education on:
    a. Starvation effects: aggravates anxiety/mood dysregulation and blocks the efficacy of antidepressants and psychotherapy
    b. Effects of L-tryptophan depletion on mood and serotonin metabolism are equivalent to the effects of dieting on the brain.
    c. Lack of efficacy of antidepressants in studies of AN
    d. Efficacy of fluoxetine for prophylaxis of AN relapse.
    e. Bupropion (Wellbutrin) is contraindicated.
3. Consider atypical antipsychotic agent.

III. Treating Comorbid Depression and BN/BED
1. Antidepressants more likely to be effective but nutritional rehabilitation also very important for effective treatment results.
2. Starvation aggravates mood symptoms, i.e., depression, irritability, lability.
3. Fluoxetine (Prozac) is the only agent found to be effective in both MDD & BN.
4. Fluvoxamine (Luvox) was not effective for BN in a large controlled trial in Europe but has reported efficacy in BED (156).
5. Sertraline (Zoloft) has been reported to be effective in BED in one study (157).

TABLE 2   Continued

6. In studies of CBT in BN, symptoms that responded significantly better to the combination of antidepressant and psychotherapy were those of major depression and anxiety.
7. CBT and IPT are proven effective in MDD (mild–moderate, nonpsychotic).
8. Bupropion (Wellbutrin) is contraindicated in BN.
9. Consider phototherapy if a fall–winter pattern of worsening symptoms is present (158).

IV. Treating Comorbid Bipolar D/O and EDs
   1. Avoid lithium, especially in those with purging of any kind, fluid restriction, or compulsive exercising: toxicity, weight gain, hypothyroidism, and kidney effects.
   2. Anticonvulsants are preferable.
   3. Bupropion (Wellbutrin) contraindicated, but anticonvulsant can be protective.
   4. Consider phototherapy, especially with seasonal pattern.
   5. Consider family therapy with focus on psychoeducation.

V. Treating Comorbid Anxiety D/O's and EDs
   1. Focus on ED first and assess change.
   2. Starvation aggravates anxiety (especially obsessive-compulsive symptoms).
   3. Use treatment guidelines for OCD, panic disorder, GAD, PTSD, and social phobia, all of which rely on cognitive–behavioral approaches involving education, challenging cognitive distortions, and exposure techniques.
   4. Use general relaxation techniques (but not progressive muscle relaxation).

A. Treating Comorbid OCD and EDs
   1. Focus on ED first and assess change.
   2. Starvation aggravates OCD symptoms.
   3. Starvation depletes serotonin which acts as inhibitor of obsessions and compulsions.
   4. Eating replenishes central serotonin.

B. Treating Social Phobia and EDs
   1. Focus on ED first and assess change.
   2. Use general relaxation techniques (but not progressive muscle relaxation).
   3. Best-proven therapies include CBT with exposure and SSRIs.
   4. Paroxetine (Paxil) and sertraline (Zoloft) have FDA indication, but all SSRIs have been found to be effective in controlled trials.

C. Treating GAD and EDs
   1. Focus on ED first and assess improvement in anxiety.
   2. SSRIs have some reported effectiveness, but may require higher doses for longer periods of time before response seen (2–5 times longer than antidepressant response).
   3. Starving/restricting undermines effectiveness of SSRIs.
   4. Venlafaxine (Effexor), buspirone (Buspar), and paroxetine (Paxil) have FDA indication.
   5. Avoid chronic benzodiazepines, if possible.

TABLE 2   Continued

VII.   Treating Substance Use D/O's and EDs
    1.   Perform a complete medical and psychiatric evaluation.
    2.   Focus on Both ED and SUD concurrently, but emphasize most the lethal or dangerous condition.
    3.   May need inpatient hospitalization for detoxification and/or nutritional rehabilitation, require longer stays, and/or be less compliant.
    4.   Assess for trauma history/PTSD and explore links.
    5.   Assess for motivational/functional links, e.g., appetite suppression, mood/anxiety regulation, and numbing/avoidance of trauma-related memories and emotions.
    6.   Alcoholic patients need a multivitamin including thiamine, folic acid, vitamin B_{-12} to avoid Wernicke–Korsakoff syndrome, neuropathy, and anemia.
    7.   Consider 12-step approach (AA, NA, OA).
VIII.   Treating Self-injurious Behaviors and EDs
    1.   Self-injurious or parasuicidal behaviors should be treated as unhealthy coping mechanisms.
    2.   Do a functional analysis; in other words, what function does the unhealthy coping mechanism have (e.g., relief of trauma related dysphoria, self-punishment).
    3.   Contract for therapy with consequences outlined. Reinforce and reward responsible behavior.
    4.   Devote enough attention to identify the NEED that is not being satisfied in a more appropriate manner.
    5.   Teach and model healthy coping mechanisms.
    6.   Integrate dialectical behavior therapy (DBT) concepts and interventions into the overall treatment plan (see Chapter 20).
IX.   Treating ADHD and EDs
    1.   ADHD and the EDs do co-occur with each other. Stimulants not only can be used in patients with BN or BED to treat the ADHD, they may also be helpful for the binge eating as well.
    2.   A major danger in this area is misdiagnosis. Other comorbidity that can be associated with alterations in attention, concentration and/or arousal, such as MDD, PTSD, and dissociative disorders, can be misdiagnosed as ADHD, particularly in children.
X.   Treating Schizophrenia and EDs
    1.   Schizophrenia and an ED occasionally also co-occur with each other, which presents particular challenges given the propensity of atypical antipsychotic agents to stimulate appetite, binge eating and subsequent weight gain (156). CBT may be particularly necessary and useful in this clinical combination.

TABLE 3 Specific Agents in the Management of EDs with Comorbidity

A. Specific Antidepressants and EDs

Fluoxetine: is the best studied of the selective serotonin reuptake inhibitors (SSRIs) in the treatment of EDs. It is proven effective for the acute and prophylactic treatment of BN and for the prophylactic treatment of AN. It is the only SSRI with an FDA indication for BN. It is also indicated for MDD, OCD, panic disorder (PD), and premenstrual dysphoric disorder (PMDD).

Sertraline: has not been studied in BN or AN, but there has been one positive study in BED (157). Sertraline has FDA indications for MDD, OCD, PD, social anxiety disorder, PTSD, PMDD.

Paroxetine: has not been studied in EDs. It has FDA indications for MDD, OCD, panic D/O, social anxiety disorder, and PTSD. Reportedly SSRI is associated with the most long-term weight gain and also potentially severe withdrawal. For this reason the sustained release form is the best choice.

Fluvoxamine: One negative study in BN; one positive study in BED (1587); FDA indication for OCD only.

Citalopram and *escitalopram*: have not been studied in the EDs, but are the most potent and specific SSRIs. Both agents have an FDA indication for MDD.

Venlafaxine: is a Serotonin-norepinephrine reuptake inhibitor (SNRI), but it has not been studied in the EDs. It has FDA indications for MDD, GAD, and social anxiety disorder; good in refractory MDD and comorbid depression–anxiety. Sustained release form best. Can raise blood pressure. May have antiobsessional effects, but a DBPC study has not been reported (159).

Nefazodone: is a serotonin antagonist and serotonin–norepinephrine reuptake inhibitor (SASNRI), which has also not been studied in the EDs. However, nefazodone is an excellent medication for the treatment of PTSD as well as anxious depression. FDA indication for MDD; Good in anxious depression; positive effects in PTSD; normalizes sleep; little or no sexual side effects or activation. Recent reports of liver failure during first 6 months of treatment have discouraged the use of this antidepressant. Total dose can effectively be given at bedtime.

Mirtazapine: is a serotonin antagonist norepinephrine agonist reuptake inhibitor (SANARI) that also has not been studied in the EDs; FDA indication for MDD; increases appetite; sedative. Effects on obsessionality not studied but not promising.

Bupropion: is a norepinephrine–dopamine reuptake inhibitor (NDRI), which is contraindicated in the EDs due to a high rate of seizures in BN trials. It has little or no antianxiety or antiobsessional effects. Recent DBPC study shows significant weight loss in obesity (160).

Reboxitene: is a norepinephrine reuptake inhibitor (NRI) that has not been studied in the EDs, although there are case reports (161). Although not on the market in the United States, it is available in more than 50 countries.

Phototherapy: or light therapy may potentiate both the antidepressant and antibulimic efficacy of antidepressants in selected ED patients with seasonal affective disorder (SAD) or a seasonal pattern of ED symptomatology (162).

Atomoxetine: is a new serotonin–norepinephrine reuptake inhibitor (SNRI) marked for the management of ADHD, which has not been studied in the EDs. FDA indication for ADHD.

TABLE 3 Continued

B. Antipsychotics and EDs
1. Useful in comorbid psychotic states (psychotic depression, bipolar mania, schizophrenia), severe PTSD/dissociative states, severe aggressive or impulsive behaviors, BPD.
2. Typical v. atypical agents: Atypical antipsychotic agents are associated with weight gain and moderate to marked sedation. However, they may have powerful antianxiety, antidepressant, antimanic, antiaggression and antidissociative effects, and can be used effectively in combination with antidepressants for a variety of conditions and symptoms. On the negative side these agents, particularly those that stimulate appetite the most, may destabilize BN. We reported on one patient who had paranoid schizophrenia, OCD, and bulimia nervosa and who was stable on thiothixene but then became acutely and severely bulimic again following a switch to clozapine (156).
3. Atypical agents include:
    a. Clozapine: has marked appetite-stimulating effects.
    b. Risperidone: has moderate appetite-stimulating effects, but more likely to cause EPS.
    c. Olanzapine: has marked appetite-stimulating effects.
    d. Quetiapine: has mild appetite-stimulating effects.
    e. Ziprasidone: has mild appetite-stimulating effects, but can cause QTc elongation on ECG.
    f. Aripiprazole: has mild appetite stimulating effects.
C. Anticonvulsants and EDs
1. Useful in comorbid bipolar disorder, other psychotic conditions, epilepsy, severe or refractory PTSD/dissociation, aggression and impulsivity, and the mood dysregulation of BPD.
2. Preferred agents:
    a. Topiramate: recent studies show independent efficacy in BN, BED and obesity (163 unpublished results),; blood levels not required.
    b. Valproic acid: FDA approved for bipolar disorder; blood levels required; associated with weight gain; associated with ovarian cysts in epileptic patients.
    c. Carbamazepine: blood levels required; less weight gain than with valproic acid; possible leukopenia.
    d. Oxcarbamazepine: better tolerated than carbamazepine; relatively weight gain neutral; blood levels not required.
    e. Lamotrigine: FDA approved for bipolar disorder; danger of severe life-threatening rash, including Stevens–Johnson syndrome and toxic epidermal necrolysis especially in children and adolescents; relatively weight gain neutral; blood levels not required.
    f. Gabapentin: not effective for bipolar disorder in DBPC trials, but may be helpful for anxiety and pain syndromes; blood levels not required; may cause weight gain.
D. Opiate Antagonists and EDs
1. Naltrexone:
    a. May have some effect in BN and AN, especially adjunctively with SSRI's (164,165).

TABLE 3 Continued

      b.   Useful for impulsive, self-mutilative, or self-destructive behaviors, e.g., cutting, burning, skin picking, hair pulling.

      c.   Useful for alcohol craving, opiate abuse, and bulimic behaviors.

E.   Benzodiazepines and EDs

   1.   *Lorazepam* and *clonazepam*: can be useful for the *short-term* management of severe eating-related anxiety, panic attacks or symptoms, and severe non-eating-related anxiety unresponsive to anxiety reduction techniques, supportive and cognitive–behavioral psychotherapy and antidepressants.

   2.   Careful monitoring of overuse is warranted given the potential to induce dependence with long-term use.

   3.   Avoid, if possible, in patients with SUDs or high impulsivity histories (personal and family).

   4.   Not useful in acute PTSD; can be countertherapeutic, especially during CBT with exposure.

F.   Stimulants and EDs:

   1.   One of the major problems with the use of stimulants is their propensity to decrease appetite and weight, particularly in the short term, which can be problematic for the AN patient but immensely helpful in the comorbid ADHD patient with a bulimic disorder or symptoms. Stimulants may augment antidepressant effects of antidepressant medications and can potentially aggravate a manic or psychotic process. Comorbid patients with SUDs or risk of SUD should be monitored closely but not necessarily denied from treatment. Studies show proper stimulant use in ADHD actually leads to a subsequent decreased risk of SUD (166).

   2.   Available agents include:

      a.   Methylphenidate: is a stimulant that, unlike the amphetamines, produces no increase in serotonin transmission; it exerts many of its effects through dopamine uptake blockade, in contrast to the amphetamines that primarily release dopamine (see Chapter 11).

      b.   Amphetamine Salts: amphetamines exert many of their effects through primary release of dopamine, but they can also increase serotonergic neurotransmission.

      c.   Methamphetamine

      d.   Dexedrine

      e.   Atomoxetine: is a serotonin–norepinephrine reuptake inhibitor with stimulant properties that may be a good choice for ED patients prone to substance abuse. However, like other reuptake inhibitors in the treatment of AN, it is not likely to work well in underweight patients. Its antidepressant, antianxiety, antibulimic effects remain to be elucidated, and it might be considered to have anti-impulsivity effects given its effectiveness in ADHD.

supported by most practice guidelines; drug treatment is usually ineffective when used alone in ED patients, especially in those with trauma-related comorbidity. The typical psychopharmacological agents used in the management of EDs are extensively reviewed in Chapter 21, but specific aspects related to how these common agents are used to manage comorbid disorders are briefly reviewed in Table 3.

Overall, these principles and recommended guidelines might serve as a useful blueprint for building a more specific treatment plan geared to the needs of the individual patient and her particular display of comorbidity within a developmental and biopsychosocial context.

REFERENCES

1. Kessler RC, Sonnega A, Bromet E, Hughes M, Nelson CB. Posttraumatic stress disorder in the National Comorbidity Survey. Arch Gen Psychiatry 1995; 52:1048–1060.
2. Kessler RC, Davis CG, Kendler KS. Childhood adversity and adult psychiatric disorder in the US National Comorbidity Survey. Psychol Med 1997; 27:1101–1119.
3. Kessler RC. Posttraumatic stress disorder: the burden to the individual and to society. J Clin Psychiatry 2000; 61(Suppl 5):4–12; discussion 13–14.
4. Bremner JD. Does Stress Damage the Brain? Understanding Trauma-Related Disorders from a Neurological Perspective. New York: W.W. Norton & Company, 2002.
5. Felitti VJ, Anda RF, Nordenberg D, Williamson DF, Spitz AM, Edwards V, Koss MP, Marks JS. Relationship of childhood abuse and household dysfunction to many of the leading causes of death in adults. The Adverse Childhood Experiences (ACE) Study. Am J Prev Med 1998; 14:245–258.
6. Kendall-Tackett K. The health effects of childhood abuse: four pathways by which abuse can influence health. Child Abuse Neglect 2002; 26:715–729.
7   Kaufman J, Charney D. Effects of early stress on brain structure and function: implications for understanding the relationship between child maltreatment and depression. Develop Psychopathol 2001; 13:451–471.
8. Keys A, Brozek J, Henschel A, Mickelsen O, Taylor HL. The Biology of Human Starvation. Minneapolis: University of Minnesota Press, 1950.
9. Kessler RC, McGonagle KA, Zhao S, Nelson CB, Hughes M, Eshleman S, Wittchen HU, Kendler KS. Lifetime and 12-month prevalence of DSM-III-R psychiatric disorders in the United States. Results from the National Comorbidity Survey. Arch Gen Psychiatry 1994; 51:8–19.
10. Resnick HS, Kilpatrick DG, Dansky BS, Saunders BE, Best CL. Prevalence of civilian trauma and posttraumatic stress disorder in a representative national sample of women. J Consult Clin Psychol 1993; 61:984–991.
11. Duncan RD, Saunders BE, Kilpatrick DG, Hanson RF, Resnick HS. Childhood physical assault as a risk factor for PTSD, depression, and substance

abuse: findings from a national survey. Am J Orthopsychiatry 1996; 66:437–448.

12. Kendler K, Bulik C. Childhood sexual abuse and adult psychiatric and substance abuse disorders in women. Arch Gen Psychiatry 2000; 57:953–959.

13. Wonderlich SA, Brewerton TD, Jocic Z, Dansky BS, Abbott DW. The relationship of childhood sexual abuse and eating disorders: a review. J Am Acad Child Adol Psychiatry 1997; 36:1107–1115.

14. Dansky BS, Brewerton TD, O'Neil PM, Kilpatrick DG. The National Women's Study: relationship of crime victimization and PTSD to bulimia nervosa. Int J Eat Disord 1997; 21:213–228.

15. Brewerton TD, Dansky BS, Kilpatrick DG, O'Neil PM. Bulimia nervosa, PTSD and "forgetting": results from the National Women's Study. In: Williams LM, Banyard VL, eds. Trauma and Memory. Durham: Sage Publications, 1999:127–138.

16. Molinari E. Eating disorders and sexual abuse. Eating and Weight Disorders: EWD 2001; 6:68–80.

17. Smolak L, Murnen SK. A meta-analytic examination of the relationship between child sexual abuse and eating disorders. Int J Eat Disord 2002; 31:136–150.

18. Kenardy J, Ball K. Disordered eating, weight dissatisfaction and dieting in relation to unwanted childhood sexual experiences in a community sample. J Psychosom Res 1998; 44:327–337.

19. Romans SE, Gendall KA, Martin JL, Mullen PE. Child sexual abuse and later disordered eating: a New Zealand epidemiological study. Int J Eat Disord 2001; 29:380–392.

20. Gleaves DH, Eberenz KP, May MC. Scope and significance of posttraumatic symptomatology among women hospitalized for an eating disorder. Int J Eat Disord 1998; 24:147–156.

21. Matsunaga H, Kaye WH, McConaha C, Plotnicov K, Pollice C, Rao R, Stein D. Psychopathological characteristics of recovered bulimics who have a history of physical or sexual abuse. J Nerv Ment Dis 1999; 187:472–477.

22. Deep AL, Lilenfeld LR, Plotnicov KH, Pollice C, Kaye WH. Sexual abuse in eating disorder subtypes and control women: the role of comorbid substance dependence in bulimia nervosa. Int J Eat Disord 1999; 25:1–10.

23. Brown L, Russell J, Thornton C, Dunn S. Experiences of physical and sexual abuse in Australian general practice attenders and an eating disordered population. Aust N Z J Psychiatry 1997; 31:398–404.

24. Brown L, Russell J, Thornton C, Dunn S. Dissociation, abuse and the eating disorders: evidence from an Australian population. Aust N Z J Psychiatry 1999; 33:521–528.

25. Nagata T, Kiriike N, Iketani T, Kawarada Y, Tanaka H. History of childhood sexual or physical abuse in Japanese patients with eating disorders: relationship with dissociation and impulsive behaviours. Psychol Med 1999; 29: 935–942.

26. Nagata T, Kawarada Y, Kiriike N, Iketani T. Multi-impulsivity of Japanese

patients with eating disorders: primary and secondary impulsivity. Psychiatry Res 2000; 94:239–250.

27. Favaro A, Dalle Grave R, Santonastaso P. Impact of a history of physical and sexual abuse in eating disordered and asymptomatic subjects. Acta Psychiat Scand 1998; 97:358–363.

28. Striegel-Moore RH, Garvin V, Dohm FA, Rosenheck RA. Eating disorders in a national sample of hospitalized female and male veterans: detection rates and psychiatric comorbidity. Int J Eat Disord 1999; 25:405–414.

29. Lipschitz DS, Winegar RK, Hartnick E, Foote B, Southwick SM. Posttraumatic stress disorder in hospitalized adolescents: psychiatric comorbidity and clinical correlates. J Am Acad Child Adol Psychiatry 1999; 38:385–392.

30. Neumark-Sztainer D, Story M, Hannan PJ, Beuhring T, Resnick MD. Disordered eating among adolescents: associations with sexual/physical abuse and other familial/psychosocial factors. Int J Eat Disord 2000; 28:249–258.

31. Wonderlich SA, Crosby RD, Mitchell JE, Roberts JA, Haseltine B, DeMuth G, Thompson KM. Relationship of childhood sexual abuse and eating disturbance in children. J Am Acad Child Adol Psychiatry 2000; 39:1277–1283.

32. Thompson KM, Wonderlich SA, Crosby RD, Mitchell JE. Sexual victimization and adolescent weight regulation practices: a test across three community based samples. Child Abuse Neglect 2001; 25:291–305.

33. Ackard DM, Neumark-Sztainer D, Hannan PJ, French S, Story M. Binge and purge behavior among adolescents: associations with sexual and physical abuse in a nationally representative sample: the Commonwealth Fund survey. Child Abuse Neglect 2001; 25:771–785.

34. Edgardh K, Ormstad K. Prevalence and characteristics of sexual abuse in a national sample of Swedish seventeen-year-old boys and girls. Acta Paediatrica 2000; 89:310–319.

35. Swanston HY, Tebbutt JS, O'Toole BI, Oates RK. Sexually abused children 5 years after presentation: a case-control study. Pediatrics 1997; 100:600–608.

36. Grilo CM, Masheb RM. Childhood psychological, physical, and sexual maltreatment in outpatients with binge eating disorder: frequency and associations with gender, obesity, and eating-related psychopathology. Obesity Res 2001; 9: 320–325.

37. Striegel-Moore RH, Dohm FA, Pike KM, Wilfley DE, Fairburn CG. Abuse, bullying, and discrimination as risk factors for binge eating disorder. Am J Psychiatry 2002; 159:1902–1907.

38. Johnson JG, Cohen P, Kasen S, Brook JS. Childhood adversities associated with risk for eating disorders or weight problems during adolescence or early adulthood. Am J Psychiatry 2002; 159:394–400.

39. Kent A, Waller G, Dagnan D. A greater role of emotional than physical or sexual abuse in predicting disordered eating attitudes: the role of mediating variables. Int J Eat Disord 1999; 25:159–167.

40. Kent A, Waller G. Childhood emotional abuse and eating psychopathology. Clin Psychol Rev 2000; 20:887–903.

41. Kinzl JF, Mangweth B, Traweger CM, Biebl W. Eating-disordered behavior in

males: the impact of adverse childhood experiences. Int J Eat Dis 1997; 22: 131–138.

42. Favaro A, Rodella FC, Santonastaso P. Binge eating and eating attitudes among Nazi concentration camp survivors. Psychol Med 2000; 30:463–466.

43. Andrews B. Bodily shame in relation to abuse in childhood and bulimia: a preliminary investigation. Br J Clin Psychol 1997; 36(Pt 1):41–49.

44. Wonderlich S, Crosby R, Mitchell J, Thompson K, Redlin J, Demuth G, Smyth J. Pathways mediating sexual abuse and eating disturbance in children. Int J Eat Disord 2001; 29:270–279.

45. Wonderlich SA, Crosby RD, Mitchell JE, Thompson KM, Redlin J, Demuth G, Smyth J, Haseltine B. Eating disturbance and sexual trauma in childhood and adulthood. Int J Eat Disord 2001; 30:401–412.

46. Murray C, Waller G. Reported sexual abuse and bulimic psychopathology among nonclinical women: the mediating role of shame. Int J Eat Disord 2002; 32:186–191.

47. Waller G, Meyer C, Ohanian V, Elliott P, Dickson C, Sellings J. The psychopathology of bulimic women who report childhood sexual abuse: the mediating role of core beliefs. J Nerv Ment Dis 2001; 189:700–708.

48. Waller G. Perceived control in eating disorders: relationship with reported sexual abuse. Int J Eat Disord 1998; 23:213–216.

49. Brady KT, Killeen TK, Brewerton T, Lucerini S. Comorbidity of psychiatric disorders and posttraumatic stress disorder. J Clin Psychiatry 2000; 61(suppl 7): 22–32.

50. Kaplan MJ, Klinetob NA. Childhood emotional trauma and chronic posttraumatic stress disorder in adult outpatients with treatment-resistant depression. J Nerv Ment Dis 2000; 188:596–601.

51. Heim C, Nemeroff CB. The role of childhood trauma in the neurobiology of mood and anxiety disorders: preclinical and clinical studies. Biol Psychiatry 2001; 49:1023–1039.

52. Penza KM, Heim C, Nemeroff CB. Neurobiological effects of childhood abuse: implications for the pathophysiology of depression and anxiety. Arch Women's Ment Health 2003; 6:15–22.

53. Hexel M, Sonneck G. Somatoform symptoms, anxiety, and depression in the context of traumatic life experiences by comparing participants with and without psychiatric diagnoses. Psychopathology 2002; 35:303–312.

54. Gladstone G, Parker G, Wilhelm K, Mitchell P, Austin MP. Characteristics of depressed patients who report childhood sexual abuse. Am J Psychiatry 1999; 156:431–437.

55. Levitan RD, Parikh SV, Lesage AD, Hegadoren KM, Adams M, Kennedy SH, Goering PN. Major depression in individuals with a history of childhood physical or sexual abuse: relationship to neurovegetative features, mania, and gender. Am J Psychiatry 1998; 155:1746–1752.

56. Brown L. Child physical and sexual abuse and eating disorders: a review of the links and personal comments on the treatment process. Aust N Z J Psychiatry 1997; 31:194–199.

57. Safren SA, Gershuny BS, Marzol P, Otto MW, Pollack MH. History of childhood abuse in panic disorder, social phobia, and generalized anxiety disorder. J Nerv Ment Dis 2002; 190:453–456.

58. Flisher AJ, Kramer RA, Hoven CW, Greenwald S, Alegria M, Bird HR, Canino G, Connell R, Moore RE. Psychosocial characteristics of physically abused children and adolescents. J Am Acad Child Adol Psychiatry 1997; 36:123–131.

59. Stein MB, Walker JR, Anderson G, Hazen AL, Ross CA, Eldridge G, Forde DR. Childhood physical and sexual abuse in patients with anxiety disorders and in a community sample. Am J Psychiatry 1996; 153:275–277.

60. Engel CC Jr, Walker EA, Katon WJ. Factors related to dissociation among patients with gastrointestinal complaints. J Psychosom Res 1996; 40:643–653.

61. Trowell J, Ugarte B, Kolvin I, Berelowitz M, Sadowski H, Le Couteur A. Behavioural psychopathology of child sexual abuse in schoolgirls referred to a tertiary centre: a North London study. Europ Child Adol Psychiatry 1999; 8:107–116.

62. Dykman RA, McPherson B, Ackerman PT, Newton JE, Mooney DM, Wherry J, Chaffin M. Internalizing and externalizing characteristics of sexually and/or physically abused children. Integr Physiol Behav Sci 1997; 32:62–74.

63. Cochrane CE, Malcolm R, Brewerton TD. Eating disorders in cocaine abusers. Addictive Dis 1998; 23:1–7.

64. Gross H, Ebert MH, Faden VB, Goldberg SC, Kaye WH, Caine ED, Hawks R, Zinberg N. A double-blind trial of delta 9-tetrahydrocannabinol in primary anorexia nervosa. J Clin Psychopharmacol 1983; 3:165–171.

65. Kessler RC, Crum RM, Warner LA, Nelson CB, Schulenberg J, Anthony JC. Lifetime co-occurrence of DSM-III-R alcohol abuse and dependence with other psychiatric disorders in the National Comorbidity Survey. Arch Gen Psychiatry 1997; 54:313–321.

66. Dansky BS, Brewerton TD, Kilpatrick DG. Comorbidity of bulimia nervosa and alcohol use disorders: results from the National Women's Study. Int J Eat Disord 2000; 27:180–190.

67. Putnam F, Guroff JJ, Silberman EK, Barban L, Post RM. The clinical phenomenology of multiple personality disorder: a review of 100 cases. J Clin Psychiatry 1986; 47:285–293.

68. Putnam F. Dissociation in Children and Adolescents: A Developmental Perspective. New York: Guilford Press, 1997.

69. Torem MS. Dissociative states presenting as an eating disorder. Am J Clin Hypnosis 1986; 29:137–142.

70. Torem MS. Covert multiple personality underlying eating disorders. Am J Psychotherapy 1990; 44:357–368.

71. Torem MS. Eating disorders in patients with multiple personality disorder. In: Kluft RP, Fine CG, eds. Clinical Perspectives on Multiple Personality Disorder. Washington, DC: American Psychiatric Press, 1993:343–353.

72. Demitrack MA, Putnam FW, Brewerton TD, Brandt HA, Gold PW. Dis-

sociative phenomena in eating disorders: relationship to clinical variables. Am J Psychiatry 1990; 147:1184–1188.

73. Goodwin JM, Attias R. Eating disorders in survivors of multimodal childhood abuse. In: Kluft RP, Fine CG, eds. Clinical Perspectives on Multiple Personality Disorder. Washington, D.C.: American Psychiatric Press, 1993:327–341.

74. Abraham SF, Beaumont PJV. How patients describe bulimia or binge eating. Psychol Med 1984; 12:625–635.

75. Everill J, Waller G, Macdonald W. Dissociation in bulimic and non-eating-disordered women. Int J Eat Disord 1995; 17:127–134.

76. Tobin DL, Molteni AL, Elin MR. Early trauma, dissociation, and late onset in the eating disorders. Int J Eat Disord 1995; 17:305–308.

77. Valdiserri S, Kihlstrom JF. Abnormal eating and dissociative experiences. Int J Eat Disord 1995; 17:373–380.

78. Gleaves DH, Eberenz KP. Correlates of dissociative symptoms among women with eating disorders. J Psychiatr Res 1995; 29:417–426.

79. Vanderlinden J, Spinhoven P, Vandereycken W, van Dyck R. Dissociative and hypnotic experiences in eating disorder patients: an exploratory study. Am J Clin Hypnosis 1995; 38:97–108.

80. Nagata T, Kiriike N, Iketani T, Kawarada Y, Tanaka H. History of childhood sexual or physical abuse in Japanese patients with eating disorders: relationship with dissociation and impulsive behaviours. Psychol Med 1999; 29:935–942.

81. Farrington A, Waller G, Neiderman M, Sutton V, Chopping J, Lask B. Dissociation in adolescent girls with anorexia: relationship to comorbid psychopathology. J Nerv Ment Dis 2002; 190:746–751.

82. Zebre KJ. Selves that starve and suffocate: the continuum of eating disorders and dissociative phenomena. Bull Menninger Clin 1993; 57:319–327.

83. Levin AP, Kahan M, Lamm JB, Spauster E. Multiple personality in eating disorder patients. Int J Eat Disord 1993; 13:235–239.

84. Greenes D, Fava M, Cioffi J, Herzog DB. The relationship of depression to dissociation in patients with bulimia nervosa. J Psychiatr Res 1993; 27:133–137.

85. Vanderlinden J, Vandereycken W, van Dyck R, Vertommen H. Dissociative experiences and trauma in eating disorders. Int J Eat Disord 1993; 13:187–193.

86. Santonastaso P, Favaro A, Olivotto MC, Friederici S. Dissociative experiences and eating disorders in a female college sample. Psychopathology 1997; 30:170–176.

87. Meyer C, Waller G. Dissociation and eating psychopathology: gender differences in a nonclinical population. Int J Eat Disord 1998; 23:217–221.

88. Nijenhuis ER, van Dyck R, Spinhoven P, van der Hart O, Chatrou M, Vanderlinden J, Moene F. Somatoform dissociation discriminates among diagnostic categories over and above general psychopathology. Aust N Z J Psychiatry 1999; 33:511–520.

89. Bienvenu OJ, Samuels JF, Riddle MA, Hoehn-Saric R, Liang KY, Cullen BA, Grados MA, Nestadt G. The relationship of obsessive-compulsive disorder to possible spectrum disorders: results from a family study. Biol Psychiatry 2000; 48:287–293.

90. Rabe-Jablonska Jolanta J, Sobow Tomasz M. The links between body dysmorphic disorder and eating disorders. Eur Psychiatry. J Assoc Eur Psychiatrists 2000; 15:302–305.

91. Grant JE, Kim SW, Eckert ED. Body dysmorphic disorder in patients with anorexia nervosa: prevalence, clinical features, and delusionality of body image. Int J Eat Disord 2002; 32:291–300.

92. Lieb R, Zimmermann P, Friis RH, Hofler M, Tholen S, Wittchen HU. The natural course of DSM-IV somatoform disorders and syndromes among adolescents and young adults: a prospective-longitudinal community study. Eur Psychiatry J Assoc Eur Psychiatrists 2002; 17:321–331.

93. Nierenberg AA, Phillips KA, Petersen TJ, Kelly KE, Alpert JE, Worthington JJ, Tedlow JR, Rosenbaum JF, Fava M. Body dysmorphic disorder in outpatients with major depression. J Affect Dis 2002; 69:141–148.

94. Imbierowicz K, Egle UT. Childhood adversities in patients with fibromyalgia and somatoform pain disorder. Eur Journal Pain 2003; 7:113–119.

95. Roelofs K, Keijsers GP, Hoogduin KA, Naring GW, Moene FC. Childhood abuse in patients with conversion disorder. Am J Psychiatry 2002; 159:1908–1913.

96. Farley M, Patsalides BM. Physical symptoms, posttraumatic stress disorder, and healthcare utilization of women with and without childhood physical and sexual abuse. Psychol Rep 2001; 89:595–606.

97. Sansone RA, Gaither GA, Sansone LA. Childhood trauma and adult somatic preoccupation by body area among women in an internal medicine setting: a pilot study. Int J Psychol Med 2001; 31:147–154.

98. George MS, Brewerton TD, Cochrane CE. Trichotillomania, trichophagy and bulimia nervosa. N Engl J Med 1990; 322:470–471.

99. Goldman MJ. Kleptomania: making sense of the nonsensical. Am J Psychiatry 1991; 148:986–996.

100. Baum A, Goldner EM. The relationship between stealing and eating disorders: a review. Harvard Review of Psychiatry 1995; 3:210–221.

101. McElroy SL, Hudson JI, Pope HG, Keck PE. Kleptomania: clinical characteristics and associated psychopathology. Psychol Med 1991; 21:93–108.

102. Favaro A, Santonastaso P. Self-injurious behavior in anorexia nervosa. J Nerv Ment Dis 2000; 188:537–542.

103. Paul T, Schroeter K, Dahme B, Nutzinger DO. Self-injurious behavior in women with eating disorders. Am J Psychiatry 2002; 159:408–411.

104. McElroy SL, Keck PE Jr, Phillips KA. Kleptomania, compulsive buying, and binge-eating disorder. J Clin Psychiatry 1995; 56(suppl 4):14–26; discussion 27.

105. Zlotnick C, Mattia JI, Zimmerman M. Clinical correlates of self-mutilation in a sample of general psychiatric patients. J Nerv Ment Dis 1999; 187:296–301.

106. Lowenstein LF. The etiology, diagnosis and treatment of the fire-setting behaviour of children. Child Psychiatry Hum Dev 1999–1999; 19:186–194.

107. McElroy SL, Phillips KA, Keck PE Jr. Obsessive compulsive spectrum disorder. J Clin Psychiatry 1994; 55(suppl):33–51; discussion 52–53.

108. Stein DJ. Neurobiology of the obsessive-compulsive spectrum disorders. Biol Psychiatry 2000; 47:296–304.

109. Hollander E, Rosen J. Impulsivity. J Psychopharmacol 2000; 14(suppl 1, 2): S39–S44.

110. Messman-Moore TL, Long PJ, Siegfried NJ. The revictimization of child sexual abuse survivors: an examination of the adjustment of college women with child sexual abuse, adult sexual assault, and adult physical abuse. Child Maltreatment 2000; 5:18–27.

111. Humphrey JA, White JW. Women's vulnerability to sexual assault from adolescence to young adulthood. J Adol Health 2000; 27:419–424.

112. Field NP, Classen C, Butler LD, Koopman C, Zarcone J, Spiegel D. Revictimization and information processing in women survivors of childhood sexual abuse. J Anxiety Disord 2001; 15:459–469.

113. Kellogg ND, Hoffman TJ. Child sexual revictimization by multiple perpetrators. Child Abuse Neglect 1997; 21:953–964.

114. Drimmer EJ. Stimulant treatment of bulimia nervosa with and without attention-deficit disorder: three case reports. Nutrition 2003; 19:76–77.

115. Sokol MS, Gray NS, Goldstein A, Kaye WH. Methylphenidate treatment for bulimia nervosa associated with a cluster B personality disorder. Int J Eat Disord 1999; 25:233–237.

116. Schweickert LA, Strober M, Moskowitz A. Efficacy of methylphenidate in bulimia nervosa comorbid with attention-deficit hyperactivity disorder: a case report. Int J Eat Disord 1997; 21:299–301.

117. Glod CA, Teicher MH. Relationship between early abuse, posttraumatic stress disorder, and activity levels in prepubertal children. J Am Acad Child Adol Psychiatry 1996; 35:1384–1393.

118. Hinshaw SP. Preadolescent girls with attention-deficit/hyperactivity disorder: I. Background characteristics, comorbidity, cognitive and social functioning, and parenting practices. J Consult Clin Psychol 2002; 70:1086–1098.

119. Heffron WM, Martin CA, Welsh RJ, Perry P, Moore CK. Hyperactivity and child abuse. Can J Psychiatry 1987; 32:384–386.

120. Cohen AJ, Adler N, Kaplan SJ, Pelcovitz D, Mandel FS. Interactional effects of marital status and physical abuse on adolescent psychopathology. Child Abuse Neglect. 2002; 26:277–288.

121. Thompson KM, Wonderlich SA, Crosby RD, Mitchell JE. The neglected link between eating disturbances and aggressive behavior in girls. J Am Acad Child Adol Psychiatry 1999; 38:1277–1284.

122. Geist R, Davis R, Heinmaa M. Binge/purge symptoms and comorbidity in adolescents with eating disorders. Can J Psychiatry 1998; 43:507–512.

123. Ford JD, Racusin R, Ellis CG, Daviss WB, Reiser J, Fleischer A, Thomas J. Child maltreatment, other trauma exposure, and posttraumatic symptomatology among children with oppositional defiant and attention deficit hyperactivity disorders. Child Maltreatment 2000; 5:205–217.

124. Ford JD, Racusin R, Daviss WB, Ellis CG, Thomas J, Rogers K, Reiser J, Schiffman J, Sengupta A. Trauma exposure among children with oppositional

defiant disorder and attention deficit-hyperactivity disorder. J Consult Clin Psychol 1999; 67:786–789.

125. Zaider TI, Johnson JG, Cockell SJ. Psychiatric comorbidity associated with eating disorder symptomatology among adolescents in the community. Intl J Eat Disord 2000; 28:58–67.

126. Johnson JG, Cohen P, Kotler L, Kasen S, Brook JS. Psychiatric disorders associated with risk for the development of eating disorders during adolescence and early adulthood. J Consult Clin Psychol 2002; 70:1119–1128.

127. Zanarini MC, Frankenburg FR, Dubo ED, Sickel AE, Trikha A, Levin A, Reynolds V. Axis I comorbidity of borderline personality disorder. Am J Psychiatry 1998; 155:1733–1739.

128. Yen S, Shea MT, Battle CL, Johnson DM, Zlotnick C, Dolan-Sewell R, Skodol AE, Grilo CM, Gunderson JG, Sanislow CA, Zanarini MC, Bender DS, Rettew JB, McGlashan TH. Traumatic exposure and posttraumatic stress disorder in borderline, schizotypal, avoidant, and obsessive-compulsive personality disorders: findings from the collaborative longitudinal personality disorders study. J Nerv Ment Dis 2002; 190:510–518.

129. Ruchkin VV, Schwab-Stone M, Koposov R, Vermeiren R, Steiner H. Violence exposure, posttraumatic stress, and personality in juvenile delinquents. J Am Acad Child Adol Psychiatry 2002; 41:322–329.

130. Shea MT, Zlotnick C, Dolan R, Warshaw MG, Phillips KA, Brown P, Keller MB. Personality disorders, history of trauma, and posttraumatic stress disorder in subjects with anxiety disorders. Compr Psychiatry 2000; 41:315–325.

131. Kaplan AS, Garfinkel PE. Difficulties in treating patients with eating disorders: a review of patient and clinician variables. Can J Psychiatry 1999; 44:665–670.

132. Zimmerman M, Mattia JI. Axis I diagnostic comorbidity and borderline personality disorder. Compr Psychiatry 1999; 40:245–252.

133. Zanarini MC, Gunderson JG, Frankenburg FR. Axis I phenomenology of borderline personality disorder. Compr Psychiatry 1989; 30:149–156.

134. Sullivan PF, Joyce PR, Mulder RT. Borderline personality disorder in major depression. J Nerv Ment Dis 1994; 182:508–516.

135. Johnson JG, Cohen P, Brown J, Smailes EM, Bernstein DP. Childhood maltreatment increases risk for personality disorders during early adulthood. Arch Gen Psychiatry 1999; 56:600–606.

136. Bell L. Does concurrent psychopathology at presentation influence response to treatment for bulimia nervosa? Eating Weight Disord 2002, 7.168–181.

137. Agras WS, Crow SJ, Halmi KA, Mitchell JE, Wilson GT, Kraemer HC. Outcome predictors for the cognitive behavior treatment of bulimia nervosa: data from a multi-site study. Am J Psychiatry 2000; 157:1302–1308.

138. Sohlberg S, Norring C, Holmgren S, Rosmark B. Impulsivity and long-term prognosis of psychiatric patients with anorexia nervosa/bulimia nervosa. J Nerv Ment Dis 1989; 177:249–258.

139. Anderson KP, LaPorte DJ, Brandt H, Crawford S. Sexual abuse and bulimia: response to inpatient treatment and preliminary outcome. J Psychiatr Res 1997; 31:621–633.

140. Kessler RC, Nelson CB, McGonagle KA, Liu J, Swartz M, Blazer DG. Comorbidity of DSM-III-R major depressive disorder in the general population: results from the US National Comorbidity Survey. Br J Psychiatry Suppl 1996; 30:17–30.

141. Pettinati HM, Horne RL, Staats JM. Hypnotizability in patients with anorexia nervosa and bulimia. Arch Gen Psychiatry 1985; 42:1014–1016.

142. Schoemaker C, Smit F, Bijl RV, Vollebergh WA. Bulimia nervosa following psychological and multiple child abuse: support for the self-medication hypothesis in a population-based cohort study. Intl J Eat Disord 2002; 32:381–388.

143. Garner DM, Garfinkel PE, eds. Handbook of Psychotherapy for Anorexia Nervosa and Bulimia. New York: Guilford Press, 1985.

144. Vandereycken W, Kog E, Vanderlinden J, eds. The Family Approach to Eating Disorders: Assessment and Treatment of Anorexia Nervosa and Bulimia. New York: PMA Publishing Corporation, 1989.

145. Smith KA, Fairburn CG, Cowen PJ. Symptomatic relapse in bulimia nervosa following acute tryptophan depletion. Arch Gen Psychiatry 1999; 56:171–176.

146. Cochrane CE, Brewerton TD, Hodges EL, Wilson D. Alexithymia in the eating disorders. Int J Eat Disord 1993; 14:219–222.

147. Feld R, Woodside DB, Kaplan AS, Olmsted MP, Carter JC. Pretreatment motivational enhancement therapy for eating disorders: a pilot study. Int J Eat Disord 2001; 29:393–400.

148. American Psychiatric Association. Practice guideline for the treatment of patients with borderline personality disorder. Am J Psychiatry 2001; 158(suppl 10):1–52.

149. Expert consensus guidelines for the treatment of posttraumatic stress disorder. J Clin Psych 1999; 60(suppl 16):6–76.

150. Ballenger JC, Davidson JR, Lecrubier Y, Nutt DJ, Foa EB, Kessler RC, McFarlane AC, Shalev AY. Consensus statement on posttraumatic stress disorder from the International Consensus Group on Depression and Anxiety. J Clin Psychiatry 2000; 61(Suppl 5):60–66.

151. Schnicke M, Resick PA. Cognitive Processing Therapy for Rape Victims: A Treatment Manual. London: Sage Publications, 1993.

152. Foa E, Rothbaum B. Treating the Trauma of Rape: Cognitive–Behavioral Therapy for PTSD. New York: Guilford Press, 2001.

153. Keane T, Foa E, Friedman M. Effective Treatments for PTSD: Practice Guidelines from the International Society for Traumatic Stress Studies. New York: Guilford Press, 2000.

154. Heflin AH, Deblinger E. Treating Sexually Abused Children and Their Nonoffending Parents: A Cognitive Behavioral Approach. London: Sage Publications, 1996.

155. Shapiro F. Eye Movement Desensitization and Reprocessing (EMDR). 2d ed. Basic Principles, Protocols, and Procedures. New York: Guilford Press, 2001.

156. Brewerton TD, Shannon M. Possible clozapine exacerbation of bulimia nervosa. Am J Psychiatry 1992; 149:1408–1409.

157. McElroy SL, Casuto LS, Nelson EB, Lake KA, Soutullo CA, Keck PE Jr, Hudson JI. Placebo-controlled trial of sertraline in the treatment of binge eating disorder. Am J Psychiatry 2000; 157:1004–1006.

158. Ricca V, Mannucci E, Mezzani B, Moretti S, Di Bernardo M, Bertelli M, Rotella CM, Faravelli C. Fluoxetine and fluvoxamine combined with individual cognitive–behaviour therapy in binge eating disorder: a one-year follow-up study. Psychother Psychosom 2001; 70:298–306.

159. Albert U, Aguglia E, Maina G, Bogetto F. Venlafaxine versus clomipramine in the treatment of obsessive-compulsive disorder: a preliminary single-blind, 12-week, controlled study. J Clin Psychiatry 2002; 63:1004–1009.

160. Anderson JW, Greenway FL, Fujioka K, Gadde KM, McKenney J, O'Neil PM. Bupropion SR enhances weight loss: a 48-week double-blind, placebo-controlled trial. Obesity Res 2002; 10:633–641.

161. El-Giamal N, de Zwaan M, Bailer U, Lennkh C, Schussler P, Strnad A, Kasper S. Reboxetine in the treatment of bulimia nervosa: a report of seven cases. Int Clin Psychopharmacol 2000; 15:351–356.

162. Lam RW, Lee SK, Tam EM, Grewal A, Yatham LN. An open trial of light therapy for women with seasonal affective disorder and comorbid bulimia nervosa. J Clin Psychiatry 2001; 62:164–168.

163. McElroy SL, Arnold LM, Shapira NA, Keck PE Jr, Rosenthal NR, Karim MR, Kamin M, Hudson JI. Topiramate in the treatment of binge eating disorder associated with obesity: a randomized, placebo-controlled trial. Am J Psychiatry 2003; 160:255–261.

164. Marrazzi MA, Bacon JP, Kinzie J, Luby ED. Naltrexone use in the treatment of anorexia nervosa and bulimia nervosa. Int Clin Psychopharmacol 1995; 10:163–172.

165. Neumeister A, Winkler A, Wober-Bingol C. Addition of naltrexone to fluoxetine in the treatment of binge eating disorder. Am J Psychiatry 1999; 156:797.

166. Wilens TE, Faraone SV, Biederman J, Gunawardene S. Does stimulant therapy of attention deficit/hyperactivity disorder beget later substance abuse? A meta-analytic review of the literature. Pediatrics 2003; 11:179–185.

167. Saunders BE, Berliner L, Hanson RF, Eds. Child Physical and Sexual Abuse: Guidelines for Treatment Final Report, January 15, 2003. Charleston, SC: National Crime Victims Research and Treatment Center, 2003.

23

Future Directions in the Management of Eating Disorders

Joel Yager
University of New Mexico School of Medicine
Albuquerque, New Mexico, U.S.A.

Making predictions about the future is fraught with uncertainty, and humility is always in order for those foolish enough to offer more than the most general of prognostications. Professional futurologists employ a variety of specific technical methods, including trend extrapolation, genius forecasting, consensus methods, simulations, cross-impact matrix methods, scenario building, decision trees, and creative disorder (a method that relies on innovations coming from grass-roots levels). None of these methods may be capable of capturing unanticipated events, known as "wild cards," or successfully anticipating their impacts. Lacking genius, a group capable of achieving consensus, and suitable simulations, the safest statements one can offer are based on trend analyses, and some imaginative scenario building and cross-matrix thinking (1,2).

A few lessons learned from futurist studies can guide our thinking about eating disorders treatment from the start: First, technical changes always occur more rapidly than social changes. Second, futurists usually tend to be more optimistic about the occurrence and rates of change, particularly social change, than is usually born out by history. Third, futurists tend to underestimate the expenses involved in producing the changes they envision. Fourth, to help put things into perspective, Arthur Clarke's three laws of the future should always be born in mind, to wit: (a) when a distinguished but elderly scientist says that something is possible, he is almost certainly right. When he states that something is impossible, he is very probably wrong. (b) The only way to discover the limits of the possible is to go beyond them to the impossible. (c) Any sufficiently advanced technology is indistinguishable from magic (3). With respect to medicine and psychiatry, the rapid advances in neuroimaging and genomics of the past few decades might seen like magic to those working in this field a few decades ago. Where "magical" technological advances will appear and how they will manifest in the next few decades can only be imagined. Where the funds and necessary public will come from to pay for the services that are likely to be possible, even demanded, is anyone's guess.

Thinking about future treatments requires that we consider the future of diagnosis, epidemiology, etiology, and pathogenesis, and how these shifts may translate to new treatments that take account of nutritional, medical, and psychobehavioral interventions, the settings in which care will be delivered, and the systems of care in which treatments are likely to occur. With the obvious caveat that anything I say about the future may turn out to be entirely wrong, the following trends seem to me to be most likely to influence how the future management of eating disorders will shape up.

THE FUTURE OF EATING DISORDERS DIAGNOSIS

Clearly, our current diagnostic schemes are, at best, works in progress, social constructions that attempt to connect sparse data points into functional categories. The DSM-IV and ICD-10 languages now employed are very recent, and there are many dissenters whose displeasure with contemporary nomenclature is freely voiced. Controversies about how eating disorders phenomena should be correctly lumped and split into meaningful syndromes and disorders, let alone diseases, are rampant and assure that the shape of eating disorders in DSM-V, probably a decade away, and ICD-10 will differ at least to some extent from what exists today. Since evidence-based treatments are supposed to be linked to valid diagnostic entities, the shape of treatment will be strongly influenced by the evolution (if not revolution) we can anticipate in diagnostics. Furthermore, since reimbursement for treatment is linked to diagnosis, definitions of where to set the bar are of great practical significance for patients, families, and clinicians.

In any era, psychological and biological treatments closely follow contemporary conceptual models of etiology and pathogenesis. Historically, psychological models and the psychotherapies they spawn have been noted to parallel the physical sciences of their times. Thus, Freudian and early behavioral models and their associated therapy metaphors loosely paralleled those of Newtonian mechanics and physics, including hydraulic and electrical theories of the late 19th century—how libidinal energy flowed from place to place. The middle to late 20th century saw psychological models loosely based on cognitive science and information theory. Future metaphors concerning the psychopathology and management of eating disorders are likely to be informed by models based on chaos and complexity theory, involving how complex adaptive subsystems of the brain organize, communicate, and change with various stressors and genetic unfoldings. We are likely to hear of psychological "strange attractors," phase transitions, and neural nets. At present, a diagnostic system for eating disorders based on fundamental understanding at the biological or bioecological level is not in sight, nor is it certain how long the field will have to wait for such a system to be achieved. However, we might anticipate that advances in functional as well as structural neuroimaging, genetic analyses, complex systems, information processing, and related cognitive sciences may lead to more discriminating diagnostic groupings based on meaning biological differences within similar phenotypes. For the foreseeable future, however, we will still rely on diagnostic systems based on clinical and laboratory observations—phenomenology.

Already, the process of reviewing current diagnostic thinking for DSM-V has begun. Particular attention will be paid to what has been called "bioecological" perspective, focusing on the first two decades of life, when rapid changes occur in behavior, emotion, and cognition. Considerable attention will be paid to developmental neuroscience, genetics, brain imaging, postmortem studies, and animal models (4).

Well-recognized gaps exist in current categorical methods for diagnosing personality disorders and their relationship with axis I disorders, and in the limited provisions for the diagnosis of relational disorders in the current nomenclature. These gaps have led to suggestions for dimensional classifications, at least for personality disorders. Relationships between mental disorders and measures of disability and impairment are likely to be revisited. Particularly salient for eating disorders, the relationships of cultural factors to psychopathology and the main cultural variables that operate in diagnostic processes will be carefully reconsidered.

Crossing this DSM-V matrix with emerging discussions in the literature, simple trend analysis suggests how several themes of the last several years may color future discussions about eating disorders diagnoses. First, with regard to nosological criteria, controversial questions have been raised regarding whether amenorrhea, included as a diagnostic criterion for anorexia nervosa from DSM-III on, should continue to be required as a criterion for anorexia nervosa (5). Since experienced clinicians have seen many cases of otherwise frank anorexia nervosa in which some degree of menstrual bleeding manages to persist, and since this finding appears to have little if any significance regarding course or outcome, amenorrhea may not be categorically required for distinctions between "caseness" and "noncaseness" of anorexia nervosa. In addition, controversies regarding whether the syndrome of binge eating disorder merits elevation from its current lowly position, lumped in the ED-NOS category, to official diagnostic status as a distinct entity will be better informed by studies in the next decade (6).

Regarding the relationship between axis II personality disorders and axis I disorders, the recent research of Westen and Harnden-Fischer is informative. Their studies support previous work suggesting that the course of anorexia nervosa is strongly related to comorbid personality configuration. To summarize, patients with perfectionistic personalities and few other personality quirks do best, whereas those with constricted and rigid personalities associated with cluster A and C disorders, and those with chaotic patterns usually associated with cluster B disorders, have much more difficult courses and are less likely to recover (7). So long as we rely on phenomenological-based nosology, careful delineation of diagnostic prototypes melding these sorts of characteristics linked to data on treatment response and outcomes may provide better diagnostic labels in the future.

Recent literature notes other clinical features that may work their way into future diagnostic schemes. One is the distinction accorded to so-called "typical" versus "atypical" anorexia nervosa. In the former, patients maintain the idea that they are too fat, holding fast to this cognitive distortion, almost to a delusional degree. In the latter, patients acknowledge that they are too thin but feel helpless to combat their ego-alien thoughts and behaviors. These distinctions, in some fashion parallel to the "delusional" versus "nondelusional" forms of body dysmorphic disorder, have been shown by Strober et al. to have prognostic significance (8). The "atypical" patients do somewhat better over the longer term, perhaps in part due to the fact that they are more willing to accept and participate in treatment.

Related to personality dimensions, typicality versus atypicality, and to assessment of disability and impairment, diagnostic thinking in the future may more routinely incorporate information regarding patients' stages of motivation for change (9), a paradigm extensively utilized in the field of addictions. Although much additional work is required to develop reliable and valid methods for assessing these stages, incorporating such concerns into diagnostic systems should improve treatment planning and prognosticating.

Finally, several murky diagnostic entities and relationships are likely to be clarified. The relationship of binge eating disorder to obesity, particularly medically serious class II and class III obesity, will be better delineated. Various types of night-eating syndrome, nocturnal eating disorders, and related conditions will be more carefully described and a better classification system for them will be developed.

THE FUTURE OF EATING DISORDERS EPIDEMIOLOGY

How will the prevalence of eating disorders and their distribution in communities change in the future? What sorts of associations with social, cultural, and community-based factors are likely to emerge? Although clear-cut predictions are no less risky than stock market predictions, several factors are likely to contribute to trends. First, in the United States, rates of obesity have been increasing substantially in spite of huge outcries from public health officials about the importance of proper diet and exercise. To the extent that eating disorders partly result from reactions against obesity-oriented tendencies, pressures to develop eating disorders will remain strong in the community at large and continue to affect those who are most vulnerable. Second, we can think about how shifting social pressures may affect vulnerability factors such as perfectionism, anxiety disorders, and depressive disorders. Might there be relationships between the extent to which Western society continues to provide increasing opportunities for self-fulfillment and individuation for women and the extent to which perfectionistic tendencies are unleashed in those who believe that excelling is of paramount importance? To what extent does today's society select for perfectionistic traits? Among the hypotheses recently advanced to account for a seemingly significant increase in the numbers of children with Asperger's disorder in California's Silicon Valley area is one based on the observation that many of these children emerge from families in which both parents were "computer nerds" (10). The question raised is whether the selective breeding of "nerds" is more likely to breed Asperger's children. In parallel fashion, to what extent do contemporary societal pressures increase the selective and assortative mating of perfectionistic men with perfectionistic women, thereby producing higher likelihoods of perfectionistic offspring vulnerable to anorexia nervosa? Are children with anorexia nervosa more likely to emerge from homes parented by hard-driving, status-seeking couples than from others?

In another vein, Sapolsky points to factors he believes are likely to contribute to his prediction of increased rates of major depression in society. He posits that ongoing rapid rates of social change and reductions in those social structures that probably counter depressogenic tendencies, signaling breakdown of community, add considerably to the stresses likely to produce depression (and, from our perspective, potentially eating disorders as well) (11). Factors include the increasing fragmentation of families into nuclear and one-parent families that lack easily accessible grandparents, aunts, uncles, and cousins as overstressed youth raised by overtaxed parents grow up. Absent the immediate availability of extended families, youth may miss the benefits afforded by the mediating, moderating, and supportive influences these other relatives may provide regarding how to live. Studies concerning the relative risk for eating disorders among adolescents raised in proximity to large extended families versus those reared in more isolated environments may illuminate this intriguing possibility.

Finally, it seems reasonable to predict that as globalization extends the ready availability of fat-rich foods, opportunities for individuation and personal choice, and the trend-setting influences of MTV and the Style Channel, the prevalence of eating disorders is likely to increase considerably in countries where these problems are now relatively uncommon. Such trends are evident from Becker et al.'s studies of the impact of introducing television in Fiji, where negative self-evaluations concerning weight and shape emerged among adolescent girls for whom these issues were previously unimportant (12). Future implications for prevention and developing intervention services are clear.

MOLECULAR GENETIC RESEARCH IN EATING DISORDERS: FUTURE IMPLICATION FOR TREATMENT

As detailed in other chapters, several lines of evidence suggest genetic vulnerability for eating disorders. These include high rates of familial transmission. Twin studies show rates of concordance approximately three times higher in identical twins than dizygotic twins, implying that both genetic and psychosocial factors are active. Monozygotic twins have roughly a 50% concordance rate for eating disorders (13). Exactly what is being inherited remains controversial and, clearly, genetics alone is not fully responsible. Rather, genetic factors appear to predispose, probably through effects on temperament, cognitive style, personality, mood regulating tendencies, set points for weight, and predispositions toward physical activity. Furthermore, still elusive, studies imply that variations in genetically mediated serotonin regulation may be important. Another hint pointing to genetic influence is the identification of genetically derived animal models of anorexia nervosa (such as "thin sow" disease—hyperactive sows that starve themselves, emerging during breeding experiments to produce thinner hogs) (14). As a result, active searches are underway to identify specific genes that may contribute to the appearance of eating disorders. Molecular genetic research on these disorders is in its infant stages. However, promising areas for future research have already been identified. These include genes involved with 5-hydroxytryptophan (5-HT, serotonin) receptors, specifically $5\text{-}HT_{2A}$, $5\text{-}HT_{2C}$, and $5\text{-}HT_{1B}$ receptors, uncoupling protein receptors (UCP-2/UCP-3), and estrogen β

receptors. Several large-scale linkage and association studies are underway (15–19). Recent advances in unraveling the mechanisms of weight control point to a crucial role of the melanocortin-4 receptor (MC4-r) systm in regulating body weight. The orexigenic neuropeptide agouti-related protein (AGRP), an MC4-r antagonist, has a crucial role in maintaining body weight by inducing food intake (20). But overall, the percentage of occurrence explained by currently studied genetic association is quite small. Furthermore, twin studies suggest that approximately 17–46% of the variance in both anorexia nervosa and bulimia nervosa can be accounted for by nonshared environmental factors (21). Future questions will concern subtle gene–nurture interactions, which vary with different environmental conditions throughout a person's lifelong development.

These genetic studies and the ones that will follow may ultimately lead to a sophisticated form of genetic profiling—gene scans—based on single-nucleotide polymorphisms, or SNPs ("snips") (22). Such scans will be able to easily run through the hundreds of genes now known to be involved in regulating aspects of intake, satiety, physical exercise, and emotional regulation, and the thousands still to be associated with these functions. The implications for prevention and treatment are many. Conceivably, SNP profiling may facilitate more accurate predictions about risk for diseases, including eating disorders, which may lead to sophisticated psychobehavioral–social and biological preventions and interventions. A cadre of health professionals (and, no doubt, many Web-based software programs) will be developed that specialize in genetic counseling based on SNP profiling. Respect for SNP-related temperamental vulnerabilities may encourage particularly susceptible individuals toward—or away from—risky pursuits, behaviors, and environments before onset, and toward modifications of diet, pharmafoods, sleep, and other more biologically based functions, all designed to stave off illnesses such as eating disorders. Conceivably, athletic and dance coaches, employers, and others may use such profiling to select and/or deselect individuals for participation in specific sports, vocations, and avocations. Furthermore, inventive genetic engineering may produce animal models of eating disorders that more closely resemble clinical disorders and that may further illuminate issues in pathogenesis and treatment.

OTHER FUTURE BIOLOGICAL INVESTIGATIONS IN EATING DISORDERS

To date, imaging studies have offered important leads in understanding and corroborating clinical observations, but as yet no findings have firmly established preexisting functional or structural abnormalities of the brain in patients with eating disorders. Studies in adolescents with anorexia nervosa showing that gray matter deficits (23) and unusual temporal lobe vascular flow asymmetries (24) are found during semistarvation and may persist following weight restoration await extension, replication, and confirmation. As yet, brain imaging studies of pre-disordered vulnerable populations have not been conducted. Future research utilizing emerging technologies including new iterations of nuclear magnetic resonance, diffusion tensor magnetic resonance imaging (DT-MRI), and functional MRI will provide increasingly detailed information about processes in the living brain. Findings from such imaging studies may help improve diagnostic subtyping and also enable clinicians to more precisely prognosticate the time and extent of recovery in individual cases.

Other emerging clinical laboratory assessment based on proteonomics, neurosteroids, and kinins will yield improved possibilities for understanding vulnerabilities and for offering prognoses regarding brain, bone, and reproductive functions and other critical aspects of eating disorder–related physiology.

THE FUTURE OF BIOLOGICAL INTERVENTIONS FOR EATING DISORDERS

It is likely that for anorexia nervosa and bulimia nervosa the principal biological intervention will continue to be good nutrition. How nutrients can best be delivered acceptably, effectively, and efficiently will drive research and practice. For example, controversies over the potential value of supplemental nasogastric feeding should be settled by controlled studies, not argued out as a matter of religious belief (25). Conceivably, technical devices that assist patients to eat by reminding them to do so in a timely fashion every few hours and that record and transmit eating and associated behaviors to a clinician may be employed via personal digital assistants (PDAs).

Until much more is known about biological contributions to the etiology of eating disorders, speculations about specific advances in pharmacological approaches must be circumspect. Genetic profiling may enable clinicians to tailor medication types and doses to individual patients in order to maximize effectiveness, minimize side effects, and avoid deleterious drug interactions. With eating disorder patients, depending on the actual clinical added value of such studies, it should be possible to more accurately assess gastrointestinal absorption, protein binding, and shifting volume distributions to better inform medication prescribing. New forms of medication delivery, such as the use of transdermal patches now being successfully employed with the monoamine oxidase inhibitor selegiline and other agents (26), may avert tyramine reactions, dietary restrictions, and other complications related to alterations in intestinal absorption in eating disorder patients.

Questions remain to be answered regarding the potential utility of atypical antipsychotic medications (including those that do not specifically have weight gain as a metabolic side effect, such as ziprazodone) on their own, and as adjunctive treatments for mood and obsessive-compulsive disorders associated with eating disorders. In addition to assessing the role of newer thymoleptics, exciting case reports appearing in the literature suggest that other agents to be investigated should include inositol (used for depression and obsessive-compulsive disorder) (27) and tramadol (28), among others. New classes of medications being developed for mood and anxiety disorders in particular are likely to be used for patients with eating disorders, initially "off label," and then, where interesting findings are obtained, in systematic clinical trials. The pipeline for new medications is large. Emerging new medications for mood disorders that may merit investigation for eating disorders include selective noradrenergic uptake inhibitors such as reboxetine; antiglucocorticoids such as mifepristone (RU486); corticotropin-releasing factor (CRF) antagonists and other neurosteroid-modulating agents; S-adenosylmethionine; the serotonin enhancer tianeptine; substance P antagonists and other agents affecting neurokinins; and reversible monoamine oxidase inhibitors such as moclobemide. Also of interest are new anxiolytics such as pregabalin, and talipexole, a dopamine D_2 and α_2-adrenergic agonist currently used for Parkinson's disease, now being studied for managing symptoms of dissociation and hyperarousal (29).

In addition to pharmacological treatments, other biological treatments using light therapy, vagus nerve stimulation and transcranial magnetic stimulation for associated depression, and other physiologically active procedures remain to be explored for specific types of complex eating disorders (30).

THE FUTURE OF PSYCHOSOCIAL INTERVENTIONS FOR EATING DISORDERS

Psychotherapies

Several trends can be identified. It is likely that research will continue on delineating evidence-based effective individual, family, and group psychotherapies for eating disorders, and on deconstructing and reassembling the underlying effective elements to give better guidance to practitioners facing complex clinical situations. Although these studies are expensive and difficult to carry out, a number of developments may facilitate such studies in the future. These include the development of multisite and, indeed, multinational clinical trials, permitting larger studies. In addition, one can envision the organization of intraprofession or multiprofession "practice research networks," essentially aggregations of up to several thousand practitioners organized to answer specific clinical questions in their practices. Such networks have already proven effective for answering clinical and health services research questions in pediatrics, family medicine, and psychiatry (31). While psychotherapies based on cognitive–behavioral and interpersonal psychotherapy models have been dominant, fusions of these approaches as in cognitive–analytical therapies are exciting. Motivational enhancement techniques, dialectic behavior therapy for complex, multi-impulsive patients, and experimental manual-based psychotherapies based on self-psychological theories are all being studied. Of particular interest are home-based treatments in which families are carefully trained and supervised in managing their child's eating behavior (so-called Maudsley model studies by Lock and colleagues) (32). The future will likely provide better guidance as to which therapies best suit each type of patients. As previously noted, new metapsychologies and accompanying psychotherapies are likely to emerge, paralleling discoveries in cognitive neuroscience, complexity theories, and other yet-to-be-delineated scientific paradigms.

THE IMPACT OF COMPUTERS AND INFORMATION TECHNOLOGY ON EATING DISORDERS MANAGEMENT

Exciting innovations in the management of eating disorders patients are likely to emerge from the application of computer and information technology to the management of eating disorders, particularly with the increasing availability of broad-band and wireless technologies. These technologies offer substantial capacity to extend care to eating disorder patients by enhancing the "four As" of contemporary health care—accessibility, affordability, affability, and accountability. Access is enhanced by providing convenience compatible with busy lifestyles, increasing contact time between patients and providers. Services to rural areas and home-bound populations are getting better with increasing broad-band technology. Affordable business plans are now being developed. Computers are clearly "affable"—increasingly user friendly, and often increasing ease of communication. Treatment programs delivered by computer are increasingly accountable, often based on evidence-based, focused therapies.

Information age health care has been conceived as operating on six separate tiers: individual self-care, friends and family, self-help networks, health professionals as facilitators, health professionals as partners, and health professionals as authorities (33). Information-age care for eating disorders is already operating on each of these levels and will undoubtedly expand in the future.

Individuals, Families and Friends, and Self-Help On-Line

For seeking information and care, these technologies seem well suited to eating disorders, especially as large proportions of youth are already on-line. According to recent figures, among all 15- to 24-year-olds, 90% have gone on-line, and one in four (24%) has gotten "a lot" of health information from the Internet. Among the 90% of all 15- to 24-year-olds who have ever gone on-line, 75% have used the Internet at least once to find health information and about one in four has looked up information on weight issues, mental health, drugs and alcohol, and violence (34).

A huge amount of information is currently available for the "on-line seeker," and information will predictably increase. In November 2002, one of the most popular search engines, Google, listed about 1,040,000 sites pertinent to eating disorders. Numerous organizations devoted to eating disorders are on-line. The Center for Counseling and Health Resources, an on-line clearinghouse, posted about 330 links related to eating disorders. Fortunately, the "top hits" on search engines include a large number of well-regarded sites. Easily accessed, too, are many commercial sites and personal web pages, some of which are very helpful, but among which are many of uncertain quality. In mid-2002 the top eating disorder sites listed on Google included Eating Disorders Awareness and Prevention (EDAP; now becoming National Eating Disorders Association), Something Fishy, Eating Disorders Mirror Mirror (Canada), ANRED, EDReferral.com, the Eating Disorders Association (England), the Harvard Eating Disorders Center, and the Academy for Eating Disorders. Although data to estimate the extent to which these sites are accessed are hard to obtain, one site, Something Fishy, indicated more than 2.9 million hits since 1995.

How good are these sites? Many questions remain concerning what criteria should be used to evaluate them. In the future, well-respected eating disorders organizations, such as the Academy for Eating Disorders, may take on the task of defining criteria by which to judge eating disorders sites using parameters such as their use of standard diagnostic criteria, the quality of information they provide about these conditions, the range of reputable treatment options they present, and the links they offer to reputable sources and facilities.

What do these sites provide? First, they provide considerable information about diagnostic criteria, permitting individuals to do reasonably good screenings for the existence of active or subclinical disorders in themselves or others. Second, they provide considerable information about the causes and courses of eating disorders, treatment, treatment resources, research, and clinical trials. Of importance, on-line sites offer considerable social and emotional support, personal narratives, chats, stories, poems, and memorials. One year-long qualitative study of an on-line support group assessed the emotional and social support provided (alt.support.eating-disord,[ASED]). The group developed its own rules, etiquette, and norms to create safe communications and support and to explicitly reduce competitiveness. The group provided a mix of problem solving and emotional support. In contrast to face-to-face support groups, the lack of physical cues and presence seemed to reduce competition regarding who is thinnest (35). Many other general and specific eating disorders groups appear on-line. For example, the sitehttp://www.healthyplace.com/Communities/Eating_Disorders/Site/comm_calender.htm offers 12 different types of eating disorder on-line support groups with different themes, including groups for eating disorder sufferers who also self-injure and groups for parents of children with eating disorders. Clearly such groups are not always available locally.

But some sites provide misinformation and misguidance. Of note, thanks to a vigorous campaign initiated by ANAD, many former "proanorexia" sites that appeared in abundance have been eliminated. However, some pro-anorexia messages may still be encountered, and may deleteriously influence and encourage young browsers who are intrigued and enchanted by the idea of becoming anorexic.

Given the extent to which patients, families, and friends are likely to be using the internet to acquire information about eating disorders, guidelines have been developed to assist clinicians in dealing with their "wired" patients. Clinicians are advised to be open minded and diplomatic about information patients bring in from their net searches, understanding that the patient wants more knowledge. Take the information seriously, discuss accurate and questionable issues, suggest other web sites that might help, and suggest that patients not act on information without consulting the provider (36).

Health Professionals as Facilitators, Partners, and Authorities

The evidence in favor of "distance medicine" is increasing. In a recent meta-analysis, 7 of 7 controlled clinical trials in general medicine showed positive outcomes, improved performance, or significant benefits from provider-initiated computerized communication. Problems concerned Alzheimer's caregivers, cardiac rehabilitation, and diabetes management (37). Available research suggests that distance treatments may be applicable for eating disorders as well.

The instruments available for offering computer-assisted services are constantly improving and increasing. Currently, they include stand-alone computers and PDAs, computer-based interviews, CD-ROM-based programs, PDA-based tracking and reminding programs, virtual reality programs, electronic communication via email, web-based programming, chats, audio- and video-phones, and telemedicine setups using telephone line–based videophones, T1 lines, and, soon, PC-based videophones.

Several forms of clinician-patient e-interactions have been described. They include e-therapy in which ongoing helping relationships take place solely via internet communication; mental health advice in which psychotherapists respond to one question in depth with communication taking place solely via internet; adjunct services in which internet or e-mail communications are used to supplement traditional, in-person treatment; and behavioral telepsychiatry which includes sophisticated videoconferencing for remote locations, as extensions of traditional clinic or hospital care. Currently, the extent to which these methods is employed varies considerably. E-mail (regular or encrypted) is used most commonly. Some clinicians now use secure web-based messaging. A few use real-time chats. Very few now use videoconferencing and voice-over-IP (Internet phone) (International Society for Online Mental Health, www.ismho.org; www.metanoia.org, May 2002). Future shifts in cost, availability, and dissemination of these various technologies will influence patterns of use in treating eating disorder patients. What follows are some illustrative examples of innovative works in progress that are likely to influence future practice and research.

Perhaps the most developed program using technology in relation to eating disorder–related issues is "Student Bodies," an e-intervention for weight- and shape-concerned college students (who do not have frank eating disorders) organized at Stanford University and San Diego State University, involving a large number of collaborating investigators. With the aim of reducing body dissatisfaction and eating disorder–related attitudes, these investigators have conducted a number of studies using Internet-delivered, computer-assisted programs (38–40). They have explored various combinations of therapeutic elements in 8-week psychoeducational programs that have included face-to-face group sessions for orientation, interactive text, audio, video, self-monitoring journals and behavior change exercises, weekly readings (CBT based), progress notes completed at each week's log-in, encouragement for the posting of weekly entries in on-line body image journals. They have explored the benefit of anonymity in groups and have also used moderated weekly asynchronous and synchronous (real-time) on-line groups in which discussions are linked to photos and personal statements of the other participants, fostering a sense of personal familiarity and connection. Studies using random assignments have compared on-line results with those of comparison groups participating in classroom forms of the program, "Body Traps," and wait-list controls. In general, students participating in the on-line groups have improved scores regarding eating concerns, eating restraint, and drive for thinness in student bodies. Results have been modestly effective for all participants and more useful for higher risk participants. Of importance, no harm occurred to participants. Not surprising, results corresponded with adherence to the program. Results for the classroom program were comparable to wait-list controls.

The lessons derived in these studies on factors that increase participant compliance, including ease of use, structure, reminders and prompts, will be useful to others establishing distance treatment in the future. Of importance are the complex clinical safety, legal, and ethical issues emerging in the context of computer-based treatments and distant medicine. These derive in part from the fact that clinicians do not have access to patients' nonverbal/behavioral cues, lack control over the participant's environment, and cannot assure the validity or accuracy of information, among other factors. These issues resemble problems of telephone encounters. Of particular concern, the potential for miscommunication and delayed response to clinical emergencies, such as postings of suicidal ideation, requires attention (41). In part, these concerns have been addressed by reminding and reiterating that on-line communications are not effective for crises, and by assuring that clinicians have accurate home and work phone numbers for patients.

Adjunctive Use of e-Mail in Ambulatory Treatment of Eating Disorder Patients

I have explored the potential use of employing frequent contact by e-mail as adjunctive treatment for ambulatory adolescents with anorexia nervosa. My experience with several dozen patients suggests that this intervention is particularly useful for restricting anorexia nervosa patients who have obsessional and perfectionistic traits. It is also helpful, but not as consistently used, by patients with binge eating–purging types of anorexia nervosa and with bulimia nervosa. The intervention is particularly helpful for patients living a distance from treatment centers. Patients are usually asked to record and e-mail details of their daily food intake (including calorie counts) and exercise-related caloric expenditure. They often add other personal comments. Phone calls and face-to-face visits are necessary for ongoing monitoring and especially when urgent issues emerge. Health Insurance Portability and Accountability Act of 1996 (HIPAA) regulations regarding privacy must be kept in mind (42).

Pilot studies to identify and treat patients with bulimia nervosa entirely by e-mail have been conducted by P. Robinson and M. A. Sefaty at the University of London. A group of 23 subjects with a high morbidity for eating disorder and depression symptoms were recruited via an e-mail solicitation, selected for a 3-month treatment trial, asked to e-mail twice weekly, and assigned for formal CBT or eclectic approach, which included diary keeping as well as interpersonal elements. These investigators found overall modest reductions in depression and eating disorder symptom scores. They surmised that their average results were less than would be anticipated from face-to-face treatment. Of note, as a result of these interventions most participants said they desired more therapy, primarily face to face (43).

Other Emerging Treatments

At the University of North Dakota work in progress involves the treatment of several patients with bulimia nervosa via telemedicine, using a 128-kbps ISDN line, a relatively "low tech" method. Feasibility for treatment has been demonstrated at 80 miles (44). Sansone has explored establishing carefully determined patient-to-patient connections via e-mail, essentially establishing e-mail "pen pals" to provide patients with additional emotional support. Careful matching of patients requires consideration of such factors as age, degree of isolation, personality traits, eating disorder diagnosis, and marital status. Thus far, he has not connected patients with clear-cut borderline personality disorders (45). In Germany, the University of Leipzig sponsors a professionally led, on-line information and consultation service for persons with eating disorders (www.ab-server.de) supported by a consortium of academic centers. This service has received several hundred requests for information in the few years it has been in existence.

Guided self-help programs, usually based on CBT treatment models, are increasingly studied and appear to be helpful for a substantial minority of patients as an important aspect of stepped care. These programs are widely available through easily acquired published workbooks, and will be increasingly administered by means of computer-aided self help programs using workbooks, monitoring, and feedback on CD-ROM or Internet (46,47). Future research to extend these models to include elements from interpersonal therapy, self-psychology, and other approaches seems warranted.

Emerging Technologies

Wireless two-way appliances increasingly used for chronic disease management, the so-called "personal health buddy," may be employed for eating disorders, facilitating reporting of eating , exercise, mood and associated features, and responses from clinicians (http://www.healthhero.com). Research conducted by Wonderlich et al. using personal digital assistants exemplifies these developments (48). Other emerging clinical applications include computer-based body image assessments (49,50) and virtual reality–based body image assessment and treatment (51).

Computer technology may provide better ways to train larger numbers of health professionals, families, and patients about eating disorders using well-established distance education models that integrate the Internet, audiotapes and videotapes, telephone supervision, etc. Such methods are already being used internationally (A. Parker, personal communication; A. Barriguete, personal communications).

Futuristic Applications

Further into the future, a number of additional applications may be developed, limited only by imagination, funding, and zeal. Of potential value for the management of eating disorders are the following possibilities: PDA-based intelligent agents linked to patient's cognitive style; voice, face, and emotion recognition artificial intelligence systems for computer-assisted self-guided therapy; outsourcing distance psychotherapy internationally in a global market; video-telemedicine for family therapy with disconnected families. Finally, research and treatment may be aided by sophisticated simulations capable of portraying increasingly complex models of individual and family dynamics. Envision future versions of "Sim Family," including the emergence of the Sims On-Line, permitting patients and families to demonstrate and work out important issues in family relationships (www.thesims.ea.com). This is not science fiction.

A cautionary note: Use of electronic communications and information technology in applications such as those described above introduces a huge set of confidentiality, patient safety, professional boundary, liability, and related ethical and legal concerns that must be carefully addressed through informed consents and practice protocols. All those writing in these fields emphasize these issues, and several offer important ethical and legal guidelines (52).

FUTURE SYSTEMS OF CARE FOR EATING DISORDERS

Substantial concerns exist concerning what systems of care may be available to treat and to fund the treatment of persons with eating disorders in the future. While resources and funding will vary from jurisdiction to jurisdiction (and, depending on insurance coverage, from family to family), overall it can be expected that resources will rarely meet needs and that services will be lacking in many communities. As parity legislation for severe mental disorders gradually works its way through state and federal agendas in the United States, and as severe eating disorders are gradually incorporated into the list of recognized biologically based disorders, the capacity to treat patients appropriately may increase. If funding is available, new, sorely needed treatment facilities may be created to care for currently underserved patients. The political will and efforts of family members of patients with severe eating disorders will be required to keep eating disorders needs on the minds and in the programs of those influential politicians, business persons, and health care administrators whose support will always be necessary to sustain the facilities and funding infrastructure necessary for treating patients. Recent appellate-court level judicial decisions that support insurance coverage based on medical rather than psychiatric benefits for treatment of malnutrition associated with severe eating disorders may be precedent setting and help patients, families, and clinicians obtain needed services (53).

Even if decent funding were to be made available, many communities lack appropriate facilities and health providers properly trained to assess and treat patients with severe eating disorders. Responsibility for increasing the availability of training opportunities will fall to academic centers and organizations with strong eating disorders capacities, and, as alluded to above, should be enhanced by the increasing availability of distance learning. However, distance learning will never substitute for live supervised clinical experience. Funding and incentives for training providers will determine the extent to which these needs are met in the future.

Regardless of the extent to which funding may improve, it should be clear that the costs of medical care will always increase so as to consume more than the available resources. No doubt, as technologically sophisticated methods for assessing genes, brains, and fluids become increasingly available, costs of care are likely to continue to increase substantially just to pay for these tests and procedures. However, the fact that new tests and treatments become available does not assure that they will necessarily contribute materially to better outcomes. Therefore, excellent judgment will always be required to ascertain the actual value of performing new procedures and treatments.

As the various health professionals involved in assessing and treating eating disorder patients continue to carefully observe and evaluate their experiences, ongoing attention will be required for continually revising, updating, and optimizing not only the evidence-based treatments and practices that command respect but also the judgment-infused future editions of practice guidelines. One hopes that tomorrow's practice guidelines will better delineate how collaborating health providers can best employ potential tests and treatments to assure that outcomes become progressively better for patients and their families. One also hopes that tomorrow's research, on which such recommendations will be based, will be guided by an unending supply of curiosity and increasingly sophisticated questions.

REFERENCES

1. Yager J. A futuristic view of psychiatry. In: Yager J, ed. The Future of Psychiatry as a Medical Specialty. Washington, DC: American Psychiatric Press, 1989:135–159.

2. Brockman J, ed., The Next Fifty Years: Science in the First Half of the Twenty-First Century. New York: Vintage, 2002.

3. Clarke AC. Technology and the future. In: Clarke AC, ed. Report on Planet Three. New York: Signet, 1972:129–141.

4. Kupfer DJ, First MB, Regier DA, eds. A Research Agenda for DSM-V. Washington, DC: American Psychiatric Association, 2002.

5. Garfinkel PE, Lin E, Goering P, Spegg C, Goldbloom D, Kennedy S, Kaplan AS, Woodside DB. Should amenorrhoea be necessary for the diagnosis of anorexia nervosa? Evidence from a Canadian community sample. Br J Psychiatry 1996; 168:500–506.

6. Pincus HA, First M. Critical differences between binge eating and overeating. Arch Gen Psychiatry 1999; 56:951.

7. Westen D, Harnden-Fischer J. Personality profiles in eating disorders: rethinking the distinction between axis I and axis II. Am J Psychiatry 2001; 158:547–562.

8. Strober M, Freeman R, Morrell W. Atypical anorexia nervosa: separation from typical cases in course and outcome in a long-term prospective study. Int J Eat Disord 1999; 25:135–142.

9. Rieger E, Touyz SW, Beumont PJ. The Anorexia Nervosa Stages of Change Questionnaire (ANSOCQ): information regarding its psychometric properties. Int J Eat Disord 2002; 32:24–38.

10. Silberman S. The Geek Syndrome: Autism—and its milder cousin Asperger's syndrome—is surging among the children of Silicon Valley. Are math-and-tech genes to blame? Wired Dec 2001; 9(12). http://www.wired.com/wired/archive/9.12/aspergers.html.

11. Sapolsky RM. Will we still be sad fifty years from now? In: Brockman J, ed. The Next Fifty Years: Science in the First Half of the Twenty-First Century. New York: Vintage Press, 2002:105–113.

12. Becker AE, Burwell RA, Gilman SE, Herzog DB, Hamburg P. Eating behaviours and attitudes following prolonged exposure to television among ethnic Fijian adolescent girls. Br J Psychiatry 2002; 180, 509–514.

13. Gorwood P, Bouvard M, Mouren-Simeoni MC, Kipman A, Ades J. Genetics and anorexia nervosa: a review of candidate genes. Psychiatr Genet 1998; 8(1):1–12.

14. Treasure JL, Owen JB. Intriguing links between animal behavior and anorexia nervosa. Int J Eat Disord 1997; 21:307–311.

15. Levitan RD, Kaplan AS, Masellis M, Basile VS, Walker ML, Lipson N, Siegel GI, Woodside DB, Macciardi FM, Kennedy SH, Kennedy JL. Polymorphism of the serotonin 5-HT$_{1B}$ receptor gene (HTR1B) associated with minimum lifetime body mass index in women with bulimia nervosa. Biol Psychiatry 2001; 50:640–643.

16. Westberg L, Bah J, Rastam M, Gillberg C, Wentz E, Melke J, Hellstrand M, Eriksson E. Association between a polymorphism of the 5-HT$_{2C}$ receptor and weight loss in teenage girls. Neuropsychopharmacology 2002; 26:789–793.

17. Klump KL, Kaye WH, Strober M. The evolving genetic foundations of eating disorders. Psychiatr Clin North Am 2001; 24:215–225.

18. Hu X, Murphy F, Karwautz A, Li T, Freeman B, Franklin D, Giotakis O, Treasure J, Collier DA. Analysis of microsatellite markers at the UCP2/UCP3 locus on chromosome 11q13 in anorexia nervosa. Mol Psychiatry 2002; 7:276–277.

19. Eastwood H, Brown KM, Markovic D, Pieri LF. Variation in the ESR1 and ESR2 genes and genetic susceptibility to anorexia nervosa. Mol Psychiatry 2002; 7:86–89.

20. Vink T, Hinney A, van Elburg AA, van Goozen SH, Sandkuijl LA, Sinke RJ, Herpertz-Dahlmann BM, Hebebrand J, Remschmidt H, van Engeland H, Adan RA. Association between an agouti-related protein gene polymorphism and anorexia nervosa. Mol Psychiatry 2001; 6:325–328.

21. Klump KL, Wonderlich S, Lehoux P, Lilenfeld LR, Bulik CM. Does environment matter? A review of nonshared environment and eating disorders. Int J Eat Disord 2002; 31:118–135.

22. Schork NJ, Fallin D, Lanchbury JS. Single nucleotide polymorphisms and the future of genetic epidemiology. Clin Genet 2000; 58:250–264.

23. Katzman DK, Zipursky RB, Lambe EK, Mikulis DJ. A longitudinal magnetic resonance imaging study of brain changes in adolescents with anorexia nervosa. Arch Pediatr Adol Med 1997; 151:793–797.

24. Gordon I, Lask B, Bryant-Waugh R, Christie D, Timimi S. Childhood-onset anorexia nervosa: towards identifying a biological substrate. Int J Eat Disord 1997; 22:159–165.

25. Robb AS, Silber TJ, Orrell-Valente JK, Valadez-Meltzer A, Ellis N, Dadson MJ, Chatoor I. Supplemental nocturnal nasogastric refeeding for better short-term outcome in hospitalized adolescent girls with anorexia nervosa. Am J Psychiatry 2002; 159:1347–1353.

26. Bodkin JA, Amsterdam JD. Transdermal selegiline in major depression: a double-blind, placebo-controlled, parallel-group study in outpatients. Am J Psychiatry 2002; 159(11):1869–1875.

27. Levine J. Controlled trials of inositol in psychiatry. Eur Neuropsychopharmacol 1997; 7:147–155.

28. Mendelson SD. Treatment of anorexia nervosa with tramadol. Am J Psychiatry 2001; 158:963–964.

29. Boschert S. Novel antidepressant therapies near approval. Clin Psychiatry News 2002; 30(10):1–20.

30. Rush AJ, George MS, Sackeim HA, Marangell LB, Husain M, Giller C, Nahas Z, Haines S, Simpson RK Jr, Goodman R. Vagus nerve stimulation (VNS) for treatment-resistant depressions: a multicenter study. Biol Psychiatry 2000; 47:276–286.

31. Pincus HA, Zarin DA, Tanielian TL, Johnson JL, West JC, Pettit AR, Marcus SC, Kessler RC, McIntyre JS. Psychiatric patients and treatments in 1997: findings from the American Psychiatric Practice Research Network. Arch Gen Psychiatry 1999; 56:441–449.

32. Lock J, Le Grange D, Agras S, Dare C. Treatment Manual for Anorexia Nervosa: A Family-Based Approach. New York: Guilford Press, 2001.

33. Ferguson T. Health Online: How to Find Health Information, Support Groups, and Self-Help Communities in Cyberspace. Boston: Addison-Wesley, 1996.
34. Kaiser Family Foundation. How young people use the internet for health information. GenerationX.Com.,http://www.kff.org/content/2001/20011211a/GenerationRx.pdf.
35. Walstrom MK. "You know, who's the thinnest?": Combating surveillance and creating safety in coping with eating disorders online. Cyber Psychol Behav 2000; 3:761–783.
36. Chin T. Site reading: physicians grapple with recommending websites. Am Med News, Oct 23–30, 2000, 24 (http://www.ama-assn.org/sci-pubs/amnews/pick_00/tesa1023.htm).
37. Balas EA, Jaffrey F, Kuperman GJ, Boren SA, Brown GD, Pinciroli F, Mitchell JA. Electronic communication with patients. Evaluation of distance medicine technology. JAMA 1997; 278:152–159.
38. Winzelberg AJ, Eppstein D, Eldredge KL, Wilfley D, Dasmahapatra R, Dev P, Taylor CB. Effectiveness of an internet-based program for reducing risk factors for eating disorders. J Consult Clin Psychol 2000; 68:346–350.
39. Celio AA, Winzelberg AJ, Wilfley DE, Eppstein-Herald D, Springer EA, Dev P, Taylor CB. Reducing risk factors for eating disorders: comparison of an internet- and a classroom-delivered psychoeducational program. J Consult Clin Psychol 2000; 68:650–657.
40. Zabinski MF, Wilfley DE, Pung MA, Winzelberg AJ, Eldredge K, Taylor CB. An interactive internet-based intervention for women at risk of eating disorders: a pilot study. Int J Eat Disord 2001; 30:129–137.
41. Humphreys K, Winzelberg A, Klaw E. Psychologists' ethical responsibilities in the Internet-based groups: issues, strategies, and a call for dialogue. Prof Psychol Res Pract 2000; 31:493–496.
42. Yager J. E-mail as a therapeutic adjunct in the outpatient treatment of anorexia nervosa: illustrative case material and discussion of the issues. Int J Eat Disord 2001; 29:125–138.
43. Robinson PH, Sefaty MA. The use of e-mail in the identification of bulimia nervosa and its treatment. Eur. Eat Disord Rev 2001; 9:182–193.
44. Bakke B, Mitchell J, Wonderlich S, Erickson R. Administering cognitive–behavioral therapy for bulimia nervosa via telemedicine in rural settings. Int J Eat Disord 2001; 30:454–457.
45. Sansone R. Patient to patient e-mail support for clinical practices. Eat Disord Treat Prev 2001; 9:373–375.
46. Kenwright M, Liness S, Marks I. Reducing demands on clinicians by offering computer-aided self-help for phobia/panic. Feasibility study. Br J Psychiatry 2001; 179:456–459.
47. Thiels C, Schmidt U, Treasure J, Garthe R, Troop N. Guided self-change for bulimia nervosa incorporating use of a self-care manual. Am J Psychiatry 1998; 155:947–953.
48. Smyth J, Wonderlich S, Crosby R, Miltenberger R, Mitchell J, Rorty M. The use of ecological momentary assessment approaches in eating disorder research. Int J Eat Disord 2001; 30:83–95.

49. Harari D, Furst M, Kiryati N, Caspi A, Davidson M. A computer-based method for the assessment of body-image distortions in anorexia-nervosa patients. IEEE Trans Inform Technol Biomed 2001; 5:311–319.
50. Leit RA, Gray JJ, Pope HG Jr. The media's representation of the ideal male body: a cause for muscle dysmorphia? Int J Eat Disord 2002; 31:334–338.
51. Riva G, Bacchetta M, Baruffi M, Molinari E. Virtual-reality-based multidimensional therapy for the treatment of body image disturbances in binge eating disorders: a preliminary controlled study. IEEE Trans Inform Technol Biomed. 2002; 6:224–234.
52. Hsiung R. Suggested principles of professional ethics for the online provision of mental health services. Telemed J E-Health 2001; 7:39–45.
53. Simons v. Blue Cross and Blue Shield of Greater New York, 144 A.D.2d 28, 536 N.Y.S.2d 431, 1989.

Index

ISBN 0-8247-4867-0

90000